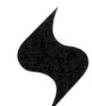

Stedman's

PSYCHIATRY
WORDS

THIRD EDITION

To MTs around the world

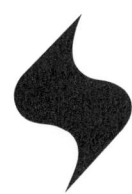

Stedman's

PSYCHIATRY
WORDS

THIRD EDITION

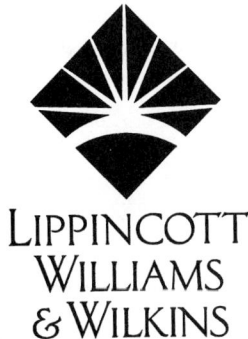

LIPPINCOTT
WILLIAMS
& WILKINS

Publisher: Rhonda M. Kumm, RN, MSN
Senior Manager: Julie K. Stegman
Senior Managing Editor: Nancy S. Wachter
Associate Managing Editor: Trista A. DiPaula
Art Program Project Manager: Jennifer Clements
Assistant Production Manager: Kevin Iarossi
Typesetter: Peirce Graphic Services, Inc.
Printer & Binder: Malloy Litho, Inc.

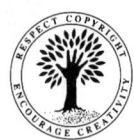
Printed in the United States of America

Third Edition, 2003

Library of Congress Cataloging-in-Publication Data

Stedman's psychiatry words.— 3rd ed.
    p. ; cm.
    Rev. ed. of: Stedman's psychiatry/neurology/neurosurgery words. c1999.
    Developed from the database of Stedman's Medical dictionary, 27th ed. and
supplemented by terminology found in current medical literature.
    Includes bibliographical references.
    ISBN 0-7817-3837-7 (alk. paper)
    1. Psychiatry—Dictionaries. 2. Neurology—Dictionaries. 3. Neurosurgery—
Dictionaries. I. Title: Psychiatry words. II. Stedman, Thomas Lathrop, 1853–1938.
III. Stedman, Thomas Lathrop, 1853–1938. Medical dictionary. IV. Stedman's
psychiatry/neurology/neurosurgery words.
    [DNLM: 1. Psychiatry—Terminology—English. WM 15 S812 2003]
RC437 .S753 2003
616.89′001′4—dc21

2002034062

01
1 2 3 4 5 6 7 8 9 10

Contents

Acknowledgments

An important part of our editorial process is the involvement of medical transcriptionists—as advisors, reviewers, and/or editors.

We extend special thanks to Pat Forbis, CMT, CTM, and Linda Byrne, CMT, for editing the manuscript, helping resolve many difficult questions, and contributing material for the appendix sections. We are grateful to our MT Editorial Advisory Board members, including Janet Stiles, BSN, CMA-C; Claudia Crickmore, CMT; Patty Gibson; and Laurel Eiler, RMR, CCR who were instrumental in the development of this reference. They shared their valuable judgment, insight, and perspective.

We also extend thanks to Pat Forbis and Darcy Johnson for working on the appendices. Additional thanks to Helen Littrell for performing the final prepublication review. Other important contributors to this edition include Peg Hughes, CMT, and Diane Heath, CMT, whose ongoing search for and distribution of new terms is invaluable.

And, as always, Barb Ferretti played an integral role in the process by reviewing the content files for format, updating the database, and providing a final quality check. Special thanks also go to Kathy Cadle and Lisa Fahnestock for their assistance with the database work.

As with all our *Stedman's* word references, this resource incorporates the suggestions and expertise of our many contacts in the medical transcriptionist community. Thanks to all of our advisory board participants, reviewers, and editors; AAMT meeting attendees; and others who have written us with requests and comments—keep talking, and we'll keep listening.

Editor's Preface

My thanks to Lippincott Williams & Wilkins and Stedman's and to their amazing staff for providing the opportunity to re-create the psychiatry word book. Special thanks go to Rhonda Kumm and Julie Stegman for listening to my ideas and to Nancy Wachter for her leadership and support. Have no doubt, Stedman's staff cares about the needs of medical transcriptionists. I am also grateful to the individuals named on the *Acknowledgments* page for their commitment to creating a quality product.

The practice of psychiatry is considered to have one of the most limited vocabularies of all medical specialties. However, its broad range of terminology is challenging and ever changing, new words and phrases often being introduced in a subtle manner. For example, street slang changes routinely, defined by geography, user age, and the knowledge by authority figures of its common use. The language of the street is so extensive that a limited number of terms and phrases are included here.

Catastrophic events and changes in the world's environment introduce new words and phrases into the psychiatric vocabulary. The events of September 11, 2001, have given clearer definition to words such as *bioterrorism* and *anthrax anxiety.* Technology has made some of us *technophobic* while others suffer from *computer addiction.*

The names of psychiatric and psychologic tests are often changed by a simple but important word such as *Revised* or *2nd Edition,* and the names of tests may be preceded by eponyms that are difficult to find in other word books. A *Psychiatric and Psychological Tests* appendix has been created to help with this challenge.

Other appendices are the DSM-IV Diagnoses and Codes, as well as sample psychiatric and psychologic reports. It appears that we are a society of fearful individuals. The plethora of phobias appear in their own appendix, identified by clinical name and by the common name of the abnormal fear.

Finally, I must share a personal thought. Logomaniac might be a coined term that best describes authors and editors of medical word books. Their love of words and the need for sharing them in the most accurate way is undeniable. Logomaniacs may also be characterized as the pack rats of etymology. They are euphoric when a new word is found or an elusive spelling is confirmed and reluctant to discharge a word as obsolete.

Pat Forbis, CMT

Publisher's Preface

Stedman's Psychiatry Words, Third Edition, offers an authoritative assurance of quality and exactness to the wordsmiths of the healthcare professions—medical transcriptionists, medical editors and copyeditors, health information management personnel, court reporters, and the many other users and producers of medical documentation.

We have received many requests to update this title. As a result, this new edition contains new terminology, street slang, phobias, drugs, and tests, and the neurology and neurosurgery terminology found in the second edition has been removed. *Stedman's Psychiatry Words, Third Edition,* covers hard-to-find terms, as well as standard terminology, meeting the needs of both beginning and experienced medical language specialists. The appendices feature street slang terms with short definitions, phobias listed alphabetically by clinical name, phobias listed alphabetically by fear, psychiatric and psychological tests, DSM-IV diagnoses and codes, sample reports, common terms by procedure, drugs by indication, and the general A-to-Z.

This compilation of more than 80,000 entries, fully cross-indexed for quick access, was built from a base vocabulary of approximately 50,000 medical words, phrases, abbreviations, and acronyms. The extensive A-Z list was developed from the database of *Stedman's Medical Dictionary, 27th Edition,* and supplemented by terminology found in current medical literature (see References on page xvi).

We at Lippincott Williams & Wilkins strive to provide you with the most up-to-date and accurate word references available. Your use of this word book will prompt new editions, which we will publish as often as updates and revisions justify. We welcome your suggestions for improvements, changes, corrections, and additions—whatever will make this *Stedman's* product more useful to you. Please complete the postpaid card in this book, and send your recommendations care of "Stedman's" at Lippincott Williams & Wilkins.

Explanatory Notes

Medical transcription is an art as well as a science. Both approaches are needed to correctly interpret the dictation of a physician, whose language is a product of education, training, and experience. This variety in medical language means that there are several acceptable ways to express certain terms, including jargon. *Stedman's Psychiatry Words, Third Edition,* provides variant spellings and phrasings for many terms. These elements, in addition to complete cross-indexing, make *Stedman's Psychiatry Words, Third Edition,* a valuable resource for determining the validity of terms as they are encountered.

Alphabetical Organization

Alphabetization of main entries is letter by letter as spelled, ignoring punctuation, spaces, prefixed numbers, accents, or other characters. For example:

affect-related
afferent
Age Discrimination in Employment Act

Terms beginning or ending with Greek letters show the Greek letters spelled out and listed alphabetically. For example:

alpha, α
    a. antagonist

In subentry alphabetization, the abbreviated singular form or the spelled-out plural form of the noun main entry word is ignored.

Format and Style

All main entries are in **boldface** to expedite locating a sought-after term, to enhance distinction between main entries and subentries, and to relieve the textual density of the pages.

Irregular plurals and variant spellings are shown on the same line as the singular or preferred form of the word. For example:

barognosis (*var. of* baragnosis)
capita (*pl. of* caput)

Hyphenation

As a rule of style, multiple eponyms (e.g., Barron-Walsh Art Scale) are hyphenated. Also, hyphens have been added between a manufacturer and one or more eponyms (e.g., Vital-Metzenbaum dissecting scissors). Please note that, in many cases, hyphenation is a question of style, not of accuracy, and thus is a matter of choice.

Possessives

Possessive forms have been dropped in this reference for the sake of consistency and conformance with the guidelines of the American Association for Medical Transcription (AAMT) and other groups. Please note, however, that in many cases, retaining the possessive, like hyphenating, is a question of style, not of accuracy, and thus is a matter of choice. To form the possessive of a word, simply add the apostrophe or apostrophe "s" to the end of the word.

Cross-indexing

The word list is in an index-like main entry-subentry format that contains two combined alphabetical listings:

(1) A *noun* main entry-subentry organization, which is typical of the A-Z section of medical dictionaries like *Stedman's:*

barrier
   architectural b.
   b. to intervention
   social b.

dance
   song and d.
   St. Vitus d.
   d. therapy

(2) An *adjective* main entry-subentry organization, which lists words and phrases as you hear them. The main entries are the adjectives or modifiers in a multiword term. The subentries are the nouns around which the terms are constructed and to which the adjectives or modifiers pertain:

delusional
   d. anxiety
   d. behavior
   d. belief

dopaminergic
   d. drug
   d. effect
   d. hyperactivity

This format provides the user with more than one way to locate and identify a multiword term. For example:

emergency
    e. intervention

intervention
    emergency i.

behavior
    explicit b.

explicit
    e. behavior.

It also allows the user to see together all terms that contain a particular descriptor, as well as all types, kinds, or variations of a noun entity. For example:

motor
    m. cortex
    m. cortical center
    m. deficit.

outburst
    aggressive o.
    angry o.
    Impulsive o.

Wherever possible, abbreviations are separately defined and cross-referenced. For example:

DSD
    depressive spectrum disorder
depressive
    d. spectrum disorder (DSD)
disorder
    depressive spectrum d. (DSD)

References

In addition to the manufacturers' literature we gather at various medical meetings, scientific reports from hospitals, and the lists of our MT Editorial Advisory Board members (from their daily transcription work), we used the following sources for new terms in *Stedman's Psychiatry Words, Third Edition.*

Books

American Heritage Dictionary of the English Language. 4th Edition. Boston: Houghton Mifflin, 2000.

Beers MH, Berkow R, Burs M, eds. Merck Manual of Diagnosis & Therapy. Whitehouse Station, NJ: Merck & Co., 1999.

Dorland's Illustrated Medical Dictionary, 29th Edition. Philadelphia: Saunders, 2000.

Drake E, Drake R. Saunders Pharmaceutical Word Book. Philadelphia: Saunders, 2002.

Drake R, et al. Saunders Pharmaceutical Xref Book. Philadelphia: Saunders, 2002.

Forbis P. The Psychiatry Word Book with Street Talk Terms. Philadelphia: FA Davis, 1993.

Keltner NL, Folks DG. Psychotropic Drugs, 3rd Edition. St. Louis, MO: Mosby, 1998

Kohut J. The Little Book of Phobias. Philadelphia: Running Press, 1994

Stedman's Abbreviations, Acronyms & Symbols, 2nd Edition. Baltimore: Lippincott Williams & Wilkins; 1999

Stedman's Medical Dictionary, 27th Edition. Baltimore: Lippincott Williams & Wilkins, 2000

Stedman's Psychiatry/Neurology/Neurosurgery Words, 2nd Edition. Baltimore: Lippincott Williams & Wilkins, 1999.

Journals

Alternative Therapies in Health and Medicine. Aliso Viejo, CA: Innovision Communications, 2002.

American Journal of Psychiatry. Washington, DC: American Psychiatric Press, 2000–2002

Journal of the American Academy of Child and Adolescent Psychiatry. Baltimore: Lippincott Williams & Wilkins, 2000.

Clinical Psychiatry News. Rockville, MD: International Medical News Group, 1999–2001.

Psychiatric Annals. Thorofare, NJ: Slack, Inc., 2000–2001

The Modesto Bee (newspaper). Modesto, CA.

CD-ROMs

Stedman's Abbreviations, Acronyms & Symbols, 2nd Edition. Baltimore: Lippincott Williams & Wilkins; 1999

Stedman's Plus 2002 Medical/Pharmaceutical Spellchecker. Baltimore: Lippincott Williams & Wilkins

Websites

http://aroundrtp.com/PED84.htm

http://healthweb.org/browse.cfm?subjectid=79

http://pni.med.jhu.edu/Projects_Methods/Tools_Technology/cognitive_tests.htm

http://www.aacap.org/Web/aacap/clinical/psychLinks.htm

http://www.aagpgpa.org

http://www.apa.org

http://www.behavior.net

http://www.cfah.org/links.cfm

http://www.csuniv.edu/Academics/Behavioral/psichi/links.htm

http://www.dna.com

http://www.drbobmentalhealth.org

http://www.hoptechno.com/book48.htm

http://www.mentalhealth.com

http://www.mentalhealth.gov.au/

http://www.nami.org (National Alliance for the Mentally Ill)

http://www.nimh.nih.gov

http://www.panic-and-anxiety.com/general_4.html

http://www.psych.org/

http://www.psychiatry.ox.ac.uk/cebmh/

http://www.psycom.net/depression.central.html.org

http://www.saferchild.org/mental.htm

http://www.stoeltingco.com/tests/products2/intellearnpage.htm

http://www.uic.edu/labs/hprl/About%20Us/Professional_links.html

http://www.virtualdrugstore.com

http://www.yorku.ca/psycenter/tests/aptitude.html

a
- a deux
- a posteriori
- a priori
- a priori criterion

AA
- academic alertness
- achievement age
- Alcoholics Anonymous
- anticipatory avoidance

AAA
- acute anxiety attack

AAAP
- American Academy of Addiction Psychiatry

AABT
- Association for Advancement of Behavior Therapy

AACAP
- American Academy of Child and Adolescent Psychiatry

AACD
- American Association for Counseling & Development

AACP
- American Academy of Clinical Psychiatrists

AACRC
- American Association of Children's Residential Centers

AADPRT
- American Association of Directors of Psychiatric Residency Training

AAF
- altered auditory feedback

AAMI
- age-associated memory impairment

AAMR
- American Association of Mental Retardation

AAO
- awake, alert, and oriented

AAP
- American Academy of Psychoanalysis
- American Academy of Psychotherapists
- Association for the Advancement of Psychoanalysis
- Association for the Advancement of Psychotherapy

AAPAA
- American Academy of Psychiatrists in Alcoholism and Addictions

AAPL
- American Academy of Psychiatry and Law

AAPM
- American Academy of Pain Medicine

AAPP
- American Academy on Physician and Patient

AAPSC
- American Association of Psychiatric Services for Children

AAS
- American Association of Suicidology

AASM
- American Academy of Sleep Medicine

AB, ab
- abortion

ab
- ab initio

ABA
- applied behavioral analysis

abactio

abactus venter

A/B/A design

abalienate

abalienatio mentis

abalientated

abandon

abandoned child

abandonment
- child a.
- a. concern
- emotional a.
- feeling of a.
- imagined a.
- perceived emotional a.
- real a.

abase

abasement

abash

abasia
- atactic a.
- a. atactica
- ataxic a.
- hysterical a.
- paralytic a.
- paroxysmal trepidant a.
- spastic a.
- trembling a.
- a. trepidans

abasia-astasia

abatardissement

abate

abatement

abating

abbau

ABC
  atomic, biological, chemical
    ABC warfare
ABCs of geriatric psychiatry
Abderhalden-Fauser reaction
abdicate
abdominal
  a. migraine
  a. pain
abduct
abduction
abed
aberrancy
aberrant
  a. behavior
  a. cycle
  a. gene
  a. motivational syndrome
  a. parental characteristic
  a. parental environment
  a. regeneration
aberration
  autosomal a.
  chromosomal a.
  mental a.
  a. of perception
  semantic a.
  sexual a.
aberrometer
abet
abetted
abetting
abeyance
ABFP
  American Board of Forensic Psychiatrists
ABFPN
  American Board of Forensic Psychiatry
    and Neurology
abhor
abhorrent
abidance
abide
abiding
  law a.
abient
abilitator
  Change a.
ability
  a. to abstract and calculate
  abstracting a.
  abstractive a.
  attentional a.
  attention shift a.
  auditory a.
  a. battery
  cognitive a.
  communication a.
  a. to con

conceptual a.
concrete abstractive a.
construction a.
coping a.
crystallized a.
disturbance in perceptual motor a.
drawing a.
eidetic a.
focal a.
general learning a.
impaired concentration a.
impaired thinking a.
intellectual a.
language a.
learning a.
a. to manage money
mathematical a.
memory a.
mental a.
money management a.
motor a.
nonverbal abstractive a.
nonverbal synthesizing a.
occupational a.
oral sensory a.
parenting a.
perceptual motor a.
poor reasoning a.
primary mental a.
psychic a.
psycholinguistic a.
reality testing a.
reasoning a.
reduced attention a.
sequencing a.
shift a.
spatial a.
synthesizing a.
a. to take criticism
a. test
test of syntactic a. (TSA)
thinking a.
thoroughness, reliability, efficiency,
  analytic a. (TREA)
verbal conceptualization a.
visuoconstructional a.
visuomotor a.
word-finding a.
writing a.
abiotic
abiotrophy
abject
ablate
ablation
  amytal a.
ABLB
  alternate binaural loudness balance
able-bodied

ablution
ablutomania
abnegate
abnegation
abnormal
    a. asymmetry
    a. behavior during sleep
    a. brain structure
    a. circumstance
    a. dermatoglyphic
    a. development
    a. EEG
    a. EEG tracing
    a. gait
    a. illness behavior
    a. involuntary movement disorder
    (AIMD)
    a. metabolism
    a. mood
    a. muscle response (AMR)
    a. pathologic condition
    a. perception
    a. personality
    a. physiological event during sleep
    a. position of distal limbs
    a. psychology
    a. reaction
    a. response
    a. responsiveness
    a. sleep-wake schedule
    a. stoppage of sound
    a. tactile sensation
    a. thinking
    a. trait
abnormality
    a. of affect
    attentional a.
    autosomal a.
    behavioral a.
    brain a.
    chromosomal a.
    electrolyte a.
    eye movement a.
    food intake a.
    gait a.
    immunologic a.
    inherited a.
    insulin a.
    laboratory a.
    lateralizing a.
    mental a.
    metabolic a.

    morphometric a.
    motoric a.
    movement a.
    nonspecific a.
    perceptual a.
    performance a.
    personality a.
    psychomotor a.
    pursuit a.
    sleep a.
    sleep-wake a.
    a.'s in sleep-wake timing
    mechanism
    startle a.
    structural brain a.
    subcortical-frontal lobe a.
    trait-level region a.'s
    vocal pitch a.
aboiement
abolish
abominable
abomination
aboriginal therapy
abort
abortifacient
abortion (AB, ab)
    criminal a.
    elective a.
    induced a.
    missed a.
    spontaneous a.
    therapeutic a. (TAB)
aboulia (*var. of* abulia)
about
    bandy a.
    a. face
    set a.
above-average
    a.-a. intelligence
    a.-a. student
aboveboard
ABP
    American Board of Psychiatry
ABPN
    American Board of Psychiatry and
    Neurology
ABR
    auditory brainstem response
    ABR audiometry
abracadabra
abradant
Abraham view of depressive disorder

NOTES

abrasive
abreact
abreaction
    hypnotic a.
    motor a.
abreactive drug
abrogate
abrosia
abrupt
    a. onset
    a. shift in affective expression
    a. topic shift
ABS
    acute brain syndrome
    aloin, belladonna, strychnine
abscess
    brain a.
abscise
abscissa
abscission
abscond
absence
    atypical a.
    automatic a.
    complex a.
    a. of depressed mood
    a. of eating plan
    a. of elevated mood
    a. of emotional responsiveness
    enuretic a.
    a. epilepsy
    epileptic a.
    a. episode
    fantasy a.
    a. of feeling
    hypertonic a.
    a. of insight
    leave of a. (LOA)
    myoclonic a.
    pure a.
    retrocursive a.
    a. seizure
    simple a.
    a. status
    sternutatory a.
    subclinical a.
    a. syndrome
    tussive a.
    typical a.
    unauthorized a. (UA)
    vasomotor a.
absent
    a. ataxia
    a. drive
    a. minded
    a. parent
    a. sexual desire
    a. speech

    a. state
    a. without leave (AWOL)
absenteeism
absentia
    a. epileptica
    in a.
absentminded
absentmindedness
absinthe, absinth
    a. addiction
    a. dependence
absinthism
absolute
    a. agraphia
    a. bliss
    a. diet
    a. field
    a. flow
    a. impression
    a. inversion
    a. measurement
    a. metabolic activity
    a. pitch
    a. quantity
    a. rating scale
    a. scotoma
    a. sensitivity
    a. threshold
    a. unconsciousness
absolution
absolutism
    cultural a.
    phenomenal a.
absolve
absorb
absorbance
absorbed mania
absorbefacient
absorbent
absorption
    erratic a.
    a. of inhalant
    intramuscular a.
    transdermal a.
abstain
abstainer
abstemious
abstention
abstinence
    alcohol a.
    alimentary a.
    caffeine a.
    a. delirium
    drug a.
    long-term a.
    nicotine a.
    opiate a.
    a. phenomenon

rule of a.
sexual a.
a. symptom
a. syndrome
total a.
abstinent
a. days
a. days per month
a. tobacco smoker
abstract
a. attitude
a. concept
a. conceptualization
a. expression
a. idea
a. intelligence
a. interpretation
a. logical thought
a. modeling
a. perception
a. reasoning
a. term
a. theory
a. thinking
a. wit
abstracting
a. ability
a. disability
abstraction
a. ladder
level of a.
a. skills
abstractive ability
abstract-versus-representational
  dimension
abstruse
absurd
absurdities test
absurdity
abubble
abulia, aboulia
cyclic a.
social a.
abulic mental change
abulomania
abundance
abundant motive
abuse
adolescent a.
adult a.
aerosol spray a.
a. of the aged

alcohol a.
amphetamine a.
amyl nitrate a.
animal a.
antidepressant a.
anxiolytic a.
barbiturate a.
benzodiazepine a.
caffeine a.
cannabis a.
a. case (AC)
cathartic a.
chemical a.
chemicals of use and a.
a. in childhood
childhood sexual a.
child sexual a.
chronic alcohol a.
chronic drug a.
cocaine a.
comorbid substance a.
concurrent alcohol and substance a.
continued a.
a. counseling
credit card a.
a. criterion
diet drug a.
drug a.
drugs of a.
early a.
elder a.
emotional a.
episodic substance a.
ethanol a.
exposure to a.
extent of a.
extrafamilial sexual a.
a. field
geriatric a.
hallucinogen a.
history of a.
hypnotic a.
illicit drug a.
index episode of sexual a.
inhalant a.
intrafamilial sexual a.
I.V. drug a.
laxative a.
a. of leave time
liability a.
long-term course of a.
maladaptive pattern of substance a.

NOTES

abuse *(continued)*
maternal a.
a. measure
medication a.
mental a.
methamphetamine a.
mixed substance a.
narcotic a.
newborn a.
nicotine a.
nondependent adult a.
a. of nonprescribed drug
nonprescription drug a.
opioid a.
parent a.
parental a.
patent medicine a.
paternal a.
patient a.
peer a.
perpetuator of a.
pharmacology of a.
physical a.
polydrug a.
polysubstance a.
a. potential
prescription drug a.
problems related to a.
psychoactive drug a.
psychoactive substance a.
psychological a.
recurrent a.
repeated a.
ritual a.
sadistic sexual a.
sedative a.
sexual a.
spousal a.
spouse a.
12-step program for substance a.
stimulant a.
substance a.
survivor of a.
sympathomimetic a.
tobacco a.
tranquilizer a.
traumatic childhood a.
verbal a.
victim a.
vocal a.
abused
being a.
abused-child
a.-c. hotline
a.-c. syndrome
abused-wife hotline
abuse/neglect
suspected child a. (SCAN)

abuser
anxious substance a.
child a.
drug a.
ethanol a.
remitted substance a.
repeat a.
spouse a.
substance a.
abusive
being a.
a. dating behavior
a. father
a. parent
a. partner
abysm
abyss
emotional a.
AC
abuse case
alcoholic cirrhosis
alternating current
a.c.
before meals
academic
a. alertness (AA)
a. difficulty
a. dysfunction
a. failure
a. inhibition
a. inventory
a. medical center
a. orientation (AO)
a. performance
a. preparation
a. problem
a. psychiatrist
a. psychiatry
a. skills disorder
a. underachievement disorder
academician
Academy of Psychosomatic Medicine (APM)
acalculia
aphasic a.
visual-spatial a.
acanthesthesia
acatalepsia
acatamathesia
acataphasia
acatastasia
acatastatic
acathexis
acathisia *(var. of* akathisia)
ACCA
American College Counseling Association
accede

accelerant
accelerated
    a. heart rate
    a. interaction
    a. reaction
    a. speech
acceleration
    educational a.
    positive a.
accelerator
accelerometer
accentuation
acceptable
    a. behavior
    a. treatment plan
acceptance
    group a.
    a. of self
    a. strategy
acceptant
acceptation
accepted
    a. behavior
    a. belief
    a. ritual
access
    a. to guns
    a. to health care services
accessing cue
accession
accessory
    a. chromosome
    a. cramp
    a. to crime
    a. sign
    a. symptom
accident
    alcohol-related risk for a.
    a. behavior
    fatal a.
    a. neurosis
    a. prevention
    a. prone
    a. reduction
    a. repeater
    a. risk
    a. victim
accidental
    a. affair
    a. crisis
    a. death
    a. error

    a. experience
    a. hanging
    a. hypothermia
    a. image
    a. injury
    a. overdose
    a. pregnancy
    a. psychosis
    a. shooting
    a. stimuli
    a. suicide
accident-prone behavior
acclaim
acclamation
acclimate
acclimation
    cold a.
acclimatize
accolade
accommodate
accommodation
    auditory a.
    interpersonal a.
    a. of nerve
    passive a.
    visual a.
accommodationist
accommodative
accompaniment
    psychopathologic a.
accompli
    fait a.
accomplished suicide
accomplishment quotient (AQ)
accord
accordance
accost
accoucheur's hand
account
    narrative a.
accountability
accountable for actions
accredit
accreditation
accretion
accrual
accrue
acculturate
acculturation
    a. difficulty
    a. problem

NOTES

acculturation (*continued*)
   a. problem with expression of customs
   a. problem with expression of habits
   a. problem with expression of political value
   a. problem with expression of religious value
   psychological a.
accumulated
accumulation
accuracy
   a. of memory
   a. test
accurate empathy (AE)
accursed
accusation
   false a.
accusative
accusatory hallucination
accuse
accustom
AC/DC
   alternating current or direct current
   bisexual
ACE
   acute care of the elderly
ace
acedia
acenesthesia
acerb
acerbate
acervuline
acervulus
acetaminophen poisoning
acetanilid
acetate
   amyl a.
acetone
acetonemia
acetonemic
acetous
acetum
acetylcholine
   a. as neurotransmitter
   a. cholinergic receptor
acetylcholinesterase (AChE)
acetylmethadol
achalasia
AChE
   acetylcholinesterase
ache
   brain a.
acheiria
achievement
   a. age (AA)
   assessment of academic a.

   a. battery
   a. behavior
   a. checklist (ACL)
   a. drive
   educational a.
   a. ethics
   exaggerated a.
   expected level of a.
   a. identification measure
   math a.
   a. motivation
   a. motive
   motive a.
   a. need (n-Ach)
   a. quotient (AQ)
   a. ratio (AR)
   reading a.
   school a.
   a. test (AT)
   a. through counseling and treatment (ACT)
   vocational a.
achievement-oriented
Achilles
   A. heel
   A. jerk
achromatic
   a. color
   a. color response
achromatic-chromatic scale
achromatism
acid
   aspartic a.
   deoxyribonucleic a. (DNA)
   a. flashback
   gamma-aminobutyric a. (GABA)
   5-hydroxyindoleacetic a. (5-HIAA)
   lysergic a.
   ribonucleic a. (RNA)
   a. rock
   a. test
acid-base
   a.-b. balance
   a.-b. disturbance
acidic
acidifiable
acidification treatment
acidify
acidism
acidity
acidogenic
acidosis
   lactic a.
   metabolic a.
acidulate
acidulous
aciduria
acknowledge

acknowledgment
ACL
    achievement checklist
    adjective checklist
acme
acmesthesia
ACN
    acute conditioned neurosis
acne
ACO
    alert, cooperative, and oriented
ACOA
    adult child of alcoholic
acoasm, akoasm
acolasia
acolyte
aconative
aconite
aconitine
aconuresis
acoria
acosmia
Acosta
    A. disease
    A. syndrome
acouasm (*var. of* acousma)
acouesthesia
acoupedic rehabilitation
acousma, acouasm
acousmatagnosis
acousmatamnesia
acoustic
    a. agnosia
    a. agraphia
    a. ambiguity
    a. analysis
    a. aphasia
    a. area
    a. center
    a. energy
    a. evoked potential
    a. feedback
    a. immittance measurement test
    a. input
    a. interface
    a. irritability
    a. nerve
    a. neurasthenia
    a. phonetics
    a. pressure
    a. radiation
    a. reflex threshold

    a. resonance
    a. signal
    a. spectrum
    a. startle
    a. stria
    a. trauma
    a. trauma deafness
acousticomotor epilepsy
acousticooptics
acoustics
ACP
    American College of Psychiatrists
acquaint
acquaintance
acquiesce
acquiescence
    response a.
    social a. (SA)
acquiescent-response set
acquirable
acquired
    a. agraphia
    a. character
    a. drive
    a. dyslexia
    a. epilepsy
    a. epileptic aphasia
    a. fluent aphasia
    a. folie morale
    a. immunodeficiency syndrome (AIDS)
    a. knowledge
    a. paranoia
    a. reflex
    a. sexual disorder
    a. sexual dysfunction
    a. situational narcissism
acquisition
    psychosocial skill a.
    reading skills a.
acquisitive
    a. instinct
    a. spirit
acquittal
acrai
acrasia
acrescentism
acrid
acrimicria
acrimonious
acrimony
acroagnosis

NOTES

acroanesthesia
acroataxia
acrocentric chromosome
acrocinesia
acrocinesis
acrocinetic
acrocyanosis
acrodynia
acrodysesthesia
acroesthesia
acrognosis
acrolein
acromania
acromegaloid personality
acromegaly, acromegalia
acromial reflex
acroparesthesia syndrome
across identity state
ACS
    acute confusional state
ACT
    achievement through counseling and
      treatment
    adaptive control of thought
    American College of Testing
    anxiety control training
act
    aggressive a.
    assaultive a.
    biologic a.
    compulsive a.
    consummatory a.
    criminal sexual a.
    a. ending
    frequency of violent a.
    future suicidal a.
    a. of God
    habitual a.
    Harrison Antinarcotic A.
    heinous a.
    imperious a.
    impulsive a.
    innocent a.
    instrumental avoidance a.
    intervening a.
    mental a.
    motive for violent a.
    past suicidal a.
    predisposition to suicidal a.'s
    promiscuous a.
    psychology a.
    rape a.
    reflex a.
    sadistic rape a.
    self-harming a.
    sensorimotor a.
    serious assaultive a.
    speech a.

    suicidal a.
    suicide a.
    symptomatic a.
    trivial a.
    a. up
    a. utilitarianism
    a.'s of violence
    violent a.
    a. and volition
acting
    a. in
    a. out
    a. out behavior
    a. out defense mechanism
    a. out potential
    a. out tendency
    play a.
    a. up
action
    accountable for a.'s
    aggressive a.
    amphetamine-like a.
    antiaggressive a.
    antigonadal a.
    antipsychotic a.
    a. of arrest
    automatic a.
    calorigenic a.
    chance a.
    chemical a.
    coercive legal a.
    compulsive a.
    consensual a.
    consequences of a.
    cumulative drug a.
    a. current
    disciplinary a.
    drug a.
    dual mechanism of a.
    duration of drug a.
    effective a.
    a. group
    a. guide
    hypnotic a.
    independent a.
    a. instrument
    intensified a.
    a. interpretation
    irrational a.
    a. level
    local vasoconstrictive a.
    a. location
    missing in a. (MIA)
    morphine-like a.
    a. organization
    a. painting
    a. pattern
    a. potential

pseudo-irreversible mechanism of a.
raptus a.
a. recipient
a. research
seriously wounded in a. (SWA)
a. system
tendency of a.
thermogenic a.
toxic a.
a. tremor
uncontrollable a.
vasoconstrictive a.
willed a.
wounded in a.

action-group process
actionless
action-oriented personality
activa
 oneirodynia a.
activated
 a. epilepsy
 a. sleep
 a. state
activating condition
activation
 amygdala a.
 brain a.
 cerebellar a.
 disturbance of behavioral a.
 EEG a.
 emotion-related a.
 functional a.
 hippocampal a.
 limbic a.
 metabolic a.
 neural a.
 neuronal a.
 a. pattern
 phasic a.
 prefrontal cortex a.
 semantic a.
 a. technique
 a. theory of emotion
 transient channel a.
activation factor
activator
active
 a. algolagnia
 a. analysis
 a. analytic psychotherapy
 a. antidepressant medication
 a. bilingualism

a. castration complex
a. compound
a. concretization
a. daydream technique
a. delirium
a. desire
a. displacement of emotive energy
a. euthanasia
a. fantasizing
a. filter
a. friendliness
a. general medical condition
a. hostility index (AHI)
a. imagining
a. immunity
a. incontinence
a. intervention
a. metabolite
a. mode of consciousness
a. modification
a. movement
a. negativism
a. nymphomania
a. passivity
a. pathophysiologic process
a. phase
a. phase of schizophrenia
a. placebo
a. psychoanalysis
a. psychosis
a. psychotic symptom
a. recreation
a. sleep
a. state
a. therapist
a. therapy
a. transport
a. treatment
a. trigger
a. vocabulary
a. voice
actively
 a. aggressive reaction type
 a. phrased question
 a. suicidal
active-passive model
active-phase
 a.-p. symptom
 a.-p. symptoms of schizophrenia
activism
activist

NOTES

activity

absolute metabolic a.
adolescent sexual a.
aimless motor a.
alpha a.
antisocial a.
anxiolytic a.
a. and attention disturbance
autonomic a.
a. and behavior
biochemical a.
blocking a.
brain opioid a.
brain wave a.
a. catharsis
cerebral a.
cholinergic a.
constricted a.
cortical a.
cortical-subcortical network a.
criminal a.
a.'s of daily living (ADL)
a.'s of daily living skills
dangerous a.
decreased interest in a.
delta a.
a. deprivation
diminished pleasure in
  everyday a.'s
a. displacement
disruption of normal a.
diversionary a.
a. drive
dynamic physical a.
electrooculographic a.
emotional a.
excessive motor a.
experience with criminal a.'s
experimental sexual a.'s
exposure to terrorist a.
fad a.
fast a.
fine motor a.
frenzied psychomotor a.
functional a.
gambling a.
goal-directed a.
graded a.
gross motor a. (GMA)
group a.
a. group psychotherapy
a. group therapy (AGT)
hedonistic a.
high-risk a.
hypnotic a.
impulsive a.
intellectual a.
a., interest, option (AIO)

late-night a.
leisure a.
a. level
limited a.
locomotor a.
a. log
loss of interest in usual a.
major life a.
masochistic sexual a.
masturbatory a.
mental a.
metabolic a.
motor a.
neuronal a.
nighttime a.
nonproductive a.
occupational a.
online sexual a.
orbitofrontal a.
organized a.
orogenital a.
outside a.
oxygen-depriving a.'s
paroxysmal a.
peak level of drug a.
perilous a.
peripheral cholinergic a.
persistent motor a.
physical a.
planned after-school a.
a. play therapy
a. pleasure
polyphasic a.
psychomotor a.
purposeless a.
a. quotient
random a.
rapid change in a.
a. record
religious a.
REM sleep a.
repetitious a.
repetitive motor a.
restricted a.
a. restriction
risk a.
risky sexual a.
sedative a.
seizure a.
self-care a.
sentinel a.
serotonergic a.
sexual a.
sleep a.
slow-frequency EEG a.
social a.
solitary a.
stereotyped a.

stream of mental a.
supervised after-school a.
synaptic a.
a. system
thalamocortical a.
a. theory of aging
a.'s therapist
thermoeffector a.
vacuum a.
a. of violence
voyeuristic a.
a. wheel
activity-interview group psychotherapy (A-IGP)
activity-reactivity
autonomic a.-r.
actograph
actometer
actor
bad a.
actual
a. derailment
a. mortality
a. neurosis
a. self
a. or threatened death
actualization
actuarial
actuate
actus reus
ACU
acute care unit
acuesthesia
acuity
auditory a.
sensory a.
visual a.
aculalia
acumen
acuology
acupressure
acupuncture
acupuncturist
acute
a. adolescent inpatient unit
a. affective reflex
a. alcoholic delirium
a. alcoholic mania
a. alcoholic myopathy
a. alcohol intoxication
a. alcoholism
a. amnesia

a. amphetamine poisoning
a. anxiety attack (AAA)
a. anxiety depression
a. anxiety reaction
a. ataxia
a. atrophic paralysis
a. brain syndrome (ABS)
a. care of the elderly (ACE)
a. care unit (ACU)
a. cerebral tremor
a. change in mental status
a. conditioned neurosis (ACN)
a. confusional insanity
a. confusional migraine
a. confusional migraine headache
a. confusional state (ACS)
a. danger
a. delusional psychosis
a. distress
a. drug toxicity
a. drunkenness
a. exacerbation
a. extrapyramidal event
a. foot-shock stress
a. hallucinatory mania
a. hallucinatory paranoia
a. hallucinosis
a. head trauma
a. hysterical psychosis
a. idiopathic polyneuritis
a. infective psychosis
a. ingestion
a. intensive treatment (AIT)
a. lead poisoning
a. maladjustment situation
a. maladjustment situational reaction
a. manic episode
a. melancholia
a. neuropsychologic disorder
a. onset
a. organic brain syndrome
a. organic reaction
a. paranoid disorder
a. paranoid reaction
a. paranoid reaction nonorganic psychosis
a. paranoid schizophrenic reaction (APSR)
a. phase
a. posttraumatic neurosis
a. posttraumatic organic psychosis
a. posttraumatic stress syndrome

NOTES

acute *(continued)*
    a. primary dementia
    a. psychiatric symptomatology
    a. psychogenic paranoid psychosis
    a. psychoorganic syndrome
    a. psychopathology
    a. psychotic aggressive behavior
    a. psychotic break
    a. psychotic episode
    a. psychotic inpatient
    a. schizophrenic attack
    a. schizophrenic episode
    a. schizophrenic reactive
    a. sedation
    a. seizure
    a. shock psychosis
    a. simple-type schizophrenia
    a. situational crisis
    a. situational depression
    a. situational disturbance
    a. stabilization
    a. stabilization inpatient care
    a. state
    a. stress disorder (ASD)
    a. stress response
    a. stress situational reaction
    a. suicide threat
    a. symptom
    a. therapy
    a. tolerance
    a. toxic encephalopathy
    a. treatment
    a. undifferentiated schizophrenia
    a. undifferentiated schizophrenic
      reaction (AUSR)
acutely
    a. abstinent tobacco smoker
    a. psychotic schizophrenic patient
    a. symptomatic
acute-phase treatment
acyanotic
acyclic
AD
    addict
    adherent
    admitting diagnosis
    Alzheimer disease
    AD Scale
ad
    ad hominem
    ad lib
    ad nauseam
ADA
    American Diabetic Association
    American Dietetic Association
    ADA diet
adage
adamant

ADAMHA
    Alcohol, Drug Abuse, and Mental Health
    Administration
Adams-Stokes
    A.-S. syndrome
adapt
adaptability
    cultural a.
    environmental a.
    a. profile
    a. to stress
adaptation
    air pollution a. (APA)
    a. approach
    autoplastic a.
    brightness a.
    cross a.
    dark a.
    disease a.
    a. disease
    a. dynamics
    failure in social a.
    a. level theory
    a. to life
    a. mechanism
    migration a.
    a. period
    positive a.
    a. reaction
    reality a.
    sexual a.
    a. skill
    social a.
    a. syndrome
    a. syndrome of Selye
    a. time
adaptational
    a. psychodynamics
adaptation-promoting therapy
adaptedness
adaptive
    a. approach
    a. behavior
    a. behavior inventory
    a. behavior scale
    a. capacity
    a. control of thought (ACT)
    a. control of thought system
    a. coping
    a. defense mechanism
    a. delinquency
    a. functioning
    a. hypothesis
    a. process
    a. response
    a. skill
    a. skill domain
    a. style

a. technique
a. testing
ADC
affective disorders clinic
AIDS dementia complex
ADD
attention deficit disorder
AD-DBD
attention deficit and disruptive behavior
disorder
ADD-HA
attention deficit disorder with
hyperactivity
addict (AD)
computer a.
drug a.
exercise a.
food a.
gambling a.
narcotic a.
object a.
sex a.
street a.
work a.
addicting drug
addiction
absinthe a.
alcohol a.
barbiturate a.
behavioral a.
biologic roots of a.
care management for chronic a.
(CMCA)
a. center
chemical a.
cocaine a.
computer a.
cross a.
drug a.
dual a.
enema a.
ethyl alcohol a.
exercise a.
food a.
gambling a.
heroin a.
iatrogenic a.
inhalant a.
Internet a.
Journal of the A.'s
laxative a.
methadone a.

methamphetamine a.
methylated spirit a.
morphine a.
narcotic a.
nicotine a.
nonprescription drug a.
object a.
online sexual a.
opiate a.
opium a.
a. organic psychosis
over-the-counter drug a.
polydrug a.
polysubstance a.
prescription drug a.
proneness to a.
a. psychiatry
psychological a.
a. relationship
relationship a.
a. root
sedative a.
a. severity
sexual a.
a. specialist
substance a.
surgical a.
sympathomimetic a.
a. syndrome
tobacco a.
a. treatment
true a.
a. withdrawal
work a.
addictionist
addiction-prone personality (APP)
addiction-related problem
addiction-type organic psychosis
addictive
a. behavior
a. disease unit (ADU)
a. disorder
a. personality
a. potential of drug
a. risk
additional drug dependence
addition articulation
additive
a. environmental influence
food a.
a. genetic influence
addle

NOTES

add-on drug
addressability
    content a.
adduce
adductor
    a. spasmodic dysphonia
ademonia
adenoid type
adenosine
    endogenous a.
    a. receptor
    a. triphosphate (ATP)
adept
adequacy
    nutritional a.
adequate
    a. care
    a. diet
    a. stimulus
    a. treatment
ADH
    antidiuretic hormone
ADHD
    attention deficit hyperactivity disorder
    ADHD rituals
ADHD-PI
    attention deficit hyperactivity disorder-
    predominantly inattentive
adherence
adherent (AD)
adhesive
    socially a.
adiadochokinesis, adiadochocinesia,
  adiadochocinesis
adiaphoria
adient behavior
Adie syndrome
adipometer
adiposis
adiposity
adiposogenitalis
    dystrophia a.
adiposogenital syndrome
adipsia, adipsy
adjective checklist (ACL)
adjudge
adjudicate
adjunct
    neuroleptic a.
    a. to treatment
adjunctive
    a. individual session
    a. medication
    a. mental health service
    a. strategy
    a. therapy
    a. treatment
    a. use

adjuration
adjure
adjustment
    attitude a.
    cultural a.
    a. depression
    a. disorder, chronic
    a. disorder with angry mood
    a. disorder with anxiety
    a. disorder with anxious mood
    a. disorder with disturbance of
    conduct
    a. disorder with mixed anxiety and
    depressed mood
    a. disorder with mixed disturbance
    of emotions
    elective mutism a.
    emotional a.
    environmental a.
    a. following migration
    a. interface disorder
    inventory a.
    a. inventory
    life-cycle a.
    marital a.
    a. measure
    a. mechanism
    a. method
    occupational a.
    partial a.
    personal a.
    premorbid a.
    a. process
    psychologic a.
    a. reaction of adolescence
    a. reaction of childhood
    a. reaction conduct disorder
    a. reaction disturbance
    a. reaction of infancy
    a. reaction of later life
    a. reaction of menopause
    a. reaction of middle age
    a. reaction physical symptom
    a. reaction physical syndrome
    school a.
    sexual a.
    a. situational reaction
    social a.
    stimulation a.
    a. therapy
    vocational a.
    withdrawal a.
adjust repetitive behavior
adjuvanticity
adjuvant therapy
ADL
    activities of daily living
    ADL scale

A

adlerian
>a. psychoanalysis
>a. psychology
>a. psychotherapy
>a. theory

Adler theory

administration
>anal a.
>avenues of a.
>chronic a.
>compulsive drug a.
>drug a.
>ECT a.
>enema drug a.
>Food and Drug A. (FDA)
>intramuscular a.
>method of a.
>methylphenidate a.
>nicotine a.
>oral a.
>parenteral drug a.
>standard dose a.
>systematic drug a.
>unsanitary drug a.

administrative
>a. psychiatry
>a. segregation
>a. therapy

administrator

admirable

admiration
>excessive a.
>need for a.

admissible
>a. admission
>a. evidence

admission
>admissible a.
>a. criterion
>elective a.
>first a.
>hospital a.
>informal a.
>involuntary a.
>prior to a. (PTA)
>psychiatric a.
>temporary a.
>voluntary a.

admitting diagnosis (AD)

admonish

admonition

ADMSEP
>Association of Directors of Medical Student Education in Psychiatry

adnata
>alopecia a.

adolescence
>adjustment reaction of a.
>anxiety disorder of a.
>avoidant disorder of a.
>crushes in a.
>a. developmental stage
>disorder of infancy, childhood, or a.
>early a.
>emancipation disorder of a.
>emotional disturbance of a.
>fearfulness disorder of a.
>gender identity disorder in a.
>identity disorder of a.
>introverted disorder of a.
>late a.
>middle a.
>oppositional disorder of a.
>overanxious disorder of a.
>reaction of a.
>relaxation training in a.
>sensitivity reaction of a.
>withdrawal reaction of a.

adolescent
>a. abuse
>alcoholic a.
>a. anger management
>antisocial a.
>a. anxiety
>a. at risk
>at-risk a.
>autistic-presymbiotic a.
>communication with a.
>a. counseling
>a. criminal
>a. crisis
>a. culture
>delinquent a.
>a. depression
>a. depression symptom
>disturbed a.
>a. diversion project
>a. drug use
>emancipated a.
>a. environment
>evaluation of a.

NOTES

17

adolescent (continued)
a. experimentation with adult behavior
a. gambler
a. gang member
a. group therapy
a. guardedness
high school a.
inner-city a.
a. inpatient unit
a. insanity
a. inventory
a. language quotient
limit-setting for a.
a. mania
middle school a.
a. negativism
a. neurotic delinquency
obese a.
a. onset
opinions toward a.'s (OTA)
out-of-control a.
a. pedophilia
a. personal identity
a. population
a. pregnancy
a. psychiatry
a. psychologist
a. psychology
a. psychopharmacology
a. psychotherapy
a. rapist
a. rebellion
a. recovery
a.'s risk for violence
self-destructive a.
a. sex offender
a. sexual activity
a. sexual change
a. sexual ideation
a. sexual identity
a. skepticism
socially dysfunctional a.
a. suicide
a. support group
a. support system
a. thinking
troubled a.
troublesome a.
a. turmoil
a. turmoil reaction
a. violence
violent a.
a. voice
a. voyeurism
adolescent-onset conduct disorder
adolescent-parent interview
adonadism

adopt
adoptable
adopted
a. child
a. father
adoptee
a. family method
putative a.
adoption study
adoptive
a. care
a. caregiver
a. family
a. father
a. parent
ADP-ribosylation
ADR
adverse drug reaction
adrenal
a. disorder
a. hyperplasia
a. segment
adrenalin
adrenaline-Mecholyl test
adrenarche
adrenergic-response state
adrenoceptor
adrenocortical insufficiency
adrenogenital syndrome (AGS)
adrenomedullary
a. component
adrenopathy
adrenopause
adrift
adroit
adromania
adromia
ADU
addictive disease unit
adulate
adult
a. abuse
a. child of alcoholic (ACOA)
consenting a.
a. depressive disorder
a. depressive episode
a. development
a. diagnostic and treatment center
a. dissociation
a. ego state
a. environment
a. foster home
gender identity disorder in a.'s
a. group therapy
a. life
a. major depression
a. motivation
nonconsenting a.

A. Protective Services (APS)
a. psychopathology
a. schizophrenia
a. self-harm behavior
a. self-injury
sexual abuse of a.
a. situational stress reaction (ASSR)
a. social dysfunction
a. socialization
stress effect on a.
a. survivor of neglect
a. unit
adult-child sex
adulterant
adulterate
adulteration
adulterer
adulterous
adultery
adultes
escala inteligencia Wechsler para a. (EIWA)
adulthood
a. developmental stage
early a.
gender identity disorder of a.
late a.
middle a.
a. psychiatry
young a.
adult-life psychosexual identity disorder
adultomorphism
adult-onset
a.-o. obesity
a.-o. proband
advance
a. directive
phase a.
sexual a.'s
unwanted sexual a.
advanced
a. dementia
a. sleep-phase pattern
a. sleep-phase syndrome
advantage
economic a.
a. by illness
law of a.
psychometric a.
take a.
therapeutic a.

adventitious
a. motor flow
a. movement
a. reinforcement
adversarial relationship
adversary model
adverse
a. autonomic response
a. background factor
a. childhood experience
a. drug effect
a. drug reaction (ADR)
a. event
a. medication effect
a. negative immunosuppressive effect
a. neurologic complication
a. psychological response
a. psychosocial environment
a. selection
adversity
advertising psychology
advice
against medical a. (AMA)
discharged against medical a. (DAMA)
face-to-face a.
medical a.
signed out against medical a. (SOAMA)
spiritual a.
advisor
school a.
spiritual a.
advocacy research
advocate
child a.
devil's a.
mental health a.
patient a.
ADW
assault with a deadly weapon
adynamia episodica hereditaria
adynamic
AE
accurate empathy
anoxic encephalopathy
aego-dystonic
AEP
auditory evoked potential
AEq
age equivalent

NOTES

aerial
aeroasthenia
aerobic exercise
aerodynamic speech analysis
aeroneurosis
aerophagia, aerophagy
aerosialophagy
aerosol
    a. inhalant
    a. spray abuse
    a. spray dependence
Aesculap ABC cervical plating system
AESP
    applied extrasensory projection
aesthetic, esthetic
    environmental a.'s
    environmentally a.
    a. pleasure
    a. value
aestheticism
aeternus
    puer a.
AF
    alleged father
affability
    surface a.
affable
affair
    accidental a.
    extramarital a.
    instrumental a.
    love a.
    unhappy love a.
    withdrawal from social a.
affect
    abnormality of a.
    ambivalent a.
    angry a.
    apathetic a.
    appropriate a.
    assessment of a.
    bland a.
    a. block
    blunted a.
    broad a.
    charge of a.
    cognitive generation of a.
    congruent a.
    constricted a.
    cooling of a.
    depressed a.
    diffuse a.
    diminution of a.
    disorder of a.
    a. displacement
    displacement of a.
    a. display
    dramatic a.

dull a.
dysphoric a.
elated a.
a. elicitation
emptiness of a.
a. energy
energy a.
euphoric a.
evoked a.
facial a.
a. fantasy
a. fixation
fixation of a.
flat a.
fluctuating a.
full a.
garrulous a.
generation of a.
a. hunger
hyperactive a.
hypoactive a.
impaired a.
inappropriate a.
incongruous a.
infantile a.
intense a.
a. intensity measure
a. intensity problem
a. inversion
isolation of a.
labile range of a.
a. memory
modulated a.
a. modulation
mood and/or a. (M/A)
negative a.
normal a.
painful a.
pervasive a.
pleasurable a.
predominant a.
preservation of a.
range of a.
removed a.
a. response
restricted range of a.
reversal of a.
schizophrenic a.
shallow a.
short-lived schizophrenic a.
silly a.
solemn a.
a. spasm
a. state
strangulated a.
superficial a.
transformation of a.
transposition of a.

a. trauma model
unstable a.
vacuous a.
a. within normal range
affectation
affect, behavior, cognition (ABCs of geriatric psychiatry)
affected
a. by feeling
germinally a.
a. individual
proportion of survivors a. (PSA)
affection
gesture of a.
masked a.
affectional
a. attachment
a. bond
a. drive
affectionate transference
affective
a. alcoholic psychosis
a. ambivalence
a. amnesia
a. arousal
a. bipolar disorder
a. blunting
a. cathexis
a. charge
a. constriction
a. depressive reaction
a. determined disorder
a. discharge
a. disease
a. disharmony
a. disorders clinic (ADC)
a. disorder syndrome
a. disturbance
a. dyscontrol
a. dysregulation
a. epilepsy
a. episode
a. experience
a. expression
a. feeble-mindedness
a. flattening
a. function
a. hallucination
a. illness
a. imagery
a. incontinence
a. insanity

a. instability
a. intensity
a. interaction
a. lability
a. melancholia
a. monomania
a. need
a. neurotic personality disorder
a. paranoid organic psychosis
a. and paranoid state
a. personality
a. process
a. processing
a. property
a. ratio
a. reaction type
a. reactivity
a. responsiveness
a. rigidity
a. schematic mental model
a. schizophreniform psychosis
a. separation
a. significance
a. slumber
a. spectrum disorder
a. stupor
a. suggestion
a. symptom
a. tone
a. value
affective-arousal theory
affectivity
characteristic pattern of a.
a. ratio
affect-laden
a.-l. delusion
a.-l. paranoia
affectomotor pattern
affect-related
a.-r. information-processing biases
a.-r. meaning
a.-r. processing
a.-r. schematic mental model
affectualization
afferent
a. feedback
a. input
a. motor aphasia
a. relation
a. stimulus interaction
a. thermosensory information

NOTES

affiliation
    a. bonding
    a. drive
    history of cult a.
    intense a.
    lifelong a.
    a. need
    political a.
    religious a.
affinal
affined
affinity
    receptor a.
affinous
affirmation
afflict
affliction
affluence
affluent
affordance
affright
affront
AFI
    amaurotic familial idiocy
aforementioned
aforethought
after
    a. glide
    a. meals
    morning a.
afteraction
aftercare
    a. group
    a. worker
aftereffect
    a. of drinking
    figural a.
afterimage
    memory a.
    positive a.
    Purkinje a.
afterlife
aftermath of trauma
afternoon (p.m.)
aftersensation
aftershock
    psychic a.
aftertaste
afterthought
afunction
against medical advice (AMA)
agape
agapism
age
    achievement a. (AA)
    adjustment reaction of middle a.
    anatomic a.

    a. at first intercourse
    a. at onset
    a. at onset of use
    basal mental a.
    a. bias
    Binet a.
    biologic a.
    bone a. (BA)
    calendar a.
    ceiling a.
    characteristic a.
    chronologic a. (CA)
    climacteric a.
    a. of consent
    a. correction
    a. correction procedure
    critical a.
    a. critique
    a. de retour
    developmental a. (DA)
    a. discrimination
    educational a. (EA)
    a. effect
    emotional a.
    a. equivalent (AEq)
    functional a.
    a. group
    legal a.
    mental a. (MA)
    middle a.
    new a.
    a. norm
    old a.
    a. peer
    physiological a.
    a. prejudice
    a. ratio
    a. of reasoning
    a. record correction
    a. regression
    relation to a.
    a. scale
    school a.
    a. score
    social a. (SA)
    stated a.
    stress effect in old a.
    test a. (TA)
    a. transition
    typical a.
    well adjusted for a.
age-appropriate
    a.-a. behavior
    a.-a. societal norm
    a.-a. strategy
age-associated memory impairment (AAMI)

A

aged
    abuse of the a.
    a. person
age-grade scaling
age-inappropriate knowledge of sexual behavior
ageism
age-level behavior
age-matched individual
agency
    A. for Health Care Policy and Research
    A. for Healthcare Research and Quality
    health systems a. (HSA)
    home-service a.
    law enforcement a.
    social service a.
agency-centered consultation
agenda
    hidden a.
    personal a.
    sociopolitical a.
agenesis
    gonadal a.
agent
    a., action, and object
    alkylating a.
    alpha receptor blocking a.
    anabolic a.
    antianxiety a.
    antidepressant a.
    antidyskinetic a.
    antihypertensive a.
    antipanic a.
    anxiolytic a.
    atypical antipsychotic a.
    beta adrenergic blocking a.
    blocking a.
    butyrophenone a.
    catalytic a.
    causative a.
    a. of change
    change a.
    chelating a.
    chemical a.
    conventional neuroleptic a.
    etiological a.
    excitatory a.
    fast-acting a.
    heterocyclic a.
    5-HT releasing a.

    hypnotic a.
    lacing a.
    MAOI-serotonergic a.
    MAOI-tricyclic a.
    mood stabilizing a.
    neuroleptic a.
    noxious a.
    offending a.
    A. Orange
    pharmacological a.
    possessing a.
    a. provacateur
    psychedelic a.
    psychopharmacologic a.
    psychotropic a.
    reinforcing a.
    second-line a.
    sedative-hypnotic a.
    serotonergic a.
    short-acting hypnotic a.
    sympathomimetic a.
    therapeutic a.
    traditional neuroleptic a.
    transforming a.
    transmissible a.
    typical antipsychotic a.
agent-action
agent-object
agerasia
age-related
    a.-r. brain change
    a.-r. cognitive decline
    a.-r. comorbidity
    a.-r. deterioration
    a.-r. developmental process
    a.-r. feature
    a.-r. hearing loss
    a.-r. pharmacodynamic change
    a.-r. pharmacodynamics
    a.-r. pharmacokinetic change
    a.-r. trend
age-specific
    a.-s. cumulative incidence rate
    a.-s. feature
    a.-s. risk factor
ageusia, ageustia
ageusic aphasia
agglutination
    image a.
agglutition
aggrandize
aggravate

NOTES

aggravated
a. assault
a. battery
aggregate
aggregation
familial a.
a. problem
aggression
a. to animals
antipredatory a.
antisocial a.
authoritarian a.
constructive a.
destructive a.
domestic a.
externally directed a.
general anger disorder with a.
general anger disorder without a.
healthy a.
hostile a.
husband-to-wife a.
identifying with a.
impulsive a.
indirect a.
instrumental a.
inward a.
juvenile a.
a. level
lifetime a.
moment of a.
parent-to-child a. (PTCA)
passive a.
pattern of a.
a. to people and animals
physical a.
a. replacement training
a. scale
self-directed a.
situational anger disorder with a.
situational anger disorder
  without a.
target of a.
territorial a.
unassertive a.
verbal a.
wife-to-husband a.
a. without provocation
aggressive
a. act
a. action
a. behavior theory
a. drive
a. fantasy
a. hostility
a. impulse
a. instinct
a. invasion
a. objectionable behavior

a. obsession
oral a.
a. outburst
a. personality
a. predatory type
a. psychotic behavior
a. psychotic inpatient
a. response
a. scale
a. thought
a. type undersocialized conduct
  disorder
a. undersocialized reaction
aggressively boisterous
aggressor
identification with the a.
aggrieved
aghast
aging
activity theory of a.
biologic changes associated with a.
cybernetic theory of a.
eversion theory of a.
a. issue
normal a.
precocious a.
a. theory
agitated
a. behavior
a. depression
a. melancholia
a. patient
a. reaction
a. state
agitation
a. catatonic schizophrenia
early manic a.
emotional a.
extreme a.
a. level
manic a.
marked motor a.
mental a.
nighttime a.
nocturnal a.
onset of a.
overlapping a.
overt a.
physical a.
psychomotor a.
purposeless a.
reduced a.
a. response
unpredictable a.
unrelieved a.
untriggered a.
violent a.
agitative feature

agitographia
agitolalia
agitophasia
agnea
agnosia
    acoustic a.
    apperceptive visual a.
    associative visual a.
    auditory a.
    autotopagnosia a.
    body-image a.
    color a.
    corporal a.
    facial a.
    finger a.
    generalized auditory a.
    ideational a.
    localization a.
    object a.
    optic a.
    position a.
    selective auditory a.
    spatial a.
    tactile a.
    time a.
    topographical a.
    verbal a.
    verbal-auditory a.
    verbal-visual a.
    visual a.
    visual-spatial a.
agnostic
    a. alexia
    a. behavior
    self-described a.
agonadal
agonadism
agonal
agonist
    dopamine a.
    5-HT a.
    inverse a.
    a. medication
    partial a.
    a. therapy
agonize
agony
    intellectual a.
    personal a.
agoramania
agoraphobia
    panic disorder with a.

    panic disorder without a.
    a. without history of panic
      disorder
agoraphobic
agrammatica
agrammatic speech
agrammatism
agrammatologia
agraphia
    absolute a.
    acoustic a.
    acquired a.
    alexia with a.
    alexia without a.
    amnemonic a.
    a. amnemonica
    aphasic a.
    apraxic a.
    atactic a.
    atactica a.
    a. atactica
    cerebral a.
    developmental a.
    jargon a.
    lexical a.
    literal a.
    mental a.
    motor a.
    musical a.
    optic a.
    phonological a.
    pure a.
    spatial a.
    verbal a.
agraphic
agreed-on
    a.-o. pattern
    a.-o. routine
agreement
    contractual a.
    reciprocal a.
    separation a.
    subject-verb a.
agriothymia hydrophobica
agrypnia
agrypnotic
AGS
    adrenogenital syndrome
    audiogenic seizure
AGT
    activity group therapy
agyria

NOTES

AH
    alcoholic hepatitis
AH1 Forms X and Y
AHI
    active hostility index
    anterior horn index
ahistorical
ahylognosia
AI
    allergy index
    anxiety index
    autoimmune
Aicardi syndrome
aid
        daily living a.
        eating a.
        electronic a.
        ergogenic a.
        first a.
        functional a.
        sexual a.
        visual a.
aide
        childcare a.
        home-health a.
        nurse's a.
aidoiomania
AIDS
    acquired immunodeficiency syndrome
        AIDS dementia complex (ADC)
        AIDS encephalopathy
        person with AIDS (PWA)
AIDS-related complex (ARC)
A-IGP
    activity-interview group psychotherapy
aigu
        delire a.
ailment
        functional a.
ailurophilia
AIM
    artificial intelligence in medicine
aim
        a. inhibition
        instinctual a.
        partial a.
        a. transference
AIMD
    abnormal involuntary movement disorder
aiming test
aimless
        a. behavior
        a. motor activity
        a. wandering
AIN
    American Institute of Nutrition
AIO
    activity, interest, option

air
        complemental a.
        a. conduction
        a. conduction deafness
        a. conduction testing
        a. drinking
        a. encephalopathy
        a. hunger
        a. pollution adaptation (APA)
        a. pollution index
        a. pollution syndrome (APS)
        a. pressure effect
        recycled a.
        a. swallowing
        tidal a.
        a. wastage
air-blade sound
airplane glue dependence
AIT
    acute intensive treatment
AK-47
AKA
        alcoholic ketoacidosis
        also known as
akataphasia
akathisia, acathisia
        neuroleptic dose-dependent a.
        neuroleptic-induced a.
        treatment-emergent a.
akinesia
        a. amnestica
        neuroleptic-induced a.
akinesia/diminished emotional expression
akinesic
akinesis
akinesthesia
akinetic
        a. apraxia
        a. autism
        a. depression
        a. epilepsy
        a. mania
        a. mutism
        a. patient
        a. psychosis
        a. seizure
        a. stupor
akinetic-abulic syndrome
akoasm (*var. of* acoasm)
aktanoesis
AL
        annoyance level
alacrity
alalia
        a. cophica
        a. organica
        a. physiologica
        a. prolongata

alalic
alanine aminotransferase (ALT)
Al-Anon
alar flutter
alarm
    a. reaction (AR)
    a. reaction stage
alarmism
alarmist
alaryngeal speech
Alateen
albedo
ALC
  alcohol
  approximate lethal concentration
alcohol (ALC)
    a. abstinence
    a. abstinence syndrome
    a. abuse
    a. abuse scale
    a. acquired (non-wilsonian) chronic
      hepatocerebral degeneration
    a. addiction
    allyl a.
    a. amnestic disorder
    a. amnestic syndrome
    amyl a.
    a. anxiety disorder
    a. as cause of seizure
    a. binge
    blood a. (BA)
    a. cerebellar degeneration
    a. consumption
    a. consumption behavior
    a. counseling
    a. craving
    a. dependence
    a. dependence syndrome
    a. dependence with tolerance
    a. dependent
    a. derivative
    a. detoxification
    a. drinking
    ethyl a. (ETOH, EtOH)
    a. habit
    a. hallucination
    a. hallucinosis
    intermediate brain syndrome due
      to a.
    a. intolerance
    a. intoxication
    a. intoxication-related disorder

    a. level
    a. metabolism
    a. misuse
    a. mood disorder
    a. offense
    a. on breath (AOB)
    a. paranoid state
    a. pathological intoxication
    pathologic reaction to a.
    a. persisting dementia
    a. poisoning
    a. problem
    a. related (AR)
    saliva screen for a.
    a. sensitivity
    a. sleep disorder
    toxic effects of a.
    a. toxicity
    a. use
    a. use disorder
    a. withdrawal delirium
    a. withdrawal hallucinosis
    a. withdrawal seizure
    a. withdrawal syndrome
    a. withdrawal tremulousness
alcohol-Antabuse reaction
alcohol-associated dementia
alcoholate
  chloral a.
alcohol-dependent
    a.-d. individual
    a.-d. sleep disorder
Alcohol, Drug Abuse, and Mental
  Health Administration (ADAMHA)
alcoholic
    a. adolescent
    adult child of a. (ACOA)
    a. amblyopia
    a. amentia
    a. amnesia
    a. amnestic disorder
    a. ataxia
    a. blackout
    a. brain syndrome
    a. cardiomyopathy
    child of a. (COA)
    a. cirrhosis (AC)
    a. classification
    closet a.
    a. coma
    a. confusional state
    a. delirium

NOTES

alcoholic (*continued*)
a. dementia
a. deterioration
detoxified a.
a. drunkenness
a. epilepsy
a. family
a. gastritis
a. hallucination
a. hallucinosis
a. hepatitis (AH)
inactive a. (IA)
a. insanity
a. jealousy
a. ketoacidosis (AKA)
a. Korsakoff psychosis
a. liver disease (ALD)
a. liver disease-type organic
psychosis
a. malabsorption syndrome
a. mania
a. myocardiopathy
a. myopathy
newly abstinent a.
a. organic mental disorder
a. pancreatitis
a. paralysis
a. paranoia
a. paranoid psychosis
a. paranoid state
a. paraplegia
a. parent
a. paresis
a. pellagra encephalopathy
a. peripheral neuropathy
a. poisoning
a. polyneuritic psychosis
a. possible pancreatic
encephalopathy
a. pseudoparesis
a. rehabilitation
a. stupor
a. symptom
a. twilight state
type I, II a.
a. withdrawal tremor
alcoholica
amblyopia a.
Alcoholics Anonymous (AA)
alcoholicum
delirium a.
alcohol-induced
a.-i. anxiety
a.-i. delirium
a.-i. depression
a.-i. hallucination
a.-i. nighttime sleep
a.-i. organic mental syndrome

a.-i. paranoid state
a.-i. peripheral neuropathy
a.-i. persisting dementia
a.-i. psychotic disorder
a.-i. psychotic disorder with
delusions
a.-i. psychotic disorder with
hallucinations
a.-i. sexual dysfunction
alcoholique
delire a.
alcoholism
acute a.
alpha a.
antisocial a.
a. associated with dementia
beta a.
chronic a.
comorbid past a.
delirium a.
delta a.
dementia associated with a.
developmentally cumulative a.
developmentally limited a.
epsilon a.
essential a.
Feighner criteria for a.
gamma a.
genetic a.
a. in isolation
mental disorder due to a.
negative-affect a.
a. organic psychosis
past a.
psychiatric disorder associated
with a.
reactive a.
regressive a.
alcoholization
alcohol-metabolizing system
alcohol-methadone interaction
alcoholomania
alcoholophilia
alcohol-positive history (APH)
alcohol-precipitated epilepsy
alcohol-related
a.-r. behavior
a.-r. birth defect (ARBD)
a.-r. diagnosis
a.-r. disorder
a.-r. harm
a.-r. insomnia
a.-r. offense
a.-r. phenotype
a.-r. physical problem
a.-r. psychiatric problem
a.-r. risk for accident
a.-r. risk for suicide

a.-r. risk for violence
a.-r. seizure
a.-r. use disorder, not otherwise
   specified
ALD
alcoholic liver disease
aldehydes
alert
a. awake state
a., cooperative, and oriented (ACO)
a. inactivity
a. and oriented
alerting
a. effect
a. mechanism
a. stimulus
alertness
academic a. (AA)
a. level
level of a.
mental a.
state of a.
visual a.
alethia
alexia
agnostic a.
a. allocheiria
anterior a.
auditory a.
central a.
cortical a.
incomplete a.
literal a.
motor a.
musical a.
optical a.
posterior a.
pure a.
sensory a.
subcortical a.
tactile a.
verbal a.
visual a.
a. with agraphia
a. without agraphia
alexic
alexithymia
alexithymic
a. behavior
a. personality
algedonic
algesia

algesic
algesichronometer
algesiogenic
algesthesia
algesthesis
algetic
algica
synesthesia a.
algogenesis
algogenic psychosyndrome
algolagnia
active a.
passive a.
algolagniac
algolagnist
algometer
algophilia, algophily
algopsychalia
algorithm
diagnostic a.
algospasm
alias
alibi
Alice in Wonderland syndrome
alien
a. obsession
a. thought
alienate
alienated
socially a.
alienatio mentis
alienation
body a.
a. coefficient
sense of a.
social a.
alienism
alienist
aliment
alimentary
a. abstinence
a. obesity
alimentation
forced a.
parenteral a.
alimentotherapy
alive
buried a.
alkali
alkaline phosphatase
alkaloid
belladonna a.

NOTES

alkaloid *(continued)*
    ergot a.
    opium a.
alkalosis
    metabolic a.
    tetany of a.
alkyl
alkylamine
alkylating agent
allachesthesia
Allah
all-American
allay
allegation
    child molestation a.
alleged father (AF)
allegiance
allegorical
allegorization
allegory
allele
allelic
allelism
allelomorph
allergen
allergenic
allergic
    a. psychogenic disorder
    a. reaction
allergy
    drug a.
    immediate a.
    a. index (AI)
alleviating
    a. violence
    a. violence in aggressive behavior
alley
    blind a.
alliance
    contractual a.
    relational a.
    therapeutic a.
    working a.
allied
    a. health professional
    a. reflex
alliterate
alliteration
allobarbital
allocentric
allocheiria
    alexia a.
allochiria, allocheiria
allocortex
allocortical cortex
allodynia
alloerotic
alloerotism, alloeroticism

alloesthesia
allogamy
allogrooming
allokinesis
allolalia
allomorph
allopath
allopathic
allopathist
allopathy
allopatric species
allophasis
allophone
alloplasty
allopsyche
allopsychic delusion
allopsychosis
all-or-none reaction
allosteric manner
allotoxin
allotriogeustia, allotriogeusia
allotriophagia, allotriophagy
allotriorhexia
allotriosmia
allotropic personality
allowable
allowance
    recommended daily a. (RDA)
Allport
    A. A-S Reaction Study
    A. group relations theory
    A. personality trait theory
Allport-Vernon-Linzey Study of Values
allude
allure
allurement
allusion in wit
allusive thinking
all-women group
allyl alcohol
alma
    perdida del a.
alogia
aloin, belladonna, strychnine (ABS)
aloneness
aloof
alopecia
    a. adnata
    androgenic a.
    a. areata
    a. celsi
    Celsus a.
    cicatricial a.
    a. cicatrisata
    a. circumscripta
    a. congenitalis
    congenital sutural a.
    a. disseminata

a. disseminate
a. dynamica
a. hereditaria
a. leprotica
male pattern a.
a. marginalis
a. medicamentosa
a. mucinosa
a. neurotic
a. neurotica
a. parviculata
a. pityrodes
postoperative pressure a.
postpartum a.
a. prematura
premature a.
a. presenilis
psychogenic a.
self-induced a.
a. senilis
stress-induced a.
a. symptomatica
syphilitic a.
a. syphilitica
a. totalis
a. toxica
traction a.
traumatic a.
trichotillomania-induced a.
a. universalis

alpha
a. activity
a. adrenergic blocking drug
a. adrenergic receptor
a. adrenergic stimulating drug
a. alcoholism
a. apparent
a. arc
a., beta, gamma hypotheses
a. block
a. blocking
a. cell
coefficient a.
a. coefficient
Cronbach a.
a. error
a. examination
a. factor
a. feedback
a. frequency
a. index
a. level

a. methyldopa
a. movement
obsessional compulsive inventory a.
a. receptor blocking agent
a. rhythm
a. state
a. verbal test
a. wave
a. wave training
alpha-2
a. adrenergic receptor
a. antagonist
alpha-arc
alphabet
initial teaching a.
alphalytic
alpha-methyldopa-induced mood disorder
alphamnimetic
alphaprodine
alpidem
alpinism
ALSD
Alzheimer-like senile dementia
alseroxylon
also known as (AKA)
ALT
alanine aminotransferase
alter
a. ego
a. ego transference
alterable
alteration
behavior a.
identity a.
a. in identity
a. of memory structure
neurocognitive a.
a. in rate of speech
reactive ego a.
receptor a.
selective speech perception a.
speech processing a.
speech tracking a.
a. in time perception
alterative
altercation
altered
a. appetite
a. auditory feedback (AAF)
a. function
a. level of consciousness
a. life circumstance

NOTES

altered *(continued)*
    a. mental status
    a. mentation
    a. mind-body perception
    a. sensation
    a. sensory perception
    a. sleep schedule
    a. state
    a. state of consciousness (ASC)
    a. tau processing
    a. time perception
    a. vision
    a. voice
alterego
alteregoism
alternate
    a. binaural loudness balance
    (ABLB)
    a. forms reliability coefficient
    a. hemianesthesia
    a. identity
    a. monaural loudness balance
    (AMLB)
    a. motion rate (AMR)
    a. response test
    a. uses test
alternating
    a. behavior
    a. bipolar disorder
    a. current (AC)
    a. current or direct current
    (AC/DC)
    a. insanity
    a. mydriasis
    a. personality
    a. perspective
    a. psychosis
    a. pulse
    a. role
    a. tremor
alternation
alternative
    a. alter ego
    a. approach
    a. behavior
    a. criterion B for dysthymic
    disorder
    a. diagnosis
    a. dimensional descriptors for
    schizophrenia
    a. explanation
    a. intervention
    least restrictive a.
    a. lifestyle
    a. lifestyle community
    a. medicine
    a. method
    a. perspective

    pharmaceutical a.
    a. psychosis
    psychotherapy a.
    a. school
    a. strategy
    a. therapy
    a. treatment
    viable a.
    a. viewpoint
altitude
    a. anoxia
    a. disease
    a. sickness
altrigenderism
altruism
altruistic
    a. behavior
    a. personality
    a. role
    a. suicide
alveolar hypoventilation syndrome
alymphoplasia
Alzheimer
    A. disease (AD)
    A. disease neuropathology
    A. Disease and Related Disorders
    Association
    A. psychosis
    A. syndrome
Alzheimer-like senile dementia (ALSD)
AM
    amplitude modulation
    attitude to medication
AMA
    against medical advice
amalgam
    emotional a.
    emotional-object a.
Amanita
    A. muscaria
    A. phalloides
amanitin
amanitoxin
amasesis
amative
amativeness
amatory
amaurosis
    epileptoid a.
    hysteric a.
    toxic a.
amaurotic
    a. axonal idiocy
    a. familial idiocy (AFI)
ambageusia
AMBHA
    American Managed Behavioral
    Healthcare Association

A

ambiance
    family a.
    sociocultural a.
ambidexterity
ambidextrism
ambidextrous
ambient
    a. air pressure
    a. behavior
    a. noise
    a. temperature
ambiguity
    acoustic a.
    diagnostic a.
    lexical a.
    role a.
    structural a.
    a. tolerance
ambiguous
    a. external stimuli
    a. figure
    a. genitalia
ambilaterality
ambilevous
ambisexual
ambisinister
ambisinistrous
ambitendency
ambitieux
    delire a.
ambivalence
    a. about living
    affective a.
    dual a.
    a. of the intellect
    post a.
    a. of the will
ambivalent
    a. affect
    a. feeling
    a. quotient
ambiversion
ambivert
amblyaphia
amblygeustia
amblyopia
    alcoholic a.
    a. alcoholica
    arsenic a.
    color a.
    hysteric a.
    nutritional a.

    tobacco a.
    toxic a.
    traumatic a.
ambulance chaser
ambulans
    paroniria a.
ambulation index
ambulatory
    a. automatism
    a. care
    a. mental health service
    a. schizophrenia
    a. status
ambush
ameboidism
ameliorate
amelioration
    tendency toward a.
amenable to treatment
amendment
amenia
amenomania
amenorrhea
    dietary a.
    dysponderal a.
    emotional a.
    nutritional a.
    pathologic a.
    physiological a.
    premenopausal a.
    secondary a.
    stress-related a.
amenorrheic
ament
amentia
    alcoholic a.
    a. attonita
    isolation a.
    nevoid a.
    a. paranoides
    phenylpyruvic a.
    primary a.
    Stearns alcoholic a.
amential
Amerasian
America
    Big Brothers of A.
    Big Sisters of A.
americamania
American
    A. Academy of Addiction
    Psychiatry (AAAP)

NOTES

American *(continued)*
  A. Academy of Child and
    Adolescent Psychiatry (AACAP)
  A. Academy of Child Psychiatry
  A. Academy of Clinical
    Psychiatrists (AACP)
  A. Academy of Pain Medicine
    (AAPM)
  A. Academy of Pediatrics Task
    Force on Violence
  A. Academy on Physician and
    Patient (AAPP)
  A. Academy of Psychiatrists in
    Alcoholism and Addictions
    (AAPAA)
  A. Academy of Psychiatry and
    Law (AAPL)
  A. Academy of Psychoanalysis
    (AAP)
  A. Academy of Psychotherapists
    (AAP)
  A. Academy of Sleep Medicine
    (AASM)
  A. Association of Children's
    Residential Centers (AACRC)
  A. Association of Community
    Psychiatrists
  A. Association for Counseling &
    Development (AACD)
  A. Association of Directors of
    Psychiatric Residency Training
    (AADPRT)
  A. Association of Emergency
    Psychiatry
  A. Association for Geriatric
    Psychiatry (AAGP)
  A. Association for Marriage and
    Family Therapy (AAMFT)
  A. Association of Mental
    Retardation (AAMR)
  A. Association of Psychiatric
    Services for Children (AAPSC)
  A. Association of Psychotherapists
  A. Association of Suicidology
    (AAS)
  A. Board of Forensic Psychiatrists
    (ABFP)
  A. Board of Forensic Psychiatry
  A. Board of Forensic Psychiatry
    and Neurology (ABFPN)
  A. Board of Medical Specialties
  A. Board of Psychiatry (ABP)
  A. Board of Psychiatry and
    Neurology (ABPN)
  A. College Counseling Association
    (ACCA)
  A. College of Neuropsychiatrists
  A. College of Psychiatrists (ACP)

  A. College of Testing (ACT)
  A. Counseling Association
  A. Diabetic Association (ADA)
  A. Diabetic Association diet
  A. Dietetic Association (ADA)
  A. Family Therapy Association
  A. Foundation for Suicide
    Prevention
  A. Institute of Nutrition (AIN)
  A. Law Institute Formulation of
    Insanity
  A. Law Institute Rule
  A. Managed Behavioral Healthcare
    Association (AMBHA)
  A. Occupational Therapy
    Association (AOTA)
  A. Orthopsychiatric Association
    (AOA)
  A. Pain Society (APS)
  A. Pharmaceutical Association
    (APhA)
  A. Physical Therapy Association
    (APTA)
  A. Psychiatric Association (APA)
  A. Psychiatry Association-Center
    for Mental Health Services
  A. Psychoanalytical Association
    (APA)
  A. Psychological Association (APA)
  A. Psychological Society (APS)
  A. Psychopathic Association
  A. Psychosomatic Society
  A. Public Health Association
    (APHA)
  A. Society of Addiction Medicine
    (ASAM)
  A. Society for Adolescent
    Psychiatry (ASAD)
  A. Society of Group Psychotherapy
    and Psychodrama (ASGPP)
  A. Society of Psychoanalytic
    Physicians (ASPP)
  The A. Academy of Psychoanalysis
americanize
ametamorphosis
amiable
amicable
amide
  lysergic acid a.
amimia
  amnesic a.
  ataxic a.
  expressive a.
amine
  biogenic a.
  tricyclic secondary a.
  tricyclic tertiary a.
amino

A

aminotransferase
    alanine a. (ALT)
    aspartate a. (AST)
amitriptyline-induced mood disorder
AMLB
    alternate monaural loudness balance
ammonium
    a. bromide
    a. salicylate
    a. valerate
amnalgesia
amnemonic
    a. agraphia
    a. aphasia
amnemonica
    agraphia a.
amnesia
    acute a.
    affective a.
    a. after trance
    alcoholic a.
    amnesic a.
    anterograde a.
    asymmetrical a.
    audioverbal a.
    auditory a.
    autohypnotic a.
    axial a.
    Broca a.
    catathymic a.
    childbirth a.
    a. in children
    chronic a.
    circumscribed a.
    complete a.
    concussion a.
    continuous a.
    cortical a.
    degree of a.
    dissociative a.
    emotional a.
    episodic a.
    epochal a.
    a. evidence
    evidence of a.
    generalized a.
    global a.
    hippocampal a.
    hypnotic a.
    hysterical a.
    ictal a.
    infantile a.

    Korsakoff a.
    lacunar a.
    localized a.
    a. loss of memory
    neurological a.
    nonpathological a.
    olfactory a.
    organic a.
    partial a.
    patchy a.
    polyglot a.
    postconcussion a.
    post-ECT a.
    postelectroconvulsive a.
    posthypnotic a.
    posttraumatic a. (PTA)
    profound a.
    psychogenic a.
    residual a.
    retroactive a.
    retroanterograde a.
    retrograde a.
    reversible a.
    selective a.
    shrinking retrograde a.
    a. for sleep and dreaming
    a. for sleep terror event
    subsequent a.
    systematized a.
    tactile a.
    toxin-provoked a.
    transient a.
    transient global a. (TGA)
    a. for trauma
    traumatic a.
    a. traumatica
    true a.
    verbal a.
    visual a.
amnesic
    a. amimia
    a. amnesia
    a. aphasia
    a. apraxia
    a. color blindness
    a. memoration
    a. patient
    a. state
    a. syndrome
amnestic
    a. aphasia
    a. apraxia

NOTES

amnestic *(continued)*
    a. confabulatory alcoholic psychosis
    a. disorder
    a. episode
    a. state
    a. syndrome
amnestica
    akinesia a.
amnestic-confabulatory syndrome
amobarbital interview
amok, amuck
amor
amoral
    a. psychopathic personality
    a. trend
amorist
amorous paranoia
amorphagnosia
amorphism
amorphosynthesis
amotivated behavior
amotivation
amotivational syndrome
amount
    maximum tolerable a.
amour
amour-propre
ampere
ampheclexis
amphetamine (AMT)
    a. abuse
    adjunctive a.
    a. challenge test
    a. delirium
    a. delusional disorder
    a. dependence
    a. inhaler
    a. intoxication
    a. intoxication, with perceptual
      disturbance
    a. look-alike
    a. overdose
    a. poisoning
    a. psychosis
    racemic a.
    substituted a.
    a. use disorder
    a. withdrawal
amphetamine-induced
    a.-i. anxiety
    a.-i. psychotic disorder with
      delusions
    a.-i. psychotic disorder with
      hallucinations
    a.-i. sexual dysfunction
amphetamine-like
    a.-l. action
    a.-l. substance

amphetamine-related disorder
amphicrania
amphierotism
amphigenesis
amphigenic inversion
amphigonadism
amphimixis
amphithymia
amphitypia
amphoriloquy
amphorophony
amphotonia, amphotony
amplification
    memory a.
    symptom a.
amplitude modulation (AM)
amputee
AMR
    abnormal muscle response
    alternate motion rate
AMS
    auditory memory span
amuck *(var. of* amok)
amulet
amusia
    expressive a.
    motor a.
    sensory a.
    vocal a.
amusing aspect
amygdala, pl. **amygdalae**
    a. activation
    a. atrophy
    a. damage
    a. nucleus group
    a. response
    a. subnucleus
    a. volume
    a. volumetric loss
amygdala-fear circuitry
amygdala-prefrontal cortex-locus ceruleus
  interaction
amygdaloid stimulation
amyl
    a. acetate
    a. alcohol
    a. chloride
    a. nitrate abuse
    a. nitrate inhalant
    a. salicylate
    a. valerate
amylase
amylene
    a. chloral
amylobarbitone
amylophagia
amyoesthesia, amyoesthesis
amyostasia

amyosthenia
amyotaxy, amyotaxia
Amytal
amytal ablation
Amytal interview
AN
    anabiosis
    anorexia nervosa
anabiosis (AN)
anabolic
    a. agent
    a. androgenic
    a. steroid
anabolism
anacatesthesia
anachronism
anachronobiology
anaclasis
anaclitic
    a. depression
    a. psychotherapy
    a. relationship
    a. therapy
Anaconda
    Operation A.
anacusis
anagogic
    a. interpretation
    a. symbolism
    a. tendency
anagogy
anal
    a. administration
    a. canal
    a. character
    a. erotism
    a. fissure
    a. humor
    a. impotence
    a. intercourse
    a. masturbation
    a. personality
    a. phase
    a. phase of infancy
    a. rape
    a. rape fantasy
    a. retentive
    a. sadism
    a. sex
    a. stage
    a. stage psychosexual development
anal-aggressive character

analectrotonic zone
analeptic
anal-expulsive stage
analgesia
    a. dolorosa
    patient-controlled a. (PCA)
analgesic
    controlled a.
    a. cuirass
    nonnarcotic a.
analgesimeter
analgetic
analis
    coitus a.
anality
analog, analogue
    a. experiment
    I-labeled cocaine a.
    libido a.
    a. marking
    a. of meperidine
    a. of phencyclidine
    prion a.
    a. study
analogic change
analogous brain mechanism
analogue (*var. of* analog)
analogy
anal-retentive personality
anal-sadistic love
analysand
analysis, pl. analyses
    acoustic a.
    active a.
    aerodynamic speech a.
    applied behavioral a. (ABA)
    auditory a.
    behavior a.
    blind a.
    cephalometric a.
    chain a.
    character a.
    child a.
    classical a.
    clinical a.
    cluster a.
    complex segregation a.
    content a.
    contrastive a.
    control a.
    conventional factor a.
    a. of coping style

NOTES

analysis *(continued)*
 cost-benefit a.
 cost-reward a.
 a. of covariance (ANCOVA)
 Cox regression a.
 critical a.
 Dasein a.
 a. in depth
 didactic a.
 discriminant a.
 distal distinctive feature a.
 distinctive feature a.
 distributive a.
 ego a.
 error a.
 existential a.
 expectant a.
 factor a.
 fate a.
 feature a.
 feeling a.
 final a.
 focused a.
 Fourier a.
 fractional a.
 functional a.
 furthest-neighbor a.
 gait a.
 grammatical a.
 group a.
 handwriting a.
 harmonic a.
 hierarchical regression a.
 holistic a.
 immunoblot a.
 impact a.
 individual a.
 intent-to-treat a.
 interaction-process a.
 item a.
 job a.
 kinesthetic a.
 kinetic a.
 latent class a.
 lay a.
 methods a.
 minor a.
 morphometric a.
 motivation a.
 multiple a.
 multivariate a.
 neurometric a.
 occupational a.
 passive a.
 pattern a.
 percept a.
 perception a.
 perceptual a.

 personal document a.
 phenomenological a.
 philosophical a.
 phonemic a.
 phonetic a.
 phonological a.
 policy a.
 post hoc a.
 preliminary a.
 principal-components a. (PCA)
 a. procedure
 regression a.
 a. of the resistance
 Schicksal a.
 script a.
 segmental a.
 sequential multiple a. (SMA)
 situs a.
 solution a.
 sound a.
 state-of-the-art a.
 substitution a.
 suprasegmental a.
 a. and synthesis
 a. by synthesis
 task performance and a.
 taxometric a.
 therapeutic group a.
 toxicological a.
 traditional phonetic a.
 training a.
 transactional a. (TA)
 a. of transference
 trial a.
 a. of variance (ANOVA)
analyst anchor test
analytic
 a. approach
 a. boundary
 a. couch
 a. exegesis
 a. frame
 a. group psychotherapy
 a. insight
 a. interpretation
 a. method
 a. neurosis
 a. object
 a. patient
 a. psychiatry
 a. psychology
 a. rule
 a. stalemate
 a. therapy
 a. treatment
analytical
 a. breakdown
 a. philosophy

a. play therapy
a. process
a. psychology
analyzer, analyzor
breath a.
noise a.
wave a.
analyzing new information disturbance
anamnesis
associative a.
anamnestic response
ananabasia
ananastasia
anancasm
anancastia
anancastic
a. depression
a. neurosis
a. personality
anandamide
anandria
anaphia, anhaphia
anaphor
anaphoric pronoun
anaphrodisia
anaphrodisiac
anaphrodite
anaphylaxis
psychiatric a.
psychic a.
anaptic
anarchic behavior
anarchism
anarithmia
anarthria
anatomic
a. age
a. correlate
a. evidence
a. impotence
a. site of pain
anatopism
anatripsis
anatriptic
anaudia
ancestral
a. spirit
a. worship
ancestry
anchone
anchor
collapsing a.

firing an a.
a. signs of withdrawal
stacking a.
stealing an a.
a. symptom
a. test
anchoring
perceptual a.
ancillary care
ANCOVA
analysis of covariance
Andes disease
Andreasen
A. positive and negative symptoms
of schizophrenia
androgen
a. insensitivity syndrome
a. level
androgenesis
androgenic
a. alopecia
anabolic a.
androgenous
androgynization
androgynoid
androgynous individual
androgyny
android
andrology
andromania
andromimetic
andromorphous
androphilia
androsterone
anecdotal
a. data
a. evidence
a. method
anecdote
clinical a.
anelectrotonic zone
anelectrotonus
anemia
anepia
anepithymia
anerethisia
anergasia
anergastic
a. organic psychosis
a. reaction
anergia
physical a.

NOTES

anergic
>a. depression
>a. schizophrenic
>a. stupor

anergy
>denial of a.

anesthesia
>block a.
>central a.
>closed a.
>combined a.
>compression a.
>conversion a.
>crossed a.
>cutaneous a.
>diagnostic a.
>dissociative a.
>a. dolorosa
>electric a.
>emotional a.
>first stage of a.
>gauntlet a.
>general a.
>girdle a.
>glove a.
>gustatory a.
>Gwathmey a.
>halogenated inhalational a.
>hypnotic a.
>hysterical a.
>infiltration a.
>inhaled a.
>insufflation a.
>insulation a.
>laryngeal a.
>mental a.
>muscular a.
>neuroleptic a.
>olfactory a.
>painful a.
>perineural a.
>peripheral a.
>pressure a.
>primary a.
>segmental a.
>sensory a.
>sexual a.
>spinal a.
>splanchnic a.
>stocking a.
>stocking-and-glove a.
>tactile a.
>thermal a.
>traumatic a.
>unilateral a.
>visceral a.

anesthetic
>a. conversion reaction

>dissociative a.
>a. variant of schizoid behavior

anethopath

anetic

A9 neuron

angel-of-death hallucination

angel's trumpet

Angelucci syndrome

anger
>a. attack
>chronic state of a.
>constant a.
>controlled a.
>difficulty controlling a.
>a. dysregulation
>externalized a.
>fit of a.
>ineffective a.
>intense a.
>internalized a.
>inwardly directed a.
>irrational a.
>a. mallet
>a. management
>marked a.
>outburst of a.
>a. outburst
>overt signs of a.
>a. reaction
>redirecting a.
>suppressed a.
>transient state of a.
>trigger for a.
>a. and violence psychiatric
>>syndrome

angiography
>digital subtraction a. (DSA)

anglicize

Anglo

anglomania

anglophile

angor
>a. animi
>a. ocularis
>a. pectoris

angry
>a. affect
>a. behavior
>a. outburst
>a. reaction
>a. reaction to minor stimuli
>a. woman syndrome
>a. word exchange

anguish
>existential a.
>personal a.
>post-binge a.

anhalonine

anhaphia (*var. of* anaphia)
anhedonia
    orgasmic a.
    pervasive a.
    social a.
anhedonia-asociality
anileridine
anilinction
anilinctus
anilingus
anility
anima
animal
    a. abuse
    aggression to a.'s
    aggression to people and a.'s
    a. companionship
    cruelty to a.'s
    history of abusing a.'s
    a. magnetism
    a. psychology
animal-assisted therapy
animalize
animal-like
animated
animation
    suspended a.
animatism
animi
    angor a.
    demissio a.
animism
animist
animistic thinking
animosity
animus
ankh
ankle
    a. clonus
    a. jerk
anlage, pl. **anlagen**
annihilation anxiety
annihilator
anniversary
    a. date
    a. excitement
    a. hypothesis
    personally significant a.
    a. reaction
annoyance level (AL)
annulment

ano
    coitus in a.
    in a.
anodyne
anoetic
anogenital
anomalotrophy
anomalous
    a. movement
    a. parental vocal pattern
    a. result
    a. sexual behavior
    a. sexual urge
anomaly
    Aristotle a.
    autosomal a.
    cranial a.
    metabolic a.
    sexual a.
anomia
    color a.
    finger a.
    tactile a.
anomic
    a. aphasia
    a. error
    a. suicide
anomie
anonacein
anonymity
Anonymous
    Alcoholics A. (AA)
    Cocaine A. (CA)
    Codependents A. (CODA)
    Gamblers A. (GA)
    Narcotics A. (NA)
    Overeaters A. (OA)
    Parents A.
    Schizophrenics A. (SA)
    Sex Addicts A. (SAA)
    Sexaholics A. (SA)
    Workaholics A. (WA)
anorchism
anorectal
    a. physiological dysfunction
    a. spasm
anorectic, anoretic
anorexia
    elective a.
    a. nervosa (AN)
    social a.
anorexiant

NOTES

anorexic
- a. behavior
- a. fast

anorexigenic

anorgasmia
- secondary a.
- SSRI-induced a.

anorgasmic

anorgasmy, anorgasmia

anosmia
- essential a.
- functional a.
- mechanical a.
- respiratory a.
- true a.

anosodiaphoria

anosognosia

anosognosic

anosphrasia

ANOVA
- analysis of variance

anoxemia

anoxia
- altitude a.
- cerebral a.
- fulminating a.
- hypokinetic a.
- metabolic a.

anoxic encephalopathy (AE)

ANS
- autonomic nervous system

Anstie
- A. rule
- A. test

answer
- bizarre a.
- irrelevant a.
- syndrome of approximate relevant a.'s
- syndrome of deviously relevant a.'s
- yes-no a.

antagonism

antagonist
- alpha-2 a.
- benzodiazepine a.
- beta-adrenergic a.
- dopaminergic a.
- a. drug
- a. medication
- narcotic a.
- opiate a.
- opioid a.

antagonistic
- a. behavior
- a. muscle strength
- a. reflex
- a. thermoeffector

antagonize

antalgic gait

antaphrodisiac

antaphroditic

antasthenic

antecedent
- early childhood identifiable a.
- a. event
- identifiable a.
- a. variable
- a.'s of violence

antecedent-consequence variable

antepartum

antergia

anterior
- a. alexia
- a. aphasia
- a. capsulotomy for treatment of OCD
- a. cingulate
- a. cingulate flow
- a. cingulate pathway
- a. cingulotomy for treatment of OCD
- a. feature English phoneme
- a. horn index (AHI)
- a. hypothalamus
- a. insula region
- a. nucleus
- a. nucleus of thalamus
- a. speech zone
- a. vermis
- a. vertical canal

anterograde
- a. amnesia
- a. loss of memory
- a. memory interference

anterotic

anthomania

anthrax
- a. anxiety
- a. exposure
- a. germ exposure

anthropocentric

anthropocentrism

anthropogenic

anthropography

anthropoid

anthropological
- a. linguistics
- a. philosophy

anthropology
- applied a.
- criminal a.
- cultural a.
- medical a.
- physical a.
- social a.

anthropometric identification

A

anthropometry
anthropomorphic
anthropomorphism
anthropomorphize
anthropopathism
anthropopathy
anthropophagus
anthropophilic
anthroposophy
anthypnotic (*var. of* antihypnotic)
anthysteric (*var. of* antihysteric)
antiabortion
antiadrenergic effect
antiaggressive
    a. action
    a. effect
antiaging
antianaphylaxis
antiandrogen therapy
antianxiety
    a. agent
    a. medication
antibody
antibrain
anticatalyst
    anticipatory a.
anticathexis
anticephalalgic
anticholinergic
    a. delirium
    a. dose
    a. drug
    a. effect
    a. medication
    a. property
    a. side effect
    a. syndrome
antichrist
anticipated emotional suffering
anticipation
    a. of role
    a. of trigger
anticipatory
    a. anticatalyst
    a. anxiety
    a. autocastration
    a. avoidance (AA)
    a. coarticulation
    a. error
    a. grief
    a. guidance

    a. response
    a. and struggle behavior
anticipatory-maturation principle
anticlimactic
anticlimax
anticonvulsant
    a. drug
    a. effect
    a. intoxication
anticonvulsive
anticrime
antidepressant
    a. abuse
    a. agent
    atypical a.
    a. compound
    heterocyclic a. (HCA)
    a. inhibition
    a. medication
    monocyclic a.
    a. response
    serotonergic a.
    somatic a.
    a. therapy
    a. treatment
    triazolopyridine a.
antidepressant-resistant
antidiuretic hormone (ADH)
antidotal
antidote
antidromic
antidyskinetic agent
antiemetic
antienergic
antiepileptic
    a. medication
antierotica
antiestablishment
antiestrogenic
antiexpectancy speech
antifeminist
antifetishism
antigen
antigen-antibody reaction
antigonadal action
anti-government feeling
antihallucinatory
antihistamine
    sedative a.
antihistaminergic effect

NOTES

antihypertensive
    a. agent
    a. medication
antihypnotic, anthypnotic
antihysteric, anthysteric
anti-impulse effect
antiinflammatory therapy
anti-instinctual force
anti-Lewisite
    British a.-L. (BAL)
antilkisis
antimanics
antimotivational syndrome
antimuscarinic effect
antimyasthenic
antinarcotic
antinauseant
antinomianism
antinomy
antioxidant therapy
antipanic agent
antipathetic
antipathetical
antipathy
antipersonnel
antiphobic
antiphony
antipoplectic
antiposia
antipredatory aggression
antipsychiatry
antipsychomotor
antipsychotic
    a. action
    atypical a.
    a. compound
    conventional dopamine receptor-
      blocking a.
    depot a.
    a. drug
    a. drug therapy
    a. drug treatment
    a. effect
    a. exposure
    a. medication
    new-generation a.
    novel a.
    a. pharmacotherapy
    a. preparation
    a. response
    second-generation a.
    a. side effect
    thioxanthene a.
    traditional a.
    tricyclic a. (TCA)
    typical a.
antipsychotic-associated sexual
  dysfunction

antipsychotic-induced weight gain
antipyretic
antiresonance
antiretroviral medication
antireward system
antiruminant
antiseizure
    a. drug
    a. medication
anti-Semite
anti-Semitic
anti-Semitism
antiserotonergic effect
antislavery
antisocial (AS)
    a. activity
    a. adolescent
    a. aggression
    a. alcoholism
    a. behavior
    a. compulsion
    a. feature
    a. juvenile
    a. lifestyle
    a. neurotic personality
    a. neurotic personality disorder
    a. patient
    a. personality (ASP)
    a. personality disorder (APD,
      ASPD)
    a. psychopathic Q factor
    a. reaction
    a. scale
    a. teenager
    a. tendency
    a. trends psychopathic
    a. trends psychopathic personality
antispasticity
antisyphilitic
antiterrorism
antiterrorist
antitetanic
antithesis
antithetical
antitonic
antitoxin
antitragus
antitrismus
antitussive
antivivisection
antiwar
Anton
    A. syndrome
antrophose
antsy
anum
    per a.
anus, pl. ani

anxietas
    a. presenilis
    a. tibiarum
anxiety
    a. adjustment disorder
    adjustment disorder with a.
    adolescent a.
    alcohol-induced a.
    amphetamine-induced a.
    annihilation a.
    anthrax a.
    anticipatory a.
    anxiolytic-induced a.
    a. attack
    authority a.
    basic a.
    caffeine-induced a.
    cannabis-induced a.
    castration a.
    catastrophic a.
    childhood separation a.
    chronic a.
    clinically significant a.
    cocaine-induced a.
    a. comorbidity
    a. control technique
    a. control training (ACT)
    covert a.
    death a.
    debilitating a.
    delusional a.
    dental a.
    a. depression
    desertion a.
    a. diagnosis
    diffuse a.
    disabling a.
    a. discharge
    disintegration a.
    a. disorder of adolescence
    a. disorder of childhood
    a. disturbance
    a. dream
    a. due to physical disorder
    a. due to a substance
    a. during pregnancy
    ego a.
    eighth-month a.
    elementary a.
    environmentally induced a.
    erotized a.
    examination a.

excessive social a.
existential a.
extreme a.
feeling of a.
a. fixation
focus of a.
free-floating a.
frequency of a.
gender differences in a.
generalized a.
heightened a.
heterosexual a.
a. hierarchy
high a. (HA)
high impulsiveness high a. (HIHA)
high impulsiveness low a. (HILA)
hypnotic-induced a.
hyposomnia associated with a.
a. hysteria
id a.
immediate a.
a. index (AI)
insomnia associated with a.
instinctual a.
intense a.
intercourse a.
intercurrent a.
internal sensations of a.
a. inventory
level of a.
a. level
low a. (LA)
a. management
a. management training (AMT)
manifest a.
marked a.
masked a.
means for a.
moral a.
morbid a.
a. neurosis
neutralized a.
noetic a.
nonpathological a.
nonpsychotic a.
normal a.
a. object
objective a.
obsessional a.
oral a.
organic a.
overwhelming a.

NOTES

anxiety *(continued)*
    pain-type a.
    panic attack neurotic a.
    a. panic reaction
    panic-type a.
    paradoxical a.
    peer a.
    performance a.
    persecutory a.
    persistent a.
    pervasive a.
    phobic a.
    physical concomitant of a.
    a. preparedness
    a. prevention
    primal a.
    primary a.
    a. profile
    profound a.
    prominent a.
    provoked a.
    psychogenic a.
    a. psychogenic disorder
    a. psychoneurosis
    a. psychoneurotic reaction
    a. rating scale
    a. reaction, mild (ARM)
    reactive depression and a.
    real a.
    reality a.
    reduced a.
    reduction of a.
    a. reduction
    relaxation-induced a. (RIA)
    a. relief response
    a. resolution
    sedative-induced a.
    self-disclosure a.
    self-reported a.
    a. sensitivity (AS)
    a. sensitivity theory
    separation a.
    severe a.
    sexual a.
    signal theory of a.
    situation a.
    sleeplessness associated with a.
    social a.
    a. source
    a. state (AS)
    a. state neurotic disorder
    a. status index (ASI)
    a. status inventory (ASI)
    stranger a.
    substance-induced a.
    superego a.
    symbolic a.
    a. symptom

    a. syndrome
    a. tension state (ATS)
    test a.
    theory of a.
    a. tolerance
    total phobic a. (TPA)
    trait a.
    transformation theory of a.
    trauma-specific a.
    traumatic a.
    true a.
    a. typology
    uncontrollable a.
    undue social a.
    urethral a.
    virginal a.
anxiety-avoiding personality disorder
anxiety-blissfulness psychosis
anxiety-depression
anxiety-induced impaired social functioning
anxiety-mood comorbidity
anxiety-provoking
    a.-p. cue
    a.-p. situation
anxiety-related
    a.-r. mental disorder
    a.-r. psychiatric syndrome
    a.-r. sensation
anxiolytic
    a. abuse
    a. activity
    a. agent
    a. amnestic disorder
    a. delirium
    a. dependence
    a. drug
    a. effect
    a. intoxication
    a. medication
    a. response
    serotonergic a.
    a. stimuli
    a. substance
    a. substance-use disorder
    a. use disorder
    a. withdrawal
anxiolytic-induced
    a.-i. anxiety
    a.-i. persisting dementia
    a.-i. psychotic disorder with delusions
    a.-i. psychotic disorder with hallucinations
    a.-i. sexual dysfunction
anxious
    a. arousal
    a. delirium

A

a. expectation
a. mania
a. mood
a. mood adjustment reaction
a. rumination
a. somatic depression
a. substance abuser
a. thought
anxious-fearful cluster
anxiousness
anxious-neurotic personality trait
anylcyclohexylamine intoxication
AO
academic orientation
avoidance of others
AO scale
AOA
American Orthopsychiatric Association
AOB
alcohol on breath
AOTA
American Occupational Therapy
Association
APA
air pollution adaptation
American Psychiatric Association
American Psychoanalytical Association
American Psychological Association
apallesthesia
apallic
a. state
a. syndrome
apandria
apanthropia, apanthropy
apareunia
apartness
apastia
apastic
apathetic
a. affect
a. withdrawal
apathetic-type personality disorder
apathic
apathism
apathy
avolition a.
euphoric a.
a. syndrome
APC
aspirin, phenacetin, caffeine

APD
antisocial personality disorder
avoidant personality disorder
aperient
aperiodic
a. reinforcement
a. wave
aperitif
apertive
apertural hypothesis
APH
alcohol-positive history
APHA
American Public Health Association
APhA
American Pharmaceutical Association
aphagia
psychogenic a.
aphasia
acoustic a.
acquired epileptic a.
acquired fluent a.
afferent motor a.
ageusic a.
amnemonic a.
amnesic a.
amnestic a.
anomic a.
anterior a.
associative a.
ataxic a.
auditory a.
Bastian a.
Benson-Geschwind classification
of a.
Broca a.
callosal disconnection syndrome a.
central a.
childhood a.
combined transcortical a.
commissural a.
complete a.
conduction a.
contiguity a.
cortical a.
developmental a.
a. disorder
dynamic a.
efferent motor a.
executive a.
expressive a.
expressive-receptive a.

NOTES

aphasia *(continued)*
 fluent a.
 frontocortical a.
 frontolenticular a.
 functional a.
 gibberish a.
 global a.
 graphic a.
 graphomotor a.
 Grashey a.
 hypophonic a.
 ideomotor a.
 impressive a.
 infantile a.
 intellectual a.
 isolation a.
 jargon a.
 Kussmaul a.
 lenticular a.
 lethica a.
 Lichtheim a.
 major motor a.
 mixed a.
 motor a.
 nominal a.
 nonfluent a.
 optic a.
 parietooccipital a.
 partial nominal a.
 pathematic a.
 pictorial a.
 pragmatic a.
 psychogenic a.
 psychosensory a.
 pure a.
 a. quotient (AQ)
 receptive a.
 a. screening test
 semantic a.
 sensory a.
 similarity disorder of a.
 simple a.
 speech reading a.
 subcortical motor a.
 syndrome a.
 syntactic a.
 tactile a.
 total a.
 transcortical a.
 traumatic a.
 true a.
 verbal a.
 visual a.
 Wernicke a.
aphasiac
aphasic
 a. acalculia
 a. agraphia

 a. disturbance
 a. error
 a. migraine
 a. migraine headache
 a. patient
 a. phonological impairment
 a. seizure
aphemesthesia
aphemia
 pure a.
aphilopony
aphonia
 conversion a.
 functional a.
 hysterical a.
 intermittent a.
 paralytica a.
 a. paranoica
 spastic a.
 tactile a.
aphonic episode
aphonous
aphorize
aphose
aphrasia paranoica
aphremia
aphrodisia
 a. phrenitica
aphrodisiac
aphthongia
aphylactic
aphylaxis
apical
apicalization
aplestia
aplomb
APM
 Academy of Psychosomatic Medicine
apneic
 a. pause
 a. period
 a. seizure
apneustic
 a. breathing
 a. period
apocalypse
apocalyptic
apocalypticism
apocryphal
apodictic
apogee
apolitical
apologetic
apopathetic behavior
apophysary point
apoplectic
 a. coma

a. dementia
a. type
apoplectica
dementia a.
apoplectiform
a. convulsion
a. seizure
apostasis
apostasy
apostate
apostatize
apotheosis
apotreptic therapy
apotropaic
APP
addiction-prone personality
apparatus, pl. **apparatus**
autonomic a.
heat-loss a.
mental a.
psychic a.
apparent
alpha a.
a. competence
a. death
apparition
appeal
a.'s court
fear a.
inspirational a.
sex a.
snob a.
appearance
asthenic a.
body a.
a. deterioration
disheveled a.
emaciated a.
haggard a.
inappropriate a.
physical a.
preoccupation with defect in a.
sloppy a.
unkempt a.
appeaser
appendicular
a. ataxia
a. ataxis
apperception
feeling a.
tendentious a.
a. test

apperceptive
a. distortion
a. visual agnosia
appersonation
appersonification
appetite
altered a.
change in a.
a. control
a. disturbance
insatiable a.
a. for life
a. loss
loss of a.
perverted a.
a. psychogenic disorder
a. suppressant
voracious a.
appetitive
a. behavior
a. center
a. disturbance
a. drive
a. phase
a. state
applicable
not a. (N/A)
application
biofeedback a.
diverse medicinal a.
ritualized makeup a.
applicator
applied
a. anthropology
a. behavioral analysis (ABA)
a. extrasensory projection (AESP)
a. psychoanalysis
a. psychology
a. relaxation (AR)
a. research
a. science
appraisal
conflict management a. (CMA)
inflated a.
manager style a.
vocational a.
apprehend
apprehensible
apprehension
a. expectation
intense a.
irresistible a.

NOTES

apprehension *(continued)*
    sensation-focused a.
    sense of a.
    a. span
    a. state
    a. test
apprehensive
apprehensiveness
    social a.
apprise, apprize
approach
    adaptation a.
    adaptive a.
    alternative a.
    analytic a.
    assertive-community treatment a.
    basal reader a.
    behavioral a.
    bottom-up a.
    carrot-and-stick a.
    categorical a.
    checklist a.
    cholinergic a.
    clinical a.
    cluster a.
    cognitive behavioral a.
    comprehensive therapeutic a.
    constructive a.
    contemporary a.
    continuous a.
    cross-culture a.
    descriptive a.
    dimensional a.
    economic a.
    empirical a.
    environmental a.
    ethical a.
    ethnographic a.
    freudian a.
    functional a.
    fundamental a.
    a. gradient
    healthy a.
    here-and-now a.
    high-risk a.
    holistic a.
    idiographic a.
    insight-oriented a.
    integrative a.
    interdisciplinary a.
    language experience a. (LEA)
    legal a.
    linguistic a.
    mechanistic a.
    mixture a.
    moisture fear-molar a.
    molar a.
    multimodal therapeutic a.

    multiple-tracer a.
    multisystemic therapy a.
    Mutt and Jeff a.
    neuroimaging a.
    nomothetic a.
    nondirective a.
    organic a.
    patient-centered a.
    pharmacological a.
    primary pharmacological a.
    psychodynamic a.
    psychotherapeutic a.
    qualitative a.
    quantitative a.
    regressive-reconstructive a.
    religious a.
    sensate focus a.
    serial problem-solving a.
    spiritual a.
    targeted a.
    task-oriented a.
    therapeutic a.
    there-and-then a.
    yawn-sign a.
approachable
approach-approach conflict
approach-avoidance
    a.-a. conflict
    a.-a. stance
approbation
appropriate
    a. affect
    a. behavior
    a. facial expression
    a. in gender
    a. relationship
    a. response
    a. treatment
appropriateness of emotional response
approval loss
approximate
    a. answers syndrome
    a. lethal concentration (ALC)
approximation
    a. conditioning
    a. method
    method of a.
    successive a.
    word a.
appurtenance
apractagnosia
apractic *(var. of* apraxic)
apragmatism
apraxia
    akinetic a.
    amnesic a.
    amnestic a.
    cerebral mapping of a.

A

classic a.
construction a.
developmental a.
disconnection a.
dressing a.
facial a.
gait a.
ideational a.
ideatory a.
ideokinetic a.
ideomotor a.
innervation a.
kinesthetic a.
Liepmann a.
limb-kinetic a.
magnetic a.
motor a.
ocular a.
oculomotor a.
oral a.
sensory a.
speech a.
transcortical a.
verbal a.
apraxic, apractic
a. agraphia
a. behavior
a. disorder
apraxis
constructional a.
aprobarbital elixir
aproctia
aprophoria
apropos
aprosexia
aprosody
speech a.
APS
Adult Protective Services
air pollution syndrome
American Pain Society
American Psychological Society
apselaphesia
apsithyria
APSR
acute paranoid schizophrenic reaction
apsychia
apsychognosia
apsychosis
APTA
American Physical Therapy Association

aptitude
a. battery
a. inventory
learning a.
mechanical a.
numerical a. (N)
A. Research Project (ARP)
spatial a.
a. test
AQ
accomplishment quotient
achievement quotient
aphasia quotient
aqueduct veil
AR
achievement ratio
alarm reaction
alcohol related
applied relaxation
arachnoid
a. layer
a. tissue
arankan
ARBD
alcohol-related birth defect
arbiter
arbitrament
arbitrary
arbitrate
arborization
ARC
AIDS-related complex
arc
alpha a.
beta a.
a. de cercle
reflex a.
sensorimotor a.
archaic
a. brain
a. inheritance
a. residue
a. thought
archaic-paralogical thinking
archenemy
archetype
archfiend
architectural barrier
architecture of the brain
Archives of General Psychiatry
Arctic hysteria
arcuate movement

NOTES

ardanesthesia
ardent
ardor
    veneris a.
arduous
area
    acoustic a.
    association a.
    auditory cortical a.
    auditory projection a.
    basic skill a.
    body surface a.
    brain a.
    Broca a.
    Brodmann a. 6
    Brodmann a. 7
    Brodmann a. 9
    Brodmann a. 24
    Brodmann a. 32
    Brodmann a. 41
    Brodmann a. 43
    Brodmann a. 44
    Brodmann a. 46
    Brodmann a. 47/11
    a. CA4-1
    callosal a.
    catchment a.
    conflict-free a.
    cortical a.
    cross-sectional a. (CSA)
    cultural a.
    dominant hemisphere parietal a.
    dominant hemisphere temporal a.
    dorsolateral prefrontal cortical a.
    Epidemiologic Catchment A. (ECA)
    formed response of colored a.
      (FC)
    frontal cortical a.
    gray matter a.
    hypothalamic a.
    language a.
    lateral rostral supplementary
      motor a.
    medial rostral supplementary
      motor a.
    mesial prefrontal cortical a.
    motor a.
    National Institute of Mental
      Health-Epidemiologic
      Catchment A. (NIMH-ECA)
    neocortical association a.
    neuropsychologic a.
    occipital association cortical a.
    orbitofrontal a.
    parabrachial a.
    paracentral gray a.
    parietal neocortical association a.
    parietotemporal a.

    periventricular gray matter a.
    prefrontal cortical a.
    premotor a.
    processing a.
    rostral supplementary motor a.
    a. sampling
    sclerotic a.
    sclerotome a.
    sensory association a.
    sensory processing a.
    septal a.
    shading response to black a.'s (Fc)
    shading response to gray a.'s (Fc)
    silent a.
    skill a.
    somatesthetic a.
    somesthetic a.
    subcortical gray matter a.
    superior temporal auditory
      cortical a.
    supplementary motor a. (SMA)
    temporal neocortical association a.
    trigger a.
    visual cortical a.
    watershed a.
    Wernicke a.
    Wernicke 22, 39, 40 a.
areata
    alopecia a.
arecoline
areflexia
arenacea
    corpora a.
    corpus a.
argentophilic plaque
argot
argument
    irrational a.
    semantic a.
argumentative
argumentativeness
aristocrat
aristogenics
aristotelian method
Aristotle anomaly
arithmetic
    a. disorder
    a. grade equivalent
    a. mean
    a. problem
    a. sign
    a. subtest
arithmetical
    a. developmental delay disorder
    a. reasoning
    a. skills learning retardation
arithmomania

ARM
anxiety reaction, mild
arm
fixed dosing a.
a. phenomenon
shot in the a.
armamentarium
clinical a.
pharmacological a.
armed combat
armistice
armor
character a.
aromatherapy
around
hang a.
kick a.
screw a.
turn a.
around-the-clock observation
arousability factor
arousal
affective a.
anxious a.
autonomic a.
a. boost
a. boost mechanism
a. category
conditional a.
confusional a.
a. detection
deviant a.
a. disorder
a. dysfunction
emotional a.
erotic a.
a. from sleep
a. function
hanging a.
high a.
hyperactive sexual a.
hypoactive sexual a.
impaired a.
increased a.
inhibited sexual a.
intense autonomic a.
a. jag
level of a.
mental a.
nonspecific a.
object of a.

oxygen-deprived sexual a.
penile a.
physiological a.
psychological-physiological a.
a. reaction
a. reduction mechanism
a. reduction technique
sense of a.
sexual a.
sleep a.
sleeplessness associated with
conditional a.
a. state
a. symptom
a. theory
aroused
a. motive
a. state of disturbed behavior
ARP
Aptitude Research Project
arranged marriage
arrangement
change in living a.
contractual a.
family sleeping a.
living a.
picture a.
task force on local a.'s
arranging
ordering and a.
array of symptoms
arrest
action of a.
cardiac a.
cardiopulmonary a.
a. of development
false a.
house a.
locomotor a.
a. reaction
a. of schizophrenia
a. of speech
speech a.
arrested development
arrhigosis
arrhythmia
cardiac a.
ventricular a.
arrival
dead on a. (DOA)
arrogance

NOTES

arrogant
    a. behavior
    a. style
arseniasis
arsenic (As)
    a. amblyopia
arsenical tremor
arsenicophagy
arsenotherapy
arsine
arson
arsonist
    incendiary a.
art
    black a.
    language a.'s
    martial a.'s
    a. test
    a. therapy
artefacta
    self-induced dermatitis a.
Artemisia vulgaris
arteriosclerotic
    a. brain disease-type organic
      psychosis
    a. brain disorder
    a. dementia confusional state
    a. depression
    a. paranoid state
    a. psychosis confusional state
artery
    a. occlusion
    a. stenosis
articular sensibility
articulate
articulation
    addition a.
    a. developmental delay disorder
    a. index
    infantile a.
    a. of speech
    a. test
articulator
articulatory
    a. loop component
    a. tic
artifact
    edge a.
    statistical a.
artifactitious
artifactual
artificial
    a. assist
    a. disorder
    a. dream
    a. fecundation
    a. insemination
    a. intelligence in medicine (AIM)

    a. language
    a. neural network
    a. neurosis
    a. penis
artificialism
artist
    escape a.
artlessness
AS
    antisocial
    anxiety sensitivity
    anxiety state
As
    arsenic
as
    also known as (AKA)
    as necessary
    as needed (prn, PRN)
    as soon as possible (ASAP)
ASAD
    American Society for Adolescent
      Psychiatry
ASAM
    American Society of Addiction Medicine
ASAP
    as soon as possible
asaphia
asapholalia
ASC
    altered state of consciousness
ascendance-submission
ascending
    a. degeneration
    a. neurotransmitter system
    a. paralysis
    a. pitch break
    a. reticular activating system
    a. technique
ascension phase
ascertainment
    method of a.
asceticism
Asch situation
ascriptive responsibility
ASD
    acute stress disorder
asemasia, asemia
    a. graphica
    a. mimica
    a. verbalis
aseptic
asexual
ASGPP
    American Society of Group
      Psychotherapy and Psychodrama
ASI
    anxiety status index
    anxiety status inventory

Asian alcohol flush reaction
aside
> set a.
> thinking a.

as-if
> a.-i. hypothesis
> a.-i. performance
> a.-i. personality
> pseudo a.-i.

asinine
asitia
asocial
> a. acting out
> a. trends psychopathic personality

asociality
> premorbid a.
> schizophrenia with premorbid a. (SPA)

asonia
asoticamania
ASP
> antisocial personality

aspartame-restricted diet
aspartate
> a. aminotransferase (AST)

ASPD
> antisocial personality disorder

aspect
> amusing a.
> associative a.
> diagnostic a.
> executive a.
> immunologic a.
> integrative a.
> ironic a.
> normative a.
> perceptual a.
> physiological a.
> prominent a.
> speech a.

Asperger
> A. disorder

aspermia
> psychogenic a. (PA)

asphalgesia
asphyctic syndrome
asphyxia
> autoerotic a.
> traumatic a.

asphyxiant
asphyxiation
aspirational group

aspiration level
aspirin
> a. combination
> a. effect
> a., phenacetin, caffeine (APC)
> a. poisoning

ASPP
> American Society of Psychoanalytic Physicians

assail
assassination
> character a.

assault
> aggravated a.
> a. and battery
> brain a.
> grievous a.
> a. gun
> indecent a.
> personal a.
> physical a.
> a. rifle
> sexual a.
> violent personal a.
> a. weapon
> a. with a deadly weapon (ADW)
> witness to a.

assaulter
> serial a.

assaultive
> a. act
> a. behavior

assay
> a. buffer
> chloride channel flux a.
> cocaethylene a.
> drug a.
> immunofluorescence a.
> immunosorbent a.

A-S scale
assembly
> cell a.
> object a. (OA)
> picture a.

assertion structured therapy
assertive
> a. behavior
> a. conditioning
> a. outreach
> a. training

assertive-community treatment approach

NOTES

assertiveness
    a. skill
    a. training
assess
assessment
    a. of academic achievement
    a. of affect
    automated a.
    baseline a.
    a. battery
    behavior a.
    behavior-oriented a.
    cognitive a.
    communication skills a.
    community a.
    a. of competence
    competency a.
    complement symptom-focused a.
    comprehensive a.
    cross-sectional a.
    cultural a.
    a. and diagnosis
    diagnostic a.
    disorganized speech a.
    environmental a.
    family a.
    fantasy a.
    functional a.
    general personality a.
    home a.
    individual comprehensive a.
    a. instrument
    a. inventory
    language a.
    longitudinal a.
    luteal phase a.
    a. in mathematics
    a. measure
    a. method
    moral a.
    multidimensional a.
    multiple-choice a.
    neuroimaging a.
    neurolinguistic a.
    neurophysiological a.
    neuropsychologic a.
    objective a.
    outcome a.
    performance a.
    personality a.
    a. procedure
    projective personality a.
    psychiatric a.
    psychosocial a. (PA)
    quality of life rehabilitation a.
    quantified cognitive a.
    a. questionnaire
    rehabilitation a.

    risk-benefit a.
    a. scale
    specialized language a.
    spiritual a.
    standardized a.
    symptom a.
    task-oriented a.
asset
assets-liabilities technique
assiduity
assign blame
assigned
    a. responsibility
    a. sex
assignment
    random a.
    sex a.
    a. therapy
    writing a.
assimilable
assimilated nasality
assimilating
    a. information
    a. information disturbance
assimilation
    cultural a.
    double a.
    a. effect
    information a.
    law of a.
    a. law
    progressive a.
    reciprocal a.
    regressive a.
    reproductive a.
    a. rule
    velar a.
    vowel a.
assimilative factor
assist
    artificial a.
assistance
    medical a.
assistant
    physician's a. (PA)
    psychiatric a.
    research a.
assisted suicide
associate
    paired a.'s
    science research a.'s (SRA)
associated
    a. descriptive feature
    a. disability
    a. disorder
    a. idea
    a. intervention
    a. laboratory finding

a. movement
a. physical examination finding
associate learning
association
   A. for Advancement of Behavior
     Therapy (AABT)
   A. for the Advancement of Gestalt
     Therapy
   A. for the Advancement of
     Psychoanalysis (AAP)
   A. for the Advancement of
     Psychotherapy (AAP)
   Alzheimer Disease and Related
     Disorders A.
   American College Counseling A.
     (ACCA)
   American Counseling A.
   American Diabetic A. (ADA)
   American Dietetic A. (ADA)
   American Family Therapy A.
   American Managed Behavioral
     Healthcare A. (AMBHA)
   American Occupational Therapy A.
     (AOTA)
   American Orthopsychiatric A.
     (AOA)
   American Pharmaceutical A.
     (APhA)
   American Physical Therapy A.
     (APTA)
   American Psychiatric A. (APA)
   American Psychoanalytical A.
     (APA)
   American Psychological A. (APA)
   American Psychopathic A.
   American Public Health A.
     (APHA)
   a. area
   backward a.
   causal a.
   a. center
   a. characteristic
   characteristic a.
   A. for Child Psychiatrists
   clang a.
   a. coefficient
   conditioned fear a.
   consequence a.
   contextual a.
   controlled a.
   co-occurring a.
   A. of Correctional Psychologists

a. cortex
a. deficit pathology
Depression and Related Affective
   Disorders A.
direct a.
A. of Directors of Medical Student
   Education in Psychiatry
   (ADMSEP)
a. disease
dominant a.
dream a.
etiological a.
false a.
fear a.
a. fluency
free a.
frequency encountered a.
freudian-free a.
guilt by a.
idea a.
indirect a.
induced a.
International Psychoanalytical A.
   (IPAA)
International Transactional
   Analysis A. (ITAA)
laws of a.
a. learning
loosening of a. (LOA)
a. mechanism
Mental Health A. (MHA)
multiple a.
National Depressive and Manic-
   Depressive A. (NDMDA)
National Mental Health A.
   (NMHA)
National Rehabilitation A.
a. neurosis
occipital a.
phoneme-grapheme a.
preceding a.
psychosis of a.
a. reaction time
schizophrenia with premorbid a.
   (SPA)
a. sensation ratio
a. of sounds and symbols
sound-symbol a.
subordinate a.
tangential a.
temporal a.
a. test

NOTES

association *(continued)*
    word a.
    World Psychiatric A. (WPA)
associationism
associative
    a. anamnesis
    a. aphasia
    a. aspect
    a. facilitation
    a. fluency
    a. inhibition
    a. learning
    a. linkage
    a. memory
    a. play
    a. reaction
    a. response to a white space on a card (Ds)
    a. shifting
    a. strength
    a. thinking
    a. visual agnosia
associativity
    criterion of a.
assonance
assortative, assortive
    a. mating, assortive mating
ASSR
    adult situational stress reaction
assuasive
assumed
    a. mean
    a. similarity
assumption
    gentle a.
    a. of new identity
    reality a.
    theoretical a.
assumptive
assurance
assuredness
AST
    aspartate aminotransferase
astasia
astasia-abasia
astatic
astemizole
astereocognosy
astereognosia
astereognosis
asteric seizure
asterixis
asthenia
    heat-induced a.
    mental a.
    neurocirculatory a.
    psychogenic a.
    treatment-emergent a.

asthenic
    a. appearance
    a. constitutional type
    a. delirium
    a. diathesis
    a. neurosis
    a. personality
    a. personality disorder
    a. reaction
asthenology
asthenopia
asthenospermia
asthma
    bronchial a.
    intrinsic a.
    nervous a.
    sleep-related a.
asthmogenic
astomia
astral
    a. body
    a. projection
astray
astrology chart
astrotravel
astute
astyphia
asyllabia
asylum
asymbolia
asymmetrical amnesia
asymmetric motor neuropathy
asymmetry
    abnormal a.
    cerebral a.
    facial a.
    functional a.
    interhemispheric a.
    leftward a.
    mental a.
    metabolic a.
    a. and order effect
    reflex a.
    skull a.
asymptomatic
    a. neurosyphilis
    a. seizure
asymptotic wish fulfillment
asynchronously
asynchrony
asyndesis
asyndetic thinking
asynergia
asynergy
asynesia
asynodia
AT
    achievement test

at
    being stared at
    at large
    at risk
    tear at
atactic
    a. abasia
    a. agraphia
    a. ataxia
atactica
    abasia a.
    agraphia a.
    a. agraphia
atactilia
ataque de nervios
ataractic drug
ataralgesia
ataraxia
ataraxic
ataraxy
atavism
atavistic regression
ataxia
    absent a.
    acute a.
    alcoholic a.
    appendicular a.
    atactic a.
    autonomic a.
    Briquet a.
    Bruns a.
    cerebellar a.
    choreic a.
    conversion a.
    crural a.
    equilibratory a.
    Friedreich a.
    hysterical a.
    intrapsychic a.
    ipsilateral cerebellar a.
    kinesigenic a.
    kinetic a.
    Leyden a.
    locomotor a.
    Marie a.
    mental a.
    mild a.
    moderate a.
    moral a.
    motor a.
    noothymopsychic a.
    optic a.

    psychogenic a.
    sensory a.
    severe a.
    spinal a.
    static a.
    trunk a.
ataxiadynamia
ataxiagram
ataxiagraph
ataxiameter
ataxiamnesic
ataxiaphasia
ataxic
    a. abasia
    a. amimia
    a. aphasia
    a. diplegia
    a. feeling
    a. gait
    a. speech
    a. writing
ataxiophemia, ataxophemia
ataxis
    appendicular a.
ataxy
atelectasis
atelesis
atelia
ateliosis
atheoretical
atheromata
athletic constitutional type
athrepsia, athrepsy
athymia
athymic
athymism
athyreosis
atman
atmosphere
    a. effect
    emotional a.
    optimistic a.
    situationally appropriate a.
    situationally optimistic a.
    therapeutic a.
    a. of trust
atmospheric
    a. condition
    a. perspective
atocia
atolide

NOTES

atom
  social a.
atomic
  a., biological, chemical (ABC)
  a., biological, chemical warfare
atomism
atomistic psychology
atone
atonement
atonia, atony
atonic
  a. absence seizure
  a. impotence
atonicity
atony (*var. of* atonia)
atopognosia, atopognosis
ATP
  adenosine triphosphate
atrabiliary
atrabilious
atraumatic
atremble
atremia
atretic
at-risk
  a.-r. adolescent
  a.-r. high school student
  a.-r. middle school student
  a.-r. patient
atrocious
atrocity
atrophedema
atrophic dementia
atrophoderma neuriticum
atrophy
  amygdala a.
  brain a.
  cerebral a.
  diffuse brain a.
  frontotemporal brain a.
  neuritic a.
  neurogenic a.
  neurotrophic a.
  nutritional type cerebellar a.
  Pick a.
  structural a.
  whole brain a.
atropine
  a. coma therapy
  a. psychosis
atropinic
ATS
  anxiety tension state
attachment
  affectional a.
  avoidant a.
  a. behavior
  a. bond

  Bowlby theory of a.
  clear-cut a.
  continuity of a.
  a. disorder
  a. disorder of infancy
  disorganized forms of a.
  disoriented forms of a.
  a. dynamic
  a. fantasy
  feeling of a.
  a. figure
  grief-based a.
  a. in infancy
  insecure a.
  a. learning
  liquidation of a.
  locality a.
  a. in the making
  maternal a.
  mother-child a.
  mother-infant a.
  object a.
  oscillations of a.
  poor a.
  predisposition to a.
  a. relationship
  resistant a.
  secure a.
  selective a.
  sense of a.
  social a.
  a. style
  suffocating a.
  symbiotic a.
  a. theory
  unstable a.
attachment-separation disorder
attack
  acute anxiety a. (AAA)
  acute schizophrenic a.
  anger a.
  anxiety a.
  attitude of a.
  bioterrorist a.
  biting a.
  bound panic a.
  character a.
  clawing a.
  cued panic a.
  dream anxiety a.
  drop a.
  full-blown panic a.
  gang a.
  glottal a.
  limited symptom a.
  nocturnal panic a.
  obsessive a.
  panic a.

physical a.
position of a.
psychomotor a.
psychotic a.
quiet biting a.
rage a.
recurrent panic a.
refreshing sleep a.
savage a.
schizophrenic a.
schizophreniform a.
situationally bound panic a.
situationally predisposed panic a.
sleep a.
spontaneous panic a.
terrorist a.
twilight a.
uncinate a.
uncontrollable sleep a.
uncued panic a.
unexpected panic a.
vagal a.
vasovagal a.
vocal a.
word a.

attacker role
attainment
educational a.
emotional a.
goal a.
attaint
attaque
attempt
a. at a.
current suicide a.
failed suicide a.
future suicide a.
hanging a.
history of suicide a.
home life, education level,
activities, drug use, sexual
activity, suicide ideation/a.'s
(HEADSS)
past suicide a.
previous a.
reconciliation a.
remote suicide a.
risk of suicide a.
suicide a. (SA)
attempter
remote a.
suicide a.

attending
a. behavior
a. to language stage
a. physician
attention
a. alertness test
center of a.
a. and concentration
controlled a.
covert visuospatial a.
a. deficit
a. deficit disorder (ADD)
a. deficit disorder, residual type
a. deficit disorder with
hyperactivity (ADD-HA)
a. deficit disorder without
hyperactivity
a. deficit and disruptive behavior
disorder (AD-DBD)
a. deficit hyperactivity disorder
(ADHD)
a. deficit hyperactivity disorder,
combined type
a. deficit hyperactivity disorder,
predominantly hyperactive-
impulsive type
a. deficit hyperactivity disorder-
predominantly inattentive (ADHD-
PI)
a. deficit symptom
a. disorder
disturbance of a.
fix and focus a.
a. fluctuation
a. focus
focus of clinical a.
focus-execute component of a.
free-floating a.
heightened a.
impaired a.
a. impairment
medical a.
need for constant a.
a. overload
a. problem
quest for a.
raptus of a.
a. reflex
selective a.
selectivity of a.
a. shift ability
a. to sound

NOTES

attention *(continued)*
    span of a.
    a. span
    state of heightened a.
    sustained a.
    a. testing
    a. time
    vigility of a.
    visual a.
    visuospatial a.
    wandering a.
attentional
    a. ability
    a. abnormality
    a. circuit
    a. control
    a. demand
    a. disturbance
    a. dysfunction
    a. failure
    a. functioning
    a. impairment
    a. measure
    a. mechanism
    a. performance
    a. problem
    a. processing
    a. skills
attention-focusing procedure
attention-getting
attention-information processing
attention-seeking behavior
attenuation
attitude
    abstract a.
    a. of active friendliness
    a. adjustment
    a. of attack
    catatonoid a.
    categorical a.
    change of a.
    complacent a.
    concrete a.
    concretizing a.
    condescending a.
    counterphobic a.
    crucifixion a.
    cultural a.
    a. to death
    defeatist a.
    a. defense
    defense a.
    deferential a.
    deviant a.
    devil-may-care a.
    Dionysian a.
    dog-eat-dog a.
    do-not-care a.

    eating a.
    emotional a.
    exposition a.
    fatalistic a.
    feminine a.
    forced a.
    gambling a.
    gender-based a.
    gender-linked a.
    holier-than-thou a.
    illogical a.
    inappropriate a.
    inflexible a.
    a. inventory
    listening a.
    masculine a.
    maternal a.
    a. to medication (AM)
    mummy a.
    negative a.
    neutral a.
    nonjudgmental a.
    object a.
    objectifying a.
    oppositional a.
    overdependent a.
    passionate a.
    a. passionelle
    paternal a.
    pessimistic a.
    phobic a.
    positive a.
    positive mental a. (PMA)
    preadaptive a.
    primary oppositional a.
    punitive psychologic a.
    a. reassessment
    referential a.
    religious a.
    a. restructuring
    rigid a.
    a. scale
    self-centered a.
    self-critical a.
    sexual a.
    spiritual a.
    stereotyped a.
    stilted a.
    a. theory
    a. therapy
    third person a.
    a. tic
    a. type
    unsympathetic a.
attitudinal
    a. group
    a. pathosis
    a. reflex

a. risk factor
a. type
attitudinize
attonita
amentia a.
cephalea a.
melancholia a.
attonity
attorney
durable power of a.
medical power of a.
attract
attraction
fatal a.
gain-loss theory of a.
magnetic a.
sexual a.
attractiveness
attributable risk
attribute-entity
attribution
environmental a.
error a.
a. error
false a.
personal a.
situational a.
social a.
a. theory
attrition rate
attune
atypia
atypical
a. absence
a. absence seizure
a. affective disorder
a. antidepressant
a. antipsychotic
a. antipsychotic agent
a. antipsychotic drug
a. antipsychotic preparation
a. anxiety disorder
a. behavior
a. bipolar disorder
a. child
a. childhood psychosis
a. conduct disorder
a. course
a. delusional experience
a. depression
a. development
a. dissociative disorder

a. eating disorder
a. factitious disorder with physical symptoms
a. feature
a. gender identity disorder
a. impulse-control disorder
a. mania
a. or mixed organic brain syndrome
a. mixed or other personality disorder
a. neuralgia
a. neurotic anxiety state
a. pain
a. paranoid disorder
a. paraphilia
a. personality disorder
a. pervasive developmental disorder
a. presentation
a. psychosexual dysfunction
a. puberty
a. schizophrenia
a. somatoform disorder
a. specific developmental disorder
a. stereotyped movement disorder
a. tic disorder
atypicality
atypism
au courant
audacious
audacity
audible
a. blocking in speech
a. speech blockade
a. thought
audience effect
audile
auding
audiobrain stimulation
audiogenic
a. epilepsy
a. seizure (AGS)
audiogram
audiometry
ABR a.
automatic a.
behavioral observation a. (BOA)
audiophile
audioverbal amnesia
audiovisual
a. stimulation
a. training

NOTES

audit
  medical a.
  patient-care a.
  personal a.
  stress a.
audition
  chromatic a.
  gustatory a.
  mental a.
auditive
auditognosis
auditory
  a. ability
  a. accommodation
  a. acuity
  a. agnosia
  a. alexia
  a. amnesia
  a. analysis
  a. aphasia
  a. aura
  a. blending
  a. brainstem response (ABR)
  a. bulb
  a. canal
  a. closure
  a. comprehension
  a. continuous performance task
  a. cortical area
  a. discrimination
  a. disorientation
  a. distance cue
  a. distortion
  electric a.
  a. evoked potential (AEP)
  a. evoked response
  a. fatigue
  a. feedback
  a. hallucination
  a. hyperalgesia
  a. hyperesthesia
  a. imagery
  a. learner
  a. localization
  a. memory
  a. memory span (AMS)
  a. nerve
  a. pathway
  a. perceptual disorder
  a. processing
  a. projection area
  a. radiation
  a. region
  a. seizure
  a. sequencing
  a. skill
  a. space perception
  a. span

  a. stimulus
  a. symptom
  a. synesthesia
  a. system
  a. threshold
  a. training
auditory-verbal dysgnosia
augment
augmentation
  a. agent overactivity in OCD
  breast a.
  drug a.
  a. strategy
  thyroid a.
augmentative communication
augury
aura, pl. **aurae**
  auditory a.
  cephalic a.
  electric a.
  epigastric a.
  epileptic a.
  gustatory a.
  a. hysterica
  hysterical a.
  a. hysterics
  intellectual a.
  a. intelligence
  a. interpretation
  jamais vu a.
  kinesthetic a.
  migraine with a. (MA)
  motor a.
  olfactory a.
  a. procursiva
  reminiscent a.
  sensory a.
  status a.
  visual a.
aural pathology
AUSR
  acute undifferentiated schizophrenic
  reaction
austere
austericity
austerity
autarky, autarchy
autemesia
autesthetic
authenticate
authentication
  patient a.
  therapist a.
authenticity
authoritarian
  a. aggression
  a. character
  a. conscience

a. leader
a. leadership pattern
a. personality
a. rejecting-neglecting parent
a. submission
authoritarianism
right wing a. (RWA)
authoritative manner
authority
a. anxiety
a. complex
a. confusion
a. figure
a. figure fixation
prescriptive a.
a. principle
rebel against a.
authorization
away without a. (AWA)
treatment a.
authorized leave
autia
autism
akinetic a.
childhood a.
early infantile a.
high-functioning a. (HFA)
infantile a.
primary a.
secondary a.
semantics of a.
autisme pauvre
autismus infantum
autistic
a. behavior
a. child
a. disorder
a. fantasy
a. isolation
a. phase
a. proband
a. psychopathy
a. psychosis
a. thinking
autistic-presymbiotic adolescent
autistic-spectrum children
autoactivation
autoaggression
autoaggressive behavior
autoanalysis
autoanamnesis
autoathography

autobiographical
a. information
a. life chart
autobiographic memory
autobiography
autocastration
anticipatory a.
autocatharsis
autochthonous
a. delusion
a. gestalt
a. idea
a. variable
autoclitic operant
autocorrelation
autocractic
autocrat
autodestruct
autodidact
autoecholalia
autoechopraxis
autoerogenous
autoerotic asphyxia
autoerotism, autoeroticism
secondary a.
autogenic training
autogenital stimulation
autogenous depression
autognosis
autognostic
autohypnosis
autohypnotic amnesia
autohypnotism
autoimmune (AI)
a. deficiency
a. illness
a. obsessive-compulsive tic disorder
autointoxication
autokinetic effect
autolesion
autologous
autolysis
automania
automanipulation
automated
a. assessment
a. clinical record
automatic
a. absence
a. action
a. audiometry
a. behavior

NOTES

automatic *(continued)*
- a. chorea
- a. drawing
- a. epilepsy
- a. gain control
- a. judgment
- a. language
- a. memory
- a. movement
- a. obedience
- a. phrase level
- a. psychological process
- a. reactivity
- a. seizure
- a. speech
- a. thought
- a. volume control
- a. writing

automaticity of performance
automation
automatism
- ambulatory a.
- chewing a.
- command a.
- epileptic a.
- facial expression a.
- gestural a.
- ictal a.
- immediate posttraumatic a.
- mumbling a.
- primary ictal a.
- swallowing a.
- verbal a.

automatograph
automaton conformity
automization
automnesia
automorphic perception
autonarcosis
autonomasia
autonomic
- a. activity
- a. activity-reactivity
- a. affective law
- a. apparatus
- a. arousal
- a. arousal disorder
- a. ataxia
- a. balance
- a. conditioning
- a. conversion reaction
- a. denervation
- a. disorganization
- a. dysfunction
- a. dysnomia
- a. dysreactivity
- a. dysregulation
- a. epilepsy
- a. function
- a. hyperactivity
- a. hyperactivity sign
- a. hyperarousal
- a. hyperreflexia
- a. hyperventilation
- a. imbalance
- a. instability
- a. motor pool
- a. nerve
- a. nervous system (ANS)
- a. neurogenic bladder
- a. neuropathy
- a. reactivity
- a. response
- a. seizure
- a. side effect
- a. sympathomimetic drug

autonomotropic
autonomous
- a. depression
- a. ego function
- a. functional component
- a. psychotherapy
- a. stage
- a. superego

autonomy
- bodily a.
- functional a.
- loss of a.
- a. loss
- a. of motives
- patient a.
- perseverative functional a.
- a. scale

autonomy-heteronomy
autopagnosia
autopathography
autopathy
autophagia
autophagic
autophagy
autophilia
autophonia
autophonomania
autoplastic
- a. adaptation
- a. change
- a. symptom

autoplasty
autopsy
- brain a.
- psychological a.
- a. study

autopsychic
- a. delusion
- a. disorientation
- a. orientation

autopsychorhythmia
autopsychosis
autopsychotherapy
autopsy-negative death
autopunition
autoscopic
    a. phenomenon
    a. psychosis
    a. syndrome
autosensitize
autosexing
autosexualism
autosexuality
autosmia
autosomal
    a. aberration
    a. abnormality
    a. anomaly
    a. dominant
    a. dominant gene
    a. dominant inheritance
    a. dominant pattern
    a. recessive
    a. trisomy
autosomatognosis
autosomatognostic
autosome
autosuggestibility
autosuggestion
autosymbolism
autosynnoia
autotelic
autotherapy
autotomia
autotopagnosia agnosia
autotoxic
autotrophic nutrition
autozygous
auxiliary
    a. ego
    a. organ
    a. solution
    a. therapist
auxoaction
auxotherapy
auxotox
availability of weapons
avalanche
    law of a.
avarice
avatar
avenge

avenues of administration
aver
average
    a. conditioning
    a. evoked response technique
    a. student
averse to risk
aversion
    a. conditioning
    a. depression
    occasional sexual a.
    a. reaction
    a. response
    risk a.
    school a.
    sexual a.
aversion-covert conditioning
aversive
    a. behavior
    a. conditioning
    a. control
    a. drive
    a. early environment
    a. incentive
    a. racism
    a. stimulus
    a. therapy
    a. training
avert
aviation medicine
aviator's
    a. disease
    a. effort syndrome
    a. neurasthenia
avid
avidity
avocation
avoidance
    anticipatory a. (AA)
    a. behavior
    a. category
    a. cluster
    cognitive a.
    a. conditioning
    conflict a.
    conscious a.
    contact a.
    emotional a.
    a. and escape learning
    a. of exposure
    eye contact a.
    a. gradient

NOTES

avoidance *(continued)*
    harm a. (HA)
    incubation of a.
    master of a.
    a. measure
    a. of others (AO)
    outside activity a.
    pain a.
    passive a.
    a. pattern
    phobic a.
    a. response
    a. score
    social situation a.
    a. speaking
    a. of speech dysfluency
    stimuli a.
    a. style
    a. symptom
    a. syndrome
    a. therapy
    a. training
    withdrawal a.
avoidance-avoidance conflict
avoidant
    a. attachment
    a. disorder of adolescence
    a. disorder of childhood
    a. feature
    a. neurotic personality disorder
    a. personality
    a. personality disorder (APD)
    a. scale
    a. symptom
avoidant-attached behavior
avoisomatognosis
avolition apathy
avouch
avow
avulsion
AWA
    away without authorization
awake
    a., alert, and oriented (AAO)
    a. state
awakening
    early a.
    nighttime a.
award
    potential external a.
aware
    keenly a.
awareness
    behavior a.
    body a.
    closed a.
    conscious a.
    contingency a.

    a. defect
    a. deficit
    emotional a.
    environmental a.
    heightened a.
    interoceptive a.
    lack of interoceptive a.
    lapse of a.
    leisure a.
    mutual pretense a.
    open a.
    phonemic a.
    postural a.
    reality a.
    sensory a. (SA)
    spiritual a.
    a. of spirituality
    state of heightened a.
    subconscious a.
    suspected a.
    a. threshold
    a. training model
away
    blow a.
    carry a.
    explain a.
    fall a.
    tear a.
    turn a.
    a. without authorization (AWA)
awestruck
awkwardness
    social a.
AWOL
    absent without leave
awry
axes (*pl. of* axis)
axial
    a. amnesia
    a. gradient
    a. hyperkinesis
    a. neuritis
    a. section
axilla
    coitus in a.
axiodrama
axiology
axis, pl. **axes**
    a. I, II conceptualization
    defensive functioning a.
    a. I, II diagnosis
    a. I, II disorder
    a. function
    a. I, II interview
    a. I, II instrument
    a. I, II item
axolysis
axonal idiocy

axonapraxia
axonometer
axonopathy
axonotmesis
axon terminal
ayahuasca
aypnia

azaloxan
azaperone
azaspirodecanedione
Azima battery
azoospermia
Azorean disease
Aztec idiocy

A

NOTES

Got a Good Idea for STEDMAN'S?

Help us keep STEDMAN'S products fresh and up-to-date with new words and new ideas! How can we make your STEDMAN'S product the best medical word reference possible? Do we need to add or revise any items? Is there a better way to organize the content? What other medical references can Stedman's provide?

Fill in the spaces provided with your thoughts and recommendations and drop the card in the mailbox (postage-paid) or visit us at **www.stedmans.com** to submit your ideas. Feel free to e-mail us with your suggestions at **stedmans@LWW.com**. Please be specific! You're our most important contributor, and we want to know what's on your mind.

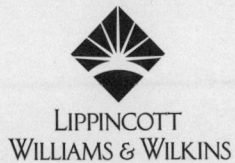

LIPPINCOTT
WILLIAMS & WILKINS

Please tell us a little about yourself.

Name/Title: _____

Company: _____

Address: _____

City/State/Zip: _____

Day Telephone No.: _____

E-mail Address: _____

Terms to be revised:

CURRENT TERM	SUGGESTED REVISION
_____	_____
_____	_____
_____	_____

New terms/words you would like us to add:

_____

_____

_____

Which of the following *Stedman's Word Book* titles need to be revised?

	NOT NECESSARY TO REVISE				REVISE NOW!
Stedman's Equipment Words	1	2	3	4	5
Stedman's OB-GYN Words	1	2	3	4	5
Stedman's Pediatric Words	1	2	3	4	5
Stedman's Endocrinology Words	1	2	3	4	5
Stedman's Cardio/Pulm Words	1	2	3	4	5

Others: _____

Additional ideas, suggestions, & comments:

_____

_____

_____

May we quote you?   ☐ Yes   ☐ No

All done? Great, just drop this card in the mail. OR visit us at **www.stedmans.com** and click on the "Got a Good Idea?" link.

Thank You!   PSYCH 738377

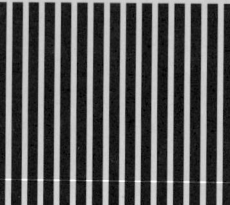

BUSINESS REPLY MAIL

FIRST CLASS   PERMIT NO. 724   BALTIMORE, MD

POSTAGE WILL BE PAID BY ADDRESSEE

ATTN: JULIE STEGMAN
LIPPINCOTT WILLIAMS & WILKINS
351 WEST CAMDEN STREET
BALTIMORE MD   21201-2436

B40
BA
  blood alcohol
  bone age
baah-ji
babble
  phonetic b.
babbling
  nonreduplicated b.
  reduplicated b.
  social b.
babel
babied
baby
  battered b.
  b. blues
  b. boomer
  b. boomlet
  b. buster
  cocaine-dependent b.
  b. talk
  war b.
baby-boom generation
baby-bust generation
babysitter
bacchanal
bacchant
bachelor
  B. of Medical Science
  B. of Social Work (BSW)
bachelorette
back
  b. down
  hang b.
  laid b.
  set b.
  snap b.
  b. talk
  turn b.
backache
  psychogenic b.
backbeat
backbite
backbone
background
  cultural b.
  ethnic b.
  b. factor
  family b.
  b. interference
  b. masking
  b. music
  b. noise
  psychotherapeutic b.
  regional b.

  religious b.
  sociocultural b.
  socioeconomic b.
backhanded
backing to velars
backlash
backon
backpedal
backseat
backslide
backstab
backstabber
back-to-back
backward
  b. association
  b. coarticulation
  b. conditioning
  b. making technique
  b. visual masking
backwards
  reading b.
bad
  b. actor
  b. blood
  b. conduct discharge (BCD)
  b. dream
  b. object
  b. self
  b. trip
badinage
bad-me
bad-mouth
bad-people fear
Bad Wildungen Metz (BWM)
baffle
bag
  b. lady
  mixed b.
baggage
  emotional b.
bagger
bagman
Bahał
bahnung
bah tschi
bail
  skip b.
bailout behavior
BAL
  blood alcohol level
  British anti-Lewisite
balance
  acid-base b.
  alternate binaural loudness b.
  (ABLB)

balance *(continued)*
    alternate monaural loudness b.
      (AMLB)
    autonomic b.
    b. control
    core body b.
    dynamic ambulatory b.
    dynamic standing b.
    electrolyte b.
    energy b.
    family structural b.
    fluid b.
    homeostatic b.
    impaired b.
    inhibition-action b.
    measure of b.
    b. mechanism
    off b.
    b. scale
    sitting b.
    spatial b.
    standing b.
    structural b.
    b. theory
    water b.
balanced
    b. diet
    b. lifestyle
    b. placebo
balanus
balbuties
balderdash
bald-faced lie
baleful
balefulness
Balint syndrome
balk
balky
ball
    eight b.
    b. of fire
    b. up
ball-and-field test
baller
ballet
    b. technique
    b. therapy
ballism
ballismus
ballistic movement
ballistics
ballistomania
ballsy
ballyhoo
balneology
balneotherapeutic
balneotherapy
bamboozle

banal
band
    b. frequency
    b. spectrum
    vocal b.
Band-Aid medicine
band-like headache
band-pass filter
bandwagon effect
bandy about
bane
baneful
banewort
bang
banger
    gang b.
banging
    head b.
    sleep-related head b.
bangungut
banish
banisterine
bank
    electronic data b.
    patient data b.
    practitioner data b.
bankrupt
bankruptcy
banter
Banting diet
baptism by fire
BAQ
    brain age quotient
baquet
bar
    dating b.
    b. hustler
    b. reflex
baragnosis, barognosis
barbaralalia
barbarian
barbaric
barbarism
barbarity
barbarize
barbarous
barbed-wire
    b.-w. disease
    b.-w. psychosis
Barbidonna No.2
barbital
    sodium b.
barbital-dependent (BD)
barbituism
barbiturate
    b. abuse
    b. addiction
    b. dependence (BD)

B

b. intoxication
long-acting b.
b. overdose
b. tolerance
ultrashort-acting b.
b. withdrawal
barbiturate-facilitated interview
barbiturate-induced
b.-i. coma
b.-i. death
barbituric acid
Bardet-Biedl syndrome
baresthesia
baresthesiometer
bargain
plea b.
bargaining
bariatrics
barking
Barnes global score
Barnum effect
BARNY
Body Awareness Resource Network
barognosis (*var. of* baragnosis)
baroreflex
barotrauma
barotropism
barracoon
barrage
barreflex
barren
barrenness
inner b.
barrier
architectural b.
communication b.
incest b.
b. to intervention
language b.
protective b.
b. response
social b.
barrier-free environment
barrio
bart
bartholinitis beseech
baryesthesia
baryglossia
barylalia
baryphonia, baryphony
barythymia

BAS
behavioral activation system
bas
de haut en b.
basal
b. diet
b. fluency
b. ganglia-cingulate gyrus-frontal
  lobe loop
b. mental age
b. metabolic rate (BMR)
b. metabolism
b. narcosis
b. pitch
b. reader approach
b. resistance level
b. temperature
base
b. component
ether b.
free b.
b. impulse
b. rate
b. rule
b. structure
b. word
baseborn
basedowian insanity
baseline (BL)
b. assessment
behavioral b.
b. cognitive functioning
b. measure
b. monitoring
b. rating
b. scan
b. severity
b. symptom
b. test
b. visit
baseline-to-endpoint change
basement
b. chemist
b. laboratory
bash
bashing
gay b.
basic
b. anxiety
b. brain mechanism
b. brain pathway
b. conflict

NOTES

basic *(continued)*
    b. diet
    b. impairment
    b. methadone service
    b. mistake
    b. mistrust
    b. personality
    b. personality type
    b. rest-activity cycle (BRAC)
    b. rule
    b. skill area
    b. skills
    b. trust
basigenous
basilect
basilic
basing
basis, pl. bases
    biologic b.
    compassionate use b.
    empirical b.
    genetic b.
    heritable b.
    outpatient b.
    pathophysiological b.
    physiological b.
    presumptive b.
    psychological b.
basophilia
    Cushing b.
    pituitary b.
basophilism
bastard
bastardize
Bastian aphasia
bastion
bathmotropic
    negatively b.
    positively b.
bathos
bathroom privileges
bathyanesthesia
bathyesthesia
bathyhyperesthesia
bathyhypesthesia
bathypnea
battacca
battalion
battalious
battarism
battarismus
batter
battered
    b. baby
    b. child
    b. child syndrome (BCS)
    b. parent
    b. spouse

    b. spouse syndrome
    b. wife
    b. woman syndrome (BWS)
    b. women's shelter
battering behavior
battery
    ability b.
    achievement b.
    aggravated b.
    aptitude b.
    assault and b.
    assessment b.
    Azima b.
    brief cognitive test b.
    chemistry screening b. I (CSB I)
    chemistry screening b. II (CSB II)
    cognitive test b.
    diagnostic b.
    educational achievement b.
    electrophysiological b.
    mental deterioration b.
    neuropsychologic b.
    b. of online test
    quantitative electrophysiological b.
    standard neuropsychological b.
    test b.
battle
    b. fatigue
    b. neurosis
    b. psychoneurosis
    B. sign
battlefront
battleground
Battley sedative
bawd
bawdry
bawdy
Bayesian technique
Bayle disease
Bayley
    B. behavior record
Baylorfast diet
BC
    behavior control
    birth control
BCD
    bad conduct discharge
BCP
    birth control pill
BCR
    behavior control room
BCS
    battered child syndrome
BCW
    biologic and chemical warfare
BD
    barbital-dependent
    barbiturate dependence

belladonna
benzodiazepine
birth date
BDAC
 Bureau of Drug Abuse Control
BDD
 body dysmorphic disorder
bdelygmia
BDID
 bystander dominates initial dominant
BDL
 below detectable levels
beads
  worry b.
BEAM
 brain electrical activity mapping
beamish
bearable
Beard disease
bearer
bearing
  grudge b.
bearish
beast fetishism
beastly
beaten
beat generation
beatific vision
beatify
beating
beau
  ideal b.
  b. monde
beauteous
bebop music
becalm
Beck
  B. view of depressive disorder
becloud
beclouded dementia
bed
  b. crisis
  out of b. (OOB)
  b. partner
bedazzle
bedevil
bedfast
bediamism
bedizen
bedlam
bedraggled
bedrest

bedridden
bedside manner
bedtime
bedwetter
bedwetting
befall
befitting
befool
before meals (a.c.)
befriend
befuddle
beggar
  emotional b.
beggary
beginner
begrudge
beguile
BEHAVE-AD
 behavioral pathology in Alzheimer
  disease
behavior
  aberrant b.
  abnormal illness b.
  abusive dating b.
  acceptable b.
  accepted b.
  accident b.
  accident-prone b.
  achievement b.
  acting out b.
  activity and b.
  acute psychotic aggressive b.
  adaptive b.
  addictive b.
  adient b.
  adjust repetitive b.
  adolescent experimentation with
   adult b.
  adult self-harm b.
  age-appropriate b.
  age-inappropriate knowledge of
   sexual b.
  age-level b.
  aggressive objectionable b.
  aggressive psychotic b.
  agitated b.
  agnostic b.
  aimless b.
  alcohol consumption b.
  alcohol-related b.
  alexithymic b.
  alleviating violence in aggressive b.

B

NOTES

behavior *(continued)*
 b. alteration
 alternating b.
 alternative b.
 altruistic b.
 ambient b.
 amotivated b.
 b. analysis
 anarchic b.
 anesthetic variant of schizoid b.
 angry b.
 anomalous sexual b.
 anorexic b.
 antagonistic b.
 anticipatory and struggle b.
 antisocial b.
 apopathetic b.
 appetitive b.
 appropriate b.
 apraxic b.
 aroused state of disturbed b.
 arrogant b.
 assaultive b.
 assertive b.
 b. assessment
 attachment b.
 attending b.
 attention-seeking b.
 atypical b.
 autistic b.
 autoaggressive b.
 automatic b.
 aversive b.
 avoidance b.
 avoidant-attached b.
 b. awareness
 bailout b.
 battering b.
 behavior b.
 binge-eating b.
 binge-purge b.
 bisexual b.
 bizarre b.
 borderline b.
 bulimic b.
 bullying b.
 catastrophic b.
 catatonic b.
 ceremonial b.
 b. chain
 change in b.
 b. characteristic
 characteristic b.
 b. checklist
 child or adolescent antisocial b.
 childhood cross-gender b.
 childish b.
 childlike b.

chronic illness b.
clinging b.
clinical b.
coercive b.
cognitive b.
collateral b.
collective b.
compelled b.
compensatory b.
competitive b.
complex motor b.
compulsive drug-taking b.
compulsive masturbatory b.
compulsive sexual b.
concealing b.
condescending b.
consensual sexual b.
consistent b.
consumer b.
contact b.
contemporaneous suicidal b.
b. contract
contractual b.
b. control (BC)
b. control room (BCR)
cooperative b.
coping b.
copulatory b.
counterphobic b.
countertransference b.
courtship b.
covert b.
criminal b.
criterion b.
cross-dressing b.
cross-gender b.
crowd b.
cuddling b.
culturally appropriate avoidant b.
culturally condoned b.
culturally sanctioned b.
cultural-related standards of
 sexual b.
cunning and hiding b.
cyclothymic-depressive b.
dangerous b.
de-escalating aggressive b.
defensive b.
defiant b.
b. deficit
delinquent b.
delusional b.
demanding b.
dementia-related b.
dependent b.
desired b.
destructive b.
b. determinant

developmentally appropriate
  avoidant b.
developmentally appropriate shy b.
deviant political b.
deviant religious b.
differential reinforcement of
  other b. (DRO)
diminution of goal-directed b.
direct self-destructive b. (DSDB)
discordant b.
discriminatory b.
disinhibited violent b.
disobedient b.
b. disorder
b. disorder of childhood
disorganized attachment b.
disoriented attachment b.
b. disruption
disruptive b.
disturbed eating b.
disturbing b.
dominant-subordinate b.
drinking b.
drive b.
driven motor b.
driving b.
drug-addictive b.
drug high-risk b.
drug-related HIV risk b.
drug risk b.
drug-seeking b.
drug use b.
b. dynamics
dysarthric b.
dysfunctional b.
dysrhythmic aggressive b.
dyssocial b.
eating b.
eccentric b.
ecstatic b.
ego-dystonic b.
elicited b.
embracing b.
emitted b.
empathic b.
employment-related b.
enraged b.
entry b.
envious b.
erotic b.
erratic b.
escape b.

ethical b.
ethnic relational b. (ERB)
evasive b.
excessive gambling b.
excitable b.
excited b.
exhibitionistic b.
experimental analysis of b.
explicit b.
exploitative-manipulative b.
exploratory b.
explosive aggressive b.
externalizing b.
extraindividual b.
extramarital b.
face-saving b.
failure to sustain consistent
  work b.
feeding b.
felony b.
fidgeting b.
b. field
finger-biting b.
fire-setting b.
flamboyant b.
flirtatious b.
following b.
food-related b.
forgotten b.
freezing b.
future suicidal b.
gambling b.
gang b.
b. genetics
goal-directed b.
grossly disorganized b.
group b.
hair-pulling b.
hallucinatory b.
haughty b.
head-banging b.
health b.
healthy adolescent b.
helping b.
help-seeking b.
heterosexual b.
hiding b.
high-risk b.
HIV risk b.
homicidal b.
homoerotic b.
homosexual b.

NOTES

behavior *(continued)*
    hostile b.
    hunting b.
    hyperactive b.
    hyperactive-impulsive b.
    hyperenergetic b.
    hysterical b.
    idiosyncratic b.
    illness b.
    imitative b.
    immediacy b.
    implicit b.
    impulsive b.
    inappropriate b.
    inattentive b.
    incoherent b.
    incompatible b.
    inconsiderate b.
    indirect self-destructive b. (ISDB)
    infantile b.
    ingratiating b.
    initiation of goal-directed b.
    innate b.
    instinctive b.
    intense sexual b.
    intentional involuntary b.
    interictal b.
    intermittent explosive b.
    interpersonal b.
    intimidating b.
    intolerable b.
    intrinsic b.
    intrusive b.
    invaluable b.
    invariable b.
    b. inventory
    involuntary b.
    irrational b.
    irresponsible work b.
    isolative b.
    kinesic b.
    kissing b.
    kleptomanic b.
    knowledge, attitude, b. (KAB)
    language b.
    b. language
    lawful b.
    leadership b.
    learned dysfunctional b.
    legal repercussion of violent b.
    life-threatening b. (LTB)
    lifetime b.
    limit-testing b.
    locality-specific pattern of
      aberrant b.
    localization of b.
    maladaptive pattern of b.
    malevolent b.

    management of assaultive b.
      (MAB)
    manipulative b.
    b. mapping
    masochistic b.
    mass b.
    masturbation b.
    maternal b.
    mating b.
    maze b.
    meddlesome b.
    medication-taking b.
    mercurial b.
    b. method
    mischievous b.
    mob b.
    modeled b.
    b. modification
    b. modification program
    b. modification therapy
    moral b.
    motor b.
    murderous predation b.
    mystifying b.
    needle-related HIV risk b.
    negative b.
    negativistic b.
    nodal b.
    nonaggressive objectionable b.
    nonparaphilic compulsive sexual b.
    nonproductive b.
    nonverbal b.
    nonviolent b.
    normative b.
    obedient b.
    objectionable b.
    obsessive b.
    obsessive-compulsive b.
    odd b.
    oedipal b.
    on-task b.
    operant b.
    operative b.
    oppositional b.
    oral b.
    orderly b.
    out-of-control b.
    overt b.
    pacing b.
    pain b.
    paranoid b.
    paraphiliac b.
    parasuicidal b.
    parental b.
    passive b.
    passive-aggressive b.
    past b.
    paternal b.

pathologic b.
b. pattern
pattern of antisocial b.
pattern of repetitive b.
peculiar b.
pedophilic b.
perplexing b.
petting b.
phobic avoidant b.
physically aggressive b.
pleasure-oriented b.
positive attention b. (PAB)
pressured b.
primary b.
problem b.
b. problem
problematic sexual b.
promiscuous sexual b.
prosocial b.
provocative b.
psychomotor b.
psychotic aggressive b.
psychotic disruptive b.
purging b.
purposeful b.
b. rating
b. rating scale
rational-emotive b.
b. reaction
real-life b.
reckless b.
b. record
b. reflex
regressive b.
rehabilitation b.
b. rehearsal
relational b.
relationship b.
religious b.
REM sleep b.
repertoire of aggressive b.
repetitious b.
repetitive checking b.
repetitive pattern of b.
repressive b.
respondent b.
responsible sexual b.
restless b.
restricted b.
restricting b.
restrictive b.
b. reversal

reward-associated b.
risk-taking b.
risky sexual b.
ritual b.
ritualistic b.
b. role
sadistic b.
b. sampling
seductive b.
self-damaging b.
self-defeating b.
self-destructive b.
self-dramatizing b.
self-harm b.
self-injurious b. (SIB)
self-mutilative b.
self-punishing b.
self-stimulatory b.
sensory-motor b.
b. setting
sex-related HIV risk b.
sex-role b.
sexual high-risk b.
sexually arousing b.
sexually inappropriate b.
sexually seductive b.
sexual predation b.
b. shaping
sissy b.
sleepwalking b.
socially acceptable b.
socially unacceptable b.
socially undesirable b.
social phobic-like b.
social stereotypical b.
sociopathic b.
spatial b.
b. specimen recording
speech b.
speech and language b.
b., speech, and other syndromes
  (BSO)
spiritual b.
splitting b.
stalking b.
standard b.
stereotyped pattern of b.
stereotypical b.
stimulation-bound b. (SBB)
structural analysis of social b.
struggle b.
subliminal b.

NOTES

behavior *(continued)*
  submissive b.
  substance-seeking b.
  substituting b.
  sucking b.
  suicidal b.
  sundowning b.
  superstitious b.
  suspicious b.
  b. system
  talking back b.
  target b.
  teenage smoking b.
  terminal achievement b.
  terrorism b.
  B. Therapy and Research Society
    (BTRS)
  threatening b.
  tic-like b.
  tomboy b.
  tool-using b.
  trancelike b.
  transference b.
  troubling b.
  b. type
  type A, B b.
  typical b.
  tyrannical b.
  unacceptable b.
  uncharacteristic b.
  uncued b.
  undersocialized conduct b.
  unethical b.
  unexpected b.
  uninhibited b.
  unlawful b.
  unpurposeful b.
  unstable b.
  unusual b.
  usual b.
  variable b.
  variety of sexual b.
  verbal b.
  violating b.
  violent criminal b.
  voluntary b.
  voyeuristic sexual b.
  water-seeking b.
  b. while driving
  wild b.
  withdrawn b.
behavioral
  b. abnormality
  b. activation system (BAS)
  b. addiction
  b. approach
  b. assessment measure
  b. avoidance test for OCD

b. baseline
b. change
b. consistency
b. contingency
b. contract
b. couples group therapy
b. criterion
b. desensitization
b. development
b. difference
b. disorder
b. disorganization in schizophrenia
b. disturbance
b. dyscontrol
b. dysfunction
b. dysfunction symptom
b. effect
b. emergency
b. endocrinology
b. expression
b. facilitation
b. flexibility
b. function
b. genetics
b. health
b. immunogen
b. inactivity
b. inhibition system (BIS)
b. input
b. intervention
b. management
b. manifestation
b. marital therapy (BMT)
b. masking
b. medicine
b. memory
b. metamorphosis
b. model
b. modeling
b. monitoring
b. neuroanatomy
b. neurobiology
b. neurochemistry
b. neurology
b. neuroscience
b. objective
b. observation
b. observation audiometry (BOA)
b. oscillation
b. outburst
b. pathogen
b. pathology in Alzheimer disease
  (BEHAVE-AD)
b. perspective
b. prosthesis
b. psychiatry
b. psychology
b. psychotherapy

B

b. rating scale
b. reaction brain syndrome
b. reciprocity
b. rehearsal
b. repertoire
b. research
b. research orientation
b. science
b. semantics
b. sensitization
b. set of disturbances
b. stability
b. support
b. technique
b. teratogenicity
b. theory
b. theory of rumination
b. toxicity
b. trajectory
b. transgression
b. treatment
b. variability
behavior-altering substance
behavior-constraint theory
behaviorism
eclectic b.
operant b.
radical b.
b. school of psychology
Tolman purposive b.
behaviorist
behavioristic psychology
behavior-oriented assessment
behead
behest
behoove
Behr
B. disorder
B. syndrome
being
b. abused
b. abusive
b. bullied
b. cognition
b. dirty
higher b.
b. locked in
b. motivation
b. stared at
supreme b.
b. tormented
b. value

bejesus
belabor
beleaguer
bel esprit
belie
belief
b. about identity
accepted b.
Christian b.
core b.
cultural b.
culture-bound b.
delusional b.
deviant b.
dominant delusional b.
dysfunctional core b.
endorsement of deviant thoughts
and b.'s
erroneous b.
exaggerated b.
false b.
fear-related b.
firmly held b.
fixed b.
formed b.
fully organized b.
b. in God
inner b.
internal world of b.
b. in life after death
loss of b.
odd b.
paranoid delusional b.
personal b.
religious b.
shared delusional b.
sustained b.
b. system of self-help
traditional b.
true b.
unreasonable b.
unshakable b.
believable
believe
make b.
belittle
belittling
continued b.
belladonna (BD)
b. alkaloid
b. and opium (B&O)
belle

NOTES

bellicose manner
belligerence
belligerent tone
bell and pad technique
bell-shaped curve
bellwether
belonging
    sense of b.
beloved
below-average student
below detectable levels (BDL)
belt
    black b.
bemar
bemegride
bemidone
bemoan
bemuse
benchmark
bench warrant
bending
    rule b.
benedict
benefactor
beneficence
beneficent
beneficial
    b. effect
    socially b.
benefit
    b. of clergy
    cognitive b.
    disability b.
    economic b.
    employee b.
    nonspecific b.
benevolence
benevolent
benighted
benign
    b. essential tremor
    b. exertional headache
    b. habit
    b. psychopathy
    b. stupor
    b. tetanus
benignant
Benson-Geschwind classification of
  aphasia
bentazepam
benthamism
bent-over neck
bent posture
ben trovato
benumb
benzisoxazole
benzoate

benzoctamine
benzodiazepine (BD, BZ)
    b. abuse
    b. antagonist
    b. dependence
    b. discontinuation syndrome
    b. overdose
    b. receptor binding
    short-acting b.
    b. tolerance
    b. withdrawal
benzodiazepine-GABA-receptor complex
benzoylmethylecgonine
BEP
    brain evoked potential
berate
berdache
berdachism
bereave
bereavement
    b. in children
    complicated b.
    conjugal b.
    b. disorder
    feigned b.
    b. support group
    symptom of b.
    traumatic b.
    uncomplicated b.
    unresolved b.
bereavement-related
    b.-r. depression
    b.-r. major depressive episode
    b.-r. mood disorder
bereft
bergsonian
bergsonism
beriberi
    wet b.
berserk
beseech
    bartholinitis b.
beset
beshrew
beside the point
besiege
besmirch
besot
bestial .
bestialis
    mixoscopia b.
bestiality
best interest of the child
bestir
besylate
beta
    b. adrenergic blocking agent
    b. adrenergic medication

b. adrenergic receptor
b. alcoholism
b. amyloid peptide
b. arc
b. blocker
b. cell
b. endorphin
b. error
b. hypothesis
b. index
b. level
b. movement
b. pattern
b. rhythm
b. stimulant
b. subunit
b. test
b. wave
b. weight
beta-adrenergic
b.-a. antagonist
b.-a. blocking drug
b.-a. medication-induced postural tremor
beta-amyloid protein
betacism
beta-hydroxylase
betaine
chloral b.
betel nut
bete noire
bethel
bethrothel
betide
betise
betray
betrayal
sense of b.
betterment
better off
betting
off-track b.
between-group variance
beverage
alcoholic b.
ceremonial b.
social b.
bewail
bewilder
bewildered
bewilderment
bewitch

bewitchery
bewitchingly
bewitchment
Bezold-Brucke phenomenon
B girl
bhakti
bhang
Bianchi syndrome
bias
affect-related information-processing b.'s
b. against the elderly
age b.
clinical b.
clinician b.
b. crime
emotional b.
ethnic b.
evaluator b.
exotic b.
experimental b.
experimenter b.
expression of b.
free recall b.
gender b.
healthcare b.
information processing b.
memory b.
negativistic b.
on-the-job b.
racial b.
selection b.
societal b.
biased
BIB
brought in by
biblicism
bibliokleptomania
bibliolatry
bibliomania
bibliophile
bibliotherapeutic strategy
bibliotherapy
Bibring view of depressive disorder
bibulous
bicarbonate
bicircadian rhythm
bicker
biconditional
BICROS
bilateral contralateral routing of signals
bicultural

NOTES

b.i.d.
> bis in die

bid deal
bide
bidialectalism
bidirectional selection study
biduous
Bidwell ghost
Bielschowsky idiocy
biennis
> Oenothera b.

bifrontal headache
bifunctional
bifurcation
Big
> B. Brothers of America
> B. Sisters of America

bigamist
bigamous
bigamy
bigot
bigoted
bigotry
bilabial
bilateral
> b. abductor paralysis
> b. adductor paralysis
> b. anterior capsule deep brain stimulation for OCD
> b. contralateral routing of signals (BICROS)
> b. ECT
> b. hermaphroditism
> b. myoclonic seizure
> b. regions
> b. speech
> b. synchrony
> b. transfer

biliary dyskinesia
bilineal family
bilingual
bilingualism
> active b.

bilious headache
bilirachia
bilirubin encephalopathy
bill
> b. of goods
> b. of health
> b. of indictment
> b. of particulars
> b. of rights

billingsgate
biloba
> *Gingko b.*

biloquialism
bimanual
bimodal distribution

binary principle
binaural shift
bind
> b. analysis date
> double b.
> b. over

binding
> benzodiazepine receptor b.
> libido b.
> nonspecific b.
> b. site

Binet age
binge
> alcohol b.
> b. buyer
> cocaine b.
> b. drinker
> b. drinking
> drug b.
> b. eater
> eating b.
> b. eating disorder
> b. eating pattern
> b. gambler
> b. and purge
> b. spender

binge-eating behavior
binge-purge behavior
binging, bingeing
binocular
> b. perception
> b. vision

binomial
> b. distribution
> b. test

Binswanger
> B. dementia
> B. encephalopathy

bioactive
bioanalysis
bioassay
bioavailability
biobehavioral shift
biocatalyst
biooccipital headache
biochemical
> b. activity
> b. exposure
> b. imbalance
> b. information
> b. pathway
> b. phenotypic marker
> b. study

biochemorphology
biocidal
biocide
bioclimatology
biocompatible

biocybernetics
biocycle
biocyclebiome
biodata
biodynamics
bioelectric potential
bioelement
bioenergetic
    b. psychotherapy
    b. therapy
bioenergetics
bioengineering
bioequivalence
bioequivalent
bioethics
biofeedback
    b. application
    b. computer
    electrodermal response b.
    electroencephalogram b.
    electromyography b.
    EMG b.
    galvanic skin response b.
    b. meter
    b. method
    temperature b.
    b. theory
    b. tones
    b. training
bioflavinoids
biogenesis
biogenetic mental law
biogenetics
biogenic
    b. amine
    b. amine hypothesis
    b. amine neurotransmitter
    b. psychosis
biogenous
biogram
biographical
    b. data
    b. memory
    b. method
biography
    reactional b.
    reactions b.
biohazard
biokinetics
biolinguistic language theory
biologic, biological
    b. act

b. age
b. basis
b. causation
b. changes associated with aging
chemical, radiological, and b.
b. and chemical warfare (BCW)
b. child
b. clock
b. consideration
b. control
b. correlate
b. data
b. determinant
b. determinism
b. diathesis
b. drive
b. dysfunction
b. dysfunction symptom
b. dysregulation
b. evidence
b. father
b. foundation
b. intelligence
b. intervention
b. issue
b. maturity
b. measure
b. mother
b. parent
b. pathogenesis
b. perspective
b. predisposition
b. process
b. psychiatrist
b. psychiatry
b. reductionism
b. research
b. research orientation
b. rhythm
b. risk factor
b. roots of addiction
b. sex
b. sibling
b. sign depression
b. status
b. stress
b. substrate
b. taxonomy
b. theory
b. therapy
b. time
b. training

NOTES

biologic *(continued)*
 b. viewpoint
 b. warfare
 b. weapon
 b. windows on CNS function
biologism
biologos
biology
 b. of affective disease
 communications in behavioral b.
 (CBB)
 b. of deceit
 developmental b.
bioluminescence
biolytic
biomathematics
biome
biomechanics
biomedical
 b. engineering
 b. model
 b. monitoring system (BMS)
 b. therapy
biomedicine
biometric result
biometry
bion
bionergy
bionic
bionomy
biophilia
biophysical
 b. life change
 b. study
 b. system
biophysics
biopotential
biopotentiality
biopsy
biopsychic
biopsychology
biopsychosocial
 b. history
 b. model
 b. paradigm
 b. variable
biopterin
bioreversible
biorhythm
bioscience
bioscopy
biosis
biosocial
 b. determinism
 b. integration
 b. theory
biosphere
biostatic

biostatistics
biosynthesis
biosystematics
Biot
 B. breathing
 B. respiration
biotaxis
biotechnology
biotelemetry
bioterrorism
 exposure to b.
 fear of b.
bioterrorist attack
biotic potential
biotin
biotoxication
biotoxicology
biotoxin
biotransformation
biotrepy
biotype
biotypology
biovular twins
biowarfare
bioweapons
biparental
biphasic symptom
bipolar
 b. I, II
 b. affective disorder
 b. affective psychosis
 b. cell
 b. depression
 b. depression disorder
 b. diathesis
 b. I, II disorder
 b. I disorder, most recent episode
 hypomanic
 b. I disorder, most recent episode
 mixed
 b. I disorder, most recent episode
 unspecified
 b. I disorder, single manic episode
 b. illness (BPI)
 b. neuron
 b. patient
 b. self
 b. spectrum disorder
 b. type currently depressed
 b. type mixed
 b. type schizoaffective disorder
bipotentiality
biracial
bird of passage
birth
 b. brain trauma organic psychosis
 b. cohort
 complete b.

b. control (BC)
b. control pill (BCP)
b. control pill contraception
b. control regimen
cross b.
b. cry
b. date (BD)
b. defect
b. family
b. father
b. injury
live b.
b. mother
multiple b.
b. name
b. order
premature b.
b. rate
b. right
season of b.
b. trauma
year of b. (YOB)
birthmark
birthplace
birthright
BIS
  behavioral inhibition system
bis in die (b.i.d.)
bisensory method
bisexual (AC/DC)
b. behavior
closet b.
b. confusion
b. libido
b. orientation
b. pedophilia
b. relationship
bisexuality
  theory of constitutional b.
bitartrate
  dihydrocodeinone b.
bitchery
bitchy
bite
bitemporal hypoperfusion
biter
  nail b.
biting
b. attack
lip b.
b. mania

nail b.
b. stage
bitter
b. end
b. humor
obsessively b.
bitterender
bitterness
bittersweet
bivariate
bizarre
b. answer
b. behavior
b. delusion
b. gesture
b. idea
b. posture
b. posturing
b. speech
b. thought process
b. variant
bizarrerie
BL
  baseline
blabbermouth
black
b. art
b. belt
b. and blue
b. book
b. box warning
b. death
b. diet
b. eye
b. hand
b. magic
b. mass
b. patch psychosis
b. patch syndrome
b. tar heroin
black-and-white thinking
blackball
blackguard
blacking out
blacklist
blackmail
  emotional b.
blackmarket medication
blackout
  alcoholic b.
  b. threshold

NOTES

bladder
    autonomic neurogenic b.
    b. continence
    b. control
    nervous b.
    neurogenic b.
    pseudoneurogenic b.
    reflex neurogenic b.
    stammering of the b.
    b. training
    uninhibited neurogenic b.
blame
    assign b.
    externalize b.
    place b.
    b. psychology
blameless
blame-placing communication pattern
blameworthy
bland
    b. affect
    b. diet
blandish
blank
    b. hallucination
    interest b.
    b. screen
    b. stare
blanket
    security b.
blasé
blaspheme
blasphemous thought
blasphemy
blatant
blather
blatherskite
blatter
bleak
blear
bleary-eyed
bleat
bleeding
    b. heart
    b. of undetermined origin (BUO)
blemish
blended family
blending
    auditory b.
    sound b.
blepharedema
blepharoplegia
blepharospasm, blepharospasmus
Bleuler diagnostic system
bleulerian type 2
blight
blind
    b. alley

    b. analysis
    color b.
    b. date
    double b.
    b. drunk
    b. faith
    b. headache
    b. matching technique
    b. spot
    b. study
    b. test
    b. trust
blindism
blindness
    amnesic color b.
    cerebral b.
    concussion b.
    conversion b.
    cortical psychic b.
    developmental word b.
    functional b.
    hysterical b.
    legal b.
    letter b.
    mind b.
    music b.
    note b.
    object b.
    psychic b.
    sign b.
    smell b.
    soul b.
    taste b.
    text b.
    transient b.
    word b.
blink
    eye b.
    b. response
bliss
    absolute b.
blister
blithe
blithely ignored need
blithesome
bloat
bloated
bloc
    en b.
block
    affect b.
    alpha b.
    b. anesthesia
    b. design
    b. design subtest
    b. design test
    genetic b.
    mental b.

methadone b.
monolithic adult b.
b. sampling

blockade
audible speech b.
central cholinergic b.
D_2 b.
emotional b.
muscarine b.
muscarinic receptor b.
narcotic b.
nicotinic receptor b.
reuptake b.
silent speech b.
thought b.

blockage
blocked speech
blocker
beta b.

blocking
b. activity
b. agent
alpha b.
emotional b.
evidence of b.
b. evidence
b. procedure
thought b.

blood
b. alcohol (BA)
b. alcohol concentration
b. alcohol concentration content (BAC)
b. alcohol content
b. alcohol level (BAL)
bad b.
b. brotherhood
b. component
b. count
b. crossmatch
b. drug screen
b. dyscrasia
b. flow change
full b.
b. group
b. level
occult b.
b. poisoning
b. pressure
b. psychogenic disorder
b. screen for drugs test
b. smear

b. sugar
b. transfusion
b. type
b. urea nitrogen (BUN)
b. volume

blood-injection-injury type
bloodless decerebration
bloodletting
bloodline
bloodshed
bloodshot
bloodstain
bloodstream
bloomer
Blos developmental model
blow
b. away
death b.
lethal b.
b. off
b. over

blow-by-blow
blowhard
blue
baby b.'s
black and b.
code b.
b. collar crime
b. edema
maternity b.'s
out of the b.
paternity b.'s
postpartum b.'s
postpartum b.'s
b. velvet syndrome

blue-blooded
blue-collar worker
blue-nose
blues
bluff
blunder
blunted
b. affect
b. emotional expression
b. response

blunting
affective b.
emotional b.

blur
blurred vision
blurring
b. of vision

NOTES

blurry
blush
blushing
bluster
BMI
    body mass index
BMR
    basal metabolic rate
BMS
    biomedical monitoring system
BMT
    behavioral marital therapy
BO
    body odor
BOA
    behavioral observation audiometry
board
    b. certified psychiatrist
    conversation b.
    direct selection communication b.
    b. eligible psychiatrist
    encoding communication b.
    gender identity b.
    institutional review b.
    Ouija b.
    room and b.
    scanning communication b.
    sounding b.
board-and-care
    b.-a.-c. facility
    b.-a.-c. home
boarders
    phantom b.
boarding home
boarding-out system
boast
boasting
bobbing
    head b.
    ocular b.
bodacious
bodement
bodhisattva
bodily
    b. autonomy
    b. disease
    b. illusion
    b. movement
    b. symptom
body
    b. alienation
    b. appearance
    astral b.
    b. awareness
    B. Awareness Resource Network
    (BARNY)
    b. boundary
    b. buffer zone

b. build
b. cathexis
b. composition
b. concept-exploration maneuver
b. conceptualization disturbance
b. contact-exploration maneuver
b. dipping
b. dissatisfaction
b. dysgnosia
b. dysmorphic defect
b. dysmorphic disorder (BDD)
b. dysphoria
b. dystonia
b. ego
b. ego concept
b. ego damage
emaciated b.
b. fat
fat b.
feeling of being detached from
    one's b.
b. fluid
foreign b.
b. functioning
b. gesture
hitting own b.
b. ideal
b. identity
b. image
immune b.
intraneuronal argentophilic Pick
    inclusion b.
b. language
b. mass index (BMI)
b. mechanics
b. memory
b. modification
b. monitor
b. movement
muscular b.
b. narcissism
obese b.
b. odor (BO)
b. orifice
b. percept
perception localized within the b.
b. piercing
pineal b.
b. position
b. posture
b. protest
b. rocking
b. schema
b. shape
b. snatching
b. surface area
b. swaying
b. therapy

b. tic
b. type
b. water
Winkler b.
body-image
b.-i. agnosia
b.-i. distortion
b.-i. disturbance
b.-i. hallucination
b.-i. perception
b.-i. recall
body-mind dichotomy
body-related obsessive-like symptom
boggle
bogus
boisterous
aggressively b.
Bolam Principle
bolasterone
bold-faced
bolster
bolus
bomb
homemade pipe b.
bombard
bombarding
bombast
bombed
bombesin
bona fide
bond
affectional b.
attachment b.
disruption of affective b.'s
emotional b.
father-child b.
high-energy b.
incapacity to sustain social b.'s
male b.
mother-child b.
pair b.
parent-child b.
parent-offspring b.
sibling b.
bondage
b. and discipline
physical b.
sensory b.
bonding
affiliation b.
human-pet b.
b. in infancy

mother-infant b.
parent-infant b.
bondsman
bone
b. age (BA)
b. conduction deafness
magic b.
parietal skull b.
pointing of the b.
b. pointing
b. sensibility
bonhomie
Bonnevie-Ullrich syndrome
Bonnier syndrome
book
black b.
closed b.
bookish
boomer
baby b.
boomlet
baby b.
boorish
boost
arousal b.
boot camp
boozer
bordello
border
Doctors Without B.'s
borderline
b. behavior
b. composite description
b. diagnosis prototype
b. dull
b. intellectual functioning
b. mental retardation
b. neurotic personality disorder
b. pathology
b. patient
b. personality
b. personality disorder (BPD)
b. personality disorder with histrionic feature
b. personality organization
b. personality style
b. personality style score
b. psychosis
b. psychosis of childhood
b. range
b. scale
b. schizophrenia (BS)

NOTES

B

borderline *(continued)*
    b. state
    b. subfactor
boredom
    feeling of b.
Borjeson-Forssman-Lehmann syndrome
borne
born worriers
bossy
Boston
    B. opium
    B. University Model of Psychiatric Rehabilitation
botch
bothersome
bottomless
bottom-up approach
boufee delirante
bouleversement
bound
    out of b.'s
    b. panic attack
    situationally b.
    upper b.
boundary
    analytic b.
    body b.
    b. case
    diagnostic b.
    ego b.
    b. enforcement
    external b.
    b.'s and gender
    group b.
    b. issue
    language b.
    loss of ego b.
    b.'s in postanalytic supervision
    posttermination b.
    b.'s posttermination
    b.'s in psychoanalysis
    role b.
    subsystem b.
    b. violation
    whole brain b.
boundless energy
bourgeois
bourgeoisie
bout of insomnia
bovarism
bovine spongiform encephalopathy
bowel
    b. control
    b. disorder
    b. incontinence
    irritable b.
    reactive b.

    stress-induced reactive b.
    b. training
Bowen
    B. model
Bower model of mood-congruent memory
Bowlby
    B. developmental model
    B. theory of attachment
box
    Goodman Lock b.
    obstruction b.
    Skinner b.
boxer's
    b. dementia
    b. encephalopathy
boy
    good old b.
boyfriend
    former b.
BPD
    borderline personality disorder
BPI
    bipolar illness
BPRS
    brief psychiatric rating scale
    brief psychiatric reacting scale
        BPRS anxiety-depression score
        BPRS anxiety-depression subscale
        BPRS total score
        BPRS withdrawal/retardation score
BRAC
    basic rest-activity cycle
brace
bracer
brachybasia
brachymorph
bradycardia
bradycinesia *(var. of* bradykinesia)
bradyesthesia
bradyglossia
bradykinesia, bradycinesia
    functional b.
bradykinetic syndrome
bradykinin
bradylalia
bradylexia
bradylogia
bradyphagia
bradyphasia
bradyphemia
bradyphrasia
bradyphrenia
bradypnea
bradypragia
bradypsychia
bradyrhythmia
bradyspermatism

bradyteleokinesis
brag
braggart
brahmanism
braid-cutting
braidism
braille
brain

b. abnormality
b. abscess
b. ache
b. activation
b. age quotient (BAQ)
archaic b.
architecture of the b.
b. area
b. assault
b. atrophy
b. autopsy
b. blood flow
b. cell damage
b. cicatrix
b. circuitry
compression of b.
b. concussion
concussion of b.
b. congestion
contrecoup injury of b.
b. control
b. contusion
b. convulsion
coup injury of b.
b. damage language disorder
b. death
b. degeneration
b. depressant
b. development
b. differentiation
b. dimorphism
b. disease
b. disease organic psychosis
b. dopamine
b. dopaminergic pathway
b. dopaminergic system
b. dysfunction
b. dysmorphology
b. edema
electrical activity of b.
b. electrical activity map
b. electrical activity mapping
  (BEAM)

electric stimulation of the b.
  (ESB)
b. evoked potential (BEP)
evolution of b.
b. fog
b. function
b. functional failure
b. function disruption
functioning b.
b. functioning
b. glucose metabolism
b. illness
b. imaging
b. imaging method
b. imaging study
b. infection organic psychosis
b. injury
b. involvement
b. lactate
b. location
b. mapping
b. metabolic effect
b. metabolic mechanism
b. metabolic response
b. metabolism
b. model
b. murmur
b. opioid activity
b. pathology
phencyclidine mixed organic b.
b. potential
b. potential study
prefrontal cortex of the b.
b. process
b. psychoorganic syndrome
b. region
b. research
b. scan
b. seizure
somatosensory cortices of the right
  hemisphere of the b.
b. space
b. spectin
b. SPECT scan
split b.
b. stem
b. stimulation
b. structure
b. structure study
b. substrate
b. swelling
b. test

NOTES

brain *(continued)*
   b. trauma
   b. trauma organic psychosis
   ventromedial prefrontal cortex of
     the b.
   b. volume
   water on the b.
   b. wave
   b. wave activity
   b. wave complex
   b. wave cycle
   b. weight
brain-behavior relationship
brain-derived
   b.-d. HVA concentration
   b.-d. neurotrophic
BrainMap
   Couples B.
brain-splitting
brainstem
   b. auditory evoked potential
   b. auditory evoked response
   b. control
   b. disease
   b. displacement
   b. dysfunction
   b. function
   b. reticular formation
   b. sign
brainstorm
brain-to-plasma ratio
brainwash
brainwashing
branching
   b. steps in therapy
   b. tree diagram
brand
Brasdor method
bravado
Bravais-jacksonian epilepsy
bravery
bravura
Brawner
   B. decision
   United States vs. B.
breach
   confidentiality b.
   b. of confidentiality
   security b.
   b. of security
breadwinner
   loss of b.
break
   acute psychotic b.
   ascending pitch b.
   major b.
   psychotic b.
   b. shock

   b. state
   b. with reality
breakaway phenomenon
breakdown
   analytical b.
   nervous b.
breaker
   law b.
   rule b.
breakoff phenomenon
breakthrough
   depressive b.
   b. tearfulness
breakup
breast
   b. augmentation
   b. complex
   b. envy
   b. feeding
   b. implant
breast-phantom phenomenon
breath
   alcohol on b. (AOB)
   b. analyzer
   b. chewing
   shortness of b.
   b. stream
   b. work
Breathalyzer
breathe
breath-holding
breathing
   apneustic b.
   Biot b.
   Cheyne-Stokes b.
   controlled b.
   crescendo-decrescendo b.
   daytime mouth b.
   diaphragmatic b.
   b. disorder
   opposition b.
   b. retraining
   sleep disordered b. (SDB)
   b. technique
   b. tic
breathing-related sleep disorder
breathy voice
bredouillement
bride
   war b.
bridge
   crossing a b.
brief
   b. cognitive test battery
   b. delusional experience
   b. depressive reaction
   b. dynamic psychotherapy
   b. episode

b. group therapy
b. posttraumatic stress disorder
b. psychiatric rating scale (BPRS)
b. psychiatric reacting scale (BPRS)
b. psychotic disorder
b. psychotic reaction
b. pulse bilateral ECT
b. pulse unilateral ECT
b. pulse waveform
b. reactive dissociative disorder
b. reactive psychosis
b. reactive psychosis with marked stressor
b. situational depression
b. stimuli technique
b. stimulus therapy (BST)

Brieger cachexia
Brigance
Briggs law
brightening
mood b.
brightness
b. adaptation
b. constancy
b. contrast
b. discrimination
b. threshold
bright normal range
bring to closure
Briquet
B. ataxia
B. disorder
B. syndrome
brisk reflex
Brissaud
B. disease
B. infantilism
Brissaud-Marie syndrome
Bristowe syndrome
British
B. anti-Lewisite (BAL)
B. Journal of Psychiatry
B. Manual of the Classification of Occupations
broad
b. affect
b. heritability
broadcasting
thought b.
Broca
B. amnesia

B. aphasia
B. area
B. center
Brodie disease
Brodmann
B. area 6
B. area 7
B. area 9
B. area 24
B. area 32
B. area 41
B. area 43
B. area 44
B. area 46
B. area 47/11
brofoxine
broken
b. engagement
b. heart
b. home
b. promise
bromatherapy
bromatology
bromatotherapy
bromazepam
bromide
ammonium b.
decamethonium b.
b. hallucinosis
b. intoxication
b. poisoning
bromine compound
brominism
bromism
bromisovalum
bromoiodism
bromomania
bromperidol
bronchial
b. asthma
b. respiration
bronchodilator
bronchogenic
bronchospasm
brood
brooding
b. compulsion
obsessional b.
b. personality
spells of doubting and b.
brother complex

NOTES

brotherhood
> blood b.

brotherliness

brotizolam

brought in by (BIB)

Brown
> B. Schools Behavioral Health System

brownian
> b. motion
> b. movement

Brown-Sequard
> B.-S. syndrome

brows
> furrowed b.

brucine

bruise

bruising of undetermined origin (BUO)

brujeria

Bruns ataxia

brusque

brutal discipline

brutality

brute pride

bruxism
> sleep-related b.
> SSRI-induced b.

bruxomania

BS
> borderline schizophrenia

BSO
> behavior, speech, and other syndromes

BST
> brief stimulus therapy

BSW
> Bachelor of Social Work

BTRS
> Behavior Therapy and Research Society

bubo
> venereal b.

buccal
> b. intercourse
> b. onanism
> b. speech

buccarum
> morsicatio b.

buccinator muscle

buckthorn polyneuropathy

Buddhism
> Zen B.

budgeting
> functional b.

buffalo neck

buffer
> assay b.
> memory b.
> b. memory
> b. neuropathy

buffoonery
> b. psychosis
> b. syndrome

bufotenin

bug
> cocaine b.

buggery

build
> body b.
> index of body b. (IB)

building
> b. fear
> b. restriction
> team b.

bulb
> auditory b.

bulbocapnine

bulesis

bulimia
> b. nervosa
> b. nervosa, nonpurging type
> b. nervosa, purging type
> purging-type b.

bulimic
> b. behavior
> b. purge

bulimic-anorexic spectrum

bulimorexia

bullet
> silver b.

bulletin
> Psychopharmacology B.

bullied
> being b.

bullies

bullying
> b. behavior
> continued b.
> b. culture
> b. experience
> repeated b.
> b. target

bum
> skid-row b.

BUN
> blood urea nitrogen

Bunney-Hamburg
> B.-H. global psychosis rating
> B.-H. global psychosis scale
> B.-H. nurse rating

BUO
> bleeding of undetermined origin
> bruising of undetermined origin

buoyancy
> high-spirited b.

burden
> family b.
> psychological b.

bureaucrat
Bureau of Drug Abuse Control (BDAC)
buried alive
burn
    napalm b.
    B. and Rand theory
burned-out
    b.-o. anergic schizophrenia
    b.-o. schizophrenic
burning
    b. pain
    b. rubber
burnout
    caretaker b.
    parent b.
    professional b.
    b. syndrome
burr
Burundanga intoxication
Buschke
Buss-Durkee scale
buster
    baby b.
butane sniffing dependence
butaperazine
butethal
butoctamide
butterfly coil
button
    mescal b.
    panic b.

butyrophenone agent
butyrophenone-based neuroleptic drug
buyer
    binge b.
buying
    compulsive b.
    b. spree
buzz
    b. group
    b. session
buzzing sensation
buzzword
BWM
    Bad Wildungen Metz
BWS
    battered woman syndrome
by
    brought in by (BIB)
byclothymosis
by-idea
bypass
    gastric b.
by-product
bystander
    b. dominates initial
    b. dominates initial dominant
    (BDID)
BZ
    benzodiazepine

B

NOTES

CA
   cancer
   chronologic age
   Cocaine Anonymous
CA4-1
   area C.
caapi
cabal
cabin fever
cable graft
CABS
   chronic alcoholic brain syndrome
cacation
cacesthesia
cache
cachectic infantilism
cachexia
   Brieger c.
   c. hypophysiopriva
   pituitary c.
cachinnation
cackle
cacodemonomania
cacoethes
cacogenesis
cacogenic
cacogeusia
cacography
cacolalia
cacophonous
cacophony
cacophoria
cacoplasty
cacosmia
cacothenics
cacotrophy
cactus
   peyote c.
cacuminal
cadaver
cadaverous
cadence
cadent
cadherin
caducity
caelotherapy
cafard
caffeinated substance
caffeine
   c. abstinence
   c. abuse
   c. cessation
   c. consumption
   c. dependence
   c. habituation

   c. holiday
   c. ingestion
   c. intake
   c. intolerance
   c. intoxication
   c. metabolism
   c. response
   c. sequela
   c. tolerance
   c. toxicity
   c. use
   c. use disorder
   c. user
   c. withdrawal
caffeine-abstinent subject
caffeine-induced
   c.-i. anxiety
   c.-i. anxiety disorder
   c.-i. contracture
   c.-i. sleep disorder
   c.-i. vasoconstriction
caffeine-intolerant individual
caffeine-related sequela
caffeine-sensitive individual
caffeinism
cage
   population c.
Cain
   C. complex
   raise C.
Cairns stupor
cajole
calami
   lapsus c.
calcarine sulcus
calculate
   ability to abstract and c.
calculation
   calendar c.
   c. skill
   c. test
calculus, pl. **calculi**
   cerebral c.
Caldwell High Speed Magnetic Stimulator
calefacient
calendar
   c. age
   c. calculation
caliber
   .22-c. handgun
   .38-c. handgun
   .410-c. handgun
   .44-c. handgun
   .22-c. revolver

C

calibrate
calibrated loop
calibration
California
    C. Child Q-Set
    C. Q-Sort
californica
caligo
calipers
calisthenics
call
    c. girl
    obscene phone c.
caller
    obscene telephone c.
callomania
callosal
    c. area
    c. disconnection syndrome
    c. disconnection syndrome aphasia
    c. sulcus
callous
calmative
calming effect
calmodulin
calm wakefulness state
caloric
    c. intake
    c. stimulation test for vestibular
      function
calorie
calorifacient
calorigenic action
calumniate
calumny
camaraderie
camazepam
Cameron
    Rouse vs C.
camisole
camouflage
cAMP
    c. response element (CRE)
    c. response element binding protein
camp
    boot c.
    day c.
    death c.
    labor c.
camptocormia
camptocormy
camptospasm
Canadian
    C. Academy of Child Psychiatry
canal
    anal c.
    anterior vertical c.
    auditory c.

    central c.
    craniopharyngeal c.
    intramedullary c.
    medullary c.
canalization
canard
Canavan
    C. sclerosis
cancellation test
cancer (CA)
    c. reaction
cancerophobe
cancerphobia
candid
candidate-gene strategy
canine
    c. hysteria
    c. spasm
caninus
    risus c.
    spasmus c.
canities
canker
cannabidiol
cannabin
cannabinoids
    cross-reacting c.
cannabinol (CBN)
cannabis
    c. abuse
    c., cocaine and heroin
    c. delusional disorder
    c. dependence
    c. intoxication
    c. intoxication delirium
    c. intoxication-related disorder
    c. intoxication, with perceptual
      disturbance
    c. and opium
    c. organic mental disorder
    c. psychosis
    C. sativa
    c. use disorder
cannabis-induced
    c.-i. anxiety
    c.-i. anxiety disorder
    c.-i. delirium disorder
    c.-i. drowsiness10000
    c.-i. euphoria
    c.-i. mental changes
    c.-i. psychotic disorder with
      delusions
    c.-i. psychotic disorder with
      hallucinations
cannabism
cannabis-related disorder, not otherwise
  specified
cannibalism

cannibalistic
    c. fantasy
    c. fixation
Cannon-Bard
    C.-B. theory
    C.-B. theory of emotion
Cannon theory
canny
canonical correlation
cant
cantankerous
Cantelli sign
cantharis, pl. **cantharides**
CAP
    carotid Amytal procedure
capability
    cognitive c.
    metabolic c.
capable
capacitance
capacity
    adaptive c.
    channel c.
    code c.
    c. code
    cognitive c.
    contractual c.
    diminished c.
    dissociative c.
    empathic c.
    functional c. (FC)
    functional residual c. (FRC)
    hedonic c.
    hypnotic c.
    c. for independent living
    intellectual c.
    intrinsic c.
    legal c.
    c. to love
    measured c.
    mental c.
    metacognitive c.
    nonverbal intellectual c.
    orgasmic c.
    oxygen-carrying c.
    paranormal c.
    physical c.
    potential intellectual c.
    psychological c.
    self-regulatory c.
    self-soothing c.
    speaking c.

    testamentary c.
    volitional c.
caper
Capgras
    C. phenomenon
    C. syndrome
capistratus
capita (*pl. of* caput)
capital
    c. offense
    c. sin
capitalize
capitation
capitis
capitium
capping
    c. cardiotoxic
    c. technique
caprice
capricious
capsule
    drug-containing c.
    external c.
capsulothalamic syndrome
captation
captious
captivate
captivation
captive
    indoctrination while c.
captivus
    penis c.
captodiame
capture
capuride
caput, pl. **capita**
    dolor capitis
    per capita
    c. succedaneum
carbamate
carbamylcholine chloride
carbinol
carbohydrate metabolism
carbon
    c. dioxide (CO_2)
    c. dioxide intoxication
    c. dioxide poisoning
    c. dioxide therapy
    c. disulfide intoxication
    c. monoxide
    c. monoxide intoxication

C

NOTES

carbon *(continued)*
    c. monoxide poisoning
    c. tetrachloride
carbonate
carbonic anhydrase inhibitor
carbonyl modification
carcinogen
card
    associative response to a white
      space on a c. (Ds)
    diary c.
    mother c.
    Rorschach c.
    c. sorting function
    tarot c.
card-game gambling
cardiac
    c. arrest
    c. arrhythmia
    c. disorder
    c. neurosis
    c. psychosis
    c. reaction
    c. rhythm
    c. symptom
cardinal
    c. ocular movement
    c. sign
    c. sin
    c. trait
    c. virtue
cardiomyopathy
    alcoholic c.
cardioneurosis
cardiophrenia
cardiopulmonary
    c. arrest
    c. resuscitation
cardiopulmonary-obesity syndrome
cardiospasm
    psychogenic c.
cardiotoxic
    capping c.
cardiovascular
    c. neurosis
    c. psychogenic disorder
    c. seizure
card stacking
care
    acute stabilization inpatient c.
    adequate c.
    adoptive c.
    ambulatory c.
    ancillary c.
    child psychiatric c.
    clinical c.
    community c.

community mental health c.
  (CMHC)
comprehensive c.
continuing c.
continuity of c.
continuum of c.
crisis residential c.
custodial c.
elder c.
eligibility for c.
end-of-life c.
enhanced standard c.
c. ethics
excessive need for c.
extended c.
family c.
foster c. (FC)
grossly pathogenic c.
health c.
home c.
hospice c.
inappropriate dependent c.
individual c.
inpatient c.
institutional c.
level of c.
long-term c.
managed c.
c. management for chronic
  addiction (CMCA)
medical c.
mental health c.
need for c.
obesity c.
online mental health c.
optimal c.
c. organization
outpatient c.
palliative c.
parental c.
pastoral c.
paternal c.
pathogenic c.
pathologic c.
pattern of c.
personal c.
primary c.
c. and protection proceeding
psychiatric c.
psychosocial residential c.
routine clinical c.
secondary c.
c. seeker
skilled nursing c. (SNC)
specialized foster c.
standard of c.
tender loving c. (TLC)
tertiary c.

carebaria

career
  c. change
  c. choice
  c. conference
  c. counseling
  c. counselor
  c. decision making
  c. development
  c. evaluation
  c. inventory
  c. planning
  c. planning program (CPP)
  c. workshop

carefree

careful observation

caregiver
  adoptive c.
  c. depression
  c. distress
  c. education
  family c.
  primary c.

caress

caretaker
  c. burnout
  primary c.

caretaking role

careworn

cargo culture

caricature

carinatum syndrome

caring
  expression of c.
  quality of c.

carnal knowledge

carnosine

carotic

carotid
  c. Amytal procedure (CAP)
  c. ultrasound test

carping

carpipramine

carpopedal
  c. contraction
  c. spasm

carrier
  insurance c.
  trait c.

carries a gun

Carroll-Klein model of bipolar disorder

carrot-and-stick approach

carry
  c. away
  c. off
  c. on
  c. through

caruncula, pl. **carunculae**

casanthranol

cascade
  pathophysiological c.

case
  abuse c. (AC)
  basket c.
  boundary c.
  c. control experimental study
    design
  c. control study
  Dora c.
  c. ethic
  false-negative c.
  c. fatality rate
  c. finding
  c. formulation
  high-profile c.
  c. history
  c. history study
  incident c.
  c. index
  index c.
  c. load
  c. method
  c. mix
  parole violation c.
  c. in point
  c. register
  c. report
  Schreber c.
  self-reported c.
  Tarasoff c.
  test c.
  textbook c.
  typical-onset c.
  c. work

casework
  social c.

caseworker

casino gambling

cassina leaf

CASST
  child-abuse-specific treatment of trauma

caste

castigate

cast on

NOTES

castrate
castration
    c. anxiety
    c. complex
    emotional c.
    c. fear
    female c.
    male c.
casual sex
casualty
    combat c.
casuistics
casuistry
CAT
    cognitive analytic therapy
    CAT scan
catabasia
catabolic force
catabolism
catabolite
cataclysmic headache
catagenesis
catalepsy
    epidemic c.
    c. schizophrenia
    schizophrenic c.
cataleptic somnambulism
cataleptiform
cataleptoid
catalexia
catalogia
catalyst
catalytic agent
catamenia
catamite
catamnesis
catamnestic
cataphasia
cataphora
cataphoric
cataphrenia
cataplasia
cataplectic
cataplexis
cataplexy episode
catastrophe theory
catastrophic
    c. ancataplexy syndrome
    c. anxiety
    c. behavior
    c. effect
    c. event
    c. expectation
    c. illness
    c. reaction
    c. response
    c. schizophrenia
    c. stress

catathymia
catathymic
    c. amnesia
    c. crisis
catatonia
    deadly c.
    depressive c.
    lethal c.
    maniac c.
    c. mitis
    periodic c.
    c. protracta
    psychotic c.
    recurrent c.
    schizophrenic c.
    Stauder lethal c.
    stuporous c.
    treatment-refractory c.
catatonic
    c. behavior
    c. cerebral paralysis
    c. dementia
    c. disorder
    c. disorder due to a general
      medical condition
    c. drug
    c. excitation
    c. excitement
    c. feature
    c. mutism
    c. negativism
    c. patient
    c. posturing
    c. presentation
    c. rigidity
    c. schizophrenia
    c. state
    c. stupor
    c. symptom
    c. syndrome
catatonoid attitude
catatony
catchment area
cat-cry syndrome
catecholamine
    c. hypophysis
    c. neurotransmitter
    peripheral c.
    c. receptor
catecholamine-induced
    c.-i. change
    c.-i. thermogenesis
catechol-o-methyltransferase (COMT)
categorical
    c. approach
    c. attitude
    c. change
    c. classification

c. definition
c. imperative
c. model
c. personality disorder diagnosis
c. perspective
c. system
c. thinking
c. thought
categorization
symbolic c.
symptom c.
category
arousal c.
avoidance c.
diagnostic c.
disorder c.
dysphoric c.
early-onset c.
histrionic diagnostic c.
late-onset c.
c. mistake
NOS c.
reexperiencing c.
schizotypal c.
semantic c.
somatic c.
syntactic c.
catelectrotonus
catenating
catenation
catharsis
activity c.
community c.
conversational c.
emotional c.
psychodramatic c.
cathartic
c. abuse
c. event
c. method
cathectic
c. discharge
cathecticize
catheresis
cathexis
affective c.
body c.
ego c.
fantasy c.
object c.
oral-sadistic c.

positive c.
word c.
cathinone
Catholic
catochus
cat's-eye syndrome
Cattell
C. factorial theory of personality (CFTP)
Caucasian
caudate
c. nucleus overactivity in OCD
c. tissue
caumesthesia
causa
causal
c. association
c. factor
c. indication
c. link
c. mechanism
c. possibility
c. relationship
c. texture
causal-attributional theory
causalgia
causalis
indicatio c.
causality
direct c.
phenomenistic c.
presumed c.
reverse c.
causation
biologic c.
organismic c.
causative
c. agent
c. mechanism
c. stress
cause
contextual c.
c. efficient
efficient c.
c. of identification
neurobiological c.
psychological c.
substance-related c.
cause-and-effect test
cause-effect relationship

C

NOTES

caustic
    c. ingestion
    c. remark
caution
cautious
CAVD
    completion, arithmetic, vocabulary, and directions
cave
caveat
cavort
CBASP
    cognitive behavioral analysis system of psychotherapy
CBB
    communications in behavioral biology
CBC
    child behavior characteristic
CBF
    cerebral blood flow
CBGT
    cognitive behavioral group therapy
CBN
    cannabinol
CBR
    chemical, bacteriological, radiological
CBS
    chronic brain syndrome
CBT
    cognitive behavior therapy
CBW
    chemical and biological warfare
CC
    chief complaint
CCD
    charge-coupled device
CCM
    Crime Classification Manual
CCS
    concentration camp syndrome
CCTV
    closed-circuit television
CD
    character disorder
    combination drug
    communication disorder
    conduct disorder
    copying drawings
    current diagnosis
Cd
    color denial
CDC
    chemical dependency counselor
CDD
    certificate of disability for discharge
CDS-ACC
    code substitution-accuracy

code substitution-immediate recall-accuracy
CDS-EFF
    code substitution-efficiency
cease
ceaseless pacing
cecocentral scotoma
CEI
    character education inquiry
ceiling
    c. age
    c. effect
celibacy vow
celibate
cell
    alpha c.
    c. assembly
    beta c.
    bipolar c.
    detention c.
    c. differentiation
    jail c.
    locked c.
    c. nucleus
    padded c.
    pallidal c.
    photoreceptor c.
    reactive c.
    somatic c.
    wandering c.
    white blood c.
cellular
    c. immunity factor
    c. immunologic response
    c. store
cellulotoxic
celsi
    alopecia c.
Celsus alopecia
cement
cenesthesia, coenesthesia
cenesthesic, cenesthetic
    c. hallucination
cenesthopathic schizophrenia
cenotrope
censor
    freudian c.
    psychic c.
censorship
    dream c.
censure
    peer c.
census tract
center
    academic medical c.
    acoustic c.
    addiction c.
    adult diagnostic and treatment c.

appetitive c.
association c.
c. of attention
Broca c.
communal residential c.
community mental health c. (CMHC)
cortical c.
counseling c.
crisis c.
day-care c.
day reporting c.
day treatment c. (DTC)
developmental evaluation c. (DEC)
C.'s for Disease Control and Prevention
drug information c. (DIC)
ego c.
guidance c.
higher brain c.
language c.
c. median
medical c.
C. for Mental Health Services (CMHS)
methadone c.
motor cortical c.
nonpublic residential treatment c.
pleasure c.
psychocortical c.
public residential treatment c.
rape crisis c.
reflex c.
regulatory c.
residential c.
residential treatment c. (RTC)
satiety c.
speech intention c.
speech monitoring c.
C. for Stress and Anxiety Disorders
C. for Substance Abuse Treatment (CSAT)
suicide prevention c.
The C. for Mental Health Services
visual c.
Wernicke c.
word c.
work-release c.
centered
child c.
community c.
group c.
self c.
centering
center-surround response
centimorgan (cM)
central
c. alexia
c. anesthesia
c. aphasia
c. canal
c. cholinergic blockade
c. conflict
c. convulsion
c. deafness
C. European subtype
c. excitatory state
c. executive component
c. fissure
c. force
c. gray matter (CGM)
c. gray matter region
c. inhibition
c. language disorder (CLD)
c. language imbalance
c. masking
c. motive state
c. nervous system (CNS)
c. neuritis
c. neurogenic hyperventilation
c. pain
c. paralysis
c. processing dysfunction
c. reflex time
c. role
c. scotoma
c. seizure
c. sensory deficit
c. sensory loss
c. sulcus
c. tegmental nucleus
c. tendency
c. tendency measure
c. theme
c. timing process
c. trait
c. transactional core
c. vision
centralism
centralist psychology
centrality
central-limit theorem
centraphose

NOTES

C

centration
The Centre for Mental Health
  Solutions
centrencephalic
    c. epilepsy
    c. seizure
centripetal
centrokinesia
centrokinetic
centromere
centrophenoxine
centro ritual
cephalalgia, cephalgia
      histaminic c.
      orgasmic c.
cephalea attonita
cephaledema
cephalemia
cephalgia (var. of cephalalgia)
cephalic
    c. aura
    c. index
    c. seizure
    c. tetanus
cephalitis
cephalodynia
cephalogenesis
cephalometric analysis
cephalometry
cephalomotor
cephalopathy
ceptor
      chemical c.
      contact c.
      distance c.
CER
    conditioned emotional response
ceramide
cercle
      arc de c.
cerea
      flexibilitas c.
cerebellar
    c. activation
    c. ataxia
    c. cortex
    c. gait
    c. hypoperfusion
    c. metabolism
    c. nuclei
    c. pathway
    c. region
    c. rigidity
    c. seizure
    c. sign
    c. speech
    c. tremor

cerebral
    c. activity
    c. agraphia
    c. anoxia
    c. asymmetry
    c. atrophy
    c. blindness
    c. blood flow (CBF)
    c. calculus
    c. compression
    c. compromise
    c. contusion
    c. convulsion
    c. cortex
    c. cortical function
    c. death
    c. decompression
    c. decortication
    c. depressant
    c. disorder
    c. disorganization
    c. dominance
    c. dynamic imaging
    c. dysfunction
    c. dysplasia
    c. eclipse
    c. edema
    c. electrotherapy (CET)
    c. fissure
    c. glucose metabolic-type organic
      psychosis
    c. glucose metabolism
    c. hemisphere
    c. hemodynamic variation
    c. hyperesthesia
    c. hyperplasia
    c. hypoplasia
    c. impairment
    c. infarct
    c. infection
    c. injection
    c. integration
    c. irritation
    c. localization
    c. location
    c. mal
    c. malaria
    c. mapping of apraxia
    c. neurosyphilis
    c. outflow tremor
    c. oxygen consumption
    c. pacemaker
    c. perfusion pressure (CPP)
    c. porosis
    c. potential
    c. region
    c. seizure
    c. sign

c. syphilis
c. tetanus
c. thumb
c. trauma
c. voxel
cerebrate posturing
cerebration
unconscious c.
cerebri
commotio c.
lacuna c.
cerebrocranial defect
cerebropathia
cerebropsychosis
cerebrospinal
c. convulsion
c. fluid (CSF)
c. index
c. pressure
c. seizure
c. system
cerebrotonia
cerebrovascular
c. disease organic psychosis
ceremonial
c. behavior
c. beverage
c. beverage
compulsive c.
ceremonious
ceremony
secret c.
CERS
Crisis Evaluation Referral Service
certainty
certifiable
certificate
dependent adult's c.
detention c.
c. of disability for discharge
(CDD)
c. of incompetency
c. of need
certification
certified social worker (CSW)
certify
ceruloplasmin test
cervicodynia
cessation
caffeine c.
cocaine c.
gambling c.

habit c.
smoking c.
CET
cerebral electrotherapy
C factor
CFS
chronic fatigue syndrome
CFTP
Cattell factorial theory of personality
CGM
central gray matter
CGPP
comparative guidance and placement
program
CHADD
children and adults with attention deficit
disorder
chain
c. analysis
behavior c.
c. reflex
c. reproduction
c. smoker
chained reinforcement
chaining response
chair
tranquilizer c.
challenge
diagnostic c.
hostile c.
c. strategy
c. test
chamber
echo c.
gas c.
chamomile
CHAMPUS
Civilian Health and Medical Program of
the Uniformed Service
chance
c. action
c. difference
c. error
last c.
c. medley
c. response parameter
c. variation
chancre
hard c.
mixed c.
monorecidive c.
soft c.

NOTES

chancre *(continued)*
    sporotrichositic c.
    true c.
    tularemic c.
chancroid
chancrous
change
    c. abilitator
    abulic mental c.
    adolescent sexual c.
    agent of c.
    c. agent
    age-related brain c.
    age-related pharmacodynamic c.
    age-related pharmacokinetic c.
    analogic c.
    c. in appetite
    c. of attitude
    autoplastic c.
    baseline-to-endpoint c.
    c. in behavior
    behavioral c.
    biophysical life c.
    blood flow c.
    cannabis-induced mental c.'s
    career c.
    catecholamine-induced c.
    categorical c.
    chronic c.
    circumscribed c.
    cognitive c.
    compulsive c.
    cultural c.
    culture c.
    deep white matter hyperintensity c.
    dietary c.
    digital c.
    disease-related c.
    c. in energy
    environmental c.
    global c.
    c. in health
    c. of heart
    hyperintensity c.
    intrapsychic c.
    job c.
    language c.
    c. in libido
    c. of life
    life cycle c.
    lifestyle c.
    c. in living arrangement
    major life c.
    maladaptive behavioral c.
    maladaptive psychological c.
    maturational c.
    medication c.
    mental status c.

    c. in mentation
    metabolic c.
    methylphenidate-induced c.
    moment-to-moment mood c.
    mood c.
    negative c.
    neurochemical c.
    newly emergent categorical c.
    nutritional c.
    c. of pace
    pathological c.
    personality c.
    c. in personality characteristic
    pharmacodynamic c.
    pharmacokinetic c.
    physical c.
    c. point
    positive attitude c.
    psychological c.
    psychomotor c.
    psychophysiological c.
    reflex c.
    sense of bodily c.
    sex c.
    c. in sleep pattern
    socioeconomic life c.
    stoichiometric c.
    structural c.
    subjective mood c.
    c. of topic
    transitional c.
    treatment c.
    trophic c.
    unpredictable mood c.
    white matter c.
changeable versus constant
changed body image
changeover
change-up
changing
    c. clothes
    c. emotion
    c. environment
    c. need
    c. sleep-wake pattern
channel
    c. capacity
    communication c.
    c. of communication
chant
chaos
    organizational c.
chaotic
chaplain
    hospital c.
    military c.
character
    acquired c.

anal c.
anal-aggressive c.
c. analysis
c. armor
c. assassination
c. attack
authoritarian c.
compulsive c.
c. defect
c. defense
c. deficit
dependent c.
depressive c.
c. development
c. disorder (CD)
c. displacement
dominant c.
c. education inquiry (CEI)
epileptic c.
erotic c.
exploitative c.
c. flaw
genital c.
histrionic c.
hoarding c.
hysterical c.
c. impulse disorder
impulsive c.
in c.
masochistic c.
narcissistic c.
national c.
c. neurosis
obsessional c.
oral c.
oral-aggressive c.
oral-passive c.
oral-receptive c.
out of c.
paranoiac c.
c. pathology
phallic c.
phallic-narcissistic c.
phobic c.
primary sex c.
receptive c.
c. resistance
secondary sex c.
sex-conditioned c.
sex-limited c.
sex-linked c.
c. spectrum disorders

c. structure
c. trait
c. type
c. witness

characteristic
aberrant parental c.
c. age
c. association
association c.
c. behavior
behavior c.
change in personality c.
child behavior c. (CBC)
clang association c.
clinical c.
comorbid c.
consumer c.
core c.
demand c.
demographic c.
dominant c.
electrical c.
environment c.
c. feature
c. manifestation
neuropsychologic c.
objective trauma c.
overrepresented c.
c. paraphiliac focus
parental environment c.
c. pattern
c. pattern of affectivity
c. pattern of motivation
c. pattern of thought
perceived trauma c.
performance c.
personality c.
phenomenological c.
predictive c.
presenting c.
primary sex c.
psychological c.
psychometric performance c.
receiver operating c. (ROC)
secondary sex c.
sex c.
c. sign
signal-noise c.
temporal c.
trait c.
trauma c.

C

NOTES

characteristic *(continued)*
    unique c.
    c. withdrawal syndrome
characterization wit
characterological depression
characterologic disorder
characterology
charas
Charcot
    C. grand hysteria
    C. triad
    C. vertigo
charge
    c. of affect
    affective c.
    conversion sensory c.
    in c.
    sensory c.
    take c.
charge-coupled device (CCD)
charisma
charismatic
    c. personality
    c. religious experience
charlatan
charlatanry
charm
    superficial c.
Charpentier law
chart
    astrology c.
    autobiographical life c.
    expectancy c.
    flow c.
    mood c.
    pediatric growth c.
    progress c.
chary
chaser
    ambulance c.
chaste
chastise
chastisement
chastity
chat
chatterbox effect
checkerboard pattern
checking
    c. compulsion
    c. and touching rituals
checklist
    achievement c. (ACL)
    adjective c. (ACL)
    c. approach
    behavior c.
    Elgin c.
    occupational c. (OCL)
    time-sample behavioral c. (TSBC)

cheeking medication
cheerful
cheerfulness
    forced c.
    sudden c.
    unnatural c.
cheerless
cheirognostic, chirognostic
cheirokinesthesia, chirokinesthesia
cheirokinesthetic
cheirology
chelating agent
chelation therapy
chemical
    c. abuse
    c. action
    c. addiction
    c. agent
    atomic, biological, c. (ABC)
    c. aversion therapy
    c., bacteriological, radiological (CBR)
    c. and biological warfare (CBW)
    c. ceptor
    c. dependence
    c. dependence clinic
    c. dependency counselor (CDC)
    endogenous c.
    exogenous c.
    c. kinetics
    c. messenger
    c. neurotransmission
    psychoactive c.
    c., radiological, and biologic
    c., radiological, and biological warfare
    c. restraint
    c. sense
    c. signaling
    c. stimulation
    c. stimulus
    c. straitjacket
    c. sympathectomy
    c. synapse
    c. transmitter
    c. of use
    c.'s of use and abuse
    c. weapon
chemical-mechanical transduction
cheminosis
chemist
    basement c.
chemistry
    clinical c.
    mental c.
    psychiatric c.
    c. screening battery I (CSB I)
    c. screening battery II (CSB II)

chemopsychiatry
chemoreceptor trigger zone
chemoreflex
chemoresistance
chemosensitive
chemosensory
chemotherapy
chemotropism
cheromania
chest
    c. discomfort
    c. pain
    c. pulse
    c. restraint
    c. voice
chewing
    c. automatism
    breath c.
    c. method
chewing-speech relationship
Cheyne-Stokes
    C.-S. breathing
    C.-S. psychosis
    C.-S. respiration
CHI
    closed head injury
chi
    tai c.
chiaroscuro
chide
chief complaint (CC)
child
    abandoned c.
    c. abandonment
    c. abuse inventory
    c. abuser
    c. abuse syndrome
    c. or adolescent antisocial behavior
    c. and adolescent fear and anxiety treatment program
    c. and adolescent psychiatry
    adopted c.
    c. advocate
    c. of alcoholic (COA)
    c. analysis
    atypical c.
    autistic c.
    battered c.
    c. behavior characteristic (CBC)
    best interest of the c.
    biologic c.
    c. centered

conduct-disordered c.
c. counselor
c. custody
c. depression inventory
c. development clinic
c. development inventory
difficult c.
easy c.
c. endangerment
exceptional c.
c. fixation
foster c.
gifted c.
c. group therapy
c. guidance
homeless c.
c. inpatient service
c. inpatient unit
c. language development
latchkey c.
love c.
malnourished c.
c. maltreatment
manic c.
c. mental health professional
mentally retarded c.
misbehaving c.
c. molestation
c. molestation allegation
c. molester
c. neglect
neglect of c.
neglected c.
normal c.
obese c.
c. outpatient services
c. pornography
prepubertal c.
preschool c.
problem c.
c. problem tic
c. prodigy
c. psychiatric care
c. psychiatrist
c. psychiatry (CHP, CP)
c. psychologist
c. psychology (CP)
c. psychopathology
c. psychopharmacology
c. psychosis
c. raising period
c. rearing

C

NOTES

child (*continued*)
    scatter c.
    school-age c.
    sexual abuse of c.
    c. sexual abuse
    sexually abused c.
    c. snatcher
    c. support
    traumatized c.
    troubled c.
    unruly c.
    unwanted c.
    violent c.
    vulnerable c.
child-abuse-specific treatment of trauma (CASST)
childbirth
    c. amnesia
    c. organic psychosis
    psychosis in c.
childcare
    c. aide
    c. facility
    c. worker
child-focused
child-guidance
    c.-g. clinic
    c.-g. therapy
childhood
    abuse in c.
    adjustment reaction of c.
    c. anxiety disorder
    anxiety disorder of c.
    c. aphasia
    c. autism
    c. autism rating scale
    avoidant disorder of c.
    behavior disorder of c.
    c. bipolar disorder
    borderline psychosis of c.
    c. cross-gender behavior
    dementia-aphonia syndrome of c.
    developmental experimentation in c.
    c. developmental stage
    c. disease
    disinhibited-type reactive attachment disorder of infancy or c.
    c. disintegrative disorder
    disorder of c.
    early c.
    emotional disturbance of c.
    c. encephalopathy
    c. environment
    c. experience
    c. fear
    fearfulness disorder of c.
    c. figure
    gender identity disorder of c.

    hyperkinetic reaction of c.
    hyperkinetic syndrome of c.
    identity disorder of c.
    introverted disorder of c.
    lane of c.
    c. loss of a parent
    c. loss of a sibling
    c. maltreatment
    c. memory
    mid c.
    c. mistreatment history
    c. motivation
    c. obsessive-compulsive disorder
    c. onset
    oppositional disorder of c.
    overanxious disorder of c.
    problems of c.
    c. psychosexual identity disorder
    c. psychosis
    psychosis of c.
    reaction of c.
    reactive attachment disorder of infancy or early c.
    relationship problems of c.
    schizoid disorder of c.
    c. schizophrenia
    schizophrenic syndrome of c.
    second c.
    sensitivity reaction of c.
    c. separation anxiety
    separation anxiety disorder of c.
    c. sexual abuse
    shyness disorder of c.
    c. social dysfunction
    social withdrawal of c.
    c. stressor
    symbiotic psychosis of c.
    c. Tourette syndrome
    c. tradition
    transient spasm tic disorder of c.
    c. trauma
    c. trauma memory
    withdrawal reaction of c.
    c. years
childhood-onset
    c.-o. insomnia
    c.-o. obsessive-compulsive disorder
    c.-o. pervasive
    c.-o. pervasive developmental disorder
    c.-o. psychosis
    c.-o. schizophrenia
    c.-o. Tourette syndrome
childish
    c. behavior
    c. emotion
childlike
    c. behavior

c. innocence
c. mannerism
c. silliness
child-parent fixation
child-penis wish
child-placement counseling
children
c. and adults with attention deficit disorder (CHADD)
amnesia in c.
c. at risk
autistic-spectrum c.
bereavement in c.
c. development of moral thought
emotional maltreatment of c.
exploitation of c.
feral c.
gender identity disorder in c.
halfway c.
identity-disordered c.
latchkey c.
latency-age c.
prepubertal c.
relaxation training in c.
troubled c.
children's
C. Health Care Act of 2000
C. Health Study (CHS)
c. language processes
C. Protective Service (CPS)
chill
nervous c.
c. out
chill-out room
chilophagia
chimeric
c. stimulant
c. stimulation
China syndrome
Chinese ginseng
chin jerk
chirobrachialgia
chirognostic (*var. of* cheirognostic)
chirokinesthesia (*var. of* cheirokinesthesia)
chirospasm
chi-square
c.-s. distribution
c.-s. test
chlamydia, pl. **chlamydiae**
chlamydial
chlamydiosis

chloral
c. alcoholate
amylene c.
c. betaine
c. derivative
chloralism
chloride
amyl c.
carbamylcholine c.
c. channel flux assay
diphenylaminearsine c.
chlormezanone
chlorohydrocarbon dependence
chlorphentermine HCl
choice
career c.
c. choice
forced c.
laxative of c. (LOC)
narcissistic object c.
object c.
occupational c.
c. point
c. reaction
symptom-based drug c.
treatment c.
vocational c.
choking
choleric type
choline
cholinergic
c. activity
c. approach
c. neuron
c. receptor
c. side effect
c. synapse
c. therapy
c. tract
c. transmission
choo-choo phenomenon
choose
freedom to c.
chorea
automatic c.
chronic progressive c.
dancing c.
electric c.
fibrillary c.
habit c.
hysterical c.
juvenile c.

C

NOTES

chorea *(continued)*
    laryngeal c.
    c. major
    methodical c.
    mimetic c.
    c. minor
    c. nutans
    procursive c.
    rhythmic c.
    c. rotatoria
    saltatory c.
    senile c.
    tetanoid c.
choreal
choreic
    c. ataxia
    c. insanity
    c. movement
choreicus
    status c.
choreiform
    c. movement
    c. syndrome
choreoid
choreophrasia
chores
CHP
    child psychiatry
chrematomania
Christian belief
Christianity
chroma
chromaffinoma
chromaffinopathy
chromatic
    c. audition
    c. color
    c. contrast
    c. dimming
    c. flicker
    c. response
    c. scale
chromaticity
chromatid
chromatin
    sex c.
chromatin-negative
chromatinolysis
chromatin-positive
chromatography
chromatolytic
chromatopsia
chromesthesia
chromium
chromolysis
chromosomal
    c. aberration
    c. abnormality

    c. loci
    c. translocation
chromosome
    c. 4
    c. 13
    c. 18
    c. 21
    accessory c.
    acrocentric c.
    fragile X c.
    c. number
    sex c.
    c. 13, 18, 21 trisomy
    c. 21-trisomy syndrome
    X c.
    Y c.
chromotherapy
chromotopsia
chromotrichia
chromotrichial
chromotropic
chronaxia, chronaxy
chronic
    adjustment disorder, c.
    c. administration
    c. African sleeping sickness
    c. alcohol abuse
    c. alcoholic brain syndrome
    (CABS)
    c. alcoholic delirium
    c. alcoholic mania
    c. alcoholism
    c. amnesia
    c. anorexia nervosa
    c. antidepressant inhibition
    c. anxiety
    c. brain syndrome (CBS)
    c. change
    c. cocaine user
    c. course
    c. deficit state
    c. delusional state
    c. dementia
    c. disability
    c. disease score
    c. drinker
    c. drug abuse
    c. drunkenness
    c. dysthymia
    c. ethanol exposure
    c. ethanol user
    c. factitious illness
    c. familial polyneuritis
    c. fatigue
    c. fatigue syndrome (CFS)
    c. feelings of emptiness
    c. headache
    c. hyperventilation syndrome

c. hypomanic personality
c. illness behavior
c. insomnia
c. integrative deficit (CID)
c. intoxication
c. lead poisoning
c. major depression
c. melancholia
c. mental distress
c. mental illness
c. motor tic
c. motor tic disorder
c. neuropsychologic disorder
c. pain
pain disorder, c.
c. paranoid psychosis
c. paranoid reaction
c. paranoid schizophrenic reaction (CPSR)
c. pattern
c. pessimism
c. phase of stable sleep difficulty
c. posttraumatic neurosis
c. posttraumatic stress disorder
c. progressive chorea
c. psychosis
c. psychosocial turbulence
c. psychotic illness
c. response
c. sleep disturbance
c. spasm tic
c. state of anger
c. stress
c. stress reaction
c. tic
c. tissue damage
c. toxic effect
c. type
c. undifferentiated
c. undifferentiated schizophrenia
c. undifferentiated schizophrenic reaction
c. use
c. vertigo
chronically
c. depressed patient
c. disabling pattern
c. mentally ill
chronicity
chronobiological
c. disorder
c. disturbance

chronobiology
chronognosis
chronograph
chronologic age (CA)
chronological
c. drinking record
c. order
c. relationship
chronology
c. of symptom
chronometry
mental c.
chronotaraxis
CHS
Children's Health Study
chum period
chunking
chutzpah
CI
coefficient of intelligence
confidence interval
cibi
fastidium c.
CIC
crisis intervention clinic
cicatrices (*pl. of* cicatrix)
cicatricial alopecia
cicatrisata
alopecia c.
cicatrix, pl. **cicatrices**
brain c.
CICI
NL CICI
normal libido, coitus, and climax
CID
chronic integrative deficit
cilium, pl. **cilia**
cinanesthesia (*var. of* kinanesthesia)
cinchonism
cinclisis
Cinderella
C. complex
C. syndrome
cingulate
anterior c.
c. cortex
c. gyrus overactivity in OCD
posterior c.
c. response
retrosplenial c.

NOTES

cingulate *(continued)*
    c. sulcus
    c. tissue
cingulum, pl. **cingula**
cinq
    folie á c.
cintriamide
CIP
    comprehensive identification process
    critical illness polyneuropathy
circa
circadian
    c. clock
    c. marker
    c. phase of sleep
    c. quotient (CQ)
    c. realignment
    c. rhythm
    c. rhythm sleep disorder
    c. rhythm sleep disorder, delayed
      sleep phase
    c. rhythm sleep disorder, jet lag
    c. rhythm sleep disorder, shift
      work
    c. system
    c. timing
circannual rhythm
circaseptan rhythm
circle
    Papez c.
    vicious c.
circuit
    attentional c.
    convergence c.
    cortex c.
    divergence c.
    dysfunctional neural c.
    error detection c.
    frontal subcortical brain c.'s
    limbic c.
    neuroanatomic c.
    neuronal c.
    Papez c.
    reverberating c.
    traditional limbic c.
    worry c.
circuitry
    amygdala-fear c.
    brain c.
    dysfunctional c.
    frontal-cerebellar-thalamic c.
    limbic c.
    normal c.
    reciprocal c.
    reward c.
    striatofrontal c.
circulaire
    folie c.

circular
    c. dementia
    c. insanity
    c. psychosis
    c. reaction
    c. thinking
circular-pattern response
circulating leptin level
circulatory psychosis
circumambulate
circumcision
    female c.
    male c.
circumfix morpheme
circumlocution
circumplex
    multifacet c.
    c. of premorbid personality type
circumscribed
    c. amnesia
    c. change
    c. craniomalacia
    c. delusion
    c. edema
    c. pyocephalus
    c. region
circumscripta
    alopecia c.
circumscription
    monosymptomatic c.
circumspect
circumstance
    abnormal c.
    altered life c.
    clinical c.
    distressing c.
    extenuating c.
    frightening c.
    inappropriate c.
    other specified family c.
    real-life c.
circumstantial
    c. evidence
    c. migraine
    c. migraine headache
    c. speech
    c. thought process
circumstantiality
CIRP
    cooperative institutional research program
cirrhosis
    alcoholic c. (AC)
    Laennec c.
    liver c.
    syphilitic c.
    toxic c.
cirrhotic liver
cisternal puncture

cisterna magna
cisvestism
cite
Citelli syndrome
citizen
    law-abiding c.
    senior c.
citrate
city and state test
civil
    c. commitment
    c. disobedience
    c. marriage
    c. rights
    c. rights violation
civilian
    C. Health and Medical Program of the Uniformed Service (CHAMPUS)
    c. trauma
civilian-catastrophe reaction
civilization
CJD
    Creutzfeldt-Jakob disease
cladiosic
claim's review
clairaudience
clairsentience
clairvoyance
clairvoyant dream
clammy skin
clamor
clan
clandestine
clang
    c. association
    c. association characteristic
clanging
clannish
clansman
clarification
clarify
clarity
    diagnostic c.
    phonetic c.
clash
    paradigm c.
    personality c.
clasp-knife
    c.-k. effect
    c.-k. phenomenon
    c.-k. response
    c.-k. rigidity
    c.-k. spasticity
class
    closed c.
    c. conscious
    diagnostic c.
    c. discrimination
    elite c.
    c. inclusion
    c. interval
    c. limit
    middle c.
    parental socioeconomic c.
    processing word c.
    c. size
    skip c.
    social c.
    socioeconomic c.
    c. word
classic
    c. apraxia
    c. euphoric mania
    c. migraine
classical
    c. analysis
    c. conditioning
    c. depression
    c. migraine headache
    c. paranoia
    c. psychoanalytical theory
classification
    alcoholic c.
    categorical c.
    c. of depression
    dichotomous c.
    DSM-IV-R c.
    empirical c.
    Kendell c.
    c. method
    multiaxial c.
    neo-kraepelian c.
    Newcastle c.
    Paykel c.
    c. system
    c. test
classism
classless
classroom
Claude
    C. hyperkinesis sign
    C. syndrome

NOTES

clausa
    rhinolalia c.
clauses
    disturbance between c.
    disturbance within c.
claustral complex
claustrophobic
claustrum, pl. **claustra**
clavus hystericus
clawing attack
clay eater
clay-modeling
    c.-m. equipment
    c.-m. therapy
CLD
  central language disorder
clear
    c. and convincing evidence
    c. rules and consequence
    c. sensorium
    c. thinking
    c. twilight state
clearance
    dopamine c.
clear-cut
    c.-c. attachment
    c.-c. schizophrenia
clearheaded
clearheadedness
clearinghouse
    privacy c.
    self-help c.
clearly demarcated relationship
clear-sighted
clear-sightedness
cleft-palate speech
clemency
clench
clenching
    fist c.
Clerambault
    C. erotomania
    C. erotomania syndrome
Clerambault-Kandinsky complex
clergy
    benefit of c.
cleric
clerical
    c. perception (Q)
    c. response
cleverness factor
cliche
client-centered
    c.-c. psychotherapy
    c.-c. therapy
climacophobia
climacteric, climacterium
    c. age

    female c.
    c. insanity
    male c.
    c. melancholia
    c. neurosis
    c. paranoid psychosis
    c. paranoid reaction
    c. paranoid state
    c. paraphrenia
    c. psychoneurosis
climate
    emotional c.
    group c.
climax
    normal libido, coitus, and c. (NL CICI, NLC&C)
    sexual c.
climber
    social c.
clinging
    c. behavior
    c. dependence
clinic
    affective disorders c. (ADC)
    chemical dependence c.
    child development c.
    child-guidance c.
    community-based c.
    crisis intervention c. (CIC)
    guidance c.
    mental health c. (MHC)
    mental hygiene c.
    outpatient c.
    pain c.
    c. patient
    c. patient population
    research c.
    satellite c.
    sex c.
    supportive medication c.
clinical
    c. analysis
    c. anecdote
    c. approach
    c. armamentarium
    c. behavior
    c. bias
    c. care
    c. case discussion
    c. characteristic
    c. chemistry
    c. circumstance
    c. comparison
    c. comparison study
    c. conceptualization
    c. condition
    c. correlate
    c. counseling

c. course
c. data
c. decision making
c. depression
c. description
c. diagnosis
c. diagnostic practice
c. difference
c. effect
c. efficacy
c. encounter
c. equivalent
c. evaluation
c. example
c. experience
c. facilitated intervention
c. feature
c. finding
c. formulation
c. grouping
c. heterogeneity
c. history
c. immunology
c. implication
c. importance
c. impression
c. improvement
c. inference
c. intervention program
c. interview
c. inventory
c. judgment
c. laboratory
c. literature
c. management
c. manifestation
c. material
c. medicine
c. method
c. monitoring
c. monitoring technique
c. need
c. neuropsychology
c. neuroscientist
c. observation
c. outcome
c. performance score (CPS)
c. perspective
c. phenomenology
c. phenomenon
c. phenotype
c. picture

c. population
c. poverty
c. poverty syndrome
c. practice setting
c. prediction
c. presentation
c. procedure
c. profile
c. progression
c. psychiatrist
c. psychiatry
c. psychobiology
c. psychologist
c. psychology
c. psychopharmacology
c. purpose
c. reasoning
c. record review
c. relevance
c. resemblance
c. response
c. responsibility
c. scale
c. sequela
c. sign
c. significance
c. significance criterion
c. situation
c. social worker
c. sociology
c. stability
c. status
c. subtype
c. symptom
c. teaching
c. theory
c. therapeutic
c. thinking
c. training
c. trial
c. understanding
c. use
c. validity
c. variable
c. visit

clinically
c. adverse sequela
c. recommended dose
c. significant
c. significant anxiety
c. significant distress
c. significant impairment

C

NOTES

clinician
 c. bias
 evaluating c.
 c. observation
 psychiatric c.
 psychodynamic c.
 c. rating
 c. rating scale
clinician-administered
clinician-consultant
clinician-observer
clinician-rated
 c.-r. cognitive symptom
 c.-r. scale
clinicopathologic
clinodactyly
clipped speech
clipping
 peak c.
clitoral
 c. hood
 c. stimulation
clitoridis
 erector c.
 glans c.
clitoris, pl. **clitorides**
clitorism
clitoromania
cloacal theory
cloaca therapy
clock
 biologic c.
 circadian c.
 c. face test
clominorex
clone
clonic
 c. convulsion
 c. movement
 c. seizure
 c. spasm
clonicity
clonic-tonic-clonic seizure
clonism
clonospasm
clonus
 ankle c.
 subsultus c.
 toe c.
 wrist c.
clopenthixol
clophenoxate
Clopixol depot
clorazepic
close
 c. clinical monitoring
 c. observation

 c. sightedness
 c. watch restriction
closed
 c. anesthesia
 c. awareness
 c. book
 c. class
 c. group
 c. head injury (CHI)
 c. head trauma
 c. horizon
 c. juncture
 c. place
closed-circuit television (CCTV)
closed-ended question
closed-loop feedback system
close-ended query
close-knit
 c.-k. community
 c.-k. family
closemouthed
closeness
closesightedness
closet
 c. alcoholic
 c. bisexual
 c. drinker
 c. homosexual
 out of the c.
closure
 auditory c.
 bring to c.
 law of c.
 perceptual c.
 c. principle
 c. process
 visual c.
clothes
 changing c.
 plucking at c.
 pulling of c.
clothing
 inappropriate c.
 tattered c.
clotiazepam
clouded
 c. sensorium
 c. state
 c. state epilepsy
clouding of consciousness
clouds
 up in the c.
cloudy sensorium
cloverleaf
 c. skull
 c. skull syndrome
clownery

clowning
  provocative c.
clownism
cloxazolam
Clozaril National Registry
cloze procedure
CLQ
  cognitive laterality quotient
CLS
  confused language syndrome
club
  social c.
clucking
  nervous c.
  c. sound
  tongue c.
clumsiness syndrome
clumsy gesture
Clunis inquiry forensic psychiatry
cluster
  c. A, B, C disorder
  c. analysis
  anxious-fearful c.
  c. approach
  avoidance c.
  c. B trait
  c. C, D symptom
  c. characteristics in personality
    disorder
  diagnostic c.
  dissociative symptom c.
  dramatic emotional c.
  DSM c.'s
  eccentric A c.
  emotional B c.
  fearful C c.
  c. headache
  inner battery c.
  c. marriage
  c. migraine
  odd-eccentric c.
  problem behavior c.'s
  c. reduction
  situation c.
  c. of situations
  suicide c.
  c. suicide
  c. of symptom
clustering
  c. criterion
  semantic c.

clutter
  hoarding and c.
cluttering
Clytemnestra complex
cM
  centimorgan
CMA
  conflict management appraisal
CMCA
  care management for chronic addiction
CME
  continuing medical education
CMHC
  community mental health care
  community mental health center
CMHS
  Center for Mental Health Services
CMV
  cytomegalovirus
CNS
  central nervous system
    CNS depressant
    CNS disease group
    CNS stimulant
    CNS syphilis
    CNS trauma
CNT
  could not test
CNV
  conative negative variation
  contingent negative variation
CO$_2$
  carbon dioxide
    CO$_2$ inhalation
COA
  child of alcoholic
coach
co-activation
coactive strategy
coaddiction
coalcoholic
coalcoholism
coalesce
coalescence
coalition
  confusingly fluid c.
coarctated personality
coarse tremor
coarticulation
  anticipatory c.
  backward c.
coast memory

C

NOTES

cobalamin deficiency
coca
    c. bush
    c. leaf
coca bush
cocaethylene assay
cocaine
    c. abuse
    c. addiction
    C. Anonymous (CA)
    c. anxiety disorder
    c. binge
    c. bug
    c. cessation
    c. craving
    c. cue
    c. delusion
    c. delusional disorder
    c. dependence
    c. freebase
    c. habit
    c. habituation
    c. and heroin
    c. intake
    c. intoxication
    c. intoxication delirium
    c. intoxication-related disorder
    c. intoxication, with perceptual
      disturbance
    intravenous c.
    c. mood disorder
    processed c.
    c. psychosis
    c. sexual dysfunction
    c. sleep disorder
    c. use disorder
    c. user
    c. withdrawal
    c. withdrawal symptom
cocaine-dependent
    c.-d. baby
    c.-d. individual
cocaine-free
    c.-f. urine sample
    c.-f. urine screen
cocaine-heroin combination
cocaine-induced
    c.-i. anxiety
    c.-i. disorder
    c.-i. dopamine stimulation
    c.-i. psychotic disorder with
      delusions
    c.-i. psychotic disorder with
      hallucinations
    c.-i. sexual dysfunction

cocaine-related
    c.-r. disorder, not otherwise
      specified
    c.-r. response
cocainism
cocainization
cocainize
cocainomania
CocAnon
cockalorum
cockamamy
cocktail
    lytic c.
    Molotov c.
    c. party effect
    c. party paradigm
cocky
coconsciousness
coconscious personality
coconut sound
cocooning
CODA
    Codependents Anonymous
coddle
code
    c. blue
    c. capacity
    capacity c.
    c. of ethics
    genetic c.
    ICD-9 c.
    imagery c.
    model penal c.
    moral c.
    penal c.
    professional c.
    psychiatric CPT c.
    c. of silence
    c. substitution-accuracy (CDS-ACC)
    c. substitution-efficiency (CDS-EFF)
    c. substitution-immediate recall-
      accuracy (CDS-ACC)
    c. test
    V c.
    Z c.
codependence
codependency disorder
codependent personality
Codependents Anonymous (CODA)
codification
coding
codominance
coefficient
    alienation c.
    c. alpha
    alpha c.
    alternate forms reliability c.
    association c.

comparable forms reliability c.
concordance c.
contingency c.
c. of correlation
correlation c.
equivalence c.
familiar correlation c.
high alpha c.
c. of inbreeding
c. of intelligence (CI)
kappa c.
low alpha c.
odd-even method reliability c.
reliability c.
scoring c.
split half reliability c.
test-retest reliability c.
validity c.
c. of variation (CV)
coenesthesia (*var. of* cenesthesia)
coenesthesia
coenesthetic schizophrenia
coerce
coerced treatment
coercion
c. program
sexual c.
coercive
c. behavior
c. communication
c. legal action
c. persuasion
c. philosophy
c. treatment
coeundi
impotentia c.
coeur
cri de c.
coexcitation
coexist
coexistence
dysfunctional c.
c. of neurotransmitter
peaceful c.
coexistent culture
coexisting
c. disorder
c. psychopathology
coffee consumption
COGA
Collaborative Study on the Genetics of
Alcoholism

cogent
cogitate
cognate confusion
cognition
affect, behavior, c. (ABCs of
geriatric psychiatry)
being c.
constriction of c.
c. disorder
dysfunctional c.
empiric c.
frontal based c.
neurologic c.
paranormal c.
c. of semantic unit (CSU)
social c.
theory of c.
cognitive
c. ability
c. analytic therapy (CAT)
c. approaches to dreaming and
repression
c. assessment
c. avoidance
c. awareness level
c. behavior
c. behavioral analysis system of
psychotherapy (CBASP)
c. behavioral approach
c. behavioral coping skills training
group
c. behavioral factor
c. behavioral group therapy
(CBGT)
c. behavior therapy (CBT)
c. benefit
c. capability
c. capacity
c. change
c. conditioning
c. control
c. decline
c. decrement
c. defect
c. deficiency
c. deficit
c. derailment
c. deterioration
c. development
c. development stages (Period
I–IV)
c. disability

C

NOTES

cognitive *(continued)*
  c. disorder
  c. disorganization
  c. disruption
  c. dissonance
  c. dissonance theory
  c. distancing
  c. distortion
  c. disturbance
  c. domain
  c. dysfunction
  c. dysmetria
  c. element
  c. enhancement therapy
  c. fatigue
  c. flexibility
  c. function
  c. functioning
  c. generation of affect
  c. growth
  c. impairment
  c. impairment of depression
  c. impairment level
  c. improvement
  c. laterality quotient (CLQ)
  c. learning theory
  c. loss
  c. map
  c. mapping
  c. maturation
  c. maturity
  c. measure
  c. mechanism
  c. mediation
  c. method
  c. model
  c. need
  c. neuropsychology
  c. neuroscience
  c. nonability
  c. pathology
  c. performance
  c. personality trait
  c. process
  c. psychodynamics
  c. psychology
  c. psychotherapy
  c. rehabilitation
  c. rehearsal
  c. remediation
  c. remediation therapy
  c. research orientation
  c. reserve
  c. restitution
  c. restricting
  c. restructuring
  c. risk factor
  c. ritual

  c. route
  c. schema
  c. science
  c. score
  c. self-hypnosis training
  c. self-reinforcement
  c. slippage
  c. state
  c. status
  c. stimulation
  c. strategy
  c. structure
  c. style
  c. subscale
  c. subsystem
  c. symptom
  c. task
  c. technique
  c. tendency
  c. test
  c. test battery
  c. testing
  c. theory of depression
  c. theory of learning
  c. trajectory
  c. triad
  c. variable
cognitive-behavioral
  c.-b. intervention
  c.-b. psychotherapy
  c.-b. technique
  c.-b. treatment
cognitive-linguistic treatment
cognitively
  c. elicited emotion
  c. intact
cognitive-physiological therapy
cognitivist
cognizance
cognizant
cogwheel
  c. phenomenon
  c. rigidity
cohabitant
cohabitation
Cohen
  C. syndrome
  C. view of depressive disorder
coherence
coherent
  c. negative picture-caption pair
  c. positive picture-caption pair
  c. stream of thought
cohesion
  figural c.
  group c.
  law of c.

cohesive
   c. device
   c. family
   c. image
cohesiveness
   level of c.
   c. level
cohoba snuff
cohort
   birth c.
   c. effect
   c. experimental design
   c. study
coil
   butterfly c.
   induction c.
coin
   c. new phrases
   c. new slang terms
   c. new words
   c. rubbing
coinage
   word c.
coital
   c. headache
   c. orgasm
   c. position
coition
coitus
   c. analis
   c. in ano
   c. in axilla
   c. condomatus
   c. inter femora
   c. interruptus
   c. a la vache
   oral c.
   c. prolongatus
   psychogenic painful c.
   c. representation
   c. reservatus
   c. Saxonius
   c. sine ejaculatione
   c. a tergo
cold
   c. acclimation
   c. comfort
   c. effect
   c. effector
   emotionally c.
   c. exposure
   c. fear

   c. mottled insensate leg
   paradoxical c.
   c. sensitivity
   c. shoulder
   c. spot
   c. turkey
cold-blooded
coldhearted
coldness
   emotional c.
cold-pack treatment
cold-sensitive neuron
colinearity
collaborate
collaboration
collaborative
   c. relationship
   C. Study on the Genetics of
      Alcoholism (COGA)
   c. therapy
   c. treatment process
collapse delirium
collapsing anchor
collateral
   c. behavior
   c. sources
collecting
   injustice c.
   c. mania
collection
   data c.
   information c.
   statistics c.
collective
   c. behavior
   c. ego
   c. experience
   c. hypnotization
   c. hysteria
   c. monologue
   c. neurosis
   c. psychosis
   c. representation
   c. suicide
   c. transference
   c. unconscious
collectivist culture
college
   c. graduate
   invisible c.
   C. Outcome Measures Program
   c. student

C

NOTES

Collet-Sicard syndrome
colligation
colloquial
collusion
colony
    Gheel c.
color
    achromatic c.
    c. agnosia
    c. amblyopia
    c. anomia
    c. blind
    chromatic c.
    c. constancy
    c. contrast
    c. denial (Cd)
    c. discrimination
    c. in dream
    c. dream
    flashes of c.
    flight of c.
    gang c.'s
    c. hearing
    c. mixture
    c. perception
    c. preference
    primary c.
    c. response
    c. sorting test
    c. taste
    c. theory
    c. therapy
    c. weakness
    c. zone
Columbine High School shooting
columella, pl. **columellae**
column
    cortical c.
    ocular dominance c.
coma
    alcoholic c.
    apoplectic c.
    barbiturate-induced c.
    diabetic c.
    hepatic c.
    irreversible c.
    Kussmaul c.
    metabolic c.
    c. scale
    c. therapy
    thyrotoxic c.
    trance c.
    c. vigil
comatose patient
combat
    armed c.
    c. casualty
    c. exhaustion

    exposure to c.
    c. fatigue
    c. fear
    c. flashback
    hors de c.
    c. hysteria
    c. neurosis
    c. reaction
    single c.
    c. stress
    c. stress exposure
    c. tension
    c. trauma
    c. veteran
combative patient
combination
    aspirin c.
    cocaine-heroin c.
    c. drug (CD)
    frequency c.
    c. headache
    law of c.
    orthogonal c.
    paradoxical c.
    c. strategy
combination-drug dependence
combinative thinking
combined
    c. anesthesia
    c. factor
    c. predictive power
    c. sclerosis
    c. system disease
    c. therapy
    c. transcortical aphasia
combined-type
    c.-t. attention deficit hyperactivity
       disorder
    c.-t. personality disorder
combining power test (CPT)
comfort
    cold c.
    contact c.
    c. dream
    emotional c.
    c. food
    c. level
comic relief
comitial mal
command
    c. auditory hallucination
    c. automatism
    embedded c.
    c. law
    negative c.
    c. negativism
    c. style commitment
comme il faut

comment
    condescending c.
    derogatory c.
    discriminatory c.
    threatening c.
commentary
    running c.
    sexual c.
commenting
    voice c.
commiserate
Commission on Psychotherapy by Psychiatrists
commissural aphasia
commit
commitment
    civil c.
    command style c.
    conscious c.
    criminal c.
    ideological c.
    institutional c.
    involuntary civil c.
    involuntary outpatient c.
    laws of c.
    legal c.
    long-term c.
    observation c.
    c. procedure
    religious c.
    sense of c.
    short-term c.
    temporary c.
    voluntary c.
committed
    legally c.
committee
    C. on Information Systems
    C. on Standards and Survey Procedures
    utilization review c.
common
    c. central process
    c. experience
    c. goal
    c. law marriage
    c. migraine
    c. migraine headache
    c. precipitant exposure
    c. sense
    c. sense psychiatry
    c. sense therapy

    c. shared feature
    c. theme
    c. trait
commonality
commonplace
commotio
    c. cerebri
    c. spinalis
communality
communal residential center
commune
communicable
    c. disease
    c. hysteria
communicated insanity
communicating
    c. empathy
    c. epilepsy
communication
    c. ability
    augmentative c.
    c. barrier
    c.'s in behavioral biology (CBB)
    c. channel
    channel of c.
    coercive c.
    consummatory c.
    c. deviance
    c. disorder (CD)
    distortion of language and c.
    email c.
    emotional c.
    exaggeration of language and c.
    facilitation of c.
    fragmented c.
    c. function
    gestural c.
    hesitant c.
    illogical c.
    impaired effective c.
    c. impairment
    indexical c.
    inhibited c.
    irreverent c.
    language and c.
    c. magic
    manual c.
    c. network
    nonverbal c.
    nonvocal c.
    oral c.
    pathologic c.

C

NOTES

communication *(continued)*
    pathological c.
    c. pattern
    personal c.
    persuasive c.
    physician-patient c.
    privileged c.
    problem-solving c.
    qualitative impairment in c.
    reciprocal c.
    c. scale
    secure c.
    signed c.
    c. in sign language
    c. skills
    c. skills assessment
    social c.
    c. theory
    therapeutic c.
    c. therapy
    c. tool
    total c.
    unaided augmentative c.
    c. unit
    vague c.
    vehicle for c.
    verbal c.
    visual c. (VC, VIC)
    c. with adolescent
    written c.
communication/cognition treatment
communicative
    c. competence
    c. comprehension
    c. disorder
    c. function
    c. interaction
communicatively impaired
communicology
communion principle
communiquee
    folie c.
community
    c. action group
    alternative lifestyle c.
    c. assessment
    c. care
    c. catharsis
    c. centered
    close-knit c.
    c. connectedness
    c. divorce
    c. effort
    elite c.
    c. feeling
    c. functioning
    homosexual c.
    impoverished c.

    inner city c.
    integrated c.
    c. intervention
    c. mental health
    mental health c.
    c. mental health care (CMHC)
    c. mental health center (CMHC)
    C. Mental Health Construction Act
      of 1963
    middle class c.
    minority c.
    c. need
    Oneida c.
    online support c.
    c. outreach program
    c. population
    c. psychiatry
    c. psychology
    religious c.
    c. resources
    c. responsibility
    c. role
    c. safety
    segregated c.
    senior citizen c.
    sense of c.
    c. service
    c. setting
    singles c.
    c. spirit
    c. study
    suburban c.
    c. support
    c. support system
    therapeutic c. (TC)
    c. treatment and reintegration
      program
    c. violence
    working c.
community-based
    c.-b. clinic
    c.-b. mental health treatment
    c.-b. psychiatric program
community-institutional relations
community-residing patient
comorbid
    c. anxiety disorder
    c. Axis II diagnosis
    c. characteristic
    c. cluster B personality disorder
    c. condition
    c. depressive disorder
    c. mental disorder
    c. mood disorder
    c. past alcoholism
    c. psychiatric diagnosis
    c. psychiatric disorder
    c. psychopathology

c. substance abuse
c. tic
comorbidity
age-related c.
anxiety c.
anxiety-mood c.
medical c.
multiple anxiety c.
psychiatric c.
somatopsychiatric c.
substantial c.
compacta
companion
imaginary c.
phobic c.
companionate marriage
companionship
animal c.
human c.
comparable
c. finding
c. forms reliability coefficient
c. worth
comparative
c. efficacy
c. guidance and placement program (CGPP)
c. judgment
c. medicine
c. psychiatry
c. psychology
c. research
c. scanning
comparison
clinical c.
c. condition
factor c.
positive c.
post hoc c.
c. region
systematic c.
compartment
synaptic c.
compartmentalize
compassion
compassionate
c. feeling
c. marriage
c. use basis
compatibility
compatible
compelled behavior

compelling evidence
compensate
compensation
c. defense mechanism
c. neurosis
c. neurotic disorder
c. psychoneurosis
c. schizophrenia
synaptic c.
compensatory
c. behavior
c. education
c. fantasy
c. mechanism
c. mood swing
c. movement
c. technique
c. trait
compete
competence
apparent c.
assessment of c.
communicative c.
cultural c.
facade of c.
juvenile c.
c. knowledge
measure of c.
mental c.
c. motivation
presumption of c.
social c.
competency
c. assessment
high degree of c.
legal criteria for c.
low threshold of c.
maternal c.
mental c.
paternal c.
c. standard
competency-based
c.-b. examination
c.-b. instruction
competent
c. decision
c. decision making
mentally c.
c., optimal relational functioning
c. relationship
c. to stand trial
competing theories of motivation

NOTES

competition
competitive
    c. behavior
    c. motive
complacence
complacent attitude
complain
complainant-listener relationship
complainer
    help-rejecting c.
complaint
    chief c. (CC)
    frequent physical c.
    habitual c.
    hypochondriacal c.
    nuisance c.
    pain c.
    primary c.
    sleep c.
    somatic c.
    subjective insomnia c.
    unfounded c.
    vague c.
complemental air
complementarity of interaction
complementary
    c. instinct
    c. medicine
    c. role
complement symptom-focused assessment
complete
    c. amnesia
    c. aphasia
    c. birth
    c. cross-dressing
    c. genital primacy
    c. mother
    c. Oedipus
    c. treatment plan
completed suicide
complete-learning method
completion
    c., arithmetic, vocabulary, and
      directions (CAVD)
    c., arithmetic, vocabulary, and
      directions test
    picture c. (PC)
    sentence c.
    suicide c.
    task c.
    treatment c.
complex
    c. absence
    active castration c.
    AIDS dementia c. (ADC)
    AIDS-related c. (ARC)
    c. aspect of fear conditioning
    authority c.

benzodiazepine-GABA-receptor c.
brain wave c.
breast c.
brother c.
Cain c.
castration c.
Cinderella c.
claustral c.
Clerambault-Kandinsky c.
Clytemnestra c.
culture c.
c. delusion
Diana c.
c. disease
disorganized symptom c.
dorsal vagus c.
ego c.
Electra c.
c. equivalence
Eshmun c.
father c.
femininity c.
c. finger routine
Friedmann c.
function c.
GABA receptor c.
God c.
grandfather c.
Griselda c.
c. hallucination
c. hand routine
heir of the Oedipus c.
hippocampal c.
homosexual c.
hypersexual c.
c. of ideas
inferiority c.
inferior orbitofrontal c.
Jocasta c.
K c.
kernel c.
Lear c.
c. learning process
Madonna c.
Madonna-prostitute c.
martyr c.
Medea c.
messiah c.
mother c.
Mother Superior c.
c. motor behavior
c. motor tic
c. multistep task
c. noise
obscenity-purity c.
oedipal c.
Oedipus c.
organ inferiority c.

c. partial epilepsy
c. partial seizure (CPS)
particular c.
passive castration c.
persecution c.
Phaedra c.
Polycrates c.
posttraumatic stress disorder c.
c. precipitated epilepsy
c. psychological construct
c. psychological trait
c. PTSD
Quasimodo c.
c. readiness
c. relationship
robin c.
c. segregation analysis
c. sentence
small penis c.
c. social interaction
spike-and-wave c.
superiority c.
symptom c.
c. thematic pictures test
c. tone
c. type
c. vocal tic
c. whole body movement

complexion

complexity
diagnostic c.
environmental c.
etiological c.
human c.
syntactic c.

compliance
c. masking covert resistance
motor c.
overt c.
patient c.
privacy c.
c. rate
social c.
strategic c.
sustained c.
treatment c.

compliant

complicate

complicated
c. bereavement
c. grief disorder

c. migraine headache
c. relationship

complication
adverse neurologic c.
drug-induced medical c.
pregnancy and birth c.
psychiatric c.
psychosocial c.

complicity

complimentary

comply
failure to c.

component
adrenomedullary c.
articulatory loop c.
autonomous functional c.
base c.
blood c.
central executive c.
cross-sectional c.
functional c.
general c.
genetic c.
heritable c.
inotropic c.
masochistic c.
physiological c.
prominent phobic anxiety c.
slave system c.
sudomotor c.
thermogenic c.
true c.
vasomotor c.

composed

composite
c. index
narcissistic c.
c. person
c. personality
c. personality description
c. score
total battery c.

composition
body c.
group c.
mixed-sex group c.
same-sex group c.
sociodemographic c.

compos mentis

composure

compound
active c.

C

NOTES

compound *(continued)*
    antidepressant c.
    antipsychotic c.
    bromine c.
    c. medicine
    primary active c.
comprehend
comprehension
    auditory c.
    communicative c.
    c. deficit
    language c.
    passage c.
    c. span
    c. subtest
comprehensive
    c. assessment
    c. care
    C. Drug Abuse Prevention and Control Act of 1970
    c. evaluation
    c. examinaton
    c. identification process (CIP)
    c. review
    c. service
    c. solution
    c. test
    c. therapeutic approach
    c. treatment
    c. treatment planning
comprehensiveness
compression
    c. anesthesia
    c. of brain
    cerebral c.
    c. paralysis
compromise
    cerebral c.
    c. distortion
    c. formation
compromised
    c. function
    severely c.
compulsion
    antisocial c.
    brooding c.
    checking c.
    counting c.
    eating c.
    c. neurosis
    c. psychoneurosis
    repetition c.
    c. score
    sexual c.
    tapping c.
    thinking c.
compulsion-obsession

compulsive
    c. act
    c. action
    c. buying
    c. ceremonial
    c. change
    c. character
    c. defense
    c. disturbance
    c. drawing
    c. drinker
    c. drug administration
    c. drug-taking behavior
    c. eater
    c. exercise
    c. fixation on an unobtainable partner
    c. gambler
    c. gambling
    c. hoarding
    c. idea
    c. insanity
    c. laughter
    c. magic
    c. mania
    c. masturbation
    c. masturbatory behavior
    c. neurosis
    c. neurotic personality disorder
    c. orderliness
    c. personality
    c. psychasthenia
    c. psychogenic disorder
    c. psychogenic tic
    c. psychoneurotic reaction
    c. quality
    c. repetition
    c. restraint
    c. ritual
    c. scale
    c. severity
    c. sex
    c. sexual behavior
    c. spasms and tics
    c. stealing
    c. substance use
    c. swearing
    c. swearing syndrome
    c. symptom
    c. thought
    c. water drinking
    c. writing
compulsivity
compulsory
compurgation
computation
    symbolic c.
computational process

computer
    c. addict
    c. addiction
    biofeedback c.
    c. crash
    c. file
    c. game
    c. hacker
    c. literate
    c. security
computer-aided therapy
computer-assisted
    c.-a. review
    c.-a. speech device
computer-guided therapy
computerized tomography scan
COMT
    catechol-o-methyltransferase
con
    ability to c.
conarium
conation
conative
    c. appetitive striving
    c. negative variation (CNV)
conatus
concatenation
concavity
conceal
concealed handgun
concealing behavior
conceit
conceivable
conceive
concentrate
    inability to c.
concentrating
    difficulty c.
    trouble c.
concentration
    approximate lethal c. (ALC)
    attention and c.
    blood alcohol c.
    brain-derived HVA c.
    c. camp syndrome (CCS)
    c. deficit
    c. difficulty
    c. disturbance
    impaired c.
    information memory c. (IMC)
    minimum effective c. (MEC)
    time of maximum c.

concept
    abstract c.
    body ego c.
    c. of brain function
    concrete c.
    conjunctive c.
    critical band c.
    cultural c.
    feces-child-penis c.
    c. formation
    grandiose c.
    humanistic c.
    key c.
    c. learning
    lexica c.
    mall treatment c.
    medicine c.
    mental c.
    object c.
    permanence c.
    psychoanalytic c.
    psychodynamic c.
    self-derogatory c.
    self-role c.
    c. of spiritual coping
    c. of spiritual healing
    traditional psychoanalytic c.
    c. of will
    Zanarini c.
conception
    hallucination of c.
    imperative c.
concept-specific
conceptual
    c. ability
    c. disorder
    c. disorganization
    c. disturbance
    c. endeavor
    c. learning
    c. limitation
    c. nervous system
    c. planning
    c. problem
    c. quotient (CQ)
    c. reasoning
    c. skill
    c. tempo
    c. thinking
conceptualization
    abstract c.

C

NOTES

conceptualization *(continued)*
    axis I, II c.
    clinical c.
conceptualized
conceptualizing
concergent and divergent validity
concern
    abandonment c.
    dispassionate c.
    ethical c.
    interpersonal c.
    malevolent c.
    physical c.
    psychological c.
    sense of c.
    sexual c.
    social c.
    spiritual c.
    unconscious c.
    ventilate c.
concernment
conciliate
concomitant
concordance
    c. coefficient
    c. rate
    twin c.
concordant result
concrete
    c. abstractive ability
    c. attitude
    c. concept
    c. image
    c. intelligence
    c. operation
    c. operational development
    c. operational stage
    c. operation period
    c. operation stage
    c. picture
    c. representation
    c. thinking
    c. thought process
concreteness
concretistic thinking
concretization
    active c.
concretizing attitude
concubinage
concubine
concubitus
concupiscence
concurrent
    c. alcohol and substance abuse
    c. personality disorder
    c. psychiatric diagnosis
    c. psychiatric problem
    c. reinforcement

    c. review
    c. therapy
    c. validity
concussion
    c. amnesia
    c. blindness
    brain c.
    c. of brain
    c. syndrome
condemn
condemnation
condensation
condescend
condescending
    c. attitude
    c. behavior
    c. comment
    c. evaluation
    c. manner
    c. speech
    c. tone of voice
condescension
condition
    abnormal pathologic c.
    activating c.
    active general medical c.
    atmospheric c.
    catatonic disorder due to a general medical c.
    clinical c.
    comorbid c.
    comparison c.
    congenital intersex c.
    delirium due to a general medical c.
    desperate financial c.
    drug-free c.
    emotional c.
    etiological neurological c.
    experimental c.
    general medical c. (GMC)
    haloperidol c.
    heterogeneous c.
    illumination c.
    insomnia-type sleep disorder due to general medical c.
    intersex c.
    life-threatening c.
    medical c.
    mental disorder due to a general medical c.
    mood disorder due to a general medical c.
    necessary c.
    neurological c.
    neuropsychiatric c.
    noise c.

c. not attributable to a mental
　disorder
organic psychotic c.
paranoid c.
c. of parole
pathologic c.
persistent emotional c.
personality change due to a
　general medical c.
physical intersex c.
preexisting c.
proband c.
psychiatric c.
psychological factors affecting
　medical c. (PFAMC)
psychological factors affecting a
　mental c.
psychologic factor affecting
　physical c.
psychosis due to physical c.
psychotic disorder due to a general
　medical c.
respondent c.
school handicap c.
sexual dysfunction due to a
　general medical c.
sexually transmitted c. (STC)
sleep disorder due to a general
　medical c.
stimulation c.
subcortical c.
test c.
test c.
treatment c.
underlying c.

conditional
c. arousal
c. discharge
c. probability

conditioned
c. avoidance response
c. cue
c. drug response
c. emotional response (CER)
c. escape response
c. fear association
c. inhibition
c. place preference (CPP)
c. reflex (CR)
c. reflex therapy
c. reinforcer
c. stimulation

c. stimulus (CS)
c. suppression
conditioning
approximation c.
assertive c.
autonomic c.
average c.
aversion c.
aversion-covert c.
aversive c.
avoidance c.
backward c.
classical c.
cognitive c.
complex aspect of fear c.
counter c.
cross c.
decorticate c.
escape c.
esprit de corps c.
exteroceptive c.
eyelid c.
false c.
fear c.
female c.
higher order c.
instrumental c.
negative c.
operant c.
pavlovian c.
primary reward c.
respondent c.
secondary reward c.
second-order c.
simple aspect of fear c.
skinnerian c.
c. therapy
trace c.
condom
condomatus
coitus c.
condonation
condone
conducive
conduct
adjustment disorder with
　disturbance of c.
consistent pattern of c.
c. disorder (CD)
disorderly c.
c. disturbance
c. disturbance adjustment disorder

NOTES

conduct *(continued)*
    c. disturbance adjustment reaction
    moral c.
    pattern of c.
    persistent pattern of c.
    c. problem
    solitary aggressive type c.
conduct-disordered child
conduction
    air c.
    c. aphasia
    c. deafness
    c. delay
    electronic c.
    ephaptic c.
    excitation and c.
    motor nerve c.
    nerve c.
conductor
conduit
confabulans
    paraphrenia c.
confabulate
confabulated
    c. detail response (dD)
    c. whole response (DW)
confabulation
conference
    career c.
    family c. (FC)
confession of guilt
confessor
    father c.
    mother c.
confidant
confidante
confide
confidence
    diagnostic c.
    c. interval (CI)
    lack of c.
    level of c.
    c. level
confident
    c. status
confidential
    c. documentation
    c. interview
    c. record
confidentiality
    breach of c.
    c. breach
configuration
    personality c.
    word c.
configurative culture
confinement
    c. effect

    c. fear
    home c.
    prison c.
    solitary c.
confirmation
conflict
    approach-approach c.
    approach-avoidance c.
    c. avoidance
    avoidance-avoidance c.
    basic c.
    central c.
    culture c.
    emotional c.
    escalating c.
    ethical c.
    extrapsychic c.
    family c.
    horizontal c.
    increased interpersonal c.
    inferred c.
    infrequent interpersonal c.
    inner c.
    c. of interest
    internal c.
    interpersonal c.
    intolerable inner c.
    intrafamilial c.
    intrapersonal c.
    intrapsychic c.
    c. level
    level of c.
    c. management
    c. management appraisal (CMA)
    marital c.
    c. mediation
    oedipal c.
    parent-child c.
    psychiatric c.
    psychodynamic c.
    religious c.
    c. resolution
    c. resolution skills
    c. resolution strategy
    resolve c.
    role c.
    roommate c.
    significant c.
    unconscious c.
    unresolved c.
    vertical c.
    c.'s with peers
conflicted feeling
conflict-free
    c.-f. area
    c.-f. function
    c.-f. sphere

conflicting
> c. emotion
> c. message
> c. motive

conflictual
> c. home environment
> c. relationship
> c. situation

confluence method

conformance
> functional c.

conformity
> automaton c.
> conventional role c.
> morality of conventional role c.
> social c.

confounding

confront

confrontation
> direct c.
> c. naming test
> premature c.
> reality c.
> simple c.
> c. stage
> supportive c.

confrontational experience

confrontative

Confucianism

confuse

confused
> c. delusion
> c. language syndrome (CLS)
> c. speech

confusingly fluid coalition

confusion
> authority c.
> bisexual c.
> cognate c.
> episodic c.
> gender identity c.
> identity vs. role c.
> mental c.
> nocturnal c.
> personal identity c.
> postictal c.
> psychogenic c.
> reactive c.
> c. reactive psychosis
> right-left c.
> role c.

> time c.
> c. of values

confusional
> c. arousal
> c. arousals from sleep
> c. episode
> c. insanity
> c. migraine headache
> c. psychotic reaction
> c. schizophreniform
> c. schizophreniform psychosis
> c. state presenile
> c. state presenile dementia
> c. twilight state

confusional-arousal disorder

congener

congenial

congenital
> c. adrenal hyperplasia
> c. atonic pseudoparalysis
> c. defect
> c. facial diplegia
> c. intersex condition
> c. neurosyphilis
> c. paramyotonia
> c. spastic paraplegia
> c. sutural alopecia
> c. syphilitic paralytic
> c. syphilitic paralytic dementia

congenitalis
> alopecia c.

congestion
> brain c.

congruence

congruent
> c. affect
> mood c.

conjoined
> c. nerve root
> c. twins

conjoint
> c. counseling
> c. interview
> c. synapse
> c. therapy

conjugal
> c. bereavement
> c. consequences of promiscuity
> c. paranoia
> c. psychosis
> c. tension

NOTES

conjugal *(continued)*
    c. visit
    c. visitation
conjugate
    c. gaze
    c. paralysis
conjunctive
    c. concept
    c. reinforcement
conjure
connate
connatural
connectedness
    community c.
    emotional c.
    family c.
    impaired c.
    social c.
connection
    interneuronal c.
    neuroanatomic c.
    reciprocal c.
    social c.
    therapeutic c.
connotation
consanguineous marriage
consanguinity
conscience
    authoritarian c.
    humanistic c.
conscientiousness
conscious
    c. avoidance
    c. awareness
    class c.
    c. commitment
    c. deceit
    c. decision
    c. guidance
    c. memory
    c. perception
    c. process
    c. resistance
    c. simulation
    c. state
consciously
    c. accessible process
    c. inaccessible process
consciousness
    active mode of c.
    altered level of c.
    altered state of c. (ASC)
    clouding of c.
    cosmic c.
    crowd c.
    crude c.
    declining c.
    depression of c.

    discrimination c.
    disintegration of c.
    c. disturbance
    c. disturbance stress reaction
    double c.
    effect of trauma on c.
    episodic changes of c.
    expanded c.
    c. expansion
    field of c.
    fluctuating level of c.
    fringe of c.
    group c.
    head c.
    higher level of c.
    higher state of c.
    impaired c.
    impairment of c.
    level of c. (LOC)
    loss of c. (LOC)
    marginal c.
    parasomniac c.
    passive mode of c.
    perceptual c.
    post September 11 c.
    c. raising
    reduced level of c.
    social c.
    c. state
    state of c. (SOC)
    stream of c.
    subliminal c.
    threshold of c.
    time c.
    unitary c.
consecutive insanity
consensual
    c. action
    c. gaze
    c. reaction
    c. reflex
    c. sexual behavior
    c. understanding
    c. validation
    c. validation consent
consensually
consent
    age of c.
    consensual validation c.
    c. forms
    informed c.
    mutal c.
    valid c.
    Willowbrook c.
consenting
    c. adult
    c. partner
    c. patient

consequence
    c.'s of action
    c. association
    clear rules and c.
    c.'s of decisions
    destructive social c.
    fatal c.
    harmful c.
    health-related c.
    interpersonal c.
    legal c.
    long-term c.
    neurobehavioral c.
    painful c.
    psychiatric c.
    psychological c.
    serious c.
    short-term c.
    social c.
    c.'s of war
consequent
consequentialism
consequentialist ethics
conservation
conservative
    c. cutoff score
    c. management
    c. medication
    c. treatment
conservator
conservatorship
considerable external support
considerate
consideration
    biologic c.
    developmental c.
    treatment c.
considered thought
consistency
    behavioral c.
    internal c.
    moral c.
    perceptual c.
    c. principle
consistent
    c. behavior
    c. delivery
    c. irresponsibility
    c. mood
    c. pattern of conduct
    c. relationship
    c. response

consociate
consolation dream
console
consolidated sleep
consolidation
    memory c.
Consortium on Special Psychiatric Delivery Setting
conspicuous consumption
conspiratorial
conspire
constancy
    brightness c.
    color c.
    emotional object c.
    extrinsic c.
    intrinsic c.
    law of c.
    libidinal object c.
    location c.
    object c.
    perceptual c.
    c. phenomenon
constant
    c. anger
    changeable versus c.
    Heinis c.
    relaxation c.
    c. routine
    c. worry
constantium
constellation
    family c.
    c. of grief
    self-pitying c.
    c. of signs and symptoms
consternation
constipation
    psychogenic c.
constitution
    epileptic psychopathic c.
    hyperadrenal c.
    posttraumatic psychopathic c.
    psychopathic c.
constitutional
    c. bisexuality theory
    c. depression
    c. depressive disposition
    c. disease
    c. factor
    c. insanity
    c. manic disposition

C

NOTES

constitutional *(continued)*
    c. medicine
    c. psychology
    c. psychopathic inferiority
    c. psychopathic state (CPS)
    c. psychosis
    c. type
constrain
constraint
    morality of c.
    c. of movement
    thought c.
    c. of thought
constrastimulus
constrict
constricted
    c. activity
    c. affect
    emotionally c.
    c. pupil
constriction
    affective c.
    c. of cognition
    emotional c.
    pupillary c.
    c. of thought
construct
    complex psychological c.
    core c.
    multidimensional c.
    personal c.
    psychological c.
    c. validity
construction
    c. ability
    c. apraxia
    exocentric c.
    hierarchy c.
    phrase c. (PC)
    visual field c.
constructional
    c. apraxis
    c. dyspraxia
constructive
    c. aggression
    c. approach
    c. criticism
    c. discipline
    c. feedback
    c. memory
    c. support
consultant
    juvenile court c.
    medical c.
    prescribing c.
consultation
    agency-centered c.
    crisis c.

    forensic c.
    patient-oriented c.
    psychiatric c.
    c. psychiatrist
    c. psychiatry
    psychopharmacology c.
    social service c.
consultation-liaison
    c.-l. psychiatry
    c.-l. service
consultative relationship
consulting
    c. psychiatrist
    c. psychologist
    c. room
    c. staff
consumer
    c. behavior
    c. characteristic
    c. education
    c. psychology
    c. research
consuming
    time c.
consummate
consummatory
    c. act
    c. communication
    c. reward
consumption
    alcohol c.
    caffeine c.
    cerebral oxygen c.
    coffee c.
    conspicuous c.
    daily caffeine c.
    drug c.
    nervous c.
    regular caffeine c.
contact
    c. avoidance
    c. behavior
    c. ceptor
    c. comfort
    continuity of c.
    eye c.
    frequency of c. (FOC)
    genital sexual c.
    oral-genital c.
    sexual c.
    social c.
    c. with reality
contagion
    emergency c.
    psychic c.
container
    c. exercise
    exerciser c.

containment
contaminated needle
contamination
    c. fear
    c. obsession
contemplate
contemplation
contemplative
contemporaneous suicidal behavior
contemporary
    c. approach
    c. practice
contempt
contemptible
contemptuous
contendere
    nolo c.
content
    c. addressability
    c. analysis
    blood alcohol c.
    blood alcohol concentration c.
      (BAC)
    c. of delusion
    dream c.
    grandiose c.
    c. of hallucination
    language c.
    latent c.
    manifest c.
    mood, orientation, judgment,
      affect, c. (MOJAC)
    paucity of speech c.
    positive speech c.
    poverty of c.
    c. psychology
    c. scale
    self-derogatory c.
    speech c.
    thought c.
    c. of thought
    c. thought disorder
    c. validity
contention
contentious
contentiousness
contentment
context
    cultural c.
    historical c.
    c. reframing
    social c.

    space c.
    spatial-temporal c.
    taken out of c.
    time c.
contextual
    c. association
    c. cause
    c. cue
    c. influence
    c. therapy
contextualism
contiguity
    c. aphasia
    c. disorder
    law of c.
    spatial c.
    temporal c.
contiguous voxel
continence
    bladder c.
    fecal c.
    urinary c.
continent
contingency
    c. awareness
    behavioral c.
    c. coefficient
    c. contract
    c. management
    c. model
    c. reinforcement
contingent
    c. negative variation (CNV)
    c. punishment
continua
    epilepsia corticalis c.
    epilepsia partialis c.
continuance
continuation
    c. therapy
    c. treatment
continued
    c. abuse
    c. belittling
    c. bullying
    c. stay review (CSR)
continuing
    c. care
    c. education
    c. medical education (CME)
    c. petit mal seizure

C

NOTES

continuity
    c. of attachment
    c. of care
    c. of contact
    sense of c.
    sleep c.
    worse sleep c.

continuous
    c. amnesia
    c. antipsychotic drug treatment
    c. antipsychotic medication
    c. approach
    c. bath treatment
    c. cognitive testing
    c. course
    c. daytime drowsiness
    c. epilepsy
    c. group
    c. growth
    c. infusion
    c. maintenance medication
    c. narcosis
    c. observation
    c. panel
    c. performance task-accuracy (CPT-ACC)
    c. performance task-efficiency (CPT-EFF)
    c. reinforcement
    c. reinforcement schedule
    c. sleep
    c. sleep therapy
    c. tremor
    c. variable

continuum, pl. continua, continuums
    c. of care
    hypothetical c.
    introversion-extroversion c.
    c. theory

contort

contraception
    birth control pill c.
    rhythm method of c.
    withdrawal method of c.

contraceptive
    c. device
    oral c.
    c. practice

contract
    c. against self-harm
    c. against suicide
    behavior c.
    behavioral c.
    contingency c.
    employment c.
    c. evaluation
    evaluation c.
    formal c.

    formalized c.
    group c.
    homicide-suicide protection c.
    individualized c.
    informal c.
    interactional c.
    legal c.
    marriage c.
    c. negotiation
    patient c.
    quasi c.
    c. review
    c. for safety
    sweetheart c.
    therapeutic c.
    c. therapy

contraction
    carpopedal c.
    lead pipe c.
    rhythmic c.
    tetanic c. (Te)

contraction-relaxation

contractual
    c. agreement
    c. alliance
    c. arrangement
    c. behavior
    c. capacity
    c. psychiatry
    c. psychotherapy

contractural diathesis

contracture
    caffeine-induced c.
    functional c.
    organic c.

contradict

contradiction

contradictory
    c. data
    c. information

contrafissura

contraindication
    medical c.
    medication c.

contralateral
    c. hemiplegia
    c. neglect syndrome
    c. parietal lobe
    c. parietal lobe dysfunction
    c. reflex
    c. sign

contrariness

contrary

contrasexual component of psyche

contrast
    brightness c.
    chromatic c.
    color c.

c. effect
law of c.
maximal c.
c. sensitivity
contrastimulus
contrastive
c. analysis
c. distribution
c. stress
contravolition
contrecoup injury of brain
contrectation
contretemps
contributing role
contribution
extracellular c.
intracellular c.
therapeutic c.
contributor
contributory
c. element
c. negligence
contrite
contrition
contrive
control
c. analysis
appetite c.
attentional c.
automatic gain c.
automatic volume c.
aversive c.
balance c.
behavior c. (BC)
biologic c.
birth c. (BC)
bladder c.
bowel c.
brain c.
brainstem c.
Bureau of Drug Abuse C. (BDAC)
cognitive c.
crowd c.
degree of c.
delusion of c.
c. delusion
c. device
diminished c.
disorder of impulse c.
distribution of c.
ego c.
executive c.

experimental c.
external force c.
external locus of c.
feedback c.
c. feedback
feeling of c.
fluoroscopic c.
c. frustration
c. group
gun c.
handgun c.
idiodynamic c.
image c.
immediate c.
impaired impulse c.
impulse c.
in c.
inadequate impulse c.
inner c.
internal-external c.
internal locus of c.
interpersonal c.
island of c.
lack of c.
learned autonomic c.
locus of c. (LOC)
locus of c.-chance (LOC-C)
locus of c.-external (LOC-E)
locus of c.-internal (LOC-I)
losing c.
loss of c.
mental c.
mind c.
need to c.
neurological c.
one's own c.
out of c. (OOC)
outside c.
pain c.
parental c.
personal c.
personal locus of c. (PLC)
c. picture-caption pair
poor impulse c.
c. preoccupation
psychooptical reflex c.
rate c.
reflex c.
rigid c.
secret c.
sense of c.
social c.

NOTES

C

control *(continued)*
    sociopolitical locus of c. (SLC)
    sphincter c.
    stimulus c.
    subjects as their own c.
    superego c.
    superstitious c.
    swing phase c.
    synergic c.
    taking c.
    thought c.
    tonic inhibitor c.
    vestibuloequilibratory c.
    voluntary c.
    weak ego c.
    worry c.
    yoked c.
controlled
    c. analgesic
    c. anger
    c. association
    c. attention
    c. breathing
    delusion of being c.
    c. drinking
    c. emotion
    c. environment
    c. exposure
    c. medication trial
    c. sampling
    c. substance
    C. Substances Act (CSA)
controlling
    c. external entities
    c. external spirit
    c. identity
    c. parent
    c. personality
controversial diagnosis
contumacious
contumacy
contumelious
contumely
contusion
    brain c.
    cerebral c.
    scalp c.
    wind c.
convalescence
convalescent dream
convenience
    c. dream
    c. gambling
    marriage of c.
conventional
    c. antipsychotic drug
    c. antipsychotic medication

    c. dopamine receptor-blocking
      antipsychotic
    c. factor analysis
    c. neuroleptic
    c. neuroleptic agent
    c. neuroleptic drug
    c. neuroleptic treatment
    c. pharmacotherapy
    c. role conformity
    c. sign
converge
convergence circuit
convergent thinking
conversation
    c. board
    meaningful c.
conversational
    c. catharsis
    c. voice
converse
conversing
    voice c.
conversion
    c. anesthesia
    c. aphonia
    c. ataxia
    c. blindness
    c. defense mechanism
    c. disorder
    c. disorder, mixed type
    c. disorder, motor type
    c. disorder, seizure type
    c. disorder, sensory tupe
    c. disorder with mixed presentation
    c. disorder with motor symptoms
      or deficit
    c. disorder with seizures or
      convulsion
    c. disorder with sensory symptom
      or deficit
    c. of emotion
    c. hysteria
    c. hysteria neurosis
    c. hysteria psychoneurosis
    metabolic c.
    c. paralysis
    c. psychoneurotic reaction
    c. seizure
    c. sensory charge
    c. symptom
    tonic-clonic c.
    c. type hysterical neurosis
    unconsciousness c.
    c. unconsciousness
**conversion-type neurotic hysterical
    disorder**
convert
convexobasia

conviction
    delusional c.
    inferred delusional c.
    religious c.
convince
convolute
convolution
convulsant threshold
convulsion
    apoplectiform c.
    brain c.
    central c.
    cerebral c.
    cerebrospinal c.
    clonic c.
    conversion disorder with seizures
      or c.
    coordinate c.
    drug-induced c.
    epileptic c.
    epileptiform c.
    essential c.
    hysterical c.
    immediate posttraumatic c.
    infantile c.
    jacksonian c.
    local c.
    mimic c.
    myoclonic c.
    paroxysmal c.
    psychomotor c.
    puerperal c.
    reflex c.
    repetitive c.
    salaam c.
    spasmodic c.
    spontaneous c.
    static c.
    tetanic c.
    tonic c.
    toxic c.
    uncinate c.
    uremic c.
convulsive
    c. disorder
    c. equivalent
    c. melancholia
    c. reflex
    c. seizure
    c. shock therapy
    c. state

    c. status epilepticus
    c. tic
co-occur
co-occurrence of depression
co-occurring
    c.-o. addictive disorder
    c.-o. association
    c.-o. mental disorder
cookbook
    c. diagnosis
    c. fashion
cool-headed
cooling
    c. of affect
    c. off
cooperate
cooperation
    morality of c.
cooperative
    c. behavior
    c. education
    c. institutional research program
      (CIRP)
    c. motive
    c. psychotherapy
    c. reward structure
    c. therapy
    c. training
    c. urban house
cooperativity
    criterion of c.
Cooper method
coordinate
    c. convulsion
    c. seizure
coordinated
    c. epilepsy
    c. reflex
coordination
    c. developmental delay disorder
    eye-hand c.
    fine motor c.
    fluid c.
    motor c.
    subaverage motor c.
    visual-motor c.
coordinatus
    spasmus c.
coparental divorce
COPE
    coping operations preference enquiry

C

NOTES

COPE *(continued)*
COPE computer software program
for depression therapy
cope
co-pharmacy
cophica
alalia c.
coping
c. ability
adaptive c.
c. behavior
concept of spiritual c.
detached c.
ideational style of c.
c. inventory
maladaptive c.
c. mechanism
c. operations preference enquiry
(COPE)
rational cognitive c.
resources for c.
c. response
c. skill
c. strategy
c. style
copper
coprolagnia
coprolalia
multiple tics with c.
tic convulsive with c.
coprolalomania
coprology
coprophagia, coprophagy
coprophagous
coprophagy
coprophemia disorder
coprophil, coprophilic
coprophilia
coprophrasia
copropraxia
copulate
copulation
copulatory behavior
copy
c. geometric designs test
c. intersecting pentagons test
copy-cat suicide
copying
c. drawings (CD)
c. mania
coquetting
flirting and c.
coranderismo
cordial
cordiality
core
c. belief
c. body balance

c. body temperature
central transactional c.
c. characteristic
c. cognitive disturbance
c. conflictual relationship theme
c. consensual understanding
c. construct
c. mindfulness skills
c. pain
c. problem
c. temperature
c. temperature fluctuation
c. values
Cornelia de Lange syndrome
corollary discharge
coronal
c. orientation
c. plane
c. section
coronary
corpora (*pl. of* corpus)
corporal
c. agnosia
c. punishment
corporate
c. crime
c. criminal
c. fraud
c. hierarchy
c. icon
corpse
corpulence
corpulent
corpus, pl. **corpora**
c. arenacea
corpora arenacea
c. callosum syndrome
habeas c.
corpora quadrigemina
c. striatum
correction
age c.
medical record c.
correctional
c. facility
c. psychiatry
c. psychology
c. transfer (CT)
correctitude
corrective
c. emotional experience
c. feedback
c. technique
c. therapist
c. therapy (CT)
correlate
anatomic c.
biologic c.

clinical c.
differential c.
psychophysiologic c.
correlation
canonical c.
coefficient of c.
c. coefficient
intraclass c.
item-total c.
c. method
multiple c.
negative c.
partial c.
positive c.
potential c.
product-moment c.
rank c.
rank-difference c.
c. ratio
c. redundancy
c. study
correlative
objective c.
correspondence
cross c.
email c.
encrypted c.
point-for-point c.
secure c.
corrigible
corroborate
corroborating dream
corrode
corrosion
corrosive
corrupt
corruptible
cortex, pl. **cortices**
allocortical c.
association c.
cerebellar c.
cerebral c.
cingulate c.
c. circuit
deep c.
dorsolateral prefrontal c.
entorhinal c.
extrinsic c.
frontal c. (FC)
inferior prefrontal c.
inferior temporal c. (ITC)
language associated c.

lateral orbitofrontal c.
medial frontal c.
medial orbitofrontal c.
medial prefrontal c.
mesial prefrontal c.
motor c.
occipital c.
occipitotemporal c.
orbital prefrontal c.
orbitofrontal c.
parietal c.
periamygdaloid c.
prefrontal c.
primary auditory c.
primary sensory c.
rostral medial prefrontal c.
sensory c.
sulcal prefrontal c.
supramarginal/angular c.
temporal c.
temporal cortices
ventromedial c.
visual association c.
cortical
c. activity
c. alexia
c. amnesia
c. aphasia
c. area
c. center
c. column
c. deafness
c. epilepsy
c. evoked potential
c. function
c. gray matter
c. input
c. lateralization
c. Lewy body
c. mapping
c. metabolism
c. network
c. pathology
c. potential
c. psychic blindness
c. region
c. sensibility
c. sensory loss
c. structure
c. testing
c. thumb position

C

NOTES

cortical *(continued)*
    c. volume
    c. zone
cortical-evoked response
corticalization
cortical-subcortical network activity
cortices (*pl. of* cortex)
corticis
corticoadrenal insufficiency
corticoid therapy
corticotropin-releasing hormone
cortin
cortisol
    plasma c.
    c. secretion
coruscation
corybantism
cosmetic
    c. issue
    c. reconstruction
cosmic
    c. consciousness
    c. identification
    c. sensitivity
cosmology
cost
    maximum allowable c. (MAC)
    treatment c.
Costa-McCrae factor
cost-benefit analysis
cost-reward
    c.-r. analysis
    c.-r. model
Cotard syndrome
co-therapy
cotinine
cottage plan
Cotunnius disease
couch
    analytic c.
cough
    habit c.
    psychogenic c.
could not test (CNT)
coulomb
Council on Psychiatric Services
counsel
counseling
    abuse c.
    adolescent c.
    alcohol c.
    career c.
    c. center
    child-placement c.
    clinical c.
    conjoint c.
    crisis c.
    divorce c.

    drug c.
    eclectic c.
    educational c.
    extended c.
    family c.
    followup c.
    genetic c.
    group c.
    individual c.
    Internet c.
    c. interview
    c. inventory
    c. ladder
    marital c.
    marriage c.
    mental health c.
    online c.
    parent-child conflict c.
    pastoral c.
    placement c.
    practical c.
    premarital c.
    c. process
    c. psychologist
    c. psychology
    reevaluation c.
    reinforcement c.
    relapse-prevention c.
    c. relationship
    risk-reduction c.
    c. service
    sex c.
    traditional c.
    vocational c.
    Web c.
counselor
    career c.
    chemical dependency c. (CDC)
    child c.
    couples c.
    disability c.
    drug c.
    family c.
    genetic c.
    grief c.
    group c.
    guidance c.
    individual c.
    industrial rehabilitation c.
    legal c.
    licensed professional c. (LPC)
    marital c.
    marriage c.
    mental health c.
    pastoral c.
    personal c.
    professional c.
    rehabilitation c.

school c.
spiritual c.
substance abuse c.
youth c.
counselor-centered therapy
count
c. backwards from 100 test
blood c.
radioactive c.
countenance
counter
c. conditioning
over the c. (OTC)
c. transference
counteracting impulsivity
counteraction
counteraggression
counterargue
counterbalance
countercompulsion
countercondition
counterconformity
countercriticism
counterculture
counterego
counteridentification
counterinfluence
counterintuitive
counterinvestment
counterirritant
counterphobic
c. attitude
c. behavior
countershock
countertransference
c. behavior
c. experience
c. neurosis
counterwill
counter-wish dream
counting
c. compulsion
c. money tremor
c. obsession
coup injury of brain
couple
C.'s BrainMap
c.'s counselor
c.'s group therapy
c. member
c.'s sex therapy
c. skills group

coupling
courage
Dutch c.
lack of c.
courageous
courant
au c.
course
atypical c.
chronic c.
clinical c.
continuous c.
deteriorating c.
developmental c.
episodic c.
fluctuating c.
global c.
c. of illness
c. of illness measure
life c.
longitudinal c.
long-term c.
perilous c.
planned c.
rapid-cycling c.
recurrent c.
c. specifier
tempestuous c.
temporal c.
c. of treatment
court
appeals c.
c. custody
c. of domestic relations
family c.
c. of honor
juvenile c.
c. of law
mental health c.
c. order
ruling of the c.
supreme c.
traffic c.
trial c.
court-appointed
c.-a. guardian
c.-a. psychiatrist
courteous
court-mandated
c.-m. evaluation
c.-m. treatment

C

NOTES

court-ordered involuntary outpatient treatment
court-related problem
courtroom psychology
courtship behavior
couth
couvade
covariance
>   analysis of c. (ANCOVA)
>   multivariate analysis of c. (MANCOVA)

covariate
coven
>   member of a c.

covenant
>   crapulous c.

covenantee
covenanter
covert
>   c. anxiety
>   c. behavior
>   c. feeling
>   c. hostility
>   c. message
>   c. modeling
>   c. reinforcement
>   c. resentment
>   c. resistance
>   c. response
>   c. sensitization
>   c. visuospatial attention

coverture
covetous
coward
Cox regression analysis
cozen
cozenage
CP
>   child psychiatry
>   child psychology

CPP
>   career planning program
>   cerebral perfusion pressure
>   conditioned place preference
>   cranial perfusion pressure

CPS
>   Children's Protective Service
>   clinical performance score
>   complex partial seizure
>   constitutional psychopathic state
>   cumulative probability of success

CPSR
>   chronic paranoid schizophrenic reaction

CPT
>   combining power test

CPT-ACC
>   continuous performance task-accuracy

CPT-EFF
>   continuous performance task-efficiency

CQ
>   circadian quotient
>   conceptual quotient

CR
>   conditioned reflex

crack
crackling
>   parchment c.

craft
>   c. neurosis
>   c. palsy

crafty
cramp
>   accessory c.
>   menstrual c.
>   miner's c.
>   musician's c.
>   occupational c.
>   pianist's c.
>   piano player's c.
>   seamstress c.
>   shaving c.
>   stoker's c.
>   tailor's c.
>   Wernicke c.

crania (pl. of cranium)
cranial
>   c. anomaly
>   c. nerve
>   c. perfusion pressure (CPP)

cranii
craniofacial
craniognomy
craniomalacia
>   circumscribed c.

craniopharyngeal canal
craniosinus fistula
craniostenosis
cranium, pl. crania
crapuleux
>   delire c.

crapulous
>   c. covenant

crash
>   computer c.
>   depressive c.

crass
crassitude
crave
craven
craving
>   alcohol c.
>   cocaine c.
>   cue-elicited c.
>   cue-induced c.
>   decreased c.

drug c.
food c.
nicotine c.
withdrawal-based c.
craze
crazy
CRE
   cAMP response element
creative
   c. imagination
   c. outlet
   c. self
   c. talent
   c. thinking
creativeness
creativity test
credence
credibility
   witness c.
credible
credit card abuse
credulous
creed
creeping-crawling sensation
crepuscular
crescendo-decrescendo breathing
crescendo sleep
cresomania
crestfallen
cretin
cretinism
cretinistic
cretinoid idiocy
cretinous
Creutzfeldt-Jakob
   C.-J. disease (CJD)
   C.-J. syndrome
CRF knockout mice
cri
   c. de coeur
   c. du chat syndrome
crib death
criblé
   état c.
cribrosus
   status c.
Crigler-Najjar
   C.-N. syndrome
crime
   accessory to c.
   c. against humanity
   bias c.

blue collar c.
C. Classification Manual (CCM)
C. Control Act of 1984
corporate c.
c. a deux
drug-related c.
hate c.
heinous c.
high profile c.
multiple personality c.
nonviolent c.
c. of passion
c. victim
violent c.
witness to c.
criminal
   c. abortion
   c. activity
   adolescent c.
   c. anthropology
   c. behavior
   c. commitment
   corporate c.
   c. degeneracy
   habitual c.
   high profile c.
   c. history
   c. hygiene
   c. insanity
   c. intent
   c. irresponsibility
   c. justice system
   juvenile c.
   c. past
   c. population
   c. profile
   c. psychiatry
   c. psychology
   c. record
   report c.
   c. response
   c. responsibility
   c. sexual act
   c. sexual psychopath (CSP)
criminalistics
criminality
criminally insane
criminology
cripple
   emotional c.
   social c.
crisis, pl. **crises**

C

NOTES

crisis *(continued)*
- accidental c.
- acute situational c.
- adolescent c.
- bed c.
- catathymic c.
- c. center
- c. consultation
- c. counseling
- custody c.
- c. effect
- emotional c.
- C. Evaluation Referral Service (CERS)
- existential c.
- financial c.
- c. group
- c. hotline
- hypertensive c.
- identity c.
- interpersonal c.
- c. intervention
- c. intervention clinic (CIC)
- laryngeal c.
- life c.
- magnetic c.
- c. management
- c. management strategy
- maturational c.
- mesmeric c.
- midlife c.
- normative c.
- occupational c.
- oral c.
- c. period
- periods of c.
- precipitating c.
- psychogenic oculogyric c.
- psychosexual identity c.
- rapprochement c.
- c. residential care
- c. resolution
- resolution of c.
- c. situation
- situational c.
- c. stabilization
- suicidal c.
- tabetic c.
- c. team
- teens in c.
- c. theory
- therapeutic c.
- c. therapy
- unanticipated c.
- urban c.
- widowhood c.

crisis-intervention group psychotherapy

criteria-defined borderline personality disorder

criterion, pl. **criteria**
- C. A, A2, B, C, D, E, F
- abuse c.
- admission c.
- c. of associativity
- c. behavior
- behavioral c.
- clinical significance c.
- clustering c.
- c. of cooperativity
- c. data
- death criteria
- dependence c.
- depression c.
- diagnostic criteria
- c. dimension
- DSM-IV axis II c.
- equivalent criteria
- equivalent intoxication c.
- equivalent withdrawal c.
- c. evaluation
- evaluation of c.
- exclusion criteria
- field-tested c.
- full symptom c.
- c. group
- impairment c.
- c. level
- level-of-care c.
- lifetime depression c.
- method of defining c.
- patient placement c.
- a priori c.
- psychiatric c.
- relevant diagnostic criteria
- restrictive c.
- Schooler-Kane criteria
- c. of specificity
- symptom criteria
- theta c.
- Thorndike-Lorge criteria
- c. validity
- c. variable
- von Knorring c.
- withdrawal criteria

criterion-referenced test
criterion-related validity
critical
- c. age
- c. analysis
- c. band concept
- c. flicker frequency
- c. illness polyneuropathy (CIP)
- c. judgment
- c. parent
- c. period

c. point
c. ratio
c. region
c. review
c. score
c. submodalities
c. thinking
c. value
critical-incident technique
criticism
    ability to take c.
    constructive c.
    destructive c.
    implied c.
    objective c.
    overt c.
    parental c.
    peer c.
    professional c.
    subjective c.
criticize
criticus
    status c.
critique
    age c.
crochet
    main en c.
crocodile tears
Cronbach alpha
crooked
cross
    c. adaptation
    c. addiction
    c. birth
    c. conditioning
    c. correspondence
    c. dependence
    c. dressing
    c. fostering
    c. tolerance
    c. training
    c. validation
cross-aggregation
crossbones
    skull and c.
crossbreed
cross-correlation mechanism
cross-cultural
    c.-c. difference
    c.-c. homogeneity
    c.-c. psychiatry
    c.-c. testing

cross-culture
    c.-c. approach
    c.-c. psychiatry
cross-dependence
cross-dressing
    c.-d. behavior
    complete c.-d.
    forced c.-d.
    motivation for c.-d.
    partial c.-d.
crossed
    c. adductor jerk
    c. anesthesia
    c. dominance
    c. eyes
    c. hemianesthesia
    c. hemiplegia
    c. knee jerk
    c. laterality
    c. paralysis
    c. phrenic phenomenon
cross-gender
    c.-g. behavior
    forced c.-g.
    c.-g. identification
    c.-g. interest
crossing a bridge
cross-linkage theory
crossmatch
    blood c.
cross-modal fluency
cross-modality perception
crossover
    c. mirroring
    c. study
cross-reacting cannabinoids
cross-sectional
    c.-s. area (CSA)
    c.-s. assessment
    c.-s. component
    c.-s. definition
    c.-s. evaluation
    c.-s. experimental study design
    c.-s. method
    c.-s. prevalence
    c.-s. research
    c.-s. snapshot
    c.-s. study
cross-sex role
cross-taper
cross-tolerance
Crouzon syndrome

C

NOTES

crowd
- c. behavior
- c. consciousness
- c. control
- c. fear
- milling c.

crowded place
crucial
crucifixion attitude
crucify
crude
- c. consciousness
- c. opium

cruel
- c. impulse
- c. punishment

cruelty to animals
cruising
crural ataxia
crus, pl. **crura**
crusade
crush
- c.'s in adolescence
- c. syndrome

crust
- upper c.

crusty
crutch
cry
- birth c.
- epileptic c.
- c. for help
- hue and c.
- inability to c.
- c. reflex

cryalgesia
cryanesthesia
cryesthesia
crying
- excessive c.
- frequent c.
- inappropriate c.
- c. jag
- pathological c.
- c. spell
- uncontrollable c.

crying-cat syndrome
crymodynia
cryomania
cryophobia
cryoprobe
cryospasm
cryosurgery
cryptanamnesia
cryptesthesia
cryptic
- c. depression
- c. message

cryptogenic
- c. epilepsy
- c. seizure
- c. symbolism

cryptomnesia
cryptorchidism
cryptotia
crystal
- c. ball gazing

crystalize
crystalline
crystallization
- symptom c.

crystallized
- c. ability
- c. grandiose delusion
- c. intelligence

CS
- conditioned stimulus

CSA
- Controlled Substances Act
- cross-sectional area

CSAT
- Center for Substance Abuse Treatment

CSB I
- chemistry screening battery I

CSB II
- chemistry screening battery II

CSF
- cerebrospinal fluid

CSP
- criminal sexual psychopath

CSR
- continued stay review

CSU
- cognition of semantic unit

CSW
- certified social worker

CT
- correctional transfer
- corrective therapy

cuckold
cuddling behavior
cuddly
cue
- accessing c.
- anxiety-provoking c.
- auditory distance c.
- cocaine c.
- conditioned c.
- contextual c.
- c. effect
- environmental c.
- exposure to c.
- c. exposure
- exposure to biowarfare c.
- external c.
- eye accessing c.

gambling c.
innocuous environmental c.
internal c.
interoceptive c.
kinesthetic c.
learning c.
minimal c.
nonverbal c.
obliviousness to social c.
orientation c.
perceptual c.
phase c.
real-word cocaine c.
c. reduction
response-produced c.
semantic c.
sensory c.
social c.
specific sensory c.
trauma c.
verbal c.
visual c.

cued
    c. panic attack
    c. speech
cue-elicited craving
cue-induced
    c.-i. craving
    c.-i. subjective effect
cueing
cuirass
    analgesic c.
    tabetic c.
culpability
culpable
cult
    homophobic c.
    killer c.
    c. member
    c. of personality
    personality c.
    religious c.
    satanic c.
cultural
    c. absolutism
    c. adaptability
    c. adjustment
    c. adjustment following migration
    c. anthropology
    c. area
    c. assessment
    c. assimilation

c. attitude
c. background
c. belief
c. change
c. competence
c. concept
c. context
c. deprivation
c. determinism
c. difference
c. disadvantage
c. discrimination
c. diversity
c. element
c. experience
c. factor
c. formulation
c. frame of reference
c. identity
c. inventory
c. item
c. lag
c. norm
c. parallelism
c. phenomenon
c. poison
c. process
c. psychiatry
c. reference group
c. relativism
c. role
c. roots
c. sensitivity
c. shock
c. stereotype
c. subgroup
c. testing
c. theme
c. tradition
c. training
c. transmission
c. value
c. variation
cultural-familial mental retardation
culturally
    c. appropriate avoidant behavior
    c. condoned behavior
    c. deprived
    c. different
    c. disadvantaged
    c. diverse population
    c. parallel

C

NOTES

culturally *(continued)*
    c. sanctioned
    c. sanctioned behavior
    c. sanctioned experience
    c. sanctioned response
    c. sanctioned symptom
    c. unsanctioned
    c. unsanctioned response
cultural-related standards of sexual behavior
culture
    adolescent c.
    bullying c.
    cargo c.
    c. change
    coexistent c.
    collectivist c.
    c. complex
    configurative c.
    c. conflict
    diagnosing organizational c.
    dominant c.
    drug c.
    hip-hop c.
    hippie c.
    host c.
    indigenous family c.
    industrialized c.
    c. of origin
    person's c.
    phallocentric c.
    pop c.
    popular c.
    school c.
    c. shock
    c. trait
    youth c.
culture-bound
    c.-b. belief
    c.-b. syndrome
culture-related feature
culture-specific
    c.-s. feature
    c.-s. intervention
    c.-s. syndrome
cumulative
    c. dose
    c. drug action
    c. effect
    c. incidence rate
    c. medication reduction
    c. probability of success (CPS)
    c. record
    c. response
    c. response curve
    c. scale
    c. stressor

    c. test
    c. trauma disorder
cunnilinction
cunnilinctus
cunnilinguist
cunnilingus
cunning and hiding behavior
curandero, curanderismo
curare
curarization-induced flaccidity
curativa
    indicatio c.
cure
    faith c.
    c. rate
    talking c.
    transference c.
    work c.
curfew
curiosity
    sexual c.
curled-into-fetal-position posture
current
    action c.
    alternating c. (AC)
    alternating current or direct c. (AC/DC)
    c. cognitive status
    c. defense level
    demarcation c.
    c. depression
    c. diagnosis (CD)
    C., Global, Psychiatric-Social Status
    c. of injury
    c. psychotic episode
    c. suicide attempt
    c. tic
curse
    Ondine c.
cursing magic
cursiva
    epilepsia c.
cursive epilepsy
curtailed sleep
curve
    bell-shaped c.
    cumulative response c.
    developmental c.
    distribution c.
    dose-response c.
    frequency c.
    gaussian c.
    learning c.
    logistic c.
    luetic c.
    nonlinear developmental c.
    normal c.
    paretic c.

probability c.
response c.

Cushing
C. basophilia
C. response

cuss

custodial
c. care
c. parent

custody
child c.
court c.
c. crisis
joint c.
parental c.
c. quotient
c. relinquishment
single c.
split c.
transfer of c.
c. transfer

custom
acculturation problem with
expression of c.'s
dietary c.
foreign c.

cut
visual field c.

cutaneous
c. anesthesia
c. experience
c. psychogenic disorder
c. reaction

cutoff score

cutting
self-inflicted hair c.
self-inflicted skin c.
wrist c.

CV
coefficient of variation

cyamemazine

cyanosis

cyanotic syndrome of Scheid

cybercrime

cybermedicine

cybernetic
c. theory
c. theory of aging

cybernetics

cyberporn

cyberpsych

cybersex

cyberstalker

cyberstalking
c. laws
c. victim

cybertherapy

cyclandelate

cyclazocine

cycle
aberrant c.
basic rest-activity c. (BRAC)
brain wave c.
desire phase of sexual response c.
duration duty c.
estrous c.
excitement phase of sexual
response c.
fusion-defusion c.
genesial c.
gonadal c.
introjective-projective c.
c. length
life c.
orgasmic phase of sexual
response c.
perceptual c.
c.'s per second tremor
phase shift of sleep-wake c.
resolution phase of sexual
response c.
sexual response c.
short c.
sleep c.
sleep-wake c.
vicious c.

cycler
rapid c.

cyclic
c. abulia
c. depression
c. ether
c. headache
c. history
c. illness
c. insanity
c. medication
c. mood disorder
c. mood swing
c. psychiatric disorder
c. schizophrenia
c. vomiting

cyclical
c. depression

NOTES

cyclical *(continued)*
 c. pattern of symptoms
 c. psychogenic vomiting
cycling
 mania with rapid c.
 mood disorder with rapid c.
 rapid c.
cycloid
 c. personality
 c. psychosis
cyclophrenia
cycloplegia
cyclothymia
cyclothymic, cyclothymiac
 c. personality
 c. personality disorder
cyclothymic-depressive behavior
cyclothymosis
cynanthropy

cynical humor
cynicism
cynic spasm
cynomania
cynorexia
cyophoria
cypenamine
cyprodenate
cyproximide
cytoarchitectural organization
cytochrome
 c. P-450 2E1
 c. P450 metabolic enzyme
 c. P450 metabolism
cytogenetics
cytogenic
cytomegalovirus (CMV)
cytoplasm
cytosine

D₂
D_2 blockade
D_2 occupancy
/d
per day
DA
developmental age
dabbler
d'accoucheur
main d.
DaCosta syndrome
d'action
folie d.
dactylophasia
dactylospasm
dad
deadbeat d.
daft
daily
d. caffeine consumption
d. dose
d. living
d. living aid
d. record of severity of problems (DRSP)
d. symptom rating
Dale law
dally
DAMA
discharged against medical advice
damage
amygdala d.
body ego d.
brain cell d.
chronic tissue d.
diencephalic d.
drug-related brain d.
extent of d.
hippocampal d.
intrinsic d.
liver d.
minimal brain d.
neuronal d.
property d.
dammed-up
d.-u. emotion
d.-u. feeling
d.-u. libido
damming up
damn
damnable
damnify
damning
dampen

d-amphetamine
damping effect
dampness
dance
d. education
Saint John's d.
shadow d.
song and d.
St. Vitus d.
d. therapy
dancing
d. chorea
d. disease
d. eye
d. mania
d. spasm
danger
acute d.
focus of anticipated d.
future d.
life-threatening d.
d. to others
perceived d.
physical d.
d. to self
d. situation
underestimating d.
danger-laden schema vulnerability
dangerous
d. activity
d. behavior
d. behavior reaction
d. delusion
d. drug
d. image
d. to one's self
d. to others
d. patient
sexually d.
d. situation
d. stunt
dangerousness
prediction of d.
dare
daredevil
dark
d. adaptation
d. environment
d. mood
darkening vision
D/ART
Depression: Awareness, Recognition, and Treatment
darwinian reflex

D

darwinism
    neural d.
    social d.
Dasein analysis
dashing
dastard
DAT
    dementia of Alzheimer type
data
    anecdotal d.
    biographical d.
    biologic d.
    clinical d.
    d. collection
    contradictory d.
    criterion d.
    empirical d.
    epidemiological d.
    evaluability-assessment d.
    field d.
    followup d.
    functional imaging d.
    historical d.
    identifying d.
    laboratory d.
    longitudinal d.
    longitudinal expert evaluation using
      all available d. (LEAD)
    long-term d.
    mental d.
    narrative d.
    normative d.
    nutriceutical d.
    paucity of d.
    personal followup d.
    postmortem d.
    psychiatric d.
    Q d.
    quantitative d.
    d. reanalysis strategy
    reanalyzed d.
    self-report d.
    d. set
    d. snooping
    supporting d.
    survey d.
date
    anniversary d.
    bind analysis d.
    birth d. (BD)
    blind d.
    personnel d.
    d. rape
    d. rape drug
    d. stamp
dating
    d. bar
    d. experience

    d. life
    d. relationship
dauernarkose
daughter language
daunt
dauntless
dawdle
DAWN
    Drug Abuse Warning Network
day
    abstinent d.'s
    d. camp
    d. care residential treatment
    d. dream
    drinks per drinking d.
    drug-free d.
    every other d.
    four times a d.
    d.'s of heavy drinking
    d. hospital
    d. of month test
    d. one
    packs per d. (PPD)
    per d. (/d)
    d. reporting center
    d. residue
    d. school
    three times a d.
    d. treatment center (DTC)
    d. treatment program
    d. treatment unit
    twice a d.
day-care
    d.-c. center
    d.-c. program
daydream
    hero d.
    suffering-hero d.
daydreaming
daylight
daymare
daytime
    d. drowsiness
    d. fatigue
    d. hallucination
    d. mouth breathing
    d. sedation
    d. sleep episode
    d. sleep hangover
    d. somnolence
day-to-day
    d.-t.-d. function
    d.-t.-d. stress
daze
dazzle
db
    decibel

DBT
    dialectical behavior therapy
DD
    dysthymic disorder
Dd
    unusual detail response
dD
    confabulated detail response
DDF
    difficulty describing feeling
DDNOS
    dissociative disorder not otherwise
      specified
DDS
    disability determination service
Dds
    detail response to small white space
DdW
    detail response elaborating the whole
de
        de Clerambault syndrome
        de facto
        de haut en bas
        de Lange syndrome
        de lunatico inquirendo
        de penses echo
DEA#
    Drug Enforcement Administration
      number
dead
        desire to be d.
        d. end
        d. hand
        identification with the d.
        d. on arrival (DOA)
        playing d.
        d. room
deadbeat
        d. dad
        d. mom
deadhead
deadline
deadlock
deadly
        d. catatonia
        d. nightshade
        d. nightshade poisoning
        d. sin
deadness
        emotional d.
deadpan
deaf

deaf-blind
deafferentation
deaf-mute
deafness
        acoustic trauma d.
        air conduction d.
        bone conduction d.
        central d.
        conduction d.
        cortical d.
        developmental word d.
        exposure d.
        functional d.
        high frequency d.
        hysterical d.
        midbrain d.
        music d.
        nerve d.
        occupational d.
        organic d.
        perceptive d.
        prelingual d.
        psychic d.
        psychogenic d.
        selective d.
        temporary d.
        tone d.
        word d.
deal
        bid d.
dealer
        dope d.
        drug d.
dealing
Dear John letter
death
        accidental d.
        actual or threatened d.
        d. anxiety
        apparent d.
        attitude to d.
        autopsy-negative d.
        barbiturate-induced d.
        belief in life after d.
        black d.
        d. blow
        brain d.
        d. camp
        cerebral d.
        d. of close friend
        crib d.
        d. criteria

D

NOTES

death *(continued)*
    desire for d.
    exhaustion d.
    expectation of d.
    d. expectation
    expected d.
    exposure to d.
    d. feigning
    fetal d.
    functional d.
    hastened d.
    hypoxyphilia-caused d.
    impending d.
    d. instinct
    intentional d.
    d. by lethal injection
    d. mask
    nerve cell d.
    d. neurosis
    parental d.
    pervasive desire for d.
    premature d.
    d. preoccupation
    preoccupation with d.
    d. rate
    d. rattle
    reaction to d.
    d. of relative
    d. row
    d. of self
    d. sentence
    serious desire for d.
    sniffing d.
    spousal loss through d.
    sudden d.
    suffering d.
    survivor of d.
    d. theme
    thought of d.
    d. threat
    threat of d.
    threatened d.
    time of d.
    timely d.
    d. trance
    d. trap
    traumatic d.
    d. trend
    unintentional d.
    untimely d.
    violent d.
    voodoo d.
    d. warrant
    d. wish
deathbed
deathwatch
debacle
debase

debate
debauchee
debauchery
debilitate
debilitating
    d. anxiety
    d. dysphoric symptom
    d. illness
debility
    nervous d.
debonair, debonaire
debriefing
    psychological d.
debris
    word d.
debt
    gambling d.
debug
debunk
DEC
    developmental evaluation center
decadent
decamethonium bromide
decay
    reflex d.
    d. theory
deceit
    biology of d.
    conscious d.
    determinants of d.
    facial d.
    technological detection of d.
deceitfulness
deceitful style
deceivable
deceive
    intention to d.
deceleration injury
decency
decent
decenter
decentralization
decentration
deception
    effects of d.
    d. style
decerebrate
    d. plasticity
    d. posture
    d. rigidity
decerebration
    bloodless d.
decerebrize
decibel (db)
decimate
decinormal
decision
    Brawner d.

competent d.
conscious d.
consequences of d.'s
Durham d.
Gault d.
informed d.
legal d.
limiting d.
d. making
Parham d.
philosophical d.
d. support
d. support system
Tarasoff d.
d. theory
treatment d.
d. tree
unilateral d.
decision-maker
executive d.-m.
decision-making
destructive d.-m.
d.-m. organizer
d.-m. process
rash d.-m.
d.-m. skill
decisive
declaim
declaration
dying d.
declarative
d. emotional memory processing
d. memory
d. memory process
declare
declass
declassify
decline
d. in academic functioning
age-related cognitive d.
cognitive d.
functional d.
postpubertal social d.
d. rate
declining consciousness
decode
decoding skill
decompensation
d. ego
full psychotic d.
impending d.
psychotic d.

decompensative neurosis
decomposition
d. in dreams
ego d.
d. of ego
d. of movement
decompress
decompression
cerebral d.
internal d.
d. operation
orbital d.
d. sickness
suboccipital d.
subtemporal d.
trigeminal d.
deconditioning
decontaminate
decoration scruple
decorticate
d. conditioning
d. posturing
decortication, decortization
cerebral d.
reversible d.
decorum
decreased
d. arm swing
d. craving
d. interest
d. interest in activity
d. job satisfaction
d. libido
d. memory
d. motivation
d. need for sleep
d. work performance
decreasing-decrement
decree
divorce d.
decrement
cognitive d.
work d.
decremental procedure
decrepitude
decriminalize
decrudescence
decry
decussation
pyramidal d.
DED
depressive-executive dysfunction

NOTES

D

dedifferentiation
dedolation
deduction
deductive reasoning
deefferentation
deem
de-emphasize
deep
> d. brain stimulation for mood disorder
> d. cortex
> d. depression
> d. inner resource
> d. place
> d. sensibility
> d. side
> d. sleep
> d. structure
> d. tendon reflex (DTR)
> d. trance
> d. trance identification
> d. white matter
> d. white matter hyperintensity
> d. white matter hyperintensity change
> d. white matter pathology
> d. white matter region

deep-pressure sensitivity
deep-rooted
deep-seated
de-erotize
de-escalate
de-escalating aggressive behavior
deface
defalcate
defamation
defatigation
defaulter
> drug d.

defeat
defeatist attitude
defecalgesiophobia
defecate
defecation reflex
defect
> alcohol-related birth d. (ARBD)
> awareness d.
> birth d.
> body dysmorphic d.
> cerebrocranial d.
> character d.
> cognitive d.
> congenital d.
> developmental d.
> exaggerated d.
> excessive concern for d.
> field d.
> genetic d.

> high-grade d.
> imagined appearance d.
> learning d.
> memory d.
> mental d.
> metabolic d.
> neurological d.
> organic d.
> perceptual d.
> physical d.
> polytrophic d.
> polytropic d.
> d. preoccupation
> preoccupation with d.
> retention d.
> sensory d.
> slight d.
> teratologic d.
> d. theorist
> visual field d.
> visuoperceptive d.

defected eyes
defective
> mentally d.

defeminization
defend
defense
> attitude d.
> d. attitude
> character d.
> compulsive d.
> ego d.
> heat d.
> d. hysteria
> hysterical character d.
> hysteroid d.
> immature d.
> insanity d.
> d. interpretation
> lack of mature d.
> d. level
> masochistic character d.
> mature d.
> d. mechanism
> normal heat d.
> d. organization
> perceptual d.
> d. psychoneurosis
> d. reaction
> d. reflex
> screen d.
> stormed d.
> d. strategy

defensible
> d. space

defensive
> d. adultomorphic stance
> d. behavior

d. dysregulation
d. dysregulation level
d. emotion
d. functioning axis
d. process
d. reaction
defensiveness
psychological d.
defer diagnosis
deference
deferential attitude
deferred
d. diagnosis
diagnosis or condition d. on axis I
diagnosis d. on axis II
d. obedience
d. reaction
d. shock
defiance
oppositional d.
defiant
d. behavior
d. rage
stubbornly d.
deficiency
autoimmune d.
cobalamin d.
cognitive d.
environmental d.
familial d.
hereditary d.
immune d.
literacy d.
d. love
mental d.
moral d.
d. motivation
d. motive
niacin d.
nicotinic acid d.
nutritional d.
orgasmic d.
oxygen d.
secondary mental d.
thiamine d.
vitamin d.
deficiens
ejaculatio d.
orgasmic d.
orgasmus d.

deficient
d. affective experience
mentally d. (MD)
d. sense of reality
d. sexual desire
deficit
attention d.
awareness d.
behavior d.
central sensory d.
character d.
chronic integrative d. (CID)
cognitive d.
comprehension d.
concentration d.
conversion disorder with motor symptoms or d.
conversion disorder with sensory symptom or d.
emotional memory d.
executive function d.
expressive language d.
gaze d.
global cognitive d.
gross motor d.
gross neurologic d.
gross sensory d.
information processing d.
intellectual function d.
interpersonal relationship d.
ipsilateral d.
language d.
memory function d.
mental d.
motor d.
multiple cognitive d.'s
neural d.
neurocognitive d.
neurolinguistic d.
parietotemporal perfusion d.
perception d.
perceptual d.
perseveration d.
pixelated parietotemporal perfusion d.
presynaptic functional d.
primary motor d.
d. reversal
d. schizophrenia
self-care d.
sensory d.
serotonergic d.

D

NOTES

deficit *(continued)*
    sleep d.
    social relations d.
    social skills d.
    speech-motor d.
    d. symptom
    temporal integration d.
    verbal d.
    vigilance d.
    visual perceptual d.
defile
define
definite
definition
    categorical d.
    cross-sectional d.
    diagnostic d.
    operational d.
definitive
    d. treatment
deflate
deflected eye
deflection
defloration scruple
deflower
deformation
    morphological d.
    d. of self
deformity
defraud
deft
defuse
defusion
defy
degeneracy
    criminal d.
    d. theory
degenerate
degeneration
    alcohol acquired (non-wilsonian)
      chronic hepatocerebral d.
    alcohol cerebellar d.
    ascending d.
    brain d.
    descending d.
    focal d.
    orthograde d.
    d. psychosis
    reaction of d. (RD)
    retrograde d.
    secondary d.
    senile d.
degenerative
    d. encephalopathy
    d. insanity
    d. primary dementia
    progressive d.

    d. psychosis
    d. status
degenerativus
    status d.
degradation
degrade
degrading ritual
degree
    d. of amnesia
    d. of control
    d. of dependence
    d. of disability
    d. of freedom
    d. of hopelessness
    d. of impairment
    d. of pain
    third d.
degustation
dehumanization
dehumanize
dehumanizing
dehydration
    d. reaction
    voluntary d.
dehydromorphine
dehypnotize
deictic
deify
deign
deindividuation
deinstitutionalization
deinstitutionalize
deism
deity
    spectral relationship to d.
deixis
    person d.
    place d.
    time d.
déjà
    d. entendu
    d. eprouve
    d. fait
    d. pense
    d. raconte
    d. vecu
    d. voulu
    d. vu
dejected mood
dejection
delahara
delate
delay
    conduction d.
    developmental d.
    global d.
    inhibition of d.
    orgasm d.

patient d.
phase d.
specific d.
d. therapy
delayed
    d. auditory feedback
    d. development
    d. discharge
    d. ejaculation
    d. gratification
    d. grief
    d. language
    d. memory
    d. postanoxic encephalopathy
    d. posttraumatic stress disorder
    d. reaction
    d. reaction experiment
    d. recall
    d. recall index
    d. reflex
    d. reinforcement
    d. response
    d. reward
    d. sensation
    d. shock
    d. sleep phase
    d. sleep phase syndrome
    d. speech
    d. therapy
    d. toilet training
delayed-alteration test
delayed-matching test
delectation
deleterious
deletion
    thought d.
deliberate
    d. fire-setting
    d. infliction of pain
    d. self-harm (DSH)
    d. therapy
deliberation
    ethical d.
    legal d.
    medical d.
delicacy
delicate
delicto
Delilah syndrome
delimitation
delineate
delineation

delineator
delinquency
    adaptive d.
    adolescent neurotic d.
    geriatric d.
    group d.
    juvenile d.
    neurotic d.
    recovery from d.
    socialized d.
delinquent
    d. adolescent
    d. behavior
    juvenile d.
    nonviolent d.
    predatory d.
    violent d.
    d. youth
deliquium
delirante
    boufee d.
delire
    d. aigu
    d. alcoholique
    d. ambitieux
    d. chronique a evolution systematique
    d. crapuleux
    d. d'emblee
    d. de negation
    d. de negation generalise
    d. denormite
    d. de toucher
    d. ecmnesique
    d. en partie double
    d. oneirique
    d. a quatre
    d. terminal
    d. tremblant
    d. vesanique
deliria (*pl. of* delirium)
deliriant
delirifacient
delirio
    delirium sine d.
    sine d.
deliriosa
    schizophrenia d.
delirious
    d. mania
    d. patient
    d. reaction

D

NOTES

delirious *(continued)*
  d. shock
  d. transient organic psychosis
delirium, pl. **deliria**
  abstinence d.
  active d.
  acute alcoholic d.
  alcoholic d.
  d. alcoholicum
  alcohol-induced d.
  d. alcoholism
  alcohol withdrawal d.
  amphetamine d.
  anticholinergic d.
  anxiolytic d.
  anxious d.
  asthenic d.
  cannabis intoxication d.
  chronic alcoholic d.
  cocaine intoxication d.
  collapse d.
  digitalis-induced d.
  drug-induced d.
  d. due to a general medical
    condition
  d. due to multiple etiologies
  d. ebriosorum
  ecmnesic d.
  d. epilepticum
  d. e potu
  exhaustion d.
  febrile d.
  d. ferox
  focused d.
  frank d.
  full-blown d.
  grandiose d.
  d. grave
  grave d.
  hallucinogen intoxication d.
  hypnotic d.
  hypoglycemic d.
  hysterical d.
  d. hystericum
  inhalant-induced d.
  inhalant intoxication d.
  intoxication d.
  lingual d.
  low d.
  macromaniacal d.
  manic d.
  marijuana d.
  melancholia with d.
  micromaniacal d.
  microptic d.
  d. mite
  d. mussitans
  muttering d.

  d. of negation
  occupational d.
  oneiric d.
  opioid-induced d.
  opioid intoxication d.
  organic d.
  panic d.
  partial d.
  d. of persecution
  phencyclidine intoxication d.
  posttraumatic d.
  d. in presenile dementia
  psychasthenic d.
  psychoactive substance d.
  puerperal d.
  rhyming d.
  d. schizophrenoides
  secondary d.
  sedative d.
  senile d.
  d. in senile dementia
  sine d.
  d. sine delirio
  d. state drug psychosis
  subacute d.
  substance-induced d.
  superimposed d.
  sympathomimetic d.
  thyroid d.
  toxic d.
  d. transient organic psychosis
  trauma-induced d.
  traumatic d.
  d. tremens (DT)
  d. tremens alcoholic psychosis
  unfocused d.
  d. unit
  vascular dementia with d.
  withdrawal d.
delirium-like state
delirium-related mental disorder
delitescence
deliver
delivery
  consistent d.
  method of d.
delta
  d. activity
  d. alcoholism
  d. index
  d. level
  d. opiate receptor
  d. rhythm
  d. sleep-inducing peptide
  d. wave
delta-wave sleep
delude

delusion

affect-laden d.
alcohol-induced psychotic disorder with d.'s
allopsychic d.
amphetamine-induced psychotic disorder with d.'s
anxiolytic-induced psychotic disorder with d.'s
autochthonous d.
autopsychic d.
d. of being controlled
bizarre d.
cannabis-induced psychotic disorder with d.'s
circumscribed d.
cocaine d.
cocaine-induced psychotic disorder with d.'s
complex d.
confused d.
content of d.
d. of control
control d.
crystallized grandiose d.
dangerous d.
depressive d.
disorganized d.
dysmorphic d.
encapsulated d.
erotic d.
erotomanic d.
established d.
expansion d.
expansive d.
expressive d.
first rank symptoms of d.
fixed d.
fleeting d.
fragmentary d.
d. of grandeur
grandeur d.
grandiose d.
hallucinogen-induced psychotic disorder with d.'s
hypnotic-induced psychotic disorder with d.'s
d. of ill health
infestation d.
d. of infidelity
infidelity d.
influence d.

d. of influence
inhalant-induced psychotic disorder with d.'s
insane d.
interpretation d.
isolated d.
jealous-type d.
jealousy d.
Mignon d.
mild d.
mixed-type d.
mood-congruent d.
mood-incongruent d.
multiple d.'s
d. of negation
negation d.
negative d.
nihilistic d.
nonbizarre d.
nonsystematized d.
object of a d.
observation d.
d. of observation
organic d.
d. of orientation
Othello d.
paranoid grandiose d.
partial d.
passivity d.
d. of passivity
pejorative d.
persecution d.
d. of persecution
persecutory d.
persistent d.
phencyclidine-induced psychotic disorder with d.'s
poorly systematized d.
d. of poverty
poverty d.
d. of power
primordial d.
psychotic disorder with d.'s
reference d.
d. of reference
referential d.
reformist d.
religious d.
schneiderian d.
sedative-induced psychotic disorder with d.'s
d. of self-accusation

D

NOTES

delusion *(continued)*
    sexual d.
    d. of sinfulness
    somatic d.
    d. stupor
    d. symptom
    systematized d.
    systemic d.
    thought broadcasting d.
    thought insertion d.
    unspecified-type d.
    unsystematized d.
    vascular dementia with d.'s
    d. of wealth
    well-formed d.
delusional
    d. anxiety
    d. behavior
    d. belief
    d. belief in intimacy
    d. conviction
    d. depression
    d. equivalent
    d. experience
    d. feature
    floridly d.
    d. insanity
    d. intensity
    d. jealousy
    d. loving
    d. misidentification syndrome
    d. network
    d. paranoid disorder
    d. percept
    d. projection
    d. proportion
    d. subtype
    d. syndrome drug psychosis
    d. system
    d. thinking
    d. thought
    d. thought pattern
    d. transient organic
    d. transient organic psychosis
delusion-like
    d.-l. idea
    d.-l. preoccupation
delusions of mind reading
delusive
delve
demagogue
demand
    attentional d.
    d. characteristic
    external d.
    functional d.
    internal d.
    role d.

    sexual d.
    d. of society
    unreasonable d.
demanding
    d. behavior
    d. interaction
    d. in nature
demarcated relationship
demarcation
    d. current
    d. potential
    d. in sensory testing
demarche
demasculinization
d'emblee
    delire d.
demean
demeanor
    mild eccentricity in d.
demented patient
dementia
    acute primary d.
    advanced d.
    alcohol-associated d.
    alcoholic d.
    alcohol-induced persisting d.
    alcoholism associated with d.
    alcohol persisting d.
    Alzheimer-like senile d. (ALSD)
    d. of Alzheimer type (DAT)
    d. of the Alzheimer type, with
      early onset
    d. of the Alzheimer type, with
      late onset
    anxiolytic-induced persisting d.
    apoplectic d.
    d. apoplectica
    d. associated with alcoholism
    atrophic d.
    beclouded d.
    Binswanger d.
    boxer's d.
    catatonic d.
    chronic d.
    circular d.
    confusional state presenile d.
    congenital syphilitic paralytic d.
    degenerative primary d.
    delirium in presenile d.
    delirium in senile d.
    depressed-type presenile d.
    depression in d.
    developmental d.
    dialysis d.
    driveling d.
    drug-induced d.
    d. due to Creutzfeldt-Jakob disease
    d. due to head trauma

d. due to traumatic brain injury
early phase of d.
end-stage d.
d. in epilepsy
epileptic d.
d. evaluation
exhaustion senile d.
familial d.
frontal lobe d.
frontosubcortical d.
global d.
hallucinatory d.
hebephrenic d.
Heller d.
higher d.
HIV-based d.
hypnotic-induced persisting d.
impairment of d.
infantile d.
d. infantilis
inhalant-induced persisting d.
juvenile paralytic d.
lacunar d.
language disorder in d.
d. myoclonica
old-age d.
organic d.
paralytic d.
d. paralytica
d. paralytica juvenilis (DPJ)
paranoid d.
d. paranoides
d. paranoides gravis
d. paranoides mitis
paranoid-type arteriosclerotic d.
paranoid-type presenile d.
paranoid-type senile d.
paraphrenic d.
d. paratonia progressiva
paretic d.
d. patient
persisting d.
d. phase
Pick disease d.
polyarteritis nodosa d.
postfebrile d.
posttraumatic d.
d. praecocissima
d. praecox
preexisting d.
presenile d.

d. presenilis
primary degenerative d. (PDD)
primary senile d.
d. process
profound d.
d. progression
progressive d.
psychoactive substance d.
psychobiological process of d.
puerperal d.
d. pugilistica
relative d.
remitting d.
repeated infarct d.
schizophrenic d.
secondary d.
sedative, hypnotic, or anxiolytic-
 induced persisting d.
sedative-induced persisting d.
d. sejunctiva
semantic d.
senile d.
severe d.
d. severity
simple depressive d.
simple senile d.
socialized d.
d. stage
d. state drug psychosis
static d.
subcortical d.
substance-abuse persisting d.
substance-induced persisting d.
superimposed d.
d. syndrome
d. syndrome of depression
syphilitic paralytic d.
syphilitic progressive d.
tabetic form paralytic d.
tardive d.
terminal d.
thalamic d.
toxic d.
transmissible virus d. (TVD)
traumatic d.
uncomplicated arteriosclerotic d.
uncomplicated presenile d.
uncomplicated senile d.
vascular d.
Wernicke d.
Wilson disease d.

D

NOTES

dementia-aphonia
    d.-a. syndrome
    d.-a. syndrome of childhood
dementia-related
    d.-r. behavior
    d.-r. mental disorder
    d.-r. psychiatric syndrome
dementing
    d. illness
    d. process
demerit
demigod
demimonde
demise
    untimely d.
demissio animi
demiurge
democratic leadership pattern
demographic
    d. characteristic
    d. feature
    d. risk factor
    d. variable
demography
    dynamic d.
    static d.
demolish
demon
demoniac
demonic possession
demonolatry
demonology
demonomania
demonomaniaque
    folie d.
demonstrable
demonstrate
demonstration
demonstrator
demoralization
    personal d.
demoralize
demorphinization
demote
demotivate
demulcent
demure
demutization
demystify
den
    opium d.
denarcotize
denegation
denervate
denervation
    autonomic d.
    law of d.
    d. level

deneutralization
deniable
denial
    d. of anergy
    color d. (Cd)
    d. defense mechanism
    d. of external reality
    parental d.
    psychodynamic d.
    psychotic d.
    reality d.
    d. of responsibility
    d. visual hallucination syndrome
denied grief
denigrate
denigrated self-esteem
denigration
denizen
denomination
    religious d.
denormite
    delire d.
denotation
denote
denounce
denovo
dense
    d. scotoma
    d. sensory loss
densitometry
density
    frontal lobe neuronal d.
    inside d.
    outside d.
    population d.
dental
    d. anxiety
    d. jurisprudence
    d. patient reaction
dentata
    vagina d.
denuding
    hair d.
denunciation
denutrition
deny
deodoratum
    opium d.
deodorized opium
deontologic theory
deontologism
deontologist
deontology
deoppilant
deorality
deoxyribonucleic acid (DNA)
department
    emergency d. (ED)

D. of Health and Human Services (DHHS)
D. of Mental Health (DMH)
psychiatric emergency d.

depatterning
dependence, dependency
  absinthe d.
  additional drug d.
  aerosol spray d.
  airplane glue d.
  alcohol d.
  amphetamine d.
  anxiolytic d.
  barbiturate d. (BD)
  benzodiazepine d.
  butane sniffing d.
  caffeine d.
  cannabis d.
  chemical d.
  chlorohydrocarbon d.
  clinging d.
  cocaine d.
  codeine d.
  combination-drug d.
  d. criterion
  cross d.
  degree of d.
  diet drug d.
  d. disorder
  drug d.
  emotional d.
  ethanol d.
  ether d.
  field d.
  full d.
  hallucinogen d.
  hallucinogenic drug d.
  hypnotic d.
  increased d.
  inhalant d.
  instrumental d.
  interpersonal d.
  laxative d.
  lighter fluid d.
  long-term d.
  LSD d.
  marijuana d.
  methadone d.
  methamphetamine d.
  morbid d.
  morning glory seeds d.
  morphine d.

narcotic drug d.
nicotine d.
nitrous oxide d.
d. on pornography
d. on therapy
opioid d.
opium d.
oral d.
d. organic psychosis
passive d.
peyote d.
pharmacology of abuse and d.
phencyclidine d.
physical d.
physiological d.
polysubstance d.
pornography d.
prescription drug d.
propoxyphene d.
psilocybin d.
psychedelic agent d.
psychic d.
psychoactive substance d.
psychostimulant d.
psychotomimetic agent d.
reward d. (RD)
sedative d.
social d.
solvent d.
soporific drug d.
state d.
substance abuse and d.
d. syndrome
synthetic drug d.
synthetic heroin d.
d. tendency
tetrahydrocannabinol d.
THC d.
therapeutic dose d.
tobacco d.
d. trait
tranquilizer drug d.
unmet d.
unspecified substance d.
volatile solvent d.
dependence-independence
  field d.-i.
dependence-type organic psychosis
dependency (*var. of* dependence)
dependent
  d. adult's certificate
  alcohol d.

D

NOTES

dependent *(continued)*
    d. behavior
    d. character
    dose d.
    d. edema
    d. feature
    d. neurotic personality disorder
    d. patient role
    d. personality
    d. relationship
    d. scale
    trait d.
    d. variable
dependent-passive personality disorder
dependent-protective relationship
depersonalization
    d. episode
    d. experience
    d. neurosis
    d. neurotic disorder
    neurotic state with d.
    d. psychoneurosis
    d. psychoneurotic
    d. psychoneurotic reaction
    recurrent d.
    d. syndrome
depersonalize
depersonalized image
depict
deplete
depletion
    metabolic volume d.
deplorable
deploy
depolarization
depolarizing muscle relaxant
deportment
depose
deposition
depot
    d. antipsychotic
    Clopixol d.
    fat d.
    d. form
    d. medication
    d. medication injection
    d. medication injection therapy
    Piportil D.
depot-administered antipsychotic drug
depravation
depraved
depravity
deprecate
deprecatory
depreciate
depreciated subsystem
deprementia

depressant
    brain d.
    cerebral d.
    CNS d.
    motor d.
depressed
    d. affect
    d. bipolar affective psychosis
    bipolar type currently d.
    depressive type currently d.
    d. mania
    d. manic state
    d. mood
    d. mood adjustment disorder
    d. mood adjustment reaction
    d. mood episode
    d. mood theme
    d. patient
    d. presentation
    d. reflex
    schizoaffective disorder, d.
    d. schizoaffective schizophrenia
    d. suicide victim
    d. tone
    d. type
depressed-type presenile dementia
depression
    acute anxiety d.
    acute situational d.
    adjustment d.
    adolescent d.
    adult major d.
    agitated d.
    akinetic d.
    alcohol-induced d.
    anaclitic d.
    anancastic d.
    anergic d.
    anxiety d.
    anxious somatic d.
    arteriosclerotic d.
    atypical d.
    autogenous d.
    autonomous d.
    aversion d.
    D.: Awareness, Recognition, and Treatment (D/ART)
    bereavement-related d.
    biologic sign d.
    bipolar d.
    brief situational d.
    caregiver d.
    characterological d.
    chronic major d.
    classical d.
    classification of d.
    clinical d.
    cognitive impairment of d.

cognitive theory of d.
d. of consciousness
constitutional d.
co-occurrence of d.
d. criterion
cryptic d.
current d.
cyclic d.
cyclical d.
deep d.
delusional d.
d. in dementia
dementia syndrome of d.
depression sine d. (DSD)
double d.
drug-induced d.
drug-resistant d.
d. during pregnancy
dysthymia with major d.
dysthymia without major d.
endogenomorphic d.
endogenous d.
d. in epilepsy
exaggerated d.
exogenous d.
d. factor
first episode of d. (FDE)
future d.
gamble to escape from d.
geriatric d.
d. history
holiday d.
hypersomnia associated with d.
hypersomnic d.
hyposomnia associated with d.
hysterical delirium d.
ictal d.
insomnia associated with d.
d. inventory
involutional d.
later-life d.
level of d.
light treatment for winter d.
major d.
manic d.
manifestation of d.
marked d.
masked d.
maternal d.
melancholic d.
menopausal d.
mental d.

mild d.
moderate d.
moderate-to-severe d.
monopolar d.
myxedema d.
nervous d.
neurotic d.
d. neurotic disorder
nonbipolar major d.
nonmajor d.
nonpsychotic unipolar d.
nonreactive d.
nuclear d.
overt signs of d.
overwhelming d.
paradoxical d.
paralyzing d.
d. period
physiogenetic d.
postdivorce d.
postdormital d.
posthysterectomy d.
postictal d.
postinfectious d.
postnatal d. (PND)
postpartum d. (PPD)
postpartum major d.
postpsychotic d.
postschizophrenic d.
post stroke d.
post TIA d.
prevention and treatment of d. (PTD)
prolonged situational d.
propensity for d.
psychogenic d.
psychoneurotic d.
psychotic d. (PD)
d. questionnaire
reactive clinical d.
reactive psychotic d.
recurrent episode psychotic d.
refractory d.
D. and Related Affective Disorders Association
resistant d.
retarded d.
reversible cognitive impairment of d.
d. risk
ruminative d.
d. scale

NOTES

depression *(continued)*
    d. score
    secondary d.
    self-blaming d.
    senile d.
    severe d.
    d. severity
    sign d.
    simple affective d.
    single-episode psychotic d.
    situational d.
    sleeplessness associated with d.
    somatic treatment for d.
    somatizing clinical d.
    d. spectrum disease
    sporadic d.
    spreading d.
    stuporous d.
    subjective d.
    d. subscale
    subsyndromal d.
    d. subtype
    d. symptom
    symptomatic d.
    syndromic d.
    d. treatment
    treatment-refractory d.
    treatment-resistant d.
    underlying d.
    unipolar chronic d.
    unipolar major d.
    unipolar recurrent d.
    unspecified d.
    vascular d.
    winter d.
    d. with psychotic feature
depression-related
    d.-r. mental disorder
    d.-r. psychiatric syndrome
depressive
    d. auditory hallucination
    d. breakthrough
    d. catatonia
    d. character
    d. character structure
    d. crash
    d. delusion
    d. disease
    d. disorder not otherwise specified
    d. episode
    d. equivalent
    d. experience
    manic d.
    d. mixed state
    d. neurosis
    d. olfactory hallucination
    d. personality
    d. personality disorder

    d. phase
    d. position
    d. pseudodementia
    psychological trauma d.
    d. psychoneurotic reaction
    d. psychotic reaction
    d. situational reaction
    d. spectrum disorder (DSD)
    d. state
    d. stupor
    d. symptom
    d. symptomatology
    d. syndrome
    d. transient organic psychosis
    d. turmoil
    d. type currently depressed
    d. visual hallucination
depressive-dysphoric personality disorder
depressive-executive dysfunction (DED)
depressive-type
    d.-t. nonorganic psychosis
    d.-t. psychoneurosis
    d.-t. psychoorganic syndrome
depressor
deprivation
    activity d.
    cultural d.
    early parental d.
    emotional d.
    environmental d.
    food d.
    masked d.
    maternal d.
    oxygen d.
    paternal d.
    perceptual d.
    psychological d.
    psychosocial d.
    role d.
    sensory d.
    severe environmental d.
    sleep d.
    social d.
    d. syndrome
    thought d.
    water d.
deprived
    culturally d.
    d. early life
    educationally d.
depth
    analysis in d.
    d.'s of despair
    d. of mood
    d. perception
    d. psychology
    d. recording

d. of sleep
d. therapy
derailment
actual d.
cognitive d.
frequent d.
speech d.
thought d.
d. of volition
deranged
mentally d.
d. neural development
derangement
mental d.
metabolic d.
derealization
dereflection
dereism
dereistic thinking
derelict
skid-row d.
dereliction
deride
derision
derivation
derivative
alcohol d.
chloral d.
ergot d.
indole d.
piperidyl d.
thioxanthene d.
dermatitis, pl. **dermatitides**
factitial d.
psychogenic d.
self-induced factitial d.
dermatoglyphic
abnormal d.
dermatothlasia
dermoneurosis
derogate
derogatory
d. comment
d. remark
d. word
dervish
De Sanctis-Cacchione syndrome
desanimania
descendant
descending
d. degeneration
d. dyscontrol

d. neuritis
d. technique
description
borderline composite d.
clinical d.
composite personality d.
DSM-IV d.
graphic d.
histrionic composite d.
narrative d.
psychological d.
Q-Sort d.
d. questionnaire
schizoid composite d.
supervisory behavior d. (SBD)
SWAP-200 d.
textual d.
descriptive
d. approach
d. detail
d. feature
d. psychiatry
d. statistics
d. validity
descriptor score
descry
desecrate
desegregate
desensitization
behavioral d.
eye movement d.
imaginal d.
phobic d.
psychologic d.
reciprocal inhibition and d.
systematic d.
systemic d.
desensitize
desert
deserted place
deserter
desertion
d. anxiety
maternal d.
paternal d.
deserve
deserved
d. punishment
d. punishment theme
desexualize
desiccant
desiccate

NOTES

D

desiccation
desiderate
design
    A/B/A d.
    block d.
    case control experimental study d.
    cohort experimental d.
    cross-sectional experimental
      study d.
    environmental d.
    equipment d.
    experimental d.
    factorial d.
    geometric d.
    independent group experimental
      study d.
    interdisciplinary environmental d.
    job d.
    longitudinal experimental study d.
    memory for d. (MFD)
    mixed d.
    multiple baseline d.
    naturalistic d.
    prospective experimental study d.
    quasi-experimental d.
    randomized group d.
    retrospective experimental study d.
    study d.
    time-series d.
designate
designer
    d. drug
    d. hallucinogen
    d. label
desirability
    low social d.
    social d.
desire
    absent sexual d.
    active d.
    d. to be dead
    d. to be thin
    d. for death
    deficient sexual d.
    d. to die
    disturbance in sexual d.
    drug d.
    hyperactive sexual d.
    hypoactive sexual d.
    impaired sexual d.
    incestuous d.
    increased sexual d.
    inhibited sexual d.
    d. to instill fear
    intense d.
    irrational d.
    d. level
    low sexual d.

    morbid d.
    d. for personal gain
    d. phase of sexual response cycle
    d. for revenge
    sexual d.
    situational hypoactive sexual d.
    d. state
    stated d.
desired
    d. behavior
    d. effect
desire-for-death rating
desirous
desist
desmethylimipramine
desmodynia
DESNOS
    disorders of extreme stress not otherwise
      specified
desolate
desomorphine
despair
    depths of d.
    ego integrity versus d.
    feeling of d.
    integrity versus d.
despeciation
desperate financial condition
despicable
despise
despite
despondent
destiny
    manifest d.
destitute
destroy
destruct
destruction
    property d.
    d. of property
destructive
    d. aggression
    d. behavior
    d. criticism
    d. decision-making
    d. drive
    d. family relationship pattern
    d. instinct
    d. obedience
    d. relationship
    d. social consequence
    d. tendency
destructiveness
    withdrawal d.
destrudo
desultoriness
desultory

desynchronization
    event-related d. (ERD)
desynchronized discharge pattern
desynchronous
detached
    d. coping
    emotionally d.
    d. manner
detachment
    emotional d.
    feeling of d.
    d. from social relationship
    pattern of d.
    sense of d.
    social d.
    somnolent d.
detail
    descriptive d.
    minimization of emotional d.
    preoccupation with d.
    d. response elaborating the whole (DdW)
    d. response to small white space (Dds)
detailed
    d. dream
    d. history
detain
detect
detectability threshold
detection
    d. of adolescent killers
    arousal d.
    lie d.
    signal d.
    d. threshold
detector
    lie d.
detention (detn)
    d. cell
    d. certificate
    d. facility
    d. home
deter
deteriorated
    d. affective disorder
    d. bipolar disorder
deteriorating
    d. course
    d. function
deterioration
    age-related d.

alcoholic d.
appearance d.
cognitive d.
d. effect
emotional d.
d. epilepsy
epileptic d.
functional d.
global d.
grooming d.
habit d.
hygiene d.
d. index (DI)
intellectual d.
irradiation-induced mental d.
language function d.
manners d.
memory d.
mental d.
mood d.
motivation d.
personality d.
posttraumatic d.
d. process
progressive d.
prominent d.
psychopathologic d.
d. quotient
radiation-induced mental d.
d. reaction type
reaction-type d.
d. scale
senile d.
significant d.
simple d.
social skills d.
status d.
stepwise d.
uniformly progressive d.
determinant
behavior d.
biologic d.
d.'s of deceit
dominant d.
dream d.
environmental d.
psychological d.
determination
forensic d.
legal d.
sex d.
determining quality

D

NOTES

determinism
  biologic d.
  biosocial d.
  cultural d.
  linguistic d.
  psychic d.
  reciprocal d.
deterrence
deterrent
  d. to suicide
  d. therapy
detest
detestable
detn
  detention
detoxicate
detoxification
  alcohol d.
  protracted d.
detoxified alcoholic
detoxify
detract
detractor
d'etre
  raison d.
detriment
detrimental
detumescence
deuce
deuteropathy
deux
  a d.
  crime a d.
  egoisme à d.
  folie a d.
  semiobsession a d.
DEV
  deviant
  deviation
devaluation
devalue
devastate
devastating effect
develop
  failure to d.
developed
  poorly d.
developing psychotic disorganization
development
  abnormal d.
  adult d.
  anal stage psychosexual d.
  arrest of d.
  arrested d.
  atypical d.
  behavioral d.
  brain d.
  career d.

character d.
child language d.
cognitive d.
concrete operational d.
delayed d.
deranged neural d.
deviant pathway of d.
disturbance of intellectual d.
ego d.
egocentric stage of d.
emotional d.
expressive language d.
fetal d.
formal operational d.
gender identity psychosexual d.
impaired d.
intellectual d.
d. inventory
kohlbergian theory of moral
  reasoning d.
language d.
d. language scale
latency period psychosexual d.
late speech d.
learning d.
level of d.
libidinal d.
life span d.
mental d.   .
moral d.
motor d.
neurobiology of early childhood d.
normal childhood d.
optimal d.
oral stage psychosexual d.
personal d.
personality d.
pervasive impairment of d.
phallic stage psychosexual d.
piagetian theory of moral
  reasoning d.
postnatal d.
preoperational d.
d. profile
d. program
d. psychobiology
psychomotor d.
psychosexual d.
psychosocial d.
d. questionnaire
receptive language d.
retarded d.
rhythms of lags and spurts in d.
d. scale
sensorimotor d.
sexual d.
slow rate of language d.
social d.

standards d.
subsequent d.
task of emotional d. (TED)
d. test

developmental
d. age (DA)
d. agraphia
d. aphasia
d. apraxia
d. arithmetic disorder
d. articulation disorder
d. biology
d. consideration
d. coordination disorder
d. course
d. curve
d. defect
d. delay
d. dementia
d. disability
d. disorder associated with hyperkinesis
d. dyslexia
d. dysphasia
d. effect
d. evaluation center (DEC)
d. experience
d. experimentation in childhood
d. expressive writing
d. expressive writing disorder
d. hand-function test (DHFT)
d. hyperactivity
d. idiocy
d. imbalance
d. impact
d. influence
d. landmark
d. language disorder
d. learning problem (DLP)
d. level
d. lines
d. milestone
d. moodiness
d. pattern
d. period
d. perspective
d. phase
d. process
d. psychology
d. reading disorder
d. retardation
d. roots

d. scale
d. schedule
d. screening
d. skills
d. stage
d. task
d. theory
d. word blindness
d. word deafness

developmental-behavioral pediatrics

developmentally
d. appropriate avoidant behavior
d. appropriate self-stimulatory behaviors in the young
d. appropriate shy behavior
d. cumulative alcoholism
d. disabled
d. inappropriate social relatedness
d. limited alcoholism

developmental-vulnerability model

deviance
communication d.
psychiatric d.
psychopathic d.
role d.
secondary d.
sexual d.
social d.

deviant (DEV)
d. arousal
d. attitude
d. belief
d. language
d. pathway of development
d. political behavior
psychopathic d. (PD)
d. religious behavior
sex d.
sexual d.

deviation (DEV)
ego d.
d. from physiological norm
mean d.
personality d.
population standard d.
primary sexual d.
quartile d. (q)
d. quotient
response d.
sample standard d.
sexual d.
skew d.

D

NOTES

deviation *(continued)*
>   standard d.
>   statistical d.

device
>   charge-coupled d. (CCD)
>   cohesive d.
>   computer-assisted speech d.
>   contraceptive d.
>   control d.
>   inanimate learning d.
>   interrupter d.
>   language acquisition d. (LAD)
>   manipulative d.
>   safety d.

devil
>   d. advocate
>   d. pact
>   d. worship

devil-may-care attitude
deviltry
devious
>   d. manner

devitalize
devoid
devoir
devolution
devolutive
devolve
devote
devotion
devour
devout
>   religiously d.

devoutly spiritual
dewy-eyed
dexamphetamine
dexterity
>   manual d.

dextral
dextrality
dextrality-sinistrality
dextromanual
dextropedal
dextropropoxyphene
dextrosinistral
DHFT
>   developmental hand-function test

DHHS
>   Department of Health and Human
>   Services

DI
>   deterioration index
>   drug information
>   drug interaction

diabetic
>   d. coma
>   d. ketoacidosis

diablerie

diabolepsy
diabolic
diabolism
diacetylmorphine HCl
diachorema
diachoresis
diachronic study
diacrisis
diacritic
diadochokinesis
diagnosable
diagnosed
>   newly d.

diagnosing organizational culture
diagnosis, pl. **diagnoses (DX, Dx)**
>   admitting d. (AD)
>   alcohol-related d.
>   alternative d.
>   anxiety d.
>   assessment and d.
>   axis I, II d.
>   categorical personality disorder d.
>   clinical d.
>   comorbid Axis II d.
>   comorbid psychiatric d.
>   concurrent psychiatric d.
>   d. or condition deferred on axis I
>   controversial d.
>   cookbook d.
>   current d. (CD)
>   defer d.
>   deferred d.
>   d. deferred on axis II
>   differential d.
>   dimensional d.
>   direct d.
>   discharge d.
>   DSM d.
>   dual d.
>   entering d. (ED)
>   equivalent d.
>   d. by exclusion
>   d. ex juvantibus
>   false-negative d.
>   false-positive d.
>   final d.
>   geriatric d.
>   ICD-10 psychiatric d.
>   incorrect d.
>   laboratory d.
>   missed d.
>   narcissistic d.
>   negative d.
>   pathologic d.
>   pendulum of d.
>   personality disorder d.
>   primary d.
>   principal d.

proband d.
provisional d.
provocative d.
psychiatric d.
reliable d.
D. and Remediation of
  Handwriting Problems
schizophrenic d.
schizophreniform d.
secondary d.
serum d.
single d.
social d.
structural d.
tentative d.
unclear d.
unrelated d.
valid d.
wastebasket d.
working d.
diagnosis-related group
diagnostic
  d. algorithm
  d. ambiguity
  d. anesthesia
  d. aspect
  d. assessment
  d. battery
  d. boundary
  d. category
  d. challenge
  d. clarity
  d. class
  d. cluster
  d. complexity
  d. confidence
  d. criteria
  d. definition
  d. feature
  d. group
  d. importance
  d. impression
  d. interview
  d. inventory
  d. judgment
  d. laboratory
  d. manual
  d. measure
  d. method
  d. noise
  d. overshadowing
  d. procedure

d. process
d. profile
d. prototype
D. and Statistical Manual (DSM)
D. and Statistical Manual, Revision
  IV (DSM-IV)
d. subgroup
d. subtype
d. teaching
d. template
d. therapy
d. use of hypnosis
diagnostician
diagnostics
diagram
  branching tree d.
  scatter d.
dialectic
dialectical
  d. behavior therapy (DBT)
  d. dilemma
dialing
  random digital d. (RDD)
dialogue
  offensive chat-room d.
dialysis
  d. dementia
  d. encephalopathy syndrome
diametrically opposed
diamorphine
Diana complex
dianoetic
diaphemetric
diaphoresis
diaphragm
diaphragmatic breathing
diarrhea
  nocturnal d.
  psychogenic d.
diary
  d. card
  sleep d.
  symptom d.
diasostic
diathesis
  asthenic d.
  biologic d.
  bipolar d.
  contractural d.
  neuropathic d.
  panic d.
  psychopathic d.

D

NOTES

diathesis *(continued)*
    spasmodic d.
    stress-driven d.
diathesis-stress
    d.-s. paradigm
    d.-s. theory of schizophrenia
diatribe
dibenzepin
dibenzothiazepine
DIC
    drug information center
dichloralphenazone
dichlorotetrafluoroethane
dichotic
    d. listening task
    d. message
dichotomization of score
dichotomize
dichotomous
    d. classification
    d. scale
    d. thinking
dichotomy
    body-mind d.
    present-absent d.
dichromatic
dichromatopsia
dictatorial
diction
dictum
dicyclic
DID
    dissociative identity disorder
didactic
    d. analysis
    d. group psychotherapy
dido
die
    bis in d. (b.i.d.)
    desire to d.
    wish to d.
diehard personality
diencephalic
    d. damage
    d. epilepsy
    d. seizure
    d. stupor
diencephalon, pl. **diencephala**
diestrus
    gestational d.
    lactational d.
diet
    absolute d.
    ADA d.
    adequate d.
    American Diabetic Association d.
    aspartame-restricted d.
    balanced d.

    Banting d.
    basal d.
    basic d.
    Baylorfast d.
    black d.
    bland d.
    dietetic d.
    d. drug
    d. drug abuse
    d. drug dependence
    elemental d.
    elimination d.
    fad d.
    Feingold d.
    high-calorie d.
    high-fat d.
    high-fiber d.
    high-protein d.
    improper d.
    Jenny Craig d.
    ketogenic d.
    lactoovovegetarian d.
    lactovegetarian d.
    light d.
    limited d.
    liquid d.
    low-calorie d.
    low-fat d.
    low-salt d.
    low-tyramine d.
    macrobiotic d.
    d. management
    Nutri/System d.
    Optifast d.
    optimal d.
    Pritikin d.
    reduced sodium d.
    regular d.
    restricted d.
    salt-free d.
    soft d.
    Spartan d.
    subsistence d.
    d. treatment
    unrestricted d.
    vegan vegetarian d.
    vegetarian d.
    Weight Watchers d.
dietary
    d. amenorrhea
    d. change
    d. chaos syndrome
    d. custom
    d. excess
    d. habit
    d. modification
    d. restriction
    d. states

d. supplement
d. theory
d. toxin
diet-controlled
dietetic diet
diethylamide
diethylmalonylurea
dieting
unwise d.
dietitian
dietotherapy
dietotoxicity
DIF
difficulty identifying feeling
differ
difference
behavioral d.
chance d.
clinical d.
cross-cultural d.
cultural d.
dose-related d.
functional d.
gender d.
gender-based mental health d.'s
genetic d.
gray-white matter d.
group d.
hormonal d.
individual d.'s
just noticeable d. (JND)
d. limen
metabolic d.
morphological d.
nonsignificant d.
pharmacological d.
phase d.
qualitative d.
religious d.
significant d.
standard error of d.
true d.
different
culturally d.
differentia
differential
d. beneficial effect
d. correlate
d. diagnosis
d. diagnostic technique
d. equation
d. extinction

d. function
d. increase
d. interaction
d. prevalence
d. reinforcement
d. reinforcement of other behavior
(DRO)
d. relaxation
d. response
semantic d.
d. therapeutic
threshold d.
d. threshold
differentiate
differentiation
brain d.
cell d.
regional d.
sex d.
sexual d.
difficult
d. child
d. to manage
d. to subdue
difficulty
academic d.
acculturation d.
d. in changing response set
chronic phase of stable sleep d.
d. concentrating
concentration d.
d. controlling anger
d. describing feeling (DDF)
emotional d.
emotional and behavioral d.'s
(EBD)
gambling-related d.
d. identifying feeling (DIF)
interpersonal d.
item d.
language d.
learning d.
d. level
life d.
memory d.
moderate d.
multiple life d.
protracted d.
protracted d.
school d.
sensory d.
specific reading d. (SRD)

D

NOTES

difficulty *(continued)*
    speech d.
    stable sleep d.
    sublimation d.
    tactile sensory d.
    d. with thought
    word-finding d.
diffidence
diffident
diffuse
    d. affect
    d. anxiety
    d. brain atrophy
    d. brain dysfunction
    d. encephalopathy
    d. function
    d. phoneme
    d. sclerosis
    d. slowing of EEG
diffused reflex
diffusion
    identity d.
    identity versus role d.
    d. respiration
    role d.
diffusional state
digamy
digestible
digestive
    d. epilepsy
    d. psychogenic disorder
digit
    d. recall
    d. repetition test
    d. reversal test
    d. span (DS)
    d. span subtest
    d. stamp
    d. symbol (DS)
    d. symbol substitution
digital
    d. change
    d. subtraction angiography (DSA)
digitalgia paresthetica
digitalis-induced delirium
digit-symbol and incidental memory
dignify
dignitary
dignity
digraph
digress
digressed speech
digressive
dihybrid
dihydrochloride
dihydrocodeine
dihydrocodeinone bitartrate
dihydrolone

dihydromorphone
DIL
    drug information log
dilate
dilated pupils
dilatory
dilatory nature
dildo
dilemma
    dialectical d.
    ethical d.
    legal d.
    need-fear d.
    organic-functional d.
diligence
diligent
dilly-dally
dilution
    transference d.
dimension
    abstract-versus-representational d.
    criterion d.
    disorganization d.
    group d.
    hyperactivity-impulsivity d.
    inattention d.
    job d.'s
    micropsychotic d.
    negative symptom d.
    personality d.
    positive symptom d.
    sensory d.
    spiritual d.
    symptom d.
dimensional
    d. approach
    d. diagnosis
    d. model
    d. rating
    d. setting
    d. system
    three d.
dimensionality
dimethyltryptamine (DMT)
diminish
diminished
    d. capacity
    d. control
    d. effect
    d. emotional expression
    d. libido
    d. pleasure in everyday activities
    d. reality testing
    d. recall
    d. reflex
    d. response to pain
    d. responsibility
    d. responsiveness

d. sensation
d. sexual interest
diminution
d. of affect
d. of goal-directed behavior
d. of thought
diminutive
dimming
chromatic d.
dimorphic
sexually d.
dimorphism
brain d.
sexual d.
dimout
DIMS
disorder of initiating and maintaining sleep
ding-dong theory
dinomania
diode
Dionysian attitude
diotic
d. listening
d. message
dioxide
carbon d. (CO_2)
dioxyamphetamine
diphasic
diphenylaminearsine chloride
diphenylchlorarsine
diphosphate
diphtheritic neuropathy
diplacusis dysharmonica
diplegia
ataxic d.
congenital facial d.
facial d.
infantile d.
masticatory d.
spastic d.
diplegic idiocy
diploid
diplomacy
diploma in psychological medicine (DPM)
diplomatic
diplomyelia
diplopia
dipole tracing (DT)
dipping
body d.

dippoldism
dipropyltryptamine (DPT)
dipsesis
dipsetic
dipsomania
dipsosis
DIR
disturbed interpersonal relationship
direct
d. association
d. causality
d. causative pathophysiological mechanism
d. confrontation
d. diagnosis
d. genetic influence
d. image
d. interview
d. motor system
d. observation
d. physiological effect
d. question
d. selection communication board
d. self-destructive behavior (DSDB)
d. suggestion under hypnosis (DSUH)
d. thermogenic effect
d. threat
d. threat to life
d. treatment
directed
d. group therapy
inner d.
other d.
d. thinking
tradition d.
direction
completion, arithmetic, vocabulary, and d.'s (CAVD)
d. prognosis
psychotic d.
spiritual d.
directionality
directive
advance d.
genetic d.
d. psychotherapy
directness
direful situation
dire straits
dirigation

D

NOTES

dirt
> d. eater
> d. eating

dirtiness
> feeling of d.

dirty
> being d.
> d. linen
> d. needle
> d. pool
> quick and d.
> d. urine
> d. words

disability
> abstracting d.
> associated d.
> d. benefit
> chronic d.
> cognitive d.
> d. counselor
> degree of d.
> d. determination service (DDS)
> developmental d.
> drawing d.
> early retirement with d. (ERD)
> emotional d.
> functional d.
> general language d.
> d. insurance
> language d.
> learning d. (LD)
> d. level
> long-term d. (LTD)
> manifested d.
> memory d.
> mental d.
> mild d.
> mobility d.
> motor d.
> observable d.
> output d.
> overall d.
> partial permanent d.
> perceptual d.
> perceptual-motor d.
> permanent d.
> posttraumatic chronic d.
> progressive d.
> psychiatric d.
> reading d.
> residual d.
> sequencing d.
> service-connected d. (SCD)
> severe d.
> social role d.
> specific learning d.
> specific reading d.
> speech d.

> d. status scale (DSS)
> temporary d.
> total d.
> work d.

disabled
> developmentally d.
> emotionally disturbed/learning d. (ED/LD)
> learning d.
> mentally d.
> partially d.
> psychiatrically d.
> temporarily d.
> totally d.

disabling
> d. anxiety
> d. headache
> d. mental illness
> socially d.
> d. stress
> d. worry

disadvantage
> cultural d.
> economic d.
> educational d.
> symptomatic d.

disadvantaged
> culturally d.
> economically d.

disaggregation
disagree
disappear
disappointment
> romantic d.

disapproval
disapproving voice
disarming
disarray
disassimilation
disassociate
disassociation (*var. of* dissociation)
disassociation
disaster
> natural d.
> d. stressor
> d. trauma
> d. work
> d. worker

disaster-related
> d.-r. avoidant symptom
> d.-r. intrusive symptom

disastrous
disavow
disavowal level
disavows responsibility
disband
disbelief
discectomy

discern
discernible
discharge
    affective d.
    anxiety d.
    bad conduct d. (BCD)
    cathectic d.
    certificate of disability for d.
      (CDD)
    conditional d.
    corollary d.
    delayed d.
    d. diagnosis
    dishonorable d.
    early d.
    epileptiform d.
    exercise-induced sympathetic d.
    honorable d.
    intensity, severity, and d. (ISD)
    interference pattern of d.
    involuntary d.
    medical d.
    d. pattern
    premature d.
    rate of recovery at d.
    sympathetic d.
discharged against medical advice
    (DAMA)
dischronation
disciplinarian
disciplinary
    d. action
    d. problem
    d. segregation
discipline
    bondage and d.
    brutal d.
    constructive d.
    excessive d.
    formal d.
    harsh d.
    inadequate d.
    inconsistent parental d.
    mental d.
    physical d.
disciplined lifestyle
disclaim
disclose
disclosure
    truth d.
discombobulate
discomfiture

discomfort
    chest d.
    emotional d.
    gender role persistent d.
    d. level
    persistent d.
    physical d.
    threshold of d. (TD)
    d. threshold
    d. with emotion
    d. with gender role
discommodity
discompose
disconcert
disconnected
    d. idea
    d. thought
disconnection
    d. apraxia
    d. hypothesis
    social d.
    d. syndrome
    d. thought disorder
    d. with reality
disconnect speech
disconsolate
discontent
discontinuance
discontinuation
    drug d.
    SSRI d.
discontinuity
discord
    marital d.
discordance
    d. of movement
    d. of voice
discordant
    d. behavior
    d. facial expression
discountenance
discourage
discourse
    spontaneous narrative d.
discourteous
discredit
discreet
discrepancy scale
discrete
    d. emotional response
    d. period
    d. symptom

D

NOTES

discretion
discriminant
    d. analysis
    d. stimulus
    d. validity
discrimination
    age d.
    auditory d.
    brightness d.
    class d.
    color d.
    d. consciousness
    cultural d.
    form d.
    gender d.
    index of d.
    d. learning
    loss d.
    minority d.
    pattern d.
    pitch d.
    racial d.
    reverse d.
    right-left d.
    score d.
    sensory d.
    sexual d.
    training d.
    visual d.
    weight d.
discriminative stimulus
discriminator
discriminatory
    d. behavior
    d. comment
discursive
discuss
discussion
    clinical case d.
    heated d.
    leaderless group d. (LGD)
    open d.
    philosophical d.
discutient
disdain
disease
    Acosta d.
    d. adaptation
    adaptation d.
    affective d.
    alcoholic liver d. (ALD)
    altitude d.
    Alzheimer d. (AD)
    Andes d.
    association d.
    aviator's d.
    Azorean d.
    barbed-wire d.

Bayle d.
Beard d.
behavioral pathology in
    Alzheimer d. (BEHAVE-AD)
biology of affective d.
bodily d.
brain d.
brainstem d.
Brissaud d.
Brodie d.
childhood d.
combined system d.
communicable d.
complex d.
constitutional d.
Cotunnius d.
Creutzfeldt-Jakob d. (CJD)
dancing d.
dementia due to Creutzfeldt-
    Jakob d.
depression spectrum d.
depressive d.
disturbance associated with organic
    mental d.
drug d.
dynamic d.
emotional d.
d. etiology
d. exacerbation
d. exposure
exposure to d.
familial pure depressive d. (FPDD)
fatigue d.
feared d.
flight into d.
d. frequency
Friedreich d.
Fuerstner d.
functional d.
Gaucher d.
genetic d.
genetotrophic d.
hepatolenticular d.
human prion d.
Iceland d.
infantile Gaucher d.
International Classification of D.'s
    (ICD)
International Classification of D.'s,
    Clinical Modification, ed. 9 (ICD-
    9CM)
International Classification of D.'s,
    ed. 9 (ICD-9)
International Classification of D.'s,
    ed. 10 (ICD-10)
Janet d.
juvenile nonneuropathic Niemann-
    Pick d.

Kempf d.
kinky-hair d.
Korsakoff d.
Kraepelin d.
Kraepelin-Morel d.
laughing d.
Lewy body variant of
  Alzheimer d.
life-threatening d.
liver d.
long-term d.
maple sugar syrup urine d.
Marateaux-Lamy d.
Marchiafava-Bignami d.
mental d.
Neftel d.
nervous d.
neurodegenerative d.
occupational d.
organic brain d. (OBD)
d. prevention
prion d.
d. process
progressive d.
psychiatric d.
psychotic d.
pure depressive d.
Saint Dymphna d.
Saint Martin d.
Saint Mathurin d.
Sander d.
Sanfilippo d.
Seitelberger d.
self-induced d.
self-perpetuated d.
self-rated impact of d.
Selter d.
d. severity
sexually transmitted d. (STD)
social d.
sporadic depressive d. (SDD)
Steele-Richardson-Olszewski d.
student's d.
suspected d.
d. theme
venereal d. (VD)
von Hippel-Lindau d.
Werdnig-Hoffmann d.
Westphal d.
white matter d.

Wilson hepatolenticular
  degeneration d.
Winkelman d.
disease-related
  d.-r. change
  d.-r. fatigue
disembody
disenchant
disenfranchise
disengage
disengagement
disentangle
disequilibrium
  neurochemical d.
disesteem
disfavor
disfigure
disfigurement
  facial d.
disfluency
  d. dyskinesia
  speech d.
disgrace
disgruntle
disguise
disguised wish fulfillment
disgust
  feeling of d.
  image eliciting d.
dishabille
disharmonious state of mind
disharmony
  affective d.
  marital d.
dishearten
disheveled
  d. appearance
  d. patient
dishonest simulation of symptom
dishonesty
  professional d.
dishonor
dishonorable discharge
disillusion
disingenuous
disinhibited
  d. type of passive developmental
    disorder
  d. violent behavior
disinhibited-type reactive attachment
  disorder of infancy or childhood

D

NOTES

disinhibition
    emotional d.
    initial d.
    motor d.
    d. psychiatric syndrome
disinhibitory psychopathology
disintegrate
disintegration
    d. anxiety
    d. of consciousness
    personality d.
disintegrative
    d. childhood psychosis
    d. disorder
disinter
disinterest in eater
disjunction
disliked
disloyal
disloyalty
    feeling of d.
dismal
dismantle
dismay
dismember
dismiss
disobedience
    civil d.
disobedient behavior
disobey
disoblige
disodium
disorder
    abnormal involuntary movement d. (AIMD)
    Abraham view of depressive d.
    academic skills d.
    academic underachievement d.
    acquired sexual d.
    acute neuropsychologic d.
    acute paranoid d.
    acute stress d. (ASD)
    addictive d.
    adjustment interface d.
    adjustment reaction conduct d.
    adolescent-onset conduct d.
    adrenal d.
    adult depressive d.
    adult-life psychosexual identity d.
    d. of affect
    affective bipolar d.
    affective determined d.
    affective neurotic personality d.
    affective spectrum d.
    aggressive type undersocialized conduct d.
    agoraphobia without history of panic d.

alcohol amnestic d.
alcohol anxiety d.
alcohol-dependent sleep d.
alcoholic amnestic d.
alcoholic organic mental d.
alcohol-induced psychotic d.
alcohol intoxication-related d.
alcohol mood d.
alcohol-related d.
alcohol-related use d., not otherwise specified
alcohol sleep d.
alcohol use d.
allergic psychogenic d.
alpha-methyldopa-induced mood d.
alternating bipolar d.
alternative criterion B for dysthymic d.
amitriptyline-induced mood d.
amnestic d.
amphetamine delusional d.
amphetamine-related d.
amphetamine use d.
antisocial neurotic personality d.
antisocial personality d. (APD, ASPD)
anxiety adjustment d.
anxiety-avoiding personality d.
anxiety due to physical d.
anxiety psychogenic d.
anxiety-related mental d.
anxiety state neurotic d.
anxiolytic amnestic d.
anxiolytic substance-use d.
anxiolytic use d.
apathetic-type personality d.
aphasia d.
appetite psychogenic d.
apraxic d.
arithmetic d.
arithmetical developmental delay d.
arousal d.
arteriosclerotic brain d.
articulation developmental delay d.
artificial d.
Asperger d.
associated d.
asthenic personality d.
attachment d.
attachment-separation d.
attention d.
attention deficit d. (ADD)
attention deficit and disruptive behavior d. (AD-DBD)
attention deficit hyperactivity d. (ADHD)

attention deficit hyperactivity d.-
predominantly inattentive (ADHD-
PI)
atypical affective d.
atypical anxiety d.
atypical bipolar d.
atypical conduct d.
atypical dissociative d.
atypical eating d.
atypical gender identity d.
atypical impulse-control d.
atypical mixed or other
personality d.
atypical paranoid d.
atypical personality d.
atypical pervasive developmental d.
atypical somatoform d.
atypical specific developmental d.
atypical stereotyped movement d.
atypical tic d.
auditory perceptual d.
autistic d.
autoimmune obsessive-compulsive
tic d.
autonomic arousal d.
avoidant neurotic personality d.
avoidant personality d. (APD)
axis I, II d.
Beck view of depressive d.
behavior d.
behavioral d.
Behr d.
bereavement d.
bereavement-related mood d.
Bibring view of depressive d.
binge eating d.
bipolar affective d.
bipolar depression d.
bipolar I, II d.
bipolar spectrum d.
bipolar type schizoaffective d.
blood psychogenic d.
body dysmorphic d. (BDD)
borderline neurotic personality d.
borderline personality d. (BPD)
bowel d.
brain damage language d.
breathing d.
breathing-related sleep d.
brief posttraumatic stress d.
brief psychotic d.
brief reactive dissociative d.

Briquet d.
caffeine-induced anxiety d.
caffeine-induced sleep d.
caffeine use d.
cannabis delusional d.
cannabis-induced anxiety d.
cannabis-induced delirium d.
cannabis intoxication-related d.
cannabis organic mental d.
cannabis-related d., not otherwise
specified
cannabis use d.
cardiac d.
cardiovascular psychogenic d.
Carroll-Klein model of bipolar d.
catatonic d.
d. category
Center for Stress and Anxiety D.'s
central language d. (CLD)
cerebral d.
character d. (CD)
character impulse d.
characterologic d.
character spectrum d.'s
d. of childhood
childhood anxiety d.
childhood bipolar d.
childhood disintegrative d.
childhood obsessive-compulsive d.
childhood-onset obsessive-
compulsive d.
childhood-onset pervasive
developmental d.
childhood psychosexual identity d.
children and adults with attention
deficit d. (CHADD)
chronic motor tic d.
chronic neuropsychologic d.
chronic posttraumatic stress d.
chronobiological d.
circadian rhythm sleep d.
cluster A, B, C d.
cluster characteristics in
personality d.
cocaine anxiety d.
cocaine delusional d.
cocaine-induced d.
cocaine intoxication-related d.
cocaine mood d.
cocaine-related d., not otherwise
specified
cocaine sleep d.

D

NOTES

disorder *(continued)*

cocaine use d.
codependency d.
coexisting d.
cognition d.
cognitive d.
Cohen view of depressive d.
combined-type attention deficit
  hyperactivity d.
combined-type personality d.
communication d. (CD)
communicative d.
comorbid anxiety d.
comorbid cluster B personality d.
comorbid depressive d.
comorbid mental d.
comorbid mood d.
comorbid psychiatric d.
compensation neurotic d.
complicated grief d.
compulsive neurotic personality d.
compulsive psychogenic d.
conceptual d.
concurrent personality d.
condition not attributable to a
  mental d.
conduct d. (CD)
conduct disturbance adjustment d.
confusional-arousal d.
content thought d.
contiguity d.
conversion d.
conversion-type neurotic
  hysterical d.
convulsive d.
co-occurring addictive d.
co-occurring mental d.
coordination developmental delay d.
coprophemia d.
criteria-defined borderline
  personality d.
cumulative trauma d.
cutaneous psychogenic d.
cyclic mood d.
cyclic psychiatric d.
cyclothymic personality d.
deep brain stimulation for mood d.
delayed posttraumatic stress d.
delirium-related mental d.
delusional paranoid d.
dementia-related mental d.
dependence d.
dependent neurotic personality d.
dependent-passive personality d.
depersonalization neurotic d.
depressed mood adjustment d.
depression neurotic d.
depression-related mental d.

depressive-dysphoric personality d.
depressive personality d.
depressive spectrum d. (DSD)
deteriorated affective d.
deteriorated bipolar d.
developmental arithmetic d.
developmental articulation d.
developmental coordination d.
developmental expressive writing d.
developmental language d.
developmental reading d.
digestive psychogenic d.
disconnection thought d.
disinhibited type of passive
  developmental d.
disintegrative d.
disorganized-type schizophrenic d.
displacement d.
disruptive behavior d.
dissociative identity d. (DID)
dissociative d. not otherwise
  specified (DDNOS)
dissociative trance d.
dissociative-type neurotic
  hysterical d.
dream anxiety d.
drug dependence d.
drug-induced mental d.
drug-related d.
d. due to combined factors
dyscontrol d.
dysmorphic somatoform d.
dysphoric personality d.
dyspneic psychogenic d.
dyssocial personality d.
dysthymic d. (DD)
dysthymic neurotic d.
early childhood behavioral d.
early trauma hypothesis of
  autistic d.
eating d.
ejaculation d.
electroconvulsive therapy-induced
  mood d.
elimination d.
emaciation d.
emancipation d.
emancipatory d.
emotional d. (ED)
emotional disturbance adjustment d.
emotional dyscontrol d.
emotional instability personality d.
emotionally-based d.
emotionally unstable character d.
  (EUCD)
endocrine psychogenic d.
environmental sleep d.
epileptic d.

epileptoid personality d.
episodic affective d.
episodic behavior d.
erectile arousal d.
erotomanic d.
esophagus psychogenic d.
evidence of dissociation d.
d. of excessive sleepiness
d.'s of excessive somnolence
  (DOES)
experimental d.
explosive neurotic personality d.
explosive personality d.
expressive language development d.
expressive writing development d.
extractive d.
extrapyramidal d.
d.'s of extreme stress not
  otherwise specified (DESNOS)
eye psychogenic d.
factitious d., combined type
factitious interface d.
factitious d., physical type
factitious d., psychological type
factitious-type neurotic hysteric d.
false role d.
familial bipolar mood d.
familial hormonal d.
feeding and eating d.
feeding psychogenic d.
female hypoactive sexual desire d.
female orgasmic d.
female sexual arousal d.
fluency d.
food intake d.
formal thought d.
Freud view of depressive d.
frontal perceptual d.
functional psychogenic d.
functional voice d.
gait d.
gambling d.
gastric psychogenic d.
gastrointestinal functional
  psychogenic d.
gender identity d. (GID)
generalized anxiety d. (GAD)
genetic d.
genitourinary psychogenic d.
geriatric depressive d.
grandiose type of paranoid d.
group-type conduct d.

habit d.
hallucinogen-affective d.
hallucinogen-delusional d.
hallucinogen-induced delirium and
  anxiety d.
hallucinogen persisting perception d.
hallucinogen-related d., not
  otherwise specified
hallucinogen use d.
Hartnup d.
heart psychogenic d.
hereditary d.
heterogenous d.
histrionic neurotic personality d.
homosexual conflict d.
hyperactive d.
hyperactive-impulse attention-
  deficit d.
hyperactivity d.
hyperkinetic conduct d.
hyperkinetic impulse d.
hypersomnia d.
hypersomnia-type sleep d.
hypersomnolence d.
hyperthymic personality d.
hypnotic-dependent sleep d.
hypnotic-induced d.
hypnotic use d.
hypoactive sexual desire d.
hypochondriacal psychogenic d.
hypochondriasis neurotic d.
hypomanic d.
hypothermic d.
hypothymic personality d.
hysteria neurotic d.
hysterical gait d.
hysterical movement d.
hysterical personality d.
hysterical psychogenic d.
hysterical psychomotor d.
iatrogenic d.
identity d.
immature personality d.
immune d.
d. of impulse control
impulse control d. (ICD)
impulse control conduct d.
inadequate personality d.
inattentive-type attention deficit
  hyperactivity d.
induced delusional d.
induced paranoid d.

D

NOTES

disorder *(continued)*
>induced psychotic d.
>d. of infancy, childhood, or adolescence
>inhalant-induced d.
>inhalant-related d.
>inhalant use d.
>d. inheritability
>inhibited-type reactive attachment d.
>inhibited-type reactive attachment d. of infancy or early childhood
>d. of initiating and maintaining sleep (DIMS)
>insomnia related to another mental d.
>insomnia-type substance-induced sleep d.
>intelligence d.
>intermittent explosive d.
>Internet addiction d.
>intersensory d.
>intersexual d.
>intestinal psychogenic d.
>intracranial d.
>introverted personality d.
>intrusive sexual d.
>isolated explosive d.
>Jacobson view of depressive d.
>jealous type of paranoid d.
>jet lag sleep d.
>joint psychogenic d.
>Klein view of depressive d.
>labile personality d.
>labyrinthine d.
>language developmental delay d.
>language and speech d.
>late luteal phase dysphoric d.
>later reading d.
>learning development d.
>learning psychogenic d.
>less pervasive d.
>lifelong personality d.
>lifetime anxiety d.
>light-therapy-induced mood d.
>limbic system d.
>limb psychogenic d.
>low back pain psychogenic d.
>low-grade thought d.
>lymphatic psychogenic d.
>major affective d.
>major depressive d. (MDD)
>major mood d.
>major psychiatric d.
>male dyspareunia male erectile d.
>male erectile d.
>male hypoactive sexual desire d.
>malingering d.
>manic bipolar d.

>manic-depressive d.
>marijuana delusional d.
>masochistic personality d.
>mathematics d.
>medication-induced movement d.
>memory d.
>menstrual psychogenic d.
>mental d.
>mental psychoneurotic d.
>mental subnormality d.
>metabolic d.
>micturition psychogenic d.
>mild neurocognitive d.
>minor depressive d.
>mixed anxiety depression d. (MADD)
>mixed development developmental delay d.
>mixed personality d.
>mixed psychoneurotic d.
>mixed specific developmental d.
>monoplegic psychogenic d.
>mood d.
>mood-cyclic d.
>mood spectrum d.
>moral deficiency personality d.
>motility d.
>motor psychogenic d.
>motor skills d.
>motor tic d.
>motor-verbal tic d.
>motor-vocal tic d.
>movement d.
>multiple personality d. (MPD)
>muscle psychogenic d.
>musculoskeletal psychogenic d.
>narcissistic neurotic personality d.
>narcissistic personality d. (NPD)
>negativistic personality d.
>neurasthenia neurotic d.
>neurocirculatory psychogenic d.
>neurocognitive d.
>neurodevelopmental d.
>neuroleptic-induced acute movement d.
>neuroleptic treatment of childhood conduct d.
>neurologic d.
>neuropsychiatric movement d.
>neuropsychologic d.
>neurotic hysteric d.
>neurotic mental d.
>neurotic personality d.
>nicotine-induced d.
>nicotine organic brain d.
>nicotine-related d., not otherwise specified
>nicotine use d.

nightmare d.
nonaggressive-type undersocialized
  conduct d.
nonfearful panic d.
nonorganic steep d.
nonpsychotic mental d.
nonpsychotic psychiatric d.
nonstress-induced personality d.
nonsubstance-induced mental d.
non-tic-related obsessive-
  compulsive d.
nontranssexual cross-gender d.
no trauma personality d.
nutritional deficiency d.
obsessional personality d.
obsessive-compulsive d. (OCD)
obsessive-compulsive neurotic d.
obsessive-compulsive personality d.
  (OCPD)
obsessive personality d.
obsessive psychogenic d.
occupational neurotic d.
occupational psychogenic d.
OCD spectrum d.
opioid-induced psychotic d.
opioid use d.
oppositional d.
oppositional defiant d. (ODD)
oppression-artifact d.
organic anxiety d.
organic brain d. (OBD)
organic delusional d.
organic mental d. (OMD)
organic mood d.
organic personality d.
organic psychiatric d.
orgasmic d.
orientation d.
other type personality d.
overanxious d.
overconscientious personality d.
overreactive d.
over-the-counter drug-related d.
pain somatoform d.
panic d. (PD)
paralytic psychosomatic d.
paranoid neurotic personality d.
paranoid-schizotypal personality d.
paranoid-type schizophrenic d.
paraphiliac coercive d.
parasomnia-type substance-induced
  sleep d.

passive-aggressive neurotic
  personality d.
past lifetime d.
pathologic gambling d. (PGD)
PCP-induced anxiety d.
PCP-related d., not otherwise
  specified
perception d.
perceptual d.
periluteal phase dysphoric d.
permissive hypothesis of
  affective d.'s
persecutory delusional d.
persecutory type of paranoid d.
persistent vegetative state d.
persisting d.
personality d. (PD)
personality change d.
personality neurotic d.
pervasive anger d.
pervasive developmental d. (PDD)
pervasive disinhibited type of
  developmental d.
phencyclidine delusional d.
phencyclidine-induced d.
phencyclidine-related d.
phencyclidine use d.
phobic neurotic d.
phobic psychogenic d.
phonological d.
physical comorbid d.
physical psychogenic d.
pica d.
polysubstance-related d.
polysubstance use d.
positive thought d.
possession trance d.
postconcussion d.
posthallucinogen perception d.
postpsychotic depressive d.
posttraumatic dissociative d.
posttraumatic personality d.
posttraumatic stress d. (PTSD)
preexisting mental d.
premenstrual dysphoric d. (PMDD)
prescription drug-related d.
presenile mental d.
primary affective d. (PAD)
primary anxiety d.
primary behavior d.
primary care evaluation of
  mental d.'s (PRIME-MD)

NOTES

disorder *(continued)*

primary mood d.
primary psychiatric d.
primary thought d.
processing d.
prolonged posttraumatic stress d.
pruritic psychosomatic d.
pseudosocial personality d.
psychiatric comorbid d.
psychiatric system interface d.
psychic d.
psychoactive substance abuse d.
psychoactive substance-induced
  organic mental d.
psychoactive substance use d.
psychoaffective d. (PAD)
psychogenic learning d.
psychogenic limb d.
psychogenic motor d.
psychogenic muscle d.
psychogenic musculoskeletal d.
psychogenic neurocirculatory d.
psychogenic obsessional d.
psychogenic pain d.
psychogenic phobic d.
psychogenic respiratory d.
psychogenic rheumatic d.
psychogenic sexual d.
psychogenic skin d.
psychogenic sleep d.
psychogenic stomach d.
psychomotor d.
psychoneurotic mental d.
psychophysiologic d.
psychosexual gender identity d.
psychosomatic paralytic d.
psychosomatic pruritic d.
psychosomatic skin d.
psychotic mental d.
psychotic presenile mental d.
pyromania d.
Rado view of depressive d.
rapid-cycling bipolar d.
reactive attachment d.
reading developmental delay d.
receptive language d.
rectal psychogenic d.
recurrent brief depressive d.
recurrent mood d.
Reitan rules to assess learning d.
related sleep d.
REM behavior d. (RBD)
REM sleep behavior d.
REM sleep-related d.
repetitive impulse d.
residual-type schizophrenic d.
resistant mood d.
resonance d.

respiratory impairment sleep d.
respiratory psychogenic d.
retardation developmental delay d.
Rett d.
rheumatic psychogenic d.
rumination d.
sadistic personality d.
sadomasochistic personality d.
Sandler view of depressive d.
schizoaffective d.
schizoid neurotic personality d.
schizoid-schizotypal personality d.
  (SSPD)
schizophrenia spectrum d.
schizophrenic d.
schizophreniform d.
schizotypal personality d.
seasonal affective d. (SAD)
seasonal mood d.
secondary mood d.
secondary sleep d.
sedative, hypnotic, or anxiolytic-
  induced anxiety d.
sedative-induced d.
sedative use d.
seductive personality d.
self-defeating personality d.
self-perceived cognitive d.
Seligman view of depressive d.
semantic pragmatic d.
semantogenic d.
senile psychotic mental d.
separation anxiety d. (SAD)
sexual arousal d.
sexual aversion d.
sexual desire d.
sexual deviance d.
sexual deviation neurotic d.
sexual and gender identity d.
sexual pain d.
sexual psychogenic d.
sham d.
shamanistic thought d.
shared paranoid d.
shared psychotic d.
shift work-related sleep d.
shyness d.
simple deteriorative d.
situational-type female orgasmic d.
situational-type female sexual
  arousal d.
skin psychogenic d.
sleep behavior d.
sleep psychogenic d.
sleep starts d.
sleeptalking d.
sleep terror d.
sleep-wake schedule d.

sleep-wake transition d.
sleepwalking d.
social anxiety d.
socialized conduct d.
sociopathic personality d. (SPD)
solitary aggressive-type conduct d.
somatic paranoid d.
somatization neurotic d.
somatizing d.
somatoform interface d.
somatoform pain d. (SPD)
somatopsychic d.
specific developmental d. (SDD)
spectrum d.
speech developmental delay d.
speech and language d.
spoken language d.
stereotyped movement d.
stereotypic movement d. (SMD)
stereotypy and habit d.
stimulant-dependent sleep d.
stress d.
stress-induced personality d.
stress-related d.
subaffective d.
substance abuse and dependence d.
substance-induced organic mental d.
substance-induced psychotic d.
substance-related d.
substance use d.
substitution d.
subsyndromal thought d.
sympathomimetic delusional d.
tactile-perceptual d.
taxonomy of anger d.
temporal-perceptual d.
temporary personality d.
thinking d.
thought process d.
thyroid d.
tic d.
tic-related obsessive-compulsive d.
time and rhythm d.
tobacco use d.
Tourette d.
toxic d.
trance-possession d.
transient situational personality d.
transient tic d.
trauma spectrum d.
unaggressive conduct d.
underachievement d.

undersocialized d.
undifferentiated attention-deficit d.
undifferentiated somatoform d.
undifferentiated-type conduct d.
undifferentiated-type
   schizophrenic d.
unhappiness and misery d.
unipolar d.
unitary d.
unknown substance-induced
   mood d.
unsocialized aggressive d.
unspecified mental d.
violent conduct d.
visceral d.
visuospatial d.
vocal, chronic motor, or tic d.
voice d.
well-delineated psychiatric d.
withdrawal d.
withdrawal-related mood d.
writing d.
d. of written expression

disordered
d. mentally
d. mental status
d. personality
d. personality function
d. relating
d. thinking

disorderly
d. conduct
drunk and d.

disorganization
autonomic d.
cerebral d.
cognitive d.
conceptual d.
developing psychotic d.
d. dimension
d. dimension of positive
   schizophrenic symptoms
linguistic d.
mental d.
psychotic d.
spatial d.
d. syndrome
thought d.

disorganized
d. attachment behavior
d. delusion
d. factor

D

NOTES

disorganized *(continued)*
    d. factor in schizophrenia
    d. forms of attachment
    d. speech
    d. speech assessment
    d. speech in schizophrenia
    d. state
    d. subtype
    d. symptom complex
    d. thinking
disorganized-type
    d.-t. schizophrenia
    d.-t. schizophrenic disorder
disorient
disorientation
    auditory d.
    autopsychic d.
    graphic d.
    posttraumatic d.
    right-left d.
    spatial d.
    speech d.
    thought d.
    time d.
    topographical d.
    visuospatial d.
disoriented
    d. attachment behavior
    d. forms of attachment
    d. patient
disown
disparage
disparaging remark
disparity
    phase d.
    vision d.
dispassionate concern
dispel
dispensation
disperse
dispersion
    response d.
dispirited
displaceability of libido
displaced
    d. child syndrome
    d. person
displacement
    activity d.
    affect d.
    d. of affect
    brainstem d.
    character d.
    d. defense mechanism
    d. disorder
    dream d.
    geographic d.
    guilt d.

    retroactive d.
    d. substitute
    symbolic d.
    d. wit
display
    affect d.
    emotional d.
    facial d.
displease
displeasure
disposition
    constitutional depressive d.
    constitutional manic d.
    personal d.
    placid d.
    polymorphous perverse d.
    d. system
    volatile d.
dispraise
disproportion
disproportionate impairment
disprove
disputatious
dispute
disputing
disqualify
disquiet
disquietude
    patient d.
disregard for rules
disreputable
disrepute
disrespectful treatment
disrobing
    inappropriate d.
disrupt
disrupted
    d. relationship
    d. sleep organization
disrupted, dysfunctional relational functioning
disruption
    d. of affective bonds
    behavior d.
    brain function d.
    cognitive d.
    family d.
    level of d.
    marital d.
    d. of normal activity
    sleep d.
disruptive
    d. behavior
    d. behavior disorder
    d. emotion
    d. family functioning
    d. impact
    d. psychotic patient

dissatisfaction
    body d.
    marital d.
dissectible cognitive operation
dissemble
disseminata
    alopecia d.
disseminate
    alopecia d.
dissemination
    evaluation d.
dissension
dissent
disservice
dissidence
dissident
dissimilar
dissimilation rule
dissimulation
dissimulator
dissipate
dissipation
    heat d.
dissociable
dissociate
dissociated
    d. learning
    d. sensory loss
    d. state
dissociate-dysmnesic
    d.-d. substitution
    d.-d. substitution reaction
dissociation, disassociation
    adult d.
    d. defense mechanism
    d. of learning
    d. level
    d. measure
    nonpathological d.
    pathological d.
    peritraumatic d.
    semantic d.
    d. sensibility
    sensory d.
    sleep d.
    d. syndrome
    visual-kinetic d.
dissociative
    d. amnesia
    d. anesthesia
    d. anesthetic
    d. capacity

    d. disorder not otherwise specified (DDNOS)
    d. episode
    d. experience
    d. fugue
    d. hysteria
    d. hysteria psychoneurosis
    d. identity disorder (DID)
    d. paranoia
    d. patient
    d. phenomenon
    d. psychoneurosis
    d. psychoneurotic reaction
    d. response
    d. state
    d. symptom
    d. symptom cluster
    d. tendency
    d. trance
    d. trance disorder
dissociative-type
    d.-t. hysterical neurosis
    d.-t. neurotic hysteria
    d.-t. neurotic hysterical disorder
dissolute
dissolution
dissonance
    cognitive d.
dissonant
dissuade
dissuasive
distal distinctive feature analysis
distance
    d. ceptor
    emotional d.
    functional d.
    optimal interpersonal d.
    d. perception
    professional d.
    d. receptor
    social d.
    sociometric d.
distancing
    cognitive d.
distant
    emotionally d.
distasteful
distension
distinct
    d. depressed presentation
    d. dysphoric presentation
    d. euphoric presentation

D

NOTES

distinction
    primary-secondary d.
distinctive feature analysis
distingue
distinguish
distort
distorted
    d. body image
    d. communication in schizophrenia
    d. grief
    d. ideas of reference
    d. inferential thinking
    d. language in schizophrenia
    d. perception
    d. perception of reality
distortion
    apperceptive d.
    auditory d.
    body-image d.
    cognitive d.
    compromise d.
    ego d.
    figure-ground d.
    inferential behavioral monitoring d.
    d. of inferential behavioral
      monitoring
    inferential perception d.
    d. of inferential thinking
    d. of interpretation
    intrapsychic d.
    language and communication d.
    d. of language and communication
    memory d.
    metonymic d.
    nonlinear d.
    paratactic d.
    parataxic d.
    perceptual d.
    psychological d.
    psychotic d.
    reality d.
    social avoidance and d.
    spatial d.
    subjective d.
    time d.
    transient d.
    visual d.
    visual-spatial d.
distract
    easy to d.
distracted easily
distractibility
    easy d.
distractible speech
distracting stimuli
distraction
distraught
    d. former lover

    d. former partner
    d. spouse
distress
    acute d.
    caregiver d.
    chronic mental d.
    clinically significant d.
    emotional d.
    event-related d.
    general psychological d.
    global index of d.
    intense psychological d.
    intrapsychic d.
    menopausal d.
    mental d.
    physical symptom d.
    posttraumatic d.
    present d.
    psychic d.
    psychological d.
    separation d.
    sexual orientation d.
    social avoidance and d. (SAD)
    spiritual d.
    subjective d.
    d. thought
    d. tolerance skills
    unconscious d.
distressing
    d. circumstance
    d. dream
    d. thought
distributed
    d. effort
    d. memory
    d. processing
distribution
    bimodal d.
    binomial d.
    chi-square d.
    contrastive d.
    d. of control
    d. curve
    fixed d.
    frequency d.
    gaussian d.
    illicit drug d.
    noncontrastive d.
    normal d.
    Poisson d.
    d. of power
    regional d.
    d. of responsibility
    skew d.
    unequal d.
distributive
    d. analysis
    d. analysis and synthesis

district
    red-light d.
distrust
    interpersonal d.
    malevolent d.
    pervasive d.
disturbance
    acid-base d.
    activity and attention d.
    acute situational d.
    adjustment reaction d.
    affective d.
    amphetamine intoxication, with
        perceptual d.
    analyzing new information d.
    anxiety d.
    aphasic d.
    appetite d.
    appetitive d.
    assimilating information d.
    d. associated with conversion
        phenomenon
    d. associated with organic mental
        disease
    d. of attention
    attentional d.
    behavioral d.
    d. of behavioral activation
    behavioral set of d.'s
    d. between clauses
    body conceptualization d.
    body-image d.
    cannabis intoxication, with
        perceptual d.
    chronic sleep d.
    chronobiological d.
    cocaine intoxication, with
        perceptual d.
    cognitive d.
    compulsive d.
    concentration d.
    conceptual d.
    conduct d.
    consciousness d.
    d. in content of thought
    core cognitive d.
    domestic d.
    eating d.
    electrolyte d.
    emotional d.
    executive functioning d.
    explosive d.

fluctuating mood d.
fluency d.
fluid d.
d. in form of thinking
frequency d.
functioning d.
gait d.
habit d.
high-level perceptual d.
hyperkinetic d.
identity d.
infancy and early childhood d.
d. of intellectual development
intermittent explosive d.
isolated explosive d.
language d.
learning new information d.
level of d.
linguistic d.
d. of memory
memory d.
mental d.
metabolic d.
mixed symptom picture with
    perceptual d.
mood d.
motor skill d.
oculomotor d.
perception d.
d. of perception
perceptual motor abilities d.
d. in perceptual motor ability
personality pattern d.
personality trait d.
phencyclidine intoxication, with
    perceptual d.
physical d.
planning d.
posttraumatic d.
predominant mood d.
psychiatric d.
psychic d.
psychographic d.
psychological d.
psychomotor d.
psychotic d.
rate of fluency d.
reasoning d.
recalling new information d.
sensory d.
d. in sexual desire
sexual desire d.

D

NOTES

205

disturbance *(continued)*
    sexual orientation d.
    situational d.
    sleep continuity d.
    socialized d.
    social relatedness d.
    sociopathic personality d. (SPD)
    speech d.
    d. in speech
    speed of information processing d.
    SSRI-induced sexual d.
    stress-related d.
    d. in suggestibility
    superego d.
    thought d.
    transient emotional d.
    transient situational d.
    undersocialized socialized d.
    visual field d.
    will d.
    d. of the will
    d. within clauses
    word-finding ability d.
disturbed
    d. adolescent
    d. attachment relationship
    d. body image
    d. eating behavior
    emotionally d. (ED)
    d. home environment
    d. interpersonal relationship (DIR)
    d. orientation
    d. person
    d. personality
    d. sense of self
    d. sleep
    d. sleep pattern
    d. social relatedness
    d. ward
disturbing
    d. behavior
    d. experience
    d. feeling
    d. thought
disturb the peace
disunite
disunity
disuse principle
disutility
disvalue
ditch
    last d.
dither
diuresis
diuretic
diuretic misuse
diurnal
    d. enuresis

    d. epilepsy
    d. mood variation
diurnus
    pavor d.
divagate
divagation
diverge
divergence circuit
divergent
    d. production
    d. thinking
diverging trend
diverse
    d. group
    d. medicinal application
    d. need
diversion
diversional therapy
diversionary activity
diversity
    cultural d.
    group d.
    sensitivity to d.
diversive exploration
divest
divination
diving reflex
division
divisive
divorce
    community d.
    coparental d.
    d. counseling
    d. decree
    economic d.
    emotional consequences of d.
    legal d.
    overt behavior consequences of d.
    parental d.
    psychic d.
    d. rate
    d. therapy
divorced status
divorcee
divulge
divulsion
dixyrazine
dizygotic twins
dizziness
dizzy spell
DKA
    olanzapine-associated D.
DLP
    developmental learning problem
DMH
    Department of Mental Health
DMT
    dimethyltryptamine

DNA
> deoxyribonucleic acid
> DNA transcription factor

DNR
> do not resuscitate

do
> do not resuscitate (DNR)
> tae kwon do

d'Ocagne nomogram
docile
docility
docket
doctor
> general medical d.
> hex d.
> medical d.
> root d.
> d. shopping
> witch d.

doctor-patient relationship
Doctors Without Borders
doctrine
> dualistic d.
> Flourens d.
> neuron d.
> parental right d.

documentation
> confidential d.

doddering
dodger
doer
DOES
> disorders of excessive somnolence

dog
> guide d.
> top d.
> d. track gambling

dog-eat-dog attitude
dogged
dogma
dogmatic
do-gooder
doing
> learning by d.

dolce vita
doldrums
doleful
Dole-Nyswauder program
doll's
> d. eye reaction
> d. eye reflex
> d. eye sign

dolor capitis
dolorific
dolorimetry
dolorogenic zone
dolorology
dolorosa
> analgesia d.
> anesthesia d.
> facies d.

dolorous
domain
> adaptive skill d.
> cognitive d.
> d. of functioning
> neuropsychologic d.
> outcome d.
> spiritual d.

domestic
> d. aggression
> d. disturbance
> d. environment
> d. fight
> d. medicine
> d. quarrel
> d. violence (DV)

domesticated pride
domicile
domiciliary care home
dominance
> cerebral d.
> crossed d.
> eye d.
> feeling of d.
> d. hierarchy
> lateral d.
> left hemisphere d.
> manual d.
> mixed cerebral d.
> right hemisphere d.
> social d.
> territorial d.
> d. test
> theory of social d.
> time d.
> X-linked d.

dominant
> d. association
> autosomal d.
> bystander dominates initial d. (BDID)
> d. character
> d. characteristic

D

NOTES

dominant (*continued*)
    d. culture
    d. delusional belief
    d. determinant
    d. feature
    d. gene
    d. genotype
    d. hand
    d. hemisphere
    d. hemisphere parietal area
    d. hemisphere temporal area
    d. idea
    d. language
    d. laterality
    left-hand d.
    d. mentality
    mixed foot d.
    d. person
    d. personality
    right-hand d.
    d. spouse
    d. trait
    d. waking frequency
dominant-subordinate behavior
dominate
domination
    sexual d.
dominatrix
domineering
Don
    D. Juanism
    D. Juan syndrome
    D. Juan type
    D. Quixote
Donaldson
    O'Connor vs D.
donna
    prima d.
do-not-care attitude
do-nothing
doom
    feeling of d.
    impending d.
    sense of impending d.
doomsayer
doomsday
door
    revolving d.
door-in-the-face effect
dopamine
    d. agonist
    brain d.
    d. clearance
    d. D_2 receptor
    d. hypothesis
    mesolimbic d.
    d. metabolism
    d. metabolite

    d. neurotransmission
    d. pathway
    d. projection
    d. ratio
    d. receptor sensitivity
    d. release
    d. reuptake
    d. stimulation
    d. synthesis
    d. system
    d. transporter
    d. uptake site
dopaminergic
    d. antagonist
    d. drug
    d. effect
    d. hyperactivity
    d. inhibition
    d. medication-induced postural tremor
    d. modulation
    d. pathway
    d. stimulant
    d. synapse
    d. system
    d. tone
    d. tract
dope dealer
Doppelganger phenomenon
Doppler
    D. shift
DO psychiatrist
Dora case
doramania
Dorian love
d'orient
    mal d.
dormant
dormido
    sangue d.
dormifacient
dormitory
doromania
dorsal
    d. anterior cingulate region
    d. column stimulation
    d. gray matter
    d. limbic region
    d. neocortical region
    d. raphe nuclei
    d. reflex
    d. vagus complex
dorsolateral
    d. pathway
    d. prefrontal cortex
    d. prefrontal cortical area
dorsum

dosage
 equivalent d.
 medication d.
 neuroleptic d.
 total neuroleptic d.
dose
 anticholinergic d.
 clinically recommended d.
 cumulative d.
 daily d.
 d. dependent
 effective d.
 d. escalation
 full d.
 improper d.
 lethal d. (LD)
 lithium d.
 low d.
 maintenance d.
 marginally therapeutic d.
 maximum permissible d.
 maximum recommended human d.
  (MRHD)
 measured d.
 minimum d.
 missed d.
 modal d.
 neuroleptic d.
 optimum d.
 oral d.
 permissible d.
 priming d.
 d. range
 recommended d.
 d. reduction
 d. reduction method
 d. reduction strategy
 sequential d.
 standard d.
 steady-state d.
 subtherapeutic d.
 therapeutic d.
 tolerance d.
 toxic d.
dose-dependent effect
dose-related difference
dose-response
 d.-r. curve
 d.-r. relation
 d.-r. relationship
dosimetric medicine

dosing
 energy d.
 fixed d.
 flexible neuroleptic d.
 neuroleptic d.
 set-by-age d.
dotage
dote
dothiepin
dot-probe task
double
 d. assimilation
 d. bind
 d. blind
 d. blind experiment
 d. blind theory
 d. consciousness
 delire en partie d.
 d. depression
 d. entendre
 d. hemiplegia
 illusion of d.'s
 d. insanity
 d. masked experiment
 d. meaning
 d. orientation
 d. personality
 d. simultaneous stimulation (DSS)
 d. standard
 subjective d.'s
 d. superego
 d. take
 d. taper
 d. vision
double-agentry
double-blind drug study
double-cross
double-dealing
double-dome
double-edged
double-entendre
double-faced
double-point threshold
doublespeak
doublethink
doubling
doubly
doubt
 d.'s of loyalty
 morbid d.
 obsessive d.
 d.'s of trustworthiness

D

NOTES

doubtful
doubting
    d. insanity
    d. mania
    d. spell
douce
    mort d.
doughty
dour
doute
    folie du d.
    maladie du d.
douze
    folie á d.
dowdy
down
    back d.
    dress d.
    d. from overdose
    gunned d.
    let d.
    shoot d.
    simmer d.
    slap d.
    stare d.
    take d.
    talk d.
    tear d.
    ups and d.'s
    wear d.
    weigh d.
down-and-out
downbeat nystagmus
downcast
downfall
downgrade
downhearted
downhill
downplay
down-regulated
downright
downsizing
down-the-line
down-to-earth
downtrodden
downturned corners of the mouth
downward drift
doze
DPJ
    dementia paralytica juvenilis
DPM
    diploma in psychological medicine
DPP
    dropout prediction and prevention
DPT
    dipropyltryptamine
dr
    unusual rare detail response

drab
Dragons
    Dungeons and D.
dramatic
    d. affect
    d. behavioral swing
    d. emotional cluster
    d. interpersonal relationship
    d. interpersonal style
    d. play
    d. speech
dramatism
dramatization
dramatize
DRAMS
    drug risk analysis message system
drapetomania
drastic
drawback
drawing
    d. ability
    automatic d.
    compulsive d.
    copying d.'s (CD)
    d. disability
    mirror d.
    d. test
drawl
drawn laughter
dread
    feeling of d.
    d. of insanity
    talion d.
dreaded situation
dream, dreamer
    anxiety d.
    d. anxiety attack
    d. anxiety disorder
    artificial d.
    d. association
    bad d.
    d. censorship
    clairvoyant d.
    color d.
    color in d.
    comfort d.
    consolation d.
    d. content
    convalescent d.
    convenience d.
    corroborating d.
    counter-wish d.
    day d.
    decomposition in d.'s
    detailed d.
    d. determinant
    d. displacement
    distressing d.

dream within a d.
d. ego
d. embarrassment
embarrassment d.
erotic d.
examination d.
exhibition d.
d. experience
d. exploration
frightening d.
frustration d.
d. function
d. illusion
d. induction
d. interpretation
made-to-order d.
manifest d.
masochistic wish d.
d. pain
paired d.'s
parallel d.
perennial d.
pipe d.
prophetic d.
punishment d.
d. recall
reconstruction d.
recurrent d.
recurring d.
d. screen
secondary elaboration of d.
Sisyphus d.
speech in d.
d. state
d. stimulus
d. symbolism
telepathic d.
terror d.
d. time
d. up
veridical d.
vivid d.
wet d.
wish d.
d. work
d. world
dreamer
dreaming
    amnesia for sleep and d.
dreamland
dreamless sleep

dreamlike
    d. hallucination
    d. state
dream-work
dreamy state
dreary
dredge
dress down
dressing
    d. apraxia
    cross d.
drift
    downward d.
    genetic d.
    d. hypothesis
    observer d.
drifter
drink
    malternative d.
    mixed d.
    d.'s per drinking day
drinker
    binge d.
    chronic d.
    closet d.
    compulsive d.
    evening d.
    incurable problem d. (IPD)
    jag d.
    periodic d.
    problem d. (PD)
    repeated heavy d.
    social d.
    weekend d.
drinking
    aftereffect of d.
    air d.
    alcohol d.
    d. behavior
    binge d.
    compulsive water d.
    controlled d.
    days of heavy d.
    d. days per week
    dyssocial d.
    early onset d.
    escape d.
    evening d.
    d. history
    inveterate d.
    jag d.
    light d.

D

NOTES

drinking (continued)
    morning d.
    nonproblematic d.
    occupational d.
    paroxysmal d.
    periodic d.
    problem d.
    recreational d.
    social d.
    somatopathic d.
    state markers of heavy d.
    volitional d.
    water d.
    weekend d.

drive
    absent d.
    achievement d.
    acquired d.
    activity d.
    affectional d.
    affiliation d.
    aggressive d.
    appetitive d.
    aversive d.
    d. behavior
    biologic d.
    destructive d.
    ego d.
    elimination d.
    erotic d.
    exploration d.
    exploratory d.
    fear d.
    hedonic d.
    homonomy d.
    hunger d.
    innate d.
    internal d.
    kinetic d.
    learned d.
    libidinal d.
    manipulative d.
    maternal d.
    obstruction d.
    paternal d.
    physiological d.
    primary d.'s
    d. reduction
    d. reduction theory
    repressed instinctual d.
    secondary d.'s
    sex d.
    stimulus d. (Sd)
    subjective d.
    thermal d.
    thirst d.
drive-by shooting
drivel

driveling dementia
driven
    d. motor behavior
    treatment d.
drivenness
driver
    drunk d.
    slave d.
driver's
    d. rage
    d. seat
driving
    d. behavior
    behavior while d.
    erratic d.
    photic d.
    reckless d.
    d. under the influence (DUI)
    d. while intoxicated (DWI)
DRO
    differential reinforcement of other
      behavior
droit
droll
dromolepsy
dromomania
drone
droning speech
drool
drooping eyelid
drop
    d. attack
    knockout d.'s
    toe d.
    wrist d.
dropout
    d. prediction and prevention (DPP)
    d. rate
    school d.
    treatment d.
drowsiness
    cannabis-induced d.
    continuous daytime d.
    daytime d.
    incapacitating d.
    pathologic d.
drowsy
DRSP
    daily record of severity of problems
drub
drubbing
drudge
drudgery
drug
    abreactive d.
    d. abstinence
    d. abstinence syndrome
    d. abuse

d.'s of abuse
abuse of nonprescribed d.
d. abuser
d. abuse rehabilitation program
d. abuse scale
D. Abuse Warning Network
 (DAWN)
d. action
d. addict
addicting d.
d. addiction
addictive potential of d.
add-on d.
d. administration
d. allergy
alpha adrenergic blocking d.
alpha adrenergic stimulating d.
antagonist d.
antianxiety d.
anticholinergic d.
anticonvulsant d.
antidepressant d.
antipsychotic d.
antiseizure d.
anxiolytic d.
d. assay
ataractic d.
atypical antipsychotic d.
d. augmentation
autonomic sympathomimetic d.
beta-adrenergic blocking d.
d. binge
butyrophenone-based neuroleptic d.
catatonic d.
combination d. (CD)
d. consumption
conventional antipsychotic d.
conventional neuroleptic d.
d. counseling
d. counselor
d. court program
d. craving
d. culture
dangerous d.
date rape d.
d. dealer
d. defaulter
d. dependence
d. dependence disorder
depot-administered antipsychotic d.
designer d.
d. desire

diet d.
d. discontinuation
d. disease
dopaminergic d.
d. education
d. effect
d. efficacy
D. Enforcement Administration
 number (DEA#)
experimental d.
d. family
gateway d.
d. habit
d. half-life
hallucinatory d.
hallucinogenic d.
heterocyclic antidepressant d.
high-dose d.
d. high-risk behavior
d. holiday
d. hunger
hypnotic d.
hypnotic-sedative d.
illegal d.
illicit psychoactive d.
d. information (DI)
d. information center (DIC)
d. information log (DIL)
d. ingestion
inhalation of d.
d. insanity
d. interaction (DI)
d. intervention
d. intolerance
d. intoxication
investigational d.
investigational new d. (IND)
legal d.
d. level
licit psychoactive d.
d. maintenance
maintenance d.
d. maintenance treatment
d. management
mind-altering d.
mood-altering d.
mood-elevating d.
narcotic agonist d.
narcotic antagonist d.
narcotic blocking d.
neuroleptic d.
new-generation antipsychotic d.

D

NOTES

drug *(continued)*
  nonprescription d.
  nonpsychotropic d.
  noradrenergic d.
  nosotropic d.
  novel antipsychotic d.
  orphan d.
  d. overdose
  over-the-counter drug d.
  d. paraphernalia
  parasympathomimetic d.
  parenteral d.
  d. pathological intoxication
  d. possession
  d. preparation
  prescription d.
  psychoactive d.
  psychodysleptic d.
  psychogenic d.
  d. psychosis
  d. psychosis hallucinatory state
  psychostimulant d.
  psychotherapeutic d.
  psychotomimetic d.
  psychotropic d. (PTD)
  rave d.
  recreational d.
  d. regimen
  d. reinforcement
  d. related
  d. response rate
  d. risk analysis message system
    (DRAMS)
  d. risk behavior
  schedule d.
  d. screen
  second-generation antipsychotic d.
  sedative d.
  sedative-hypnotic d.
  self-administration of
    psychoactive d. (SAPD)
  street d.
  d. supply
  sympathomimetic d.
  d. tapering
  tertiary amine tricyclic
    antidepressant d.
  d. tetanus
  d. theft
  d. therapy
  d. tolerance
  d. toxicity
  d. trading
  d. traffic
  d. trafficking
  d. transporter
  tricyclic d.
  tricyclic antidepressant d. (TCAD)

  d. trip
  unaltered d.
  d. under investigation
  d. use behavior
  d. use frequency
  d. use history
  d. user
  d. use review (DUR)
  d. war
  war on d.
  d. washout
  d. withdrawal
  d. withdrawal seizure
  d. withdrawal syndrome
  wonder d.
drug-addictive behavior
drug-associated
  d.-a. mortality
  d.-a. weight gain
drug-containing capsule
drug-dependent
  d.-d. individual
  d.-d. insomnia
drug-facilitated interview
drug-free
  d.-f. condition
  d.-f. day
  d.-f. employee
  d.-f. patient
  d.-f. period
drug-fueled music marathon
drug-induced
  d.-i. confusional state
  d.-i. convulsion
  d.-i. delirium
  d.-i. dementia
  d.-i. depression
  d.-i. dystonia
  d.-i. floating sensation
  d.-i. hallucination
  d.-i. hallucinatory state
  d.-i. hallucinosis
  d.-i. high
  d.-i. mania
  d.-i. medical complication
  d.-i. mental disorder
  d.-i. negative symptom
  d.-i. paranoid state
  d.-i. parkinsonism
  d.-i. psychosis
  d.-i. seizure
  d.-i. semihypnotic state
  d.-i. sexual dysfunction
  d.-i. syndrome
  d.-i. treatment
drug-injecting equipment
drug-like desire state
drugmaker

drug-negative urine
drug-related
  d.-r. brain damage
  d.-r. crime
  d.-r. disorder
  d.-r. HIV risk behavior
  d.-r. incarceration
  d.-r. insomnia
  d.-r. sexual side effect
  d.-r. violence
drug-resistant depression
drug-responsive treatment
drug-seeking behavior
drug-using
  d.-u. man
  d.-u. woman
drum up
drunk
  blind d.
  d. and disorderly
  d. driver
  dry d.
  legally d.
drunkard
drunken
drunkenness
  acute d.
  alcoholic d.
  chronic d.
  ether d.
  maudlin d.
  pathologic d.
  pathological d.
  public d.
  simple alcoholic d.
  sleep d.
  sleeping d.
drunkometer
dry
  d. drunk
  d. leprosy
  d. mouth
  d. orgasm
  d. out
  d. up
dry-eye
DS
  digit span
  digit symbol
Ds
  associative response to a white space on
  a card

DSA
  digital subtraction angiography
DSD
  depression sine depression
  depressive spectrum disorder
DSDB
  direct self-destructive behavior
DSH
  deliberate self-harm
DSM
  Diagnostic and Statistical Manual
    DSM clusters
    DSM diagnosis
    DSM disorder overlap
DSM-IV
  Diagnostic and Statistical Manual,
    Revision IV
    DSM-IV axis II criterion
    DSM-IV description
DSM-IV-R classification
DSS
  disability status scale
  double simultaneous stimulation
DSUH
  direct suggestion under hypnosis
DT
  delirium tremens
  dipole tracing
  duration tetany
DTC
  day treatment center
DTR
  deep tendon reflex
dual
  d. addiction
  d. ambivalence
  d. diagnosis
  d. diagnosis patient
  d. diagnosis program
  d. leadership
  d. mechanism of action
  d. personality
  d. purpose
  d. relationship
  d. transference therapy
dual-arousal model
dual-instinct theory
dualism
  mind-body d.
  psychic d.
dualistic doctrine
dual-process theory

D

NOTES

215

dual-sex therapy
dub
dubiety
dubious
dubitable
Dubois method
Dubowitz syndrome
dud
duel
duende
due process
duffer
DUI
   driving under the influence
dulcify
dull
   d. affect
   borderline d.
   d. normal range
dullard
dullness
   emotional d.
dumbfound
dumbness
   word d.
dumbstruck
Dunedin Multidisciplinary Health and Development Study
Dungeons and Dragons
dupe
duplex transmission
duplicate
duplication of ego
duplicative reaction
duplicity
DUR
   drug use review
durable power of attorney
dural graft matrix
duraplasty
duration
   d. of drug action
   d. duty cycle
   emergency dyscontrol d.
   minimum d.
   d. of mood
   short sleep d.
   d. tetany (DT)
   treatment d.
   d. of treatment
   d. of worry
duress
   episodic dyscontrol d.
Durham
   D. decision
   D. rule
   D. test
Durkheim theory of suicide

dusky
Dutch courage
duteous
dutiful
duty
   line of d.
   neglect of d.
   omission of d.
   d. to warn
DV
   domestic violence
DW
   confabulated whole response
dwarfism
   psychosocial d.
DWI
   driving while intoxicated
DX, Dx
   diagnosis
dyad
   mother-child d.
   parent-child d.
   sister-sister d.'s
   social d.
dyadic
   D. Parent-Child Interaction Coding System
   d. psychotherapy
   d. session
   d. symbiosis
dybbuk
dying declaration
dynamic
   d. ambulatory balance
   d. aphasia
   attachment d.
   d. demography
   d. disease
   d. equilibrium
   d. formulation
   d. personality
   d. physical activity
   power d.
   d. principle
   d. psychiatry
   d. psychology
   d. psychotherapy
   d. range
   d. reasoning
   d. standing balance
   d. variable
dynamica
   alopecia d.
dynamics
   adaptation d.
   behavior d.
   family d.
   group d.

hemispheric d.
infantile d.
intermediate hemispheric d.
lateral hemispheric d.
medial hemispheric d.
narcissistic d.
personality d.
prominent narcissistic d.
religious d.
temporal d.
dynamism
lust d.
mental d.
dynamo
dynamorphany
dysacusis
dysanagnosia
dysantigraphia
dysaphia
dysaphic
dysarthric
d. behavior
d. speech
dysautonomic
d. feature
d. illness
dysbasia lordotica progressiva
dysbasis
dysbulia, dysboulia
dysbulic
dyscalculia
dyschezia
dyschronism
dyscoimesis
dyscontrol
affective d.
behavioral d.
descending d.
d. disorder
emergency d.
emotional d.
episodic d.
impulsive d.
instinctual d.
organic d.
seizure d.
temper d.
dyscrasia
blood d.
dyseneia
dysequilibrium state
dyserethesia

dyserethism
dysergastic reaction
dysergia
dysesthesia
dysesthetic
dysfluency
avoidance of speech d.
dysfunction
academic d.
acquired sexual d.
adult social d.
alcohol-induced sexual d.
amphetamine-induced sexual d.
anorectal physiological d.
antipsychotic-associated sexual d.
anxiolytic-induced sexual d.
arousal d.
attentional d.
atypical psychosexual d.
autonomic d.
behavioral d.
biologic d.
brain d.
brainstem d.
central processing d.
cerebral d.
childhood social d.
cocaine-induced sexual d.
cocaine sexual d.
cognitive d.
contralateral parietal lobe d.
depressive-executive d. (DED)
diffuse brain d.
drug-induced sexual d.
educational d.
ejaculatory d.
emotional d.
erectile d.
executive system d.
focal lateralized d.
frontal cortical d.
frontal lobe d.
functional dyspareunia
psychosexual d.
functional vaginismus
psychosexual d.
generalized sexual d.
hemispherical d.
higher cerebral d. (HCD)
higher cortical d.
household d.
hypnotic-induced sexual d.

D

NOTES

dysfunction *(continued)*
    hypothalamic d.
    hypothalamic-pituitary axis d.
    immunologic d.
    inhibited female orgasm
      psychosexual d.
    inhibited male orgasm
      psychosexual d.
    inhibited sexual desire
      psychosexual d.
    inhibited sexual excitement
      psychosexual d.
    interpersonal d.
    language d.
    lateralized d.
    lifelong sexual d.
    lobar d.
    lobe d.
    male erectile d.
    maternal d.
    midbrain d.
    minimal brain d. (MBD)
    neurodevelopmental d.
    neurological d.
    occupational d.
    opioid-induced sexual d.
    organic brain d.
    orgasm d.
    orgasmic d.
    parental d.
    parietal lobe d.
    perceived maternal d.
    perceived parental d.
    perceptual motor d.
    personality d.
    posttraumatic cortical d.
    premature ejaculation
      psychosexual d.
    primary orgasmic d.
    psychological d.
    psychosexual d.
    refractory erectile d.
    school d.
    secondary erectile d.
    secondary orgasmic d.
    sedative, hypnotic, or anxiolytic-
      induced sexual d.
    self-care d.
    sensory integration d. (SID)
    severe diffuse brain d.
    sexual d.
    situational orgasmic d.
    situational sexual d.
    sleep d.
    social d.
    speech d.
    SSRI-induced erectile d.
    striatofrontal d.

    substance-induced sexual d.
    sympathetic d.
    work d.
dysfunctional
    d. behavior
    d. circuitry
    d. coexistence
    d. cognition
    d. core belief
    d. dopamine system
    d. family
    d. family factor
    d. family style
    d. father
    d. mother
    d. neural circuit
    d. personality style
    d. relational functioning
    d. relationship
    socially d.
dysgenesis
    gonadal d.
dysgenic
dysgenitalism
dysgeusia
dysgnosia
    auditory-verbal d.
    body d.
    number d.
    visual letter d.
    visual number d.
dysgonesis
dysgrammatism
dysgraphia
dysgraphicus
    status d.
dysharmonica
    diplacusis d.
dysidentity
dysjunction
    personal d.
dyskinesia
    biliary d.
    disfluency d.
    extrapyramidal d.
    medication-induced tardive d.
    neuroleptic-induced tardive d.
    orofacial d.
    paroxysmal d.
    spontaneous d.
    tardive d.
    withdrawal d.
dyskinetic movement
dyskoimesis
dyslalia
dyslexia
    acquired d.
    developmental d.

dyslexic
dyslogia
dyslogistic
dysmaturation
    social d.
dysmegalopsia
dysmenorrhea
    psychogenic d.
dysmentia
dysmetria
    cognitive d.
dysmetric hand movement
dysmetropsia
dysmimia
dysmnesia
dysmnesic
    d. psychosis
    d. syndrome
dysmorphic
    d. delusion
    d. somatoform disorder
dysmorphogenesis
dysmorphology
    brain d.
dysmorphomania
dysmorphopsia
dysmyelination
dysmyotonia
dysnisophrenia
dysnomia
    autonomic d.
dysnystaxis
dysorexia
dysorthography
dysosmia
dysostosis multiplex
dyspallia
dyspareunia
    female d.
    functional d.
    generalized-type d.
    lifelong-type d.
    male d.
    psychogenic d.
    situational-type d.
dyspepsia
    psychogenic d.
dysperception
    metabolic d.
dysphagia
    d. globosa
    d. nervosa

dysphasia
    developmental d.
    expressive d.
    receptive d.
    Wernicke d.
dysphemia
dysphonia
    adductor spasmodic d.
    hyperkinetic d.
    spastic d.
    d. spastica
    ventricular d.
dysphoretic
dysphoria
    body d.
    gender d.
    hysteroid d.
    intense episodic d.
    d. nervosa
    neuroleptic-induced d.
    omnipresent d.
    premenstrual d.
dysphoriant
dysphoric
    d. affect
    d. category
    d. character structure
    d. mania
    d. manic state
    d. mood
    d. patient
    d. personality disorder
    d. presentation
    d. Q factor
    d. response
    d. subfactor
    d. subjective experience
dysphrasia
dysphrenia
dysphylaxia
dysplasia
    cerebral d.
    septooptic d.
dysplastic constitutional type
dyspnea response
dyspneic psychogenic disorder
dysponderal amenorrhea
dysponesis
dyspractic movement
dyspragia
dyspraxia
    constructional d.

D

NOTES

dyspraxia *(continued)*
   speech d.
   spelling d.
   d. syndrome
dysprosody
dysraphicus
   status d.
dysreactivity
   autonomic d.
dysreflexia
dysregulate
dysregulated
   d. neurotransmission
   d. stress response
dysregulation
   affective d.
   anger d.
   autonomic d.
   biologic d.
   defensive d.
   endocrine d.
   level of defensive d.
   limbic d.
   prefrontal cortical activity d.
dysrhaphic
dysrhythmic
   d. aggressive behavior
   d. movement
   d. speech
dyssocial
   d. behavior
   d. drinking
   d. personality
   d. personality disorder
   d. reaction
dyssombole
dyssomnia
   jet lag-type d.
   shift work-type d.
   sleep phase d.
   unspecified-type d.
dysspondylism

dysstasia
dyssymbiosis
dyssymbolia
dyssynergia
   d. cerebellaris myoclonica
   d. cerebellaris progressiva
dystaxia
dysteleology
dysthymia
   chronic d.
   primary d.
   d. scale
   subaffective d.
   d. with major depression
   d. without major depression
dysthymic
   d. adjustment reaction
   d. disorder (DD)
   d. neurotic disorder
dystonia
   body d.
   drug-induced d.
   idiopathic d.
   neuroleptic-induced acute d.
   nocturnal paroxysmal d.
   paroxysmal d.
   psychogenic d.
   substance-induced d.
   tardive d.
   withdrawal d.
dystonic
   d. movement
   d. posturing
   d. reaction
   d. tremor
dystopia
dystrophia
   d. adiposogenitalis
dystropy
dysuria
   psychic d.
   psychogenic d.

E

E scale
E trisomy

2E1

cytochrome P-450 2E1

e4/e4 genotype

EA

educational age

eagerness

EAP

Employee Assistance Program

ear

glue e.
listening with the third e.
e. pulling
third e.
wet behind the e.'s

early

e. abuse
e. adolescence
e. adulthood
e. awakening
e. childhood
e. childhood behavioral disorder
e. childhood identifiable antecedent
e. component waveform
e. discharge
e. environment
e. full remission
e. genital primacy
e. infantile autism
e. latency potential
e. life stressor
e. manic agitation
e. onset drinking
e. parental deprivation
e. and periodic screening,
   diagnosis, and treatment (EPSDT)
e. pharmacological intervention
e. phase of dementia
e. posttraumatic epilepsy
e. predictor
e. psychotherapeutic intervention
e. relationship
e. retirement with disability (ERD)
e. separation
e. speech impairment
e. trauma hypothesis of autistic
   disorder
e. traumatic epilepsy
e. treatment
e. warning sign

early-onset

e.-o. category

e.-o. mental illness
e.-o. schizophrenia

earner

wage e.

earth eater

earth-eating

earthy

ease

e. of fatigue
ill at e.

easily

distracted e.
e. disturbed sleep
e. provoked

Eastern

E. religion
E. subtype

easy

e. child
e. to distract
e. distractibility
e. fatigue
free and e.
e. going
e. mark
e. virtue

easygoing

eat

refusal to e.

eater

binge e.
clay e.
compulsive e.
dirt e.
disinterest in e.
earth e.
emotional e.
erratic e.
finicky e.
picky e.
starch e.

eating

e. aid
e. attitude
e. behavior
e. binge
e. compulsion
dirt e.
e. disorder
e. disorder investigation (EDI)
e. disorders not otherwise specified
   (EDNOS)
e. disturbance
e. fear
e. hair

E

eating *(continued)*
    e. and purging
    e. without satiation
eavesdropper
Ebbinghaus
EBD
    emotional and behavioral difficulties
EBM
    evidence-based medicine
Ebonics
ebriety
ebriose
ebriosorum
    delirium e.
ebrious
ebullience
ebullient
ebullition
EBV
    Epstein-Barr virus
ECA
    Epidemiologic Catchment Area
    ECA study
eccentric
    e. A cluster
    e. behavior
    e. paranoia
    e. personality
    e. projection
    e. thinking
eccentricity
ecchordosis physaliformis
ecclesiasticism
ecdemiomania
ecdemonomania
ecdysiasm
ecdysist
ecgonine
echelon
    higher e.
echeosis
echinacea
echo, pl. **echoes**
    e. chamber
    e. de pensee
    de penses e.
    e. des penses
    e. phenomenon
    e. principle
    e. reaction
    e. sign
    e. speech
    thought e.
echoacousia
echoencephalography
echographia
echoic memory

echoing
    thought e.
echokinesis, echokinesia
echolalia
    immediate e.
    mitigated e.
    unmitigated e.
echolalus
echolocation
echomatism
echomimia
echomotism
echopalilalia
echopathy
echophotony
echophrasia
echopraxia
echopraxis
eclaircissement
eclamptic symptom
eclat
eclectic
    e. behaviorism
    e. counseling
eclecticism
eclimia
eclipse
    cerebral e.
    mental e.
ECM
    external chemical messenger
ecmnesia
ecmnesic delirium
ecmnesique
    delire e.
ecnoia
ecocide
ecofreak
ecogenetics
ecological
    e. perception
    e. psychiatry
    e. study
    e. systems model
    e. validity
ecologic framework
ecomania
economic
    e. advantage
    e. approach
    e. benefit
    e. disadvantage
    e. divorce
    e. principle
    e. viewpoint
economically disadvantaged
ecopharmacology
ecopsychiatry

ecopsychology
ECOScales
ecosystem
e-counseling
ecouteur
ecouteurism
ecphorize
ECS
    electrocerebral silence
    electroconvulsive shock
    epileptic confusional state
ECST
    electroconvulsive shock therapy
    electroconvulsive shock treatment
ecstasy
    religious e.
ecstatic
    e. behavior
    e. pain
    e. trance
ECT
    electroconvulsive therapy
    electroshock therapy
    ECT administration
    bilateral ECT
    brief pulse bilateral ECT
    brief pulse unilateral ECT
    involuntary ECT
    sine wave unilateral ECT
    suprathreshold ECT
    unilateral brief pulse ECT
    unilateral nondominant-hemisphere
      ECT
    unilateral sine wave ECT
ectasy-associated malignant hyperthermia
ectoderm
ectodermogenic neurosyphilis
ectomorph
ectomorphic constitutional type
ectopic ACTH syndrome
ectoplasm
ectype
ecumenicist
ecumenics
eczema
    psychogenic e.
ED
    emergency department
    emotional disorder
    emotionally disturbed
    entering diagnosis

edema
    blue e.
    brain e.
    cerebral e.
    circumscribed e.
    dependent e.
    hunger e.
    nutritional e.
    pitting e.
    toxic e.
edeomania
edetate
edge
    e. artifact
    on e.
edgy
EDI
    eating disorder investigation
edict
Edinburgh
Edinger-Westphal nucleus
editable
ED/LD
    emotionally disturbed/learning disabled
EDNOS
    eating disorders not otherwise specified
EDR
    electrodermal response
EDS
    excessive daytime sleepiness
education
    caregiver e.
    compensatory e.
    consumer e.
    continuing e.
    continuing medical e. (CME)
    cooperative e.
    dance e.
    drug e.
    environmental e.
    formal e.
    high quality e.
    level of e.
    low e.
    online e.
    patient e.
    physical e.
    progressive e.
    psychiatric e.
    e. quotient (EQ)
    sex e.
    special e.

E

NOTES

education *(continued)*
    vocational rehabilitation and e.
      (VR&E)
educational
    e. acceleration
    e. achievement
    e. achievement battery
    e. age (EA)
    e. attainment
    e. counseling
    e. disadvantage
    e. dysfunction
    e. functioning
    e. history
    e. information
    e. intervention
    e. level
    e. measurement
    e. opportunity
    e. program
    e. psychology
    e. psychotherapy
    e. quotient (EQ)
    e. setting
    e. situation
    e. stressor
    e. test
    e. therapist
    e. treatment
    e. value
educationally
    e. deprived
    e. mentally handicapped (EMH)
    e. mentally retarded (EMR)
    e. subnormal (ESN)
educational-socialization model
education-focused session
educative intervention
educe
eduction
edulcorate
Edwards syndrome
EE
    expressed emotion
EEG
    electroencephalogram
    electroencephalograph
    electroencephalography
    abnormal EEG
    EEG activation
    EEG activity measurement
    diffuse slowing of EEG
    nonspecific abnormality on EEG
    phase lag on EEG
    phase spike on EEG
    sleep deprived EEG
    sleep spindle on EEG
    theta wave on EEG

    EEG tracing
    waking EEG
eerie
effect
    adverse drug e.
    adverse medication e.
    adverse negative
      immunosuppressive e.
    age e.
    air pressure e.
    alerting e.
    antiadrenergic e.
    antiaggressive e.
    anticholinergic e.
    anticholinergic side e.
    anticonvulsant e.
    antihistaminergic e.
    anti-impulse e.
    antimuscarinic e.
    antipsychotic e.
    antipsychotic side e.
    antiserotonergic e.
    anxiolytic e.
    aspirin e.
    assimilation e.
    asymmetry and order e.
    atmosphere e.
    audience e.
    autokinetic e.
    autonomic side e.
    bandwagon e.
    Barnum e.
    behavioral e.
    beneficial e.
    brain metabolic e.
    calming e.
    catastrophic e.
    ceiling e.
    chatterbox e.
    cholinergic side e.
    chronic toxic e.
    clasp-knife e.
    clinical e.
    cocktail party e.
    cohort e.
    cold e.
    confinement e.
    contrast e.
    crisis e.
    cue e.
    cue-induced subjective e.
    cumulative e.
    damping e.
    e.'s of deception
    desired e.
    deterioration e.
    devastating e.
    developmental e.

differential beneficial e.
diminished e.
direct physiological e.
direct thermogenic e.
door-in-the-face e.
dopaminergic e.
dose-dependent e.
drug e.
drug-related sexual side e.
effect expectancy e.
empathogenic e.
enhanced e.
enlightenment e.
environmental e.
ether e.
euphoric e.
euphorigenic e.
experimenter e.
experimenter-expectancy e.
extrapyramidal medication side e.
fetal alcohol e. (FAE)
first-pass e.
genetic e.
Glick e.
e. gradient
Halloween e.
hallucinogen toxic e.
halo e.
hangover e.
Hawthorn e.
head shadow e.
hedonic psychoactive e.
humidity e.
hypermetabolic e.
iatrogenic e.
idiosyncratic side e.
immunosuppressive e.
inhibitory e.
interaction e.
interactive e.
interviewer e.
intolerable side e.
isolation e.
kindling e.
late-emerging medical side e.
e. law
law of e.
less than maximal e.
limbic e.
limited e.
long-hot-summer e.
long-lasting drug e.

long-term e.
loss of e.
main e.
maximal e.
measurement e.
mediating e.
medical e.
medication side e.
Mellanby e.
mere-exposure e.
metabolic e.
misinformation e.
modified Stroop e.
movement disorder e.
Mozart e.
muscle-relaxing e.
negative immunosuppressive e.
neurotropic e.
nonsignificant protective e.
nonspecific e.
noradrenergic e.
off e.
on e.
Orbeli e.
partial-reinforcement e. (PRE)
passing stranger e.
peak behavioral e.
peripheral sympathomimetic e.
personal e.'s
physiological e.
placebo e.
positive e.
potential adverse e.
practice e.
primary e.
protective e.
psychiatric e.
psychoactive e.
psychodynamic e.
psychological e.
psychostimulant e.
putative e.
Pygmalion e.
rebound e.
reinforcing e.
rewarding e.
secondary e.
secure base e.
sedative e.
serotonergic side e.
sexual side e.
short-lasting drug e.

E

NOTES

effect *(continued)*
    side e.
    e. size
    specific e.
    SSRI-induced sexual side e.
    stimulant e.
    stimulation-related adverse e.
    e.'s of stress
    Stroop e.
    subjective e.
    suggestibility e.
    sundowner e.
    sympathomimetic e.
    temperature e.
    therapeutic e.
    thermogenic e.
    Thorndike law of e.
    toxic side e.
    Transylvania e.
    e.'s of trauma
    e. of trauma on consciousness
    treatment e.
    treatment-emergent extrapyramidal
      side e.
    tricyclic e.
    undifferentiated e.
    unintended e.
    untoward cholinergic e.
    Vulpian e.
    Wever-Bray e.
    wind e.
    withdrawal e.
    Zeigarnik e.
effective
    e. action
    e. dose
    e. ego
    e. level
    e. masking
    occupationally e.
    socially e.
    e. stimulus
    e. technique
    e. treatment
    vasoactive e.
effective-habit strength
effectiveness
    long-term e.
    treatment e.
effective-reaction potential
effector
    cold e.
    heat e.
    e. operation
    warm e.
effectual
effeminate homosexual
effemination

efferent
    e. feedback
    e. motor aphasia
    e. nerve
    e. relation
effervesce
effervescent
effete
efficacious
efficacy
    clinical e.
    comparative e.
    drug e.
    lack of e.
    relational e.
    e. scale
    therapeutic e.
efficiency
    good sleep e.
    index of forecasting e.
    masking e.
    neural e.
    REM sleep e.
    sleep e.
efficient
    cause e.
    e. cause
effigy
effort
    e. after meaning
    community e.
    distributed e.
    e. level
    new-work e.
    e. syndrome
effort-reward imbalance
effort-shape technique
effrontery
effulgence
effusive
E-F scale
EFT
    extended family therapy
egalitarianism
egersis
ego
    alter e.
    alternative alter e.
    e. alter theory
    e. analysis
    e. anxiety
    auxiliary e.
    body e.
    e. boundary
    e. boundary loss
    e. cathexis
    e. center
    collective e.

e. complex
e. control
decompensation e.
decomposition of e.
e. decomposition
e. defense
e. defense mechanism
e. development
e. deviation
e. distortion
dream e.
e. drive
duplication of e.
e. dystonic homosexuality
e. dystonic pseudohallucination
effective e.
e. erotism
escape from the e.
extinction of e.
e. formation
fragmentation of e.
e. function
id e.
e. ideal
ideal e.
e. identity
e. instinct
e. integration
e. integrity
e. integrity versus despair
e. involvement
e. libido
loss of boundaries of e.
e. maximation
mental e.
e. model
motor control of the e.
e. narcissism
negation of the e.
e. neurosis
e. nucleus
oral e.
perception e.
pleasure e.
preschizophrenic e.
e. proper
e. psychology
e. psychotherapy
purified pleasure e.
reality life of e.
reasonable e.
e. resistance

e. restriction
e. retrenchment
safety of e.
split in the e.
e. splitting
stability of e.
e. state
e. strength (ES)
e. strength scale
e. stress
e. structure
e. subject
e. substance
e. suffering
supportive e.
surface e.
e. syntonic
e. transcendence
e. trip
weak e.
e. weakness
ego-alien
egocentric
e. language
e. speech
e. stage of development
e. thinking
e. thought process
egocentricity
egocentrism
ego-coping skill
ego-dystonic
e.-d. behavior
e.-d. intrusion
e.-d. obsession
e.-d. orientation
e.-d. promiscuity
ego-ideal
egoism
egoisme à deux
egoity
egomania
ego-oriented individual therapy
egopathyegotism
ego-state therapy
egosyntonia
ego-syntonic gambling urge
egotism
egotistical
egotistic suicide
egotropic
egregious

NOTES

E

egress
EH
    emotional handicap
E&H
    environment and heredity
Ehret syndrome
Eichhorst neuritis
eidetic
    e. ability
    e. image
    e. imagery
    e. personification
    e. type
eidolon
eidoptometry
eight
    e. ball
    Section E.
    e. stages of man
eighth-month anxiety
EIO
    exploratory insight-oriented
    psychotherapy
Eisenlohr syndrome
either-or
    e.-o. situation
    e.-o. thinking
EIWA
    escala inteligencia Wechsler para adultes
ejaculate
    inability to e.
ejaculatio
    e. deficiens
    e. praecox
    e. retardata
    e. retardate
ejaculation
    delayed e.
    e. disorder
    female e.
    immediate e.
    e. physiology
    premature e.
    primary retarded e.
    e. reflux
    retarded e.
    retrograde e.
    secondary retarded e.
ejaculatione
    coitus sine e.
ejaculatory
    e. dysfunction
    e. impotence
    e. incompetence
    e. pain
    e. reflex
Ekbom syndrome
ekistics

EL
    elopement
elaborate dream sequence
elaboration
    secondary e.
    symbolic e.
elan vital
elasticity
elated
    e. affect
    e. mood
elation
elder
    e. abuse
    e. adult neglect
    e. care
    e. maltreatment
elderly
    acute care of the e. (ACE)
    bias against the e.
    e. depressed patient
    psychiatric disorders in the e.
    psychosis in the e.
    e. suicide
eldest
eldritch
elective
    e. abortion
    e. admission
    e. anorexia
    e. mutism
    e. mutism adjustment
    e. mutism adjustment reaction
    e. sterility
    e. therapy
Electra complex
electric
    e. anesthesia
    e. auditory
    e. aura
    e. chorea
    e. field
    e. irritability
    e. shock therapy
    e. shock treatment
    e. skin shock
    e. sleep
    e. stimulation of the brain (ESB)
    e. wine
electrical
    e. activity of brain
    e. characteristic
    e. current brain trauma organic
    psychosis
    e. habituation
    e. intracranial stimulation
    e. potential
    e. shock

e. synapse
e. transcranial stimulation (ETS)
electricity
feeling of e.
electrify
electroanalgesia
electroanalysis
electroanesthesia
electrobasograph
electrocerebral silence (ECS)
electrocoma
electrocontractility
electroconvulsive
e. shock (ECS)
e. shock therapy (ECST)
e. shock treatment (ECST)
e. therapy (ECT)
e. therapy-induced mood disorder
electrocorticogram
electrocorticography
electrode placement
electrodermal
e. response (EDR)
e. response biofeedback
electrodiagnosis
electrodiagnostic study
electroencephalogram (EEG)
e. biofeedback
flat e.
quantitative e. (QEEG)
electroencephalograph (EEG)
electroencephalographic
electroencephalography (EEG)
quantitative e. (QEEG)
electrokinetic
electrolepsy
electrolyte
e. abnormality
e. balance
e. disturbance
e. imbalance
e. replacement
electromagnetic wave
electromicturation
electromigratory
electromotive force (EMF)
electromyograph (EMG)
electromyography biofeedback
electron
electronarcosis (EN)
electroneurography

electronic
e. aid
e. conduction
e. data bank
e. disaster recovery plan
e. monitoring
electrooculographic activity
electroolfactogram (EOG)
electropathology
electrophrenic respiration
electrophysiological battery
electrophysiology
electroplexy
electroshock (ES)
maximal e.
e. therapy (ECT, EST, est)
e. threshold (EST, est)
e. treatment (EST, est)
electroshock-induced
e.-i. psychosis
e.-i. psychotic syndrome
electrosleep therapy (ETS)
electrospectrography
electrostimulation
electrostriatogram
electrosynthesis
electrotherapeutic
e. sleep
e. sleep therapy
electrotherapist
electrotherapy
cerebral e. (CET)
transcerebral e. (TCET)
electrotonus
electrovibratory massage
element
cAMP response e. (CRE)
cognitive e.
contributory e.
cultural e.
identical e.
thyroid response e. (TRE)
elemental diet
elementarily
elementary
e. anxiety
e. hallucination
e. manner
e. partial seizure
e. process
Eleutherococcus senticosus
eleutheromania

E

NOTES

229

elevated
    e. mood
    e. risk
    e. score
elevation
    mood e.
    nonfocal e.
    prolactin e.
    T score e.
elevator
    mood e.
elfin facies
Elgin checklist
elicitation
    affect e.
    emotion e.
elicited
    e. behavior
    e. imitation
eligibility for care
eliminant
elimination
    e. diet
    e. disorder
    e. drive
    process of e.
elision
elite
    e. class
    e. community
elixir
    amobarbital e.
    aprobarbital e.
    high-alcoholic e.
    potassium chloride e.
ellipsis wit
elocution
elopement (EL)
    e. ideation
    e. status (ES)
eloquence
eloquent
ELP
    estimated learning potential
Elpenor syndrome
elucidation
elude
elusion
elusive
    e. illness state
    e. syndrome
emaciated
    e. appearance
    e. body
emaciation disorder
email
    e. communication
    e. correspondence

    e. harassment
    e. relationship
emanate
emanative
emancipated
    e. adolescent
    e. minor
emancipation
    e. disorder
    e. disorder of adolescence
emancipatory
    e. disorder
    e. striving
emasculate
emasculation
embarrass
embarrassing
embarrassment
    dream e.
    e. dream
    e. psychosis
embattle
embedded command
embellish
embezzle
embezzlement
embezzler
embitter
emblazon
emblem
embodiment
embody
embolalia, embololalia
embolden
embolophasia
embolophrasia
emboloplasia
embonpoint
embracing behavior
embroil
EMDR
    eye movement desensitization and reprocessing
emergence
emergency
    behavioral e.
    e. care facility
    e. contagion
    e. department (ED)
    e. dyscontrol
    e. dyscontrol duration
    e. intervention
    medical e.
    e. medical technician (EMT)
    e. medicine
    opiate-induced e.
    psychiatric e.
    e. psychiatric setting

e. psychotherapy
e. room (ER)
e. service (ES)
e. situation
spiritual e.
suicidal e.
e. theory
e. theory of emotion
e. treatment
e. unit (EU)
emergent
e. evolution
treatment e.
emetatrophia
emetocathartic
emetomania
EMF
electromotive force
EMG
electromyograph
EMG biofeedback
EMH
educationally mentally handicapped
emigrant
emigration
forced e.
eminence
eminent
emission
nocturnal e.
e. tomography scan
emitted behavior
emotiomotor
emotiomuscular
emotion
activation theory of e.
adjustment disorder with mixed
  disturbance of e.'s
Cannon-Bard theory of e.
changing e.
childish e.
cognitively elicited e.
conflicting e.
controlled e.
conversion of e.
dammed-up e.
defensive e.
discomfort with e.
disruptive e.
e. elicitation
emergency theory of e.
expressed e. (EE)

ictal e.
image eliciting neutral e.
inability to experience e.
e. induction
James-Lange theory of e.
level of expressed e.
maladaptive pattern of e.
manifestation of e.
memory by e.
moral e.
natural e.
negative e.
Papez theory of e.
pervasive e.
pleasurable e.
positive e.
e. production
public display of e.
recall-generated e.
e. regulation training
retraining e.
roller-coaster e.
stirred-up e.
sustained e.
taboo e.
two-factor theory of e.
uncanny e.
unconscious e.
welfare e.
emotional
e. abandonment
e. abuse
e. abyss
e. activity
e. adjustment
e. age
e. agitation
e. amalgam
e. amenorrhea
e. amnesia
e. anesthesia
e. arousal
e. atmosphere
e. attainment
e. attitude
e. avoidance
e. awareness
e. baggage
e. B cluster
e. beggar
e. and behavioral difficulties (EBD)
e. bias

E

NOTES

emotional *(continued)*

e. blackmail
e. blockade
e. blocking
e. blunting
e. bond
e. castration
e. catharsis
e. cause of seizure
e. climate
e. coldness
e. comfort
e. communication
e. condition
e. conflict
e. connectedness
e. consequences of divorce
e. constriction
e. control therapy
e. cripple
e. crisis
e. deadness
e. dependence
e. deprivation
e. detachment
e. deterioration
e. development
e. difficulty
e. disability
e. discomfort
e. disease
e. disinhibition
e. disorder (ED)
e. display
e. distance
e. distress
e. disturbance
e. disturbance adjustment disorder
e. disturbance adjustment reaction
e. disturbance of adolescence
e. disturbance of childhood
e. disturbance stress reaction
e. dullness
e. dyscontrol
e. dyscontrol disorder
e. dysfunction
e. eater
e. emptiness
e. episode
e. event
e. experience
e. facial expression
e. factor
e. fatigue
e. fatigue study
e. flatness
e. flattening
e. flavor

e. flooding
e. functioning
e. handicap (EH)
e. health
e. illness
e. immaturity
e. impairment
e. incontinence
e. information processing
e. inhibition
e. inoculation
e. input
e. insanity
e. insight
e. instability
e. instability personality disorder
e. insulation
e. investment
e. involvement
e. lability
e. learning
e. maltreatment of children
e. manipulation
e. material
e. maturation
e. maturity
e. mechanism
e. memory
e. memory deficit
e. memory process
e. memory processing
e. memory score
e. misery
e. modulation
e. monomania
e. need
e. neglect
e. numbing
e. numbness
e. nutriment
e. object constancy
e. overlay
e. overreaction
e. personality
e. problem
e. range
e. reactivity
e. reciprocity
e. reeducation
e. reenactment
e. regulation
e. release
e. release therapy
e. repression
e. response
e. responsiveness
e. responsivity
e. salience

e. scars
e. security
e. shading
e. significance
e. speech
e. stability
e. state
e. stimulation
e. stimulus
e. storm
e. stress
e. stress depressive psychosis
e. stress precipitating tremor
e. stress reaction
e. stupor
e. suffering
e. supply
e. support
e. symptom
e. tension
e. thought
e. tone
e. trajectory
e. trauma
e. turmoil
e. upheaval
e. upset
e. valence
e. vulnerability
e. well-being
e. withdrawal
emotionalism
emotionality
excessive e.
labile e.
negative e.
pathologic e.
pathological e.
positive e.
emotionally
e. arousing information
e. cold
e. constricted
e. detached
e. distant
e. disturbed (ED)
e. disturbed/learning disabled (ED/LD)
e. handicapped
e. impaired
e. inhibited
e. invested

e. isolated
e. laden topic
e. loaded event memory
e. provoking stimulus
e. stable
e. unavailable
e. unstable
e. unstable character disorder (EUCD)
e. unstable immaturity
e. unstable immaturity reaction
e. unstable personality
e. upset
emotionally-based disorder
emotional-object amalgam
emotion-cognition interface
emotion-laden situation
emotionless
emotion-related
e.-r. activation
e.-r. feedback stimulus
e.-r. meaning
emotions-conduct adjustment reaction
emotive
e. energy
e. imagery
e. language
e. process
e. speech
e. stimulus
e. theory
e. therapy
empacho
empathic
e. behavior
e. capacity
e. failure
e. identification
e. index
empathize
empathogenic effect
empathy
accurate e. (AE)
communicating e.
failure to develop e.
generative e.
lack of e.
support, autonomy, fusioning, e. (SAFE)
victim e.
emphatic speech

E

NOTES

empiric
  e. cognition
  e. drug treatment
  e. risk
empirical
  e. approach
  e. basis
  e. classification
  e. data
  e. evidence
  e. finding
  e. formula
  e. law
  e. limitation
  e. process
  e. question
  e. research
  e. review
  e. self
  e. study
  e. support
  systematic, complete, objective, practical, e. (SCOPE)
  e. test
  e. validity
empirical-criterion keying
empirical-rational strategy
empiricism
  scientific e.
empiricist theory
empiric-risk figure
empleomania
employ
employable
employed
  gainfully e.
employee
  E. Assistance Program (EAP)
  e. benefit
  drug-free e.
  e. drug use
  e. evaluation
  semiskilled e.
employment
  e. contract
  e. failure
  e. interview
  e. inventory
  e. problem
  e. problem rating
  e. profile
  e. workshop
employment-related behavior
empower
empowered family
empowerment
  sense of e.
empressement

emprise
emprosthotonos
emptiness
  e. of affect
  chronic feelings of e.
  emotional e.
  e. fear
  feeling of e.
  spiritual e.
empty
  e. nest
  e. nest syndrome
  e. organism
  e. set
  e. stare
  e. word
empty-chair technique
empty-handed
empty-headed
emptying reflex
EMR
  educationally mentally retarded
EMT
  emergency medical technician
emulate
emulation
emulous
emulsion
emylcamate
EN
  electronarcosis
en
  en bloc
  en frenzy
  en masse
  en rapport
enabler
enact
enactive
  e. mode
  e. period
enactment
enanthate
enantiodromia
enantiolalia
enantiopathic
encapsulated delusion
encephalasthenia
encephalatrophic
encephalatrophy
encephalauxe
encephalemia
encephalic
encephalitogen
encephalitogenic
encephalization
encephalociastic
encephalopathia

encephalopathy
  acute toxic e.
  AIDS e.
  air e.
  alcoholic pellagra e.
  alcoholic possible pancreatic e.
  anoxic e. (AE)
  bilirubin e.
  Binswanger e.
  bovine spongiform e.
  boxer's e.
  childhood e.
  degenerative e.
  delayed postanoxic e.
  diffuse e.
  epileptogenic e.
  familial e.
  hepatic e. (HE)
  hyperkinetic e.
  hypernatremic e.
  hypertensive e.
  hypoglycemic e.
  hypoxic-ischemic e. (HIE)
  idiopathic e.
  lead e.
  mercury e.
  metabolic e.
  painter's e.
  palindromic e.
  portal systemic e. (PSE)
  postanoxic e.
  post contusion syndrome e.
  posttraumatic e.
  progressive degenerative
    subcortical e.
  progressive traumatic e.
  punch-drunk e.
  recurrent e.
  saturnine e.
  static e.
  subacute spongiform e.
  subcortical arteriosclerotic e.
  thiamine deficiency e. (TDE)
  thyrotoxic e.
  toxic e.
  traumatic progressive e.
  Wernicke fluent e.
  Wernicke-Korsakoff e.
encephalopsy
encephalopsychosis
encephalopyosis
encephalorrhagia

encephaloscopy
encephalosis
encephalothlipsis
encephalotome
encephalotrophy
enchain
enchant
enclose
enclosed space
encoding
  e. communication board
  memory e.
  e. skill
encopresis
  functional e.
  overflow e.
  primary e.
encounter
  clinical e.
  forced sexual e.
  gang e.
  e. group
  indiscriminate sexual e.
  intuitive e.
  marriage e.
  e. movement
  online e.
  physician-patient e.
  sexual e.
  stressful e.
encrypted correspondence
encrypted file
encryption
enculturate
enculturation
encumber
encumbrance
encyclical
encyprate
end
  bitter e.
  dead e.
  e. organ
  e. point
  e. point tremor
  e. product
  e. spurt
  e. state
endangerment
  child e.
endear

E

NOTES

endeavor
> conceptual e.

endemic
> e. neuritis
> e. paralytic vertigo

endemica

endergonic

endermic

ending
> act e.
> sympathetic nerve e.

endocrine
> e. disease organic psychosis
> e. dysregulation
> e. obesity
> e. psychogenic disorder
> e. therapy
> e. type organic psychosis

endocrinology
> behavioral e.

end-of-life
> e.-o.-l. care
> e.-o.-l. decision making
> e.-o.-l. issue
> e.-o.-l. question

endogamy

endogenetic

endogenic

endogenomorphic
> e. depression

endogenous
> e. adenosine
> e. brain mechanism
> e. chemical
> e. circadian pacemaker
> e. circadian period
> e. circadian rhythm phase
> e. depression
> e. factor
> e. negativity
> e. obesity
> e. opioid
> e. pain
> e. rhythm
> e. smile
> e. stimulation
> e. Zeitgeber

endogenously produced substance

endogeny

endomorph

endomorphic constitutional type

endomusia

endonuclease
> restriction e.

endoperineuritis

endopredator

endoreactive

endorphin
> beta e.

endorse

endorsement of deviant thoughts and beliefs

endoscopic

endosymbiosis

endowment
> genetic e.

endplate, end-plate

end-pleasure

endpoint CGI scores

end-stage dementia

end-state functioning

endurance level

enduring
> e. pattern
> e. pattern of inflexibility
> e. problem

enema
> e. addiction
> e. drug administration
> nutritive e.

enemator

energetic

energizer
> psychic e.

energy
> acoustic e.
> active displacement of emotive e.
> affect e.
> e. affect
> e. balance
> boundless e.
> change in e.
> e. dosing
> emotive e.
> increased e.
> intense e.
> kinetic e.
> lack of e.
> e. level
> libidinal e.
> life e.
> loss of e.
> low e.
> mental e.
> metabolic e.
> e. metabolism
> e. output
> potential e.
> psychic e.
> sexual e.
> e. swing
> vital e.

enervate

enervation

enfeedable

enfold
enforced treatment
enforcement
        boundary e.
engagement
        broken e.
        e. level
engender
engineering
        biomedical e.
        genetic e.
        human e.
        e. psychologist
        e. psychology
        social e.
English
        E. as a second language (ESL)
engrafted schizophrenia
engram
        e. entitlement
        function e.
engraphia
engrave
engrossment
engulfment
enhanced
        e. effect
        e. methadone maintenance treatment
        e. sensitivity
        e. standard care
        e. standard methadone maintenance
          treatment program
        e. standard methadone service
enhancement
enhexymal
enigma
enjoin
enkephalin
enlargement
enlighten
enlightenment effect
enlisted man
enliven
enmesh
enmeshment
enmity
ennui
enomania
enormity
enosimania
enounce

enquiry
        coping operations preference e.
          (COPE)
enrage
enraged behavior
enrapt
enrapture
enriched environment
enrichment
        environmental e.
        job e.
        e. program
ensconce
enserf
enslave
ensoul
ensure
entailment
entangle
entelechy
entendre
        double e.
entendu
        déjà e.
entering diagnosis (ED)
enterprising
entheomania
enthlasis
enthrall
enthusiasm
enthusiastic
enthymeme
entitlement
        engram e.
        e. program
        sense of e.
entity, pl. entities
        controlling external entities
        external e.
entoderm
entomomania
entopic vision
entorhinal cortex
entourage
entrainment
entrance event
entreat
entrench
entropy
entrust

E

NOTES

entry
  e. behavior
  organizational e.
enunciate
enuresis
  diurnal e.
  e. nocturna
  primary nocturnal e.
  psychogenic e.
enuretic
  e. absence
  e. event
envenom
enviable
envious behavior
environment
  aberrant parental e.
  adolescent e.
  adult e.
  adverse psychosocial e.
  aversive early e.
  barrier-free e.
  changing e.
  e. characteristic
  childhood e.
  conflictual home e.
  controlled e.
  dark e.
  disturbed home e.
  domestic e.
  early e.
  enriched e.
  facilitating e.
  free-access e.
  ghetto e.
  e. and heredity (E&H)
  holding e.
  home e.
  hostile work e.
  immediate e.
  impoverished early e.
  inadequate school e.
  individual-specific e.
  institutional e.
  interdisciplinary e.
  invalidating e.
  litigious e.
  low sensory e.
  low stimulation e.
  managed care e.
  milieu e.
  e. modification
  multicultural e.
  natural e.
  nurturing e.
  parental e.
  perception of the e.
  permissive e.

physical e.
planned learning e.
respond to e.
response to e.
secondary e.
secure e.
sensory e.
social e.
socially disruptive e.
stimulating e.
stressful e.
therapeutic e.
unawareness of e.
working e.
environmental
  e. adaptability
  e. adjustment
  e. aesthetics
  e. approach
  e. assessment
  e. attribution
  e. awareness
  e. change
  e. complexity
  e. cue
  e. deficiency
  e. deprivation
  e. design
  e. determinant
  e. disturbance of sleep
  e. education
  e. effect
  e. enrichment
  e. experimentation
  e. factor
  e. hazard
  e. influence
  e. inventory
  e. learning theory
  e. load theory
  e. manipulation
  e. medicine
  e. modification
  e. mold trait
  e. neurosis
  e. press
  e. pressure
  e. problem
  e. process
  e. psychologist
  e. psychology
  e. resistance (ER)
  e. sleep disorder
  e. stimulation (ES)
  e. stimulus
  e. stress
  e. stress theory
  e. support

e. susceptibility
e. therapy
environmentalist
environmentally
e. aesthetic
e. induced anxiety
environment-centered service
environs
envisage
envy
breast e.
penis e.
phallus e.
vaginal e.
womb e.
enzyme
cytochrome P450 metabolic e.
e. gene
e. induction
lipolytic e.
neurotransmitter synthesizing e.
E&O
evaluation and observation
EOG
electroolfactogram
eonism
eosinopenia
EOT
externally oriented thinking
EP
evoked potential
epena
ependyma
ependymitis
ephaptic conduction
epharmony
ephebiatrics
ephebic
ephebogenesis
ephebology
ephebophilia
Ephedra sinica
ephedrine
ephemera
ephemeral mania
EPI
extrapyramidal involvement
epicrisis
epicritic
e. sensation
e. sensibility
e. system

epicure
epidemic
e. catalepsy
e. of fear
e. hysteria
epidemiologic
epidemiological
e. data
e. research
e. study
Epidemiologic Catchment Area (ECA)
epidemiologist
psychiatric e.
epidemiology
pandemic e.
psychiatric e.
epidurography
epigastric aura
epigenesis
epigenetic
e. principle
e. theory
epilation
permanent e.
temporary e.
epilepsia
e. corticalis continua
e. cursiva
e. mitis
e. nutans
e. partialis continua
e. partialis continua seizure
e. vertiginosa
epilepsy
absence e.
acousticomotor e.
acquired e.
activated e.
affective e.
akinetic e.
alcoholic e.
alcohol-precipitated e.
audiogenic e.
automatic e.
autonomic e.
Bravais-jacksonian e.
centrencephalic e.
clouded state e.
communicating e.
complex partial e.

E

NOTES

epilepsy *(continued)*
    complex precipitated e.
    continuous e.
    coordinated e.
    cortical e.
    cryptogenic e.
    cursive e.
    dementia in e.
    depression in e.
    deterioration e.
    diencephalic e.
    digestive e.
    diurnal e.
    early posttraumatic e.
    early traumatic e.
    erotic e.
    essential e.
    extrapyramidal e.
    extrinsic e.
    e. fear
    focal e.
    gelastic e.
    generalized flexion e.
    generalized tonic-clonic e.
    genuine e.
    gestational e.
    grand mal e.
    hallucinatory e.
    haut mal e.
    hippocampal e.
    hysterical e.
    idiopathic e.
    impulsive petit mal e.
    inhibition e.
    inhibitory e.
    intractable grand mal e.
    Jackson e.
    jacksonian e.
    juvenile myoclonic e.
    larval e.
    larvated e.
    laryngeal e.
    latent e.
    late traumatic e.
    limbic e.
    local e.
    localized e.
    major e.
    masked e.
    matutinal e.
    minor e.
    mixed-type e.
    musicogenic e.
    myoclonic astatic e.
    myoclonus e.
    nocturnal e.
    organic e.
    e. organic psychosis

parasympathetic e.
partial e.
pattern-induced e.
pattern sensitive e.
perceptive e.
peripheral e.
petit mal e.
photic e.
photogenic e.
photosensitive e.
postanoxic e.
precipitating of e.
primary generalized e.
procursive e.
psychic e.
psychomotor e.
psychopathology of e.
psychosensory e.
reactive e.
reading e.
reflex inhibition of e.
regional e.
retropulsive e.
rolandic e.
secondary generalized e.
seizure e.
senile e.
sensorial e.
sensory-induced e.
sensory precipitated e.
serial e.
short stare e.
situation-related e.
sleep e.
sleep-related e.
somatomotor e.
somatosensory e.
somnambulic e.
startle e.
status e.
sympathetic e.
symptomatic e.
tardy e.
temporal lobe e. (TLE)
tetanoid e.
thalamic e.
tonic e.
tornado e.
traumatic e.
true e.
twilight e.
uncinate e.
vasomotor e.
vasovagal e.
vertiginous e.
visceral e.
visual e.

epileptic
- e. absence
- e. aura
- e. automatism
- e. character
- e. clouded state
- e. confusional state (ECS)
- e. convulsion
- e. cry
- e. dementia
- e. deterioration
- e. disorder
- e. equivalent
- e. focus
- e. fugue
- e. furor
- e. idiocy
- e. mania
- e. personality
- e. psychopathic constitution
- e. seizure
- e. stupor
- e. swindler
- e. syndrome (ES)
- e. transient organic psychosis
- e. twilight state
- e. variant
- e. vertigo

epileptica
- absentia e.

epilepticum
- delirium e.

epilepticus
- convulsive status e.
- furor e.
- ictus e.
- nonconvulsive status e.
- status e.

epileptiform
- e. convulsion
- e. discharge
- e. neuralgia
- e. seizure

epileptogenic
- e. encephalopathy
- e. focus
- e. stimulation
- e. stimulus
- e. zone

epileptoid
- e. amaurosis
- e. personality disorder

epiloia
epinosic gain
epiphenomenalism
epiphenomenon
epiphysiopathy
episode
- absence e.
- acute manic e.
- acute psychotic e.
- acute schizophrenic e.
- adult depressive e.
- affective e.
- amnestic e.
- aphonic e.
- bereavement-related major depressive e.
- bipolar I disorder, single manic e.
- brief e.
- cataplexy e.
- confusional e.
- current psychotic e.
- daytime sleep e.
- depersonalization e.
- depressed mood e.
- depressive e.
- dissociative e.
- emotional e.
- first psychotic e.
- florid e.
- full-blown depressive e.
- full psychotic e.
- future e.
- gray-out e.
- hypomanic mood e.
- index e.
- intoxication e.
- length of e.
- lifetime e.
- major depressive e. (MDE)
- manic-like e.
- manic mood e.
- micropsychotic e.
- mixed mania e.
- mixed mood e.
- mood e.
- neurotic state with depersonalization e.
- nocturnal sleep e.
- personal e.
- prodromal e.
- prolonged nocturnal sleep e.
- psycholeptic e.

E

NOTES

241

episode *(continued)*
    psychotic e.
    psychotic schizophrenic e.
    real-life emotional e.
    recurrent e.
    schizoaffective e.
    schizophrenic e.
    single e.
    sleep-onset e.
    sleep terror e.
    substance-induced manic e.
    unintentional daytime sleep e.
    uninterrupted e.
    unspecified mood e.
    untreated e.
    e. version

episodic
    e. affective disorder
    e. amnesia
    e. behavior disorder
    e. bilateral loss of muscle tone
    e. changes of consciousness
    e. confusion
    e. course
    e. dyscontrol
    e. dyscontrol duress
    e. dyscontrol syndrome
    e. memory
    e. memory function
    e. substance abuse

epistemophilia
epistolary
epithalamus
epithet
    national e.

epitonic
epitonos
epochal amnesia
epochs
    wakefulness e.

EPR
    evoked potential response

eprouve
    déjà e.

EPS
    exhaustion syndrome
    extrapyramidal symptom
    extrapyramidal syndrome
    extrapyramidal system

EPSDT
    early and periodic screening, diagnosis, and treatment

epsilon
    e. alcoholism
    e. movement

EPSP
    excitatory postsynaptic potential

Epstein-Barr
    E.-B. syndrome
    E.-B. virus (EBV)

EQ
    educational quotient
    education quotient

equable
equal
    e. employment opportunity
    e. interval scale

equal-and-unequal-cases method
equal-appearing-intervals method
equality
    law of e.
    e. law
    point of subjective e. (PSE)
    e. stage
    subjective e.

equalization of excitation
equanimity
equate
equation
    differential e.
    logistic regression e.
    personal e.

equatorial phase
equicaloric
equidominant
equilibration
equilibratory
    e. ataxia
    e. sense

equilibrium
    dynamic e.
    genetic e.
    Hardy-Weinberg e.
    homeostatic e.
    narcissistic e.
    nutritive e.
    sense of e.

equine gait
equipment
    clay-modeling e.
    e. design
    drug-injecting e.

equiponderant
equipotential
equipotentiality law
equitable
equity
    e. stage
    e. theory

equivalence
    e. coefficient
    complex e.

equivalent
    age e. (AEq)
    arithmetic grade e.

clinical e.
convulsive e.
e. criteria
delusional e.
depressive e.
e. diagnosis
e. dosage
epileptic e.
e. form
e. form reliability
grade e.
grammatical e.
e. group
e. intoxication criterion
masturbation e.
e. method
pharmaceutical e.
psychic e.
reading grade e.
spelling grade e.
e. symptom
e. symptomatic presentation
e. withdrawal criterion
equivocal finding
equivocate
ER
emergency room
environmental resistance
evoked response
era
juvenile e.
neomyerian e.
eradicate
ERB
ethnic relational behavior
ERD
early retirement with disability
event-related desynchronization
erectile
e. arousal disorder
e. disorder due to combined
factors
e. disorder due to psychological
factors
e. dysfunction
e. failure
e. impotence
erection
pharmacologically induced penile e.
(PIPE)
psychogenic painful e.
sleep e.

erector
e. clitoridis
e. penis
eremiomania
eremite
eremophilia
erethism
e. mercuralis
sexual e.
erethismic, erethistic, erethitic
e. idiocy
e. idiot
e. shock
erethisophrenia
ERG
existence, relatedness, and growth theory
ergasia
ergasiatry
ergasiology
ergasiomania
ergasthenia
ergastic
ergogenic aid
ergograph
ergomania
ergometer
ergonomics
ergonovine
ergot
e. alkaloid
e. derivative
ergotherapist
ergotherapy
ergotism
ergotropic
e. process
e. system
Erhardt seminar training
Erickson
E. developmental model
E. theory of latency
erigendi
impotentia e.
Erikson eight stages of man
eristic
erode
erodible
erogeneity
erogenous zone
eromania
eros
erosion of privacy

E

NOTES

erotic
- e. arousal
- e. behavior
- e. character
- e. delusion
- e. dream
- e. drive
- e. epilepsy
- e. fantasy
- e. image
- e. instinct
- e. language
- e. obsession
- e. paranoia
- e. pyromania
- e. seizure
- e. stimulus
- e. transference
- e. type
- e. zoophilism

erotica
erotic-arousal pattern
eroticism (*var. of* erotism)
eroticize
eroticized fantasy
eroticomania
erotique
- monomanie e.

erotism, eroticism
- anal e.
- ego e.
- genital e.
- lip e.
- muscle e.
- olfactory e.
- oral e.
- organ e.
- paranoid e.
- skin e.
- temperature e.
- urethral e.

erotization
erotize
erotized
- e. anxiety
- e. hanging

erotogenesis
erotogenic
- e. masochism
- e. zone

erotographomania
erotolalia
erotology
erotomania
- Clerambault e.

erotomaniac
erotomanic
- e. delusion

- e. delusional state
- e. disorder
- e. subtype
- e. type

erotopath
erotopathic
erotopathy
ERP
- event-related potential
- exposure and response prevention

errant thought
erratic
- e. absorption
- e. behavior
- e. driving
- e. eater
- e. mood
- e. parenting
- e. sleep
- e. speech rhythm
- e. thinking

erroneous
- e. belief
- e. impression

error
- accidental e.
- alpha e.
- e. analysis
- anomic e.
- anticipatory e.
- aphasic e.
- attribution e.
- e. attribution
- beta e.
- chance e.
- e. detection circuit
- experimental e.
- fundamental attribution e.
- genetic e.
- gross medical e.
- e. of measurement
- measurement e.
- motivated e.
- paraphasic e.
- perceptual e.
- perseverative e.
- probable e. (PE)
- standard e.
- subjective e.
- time e.
- trial and e.
- type I, II e.
- e. variance
- vicarious trial and e. (VTE)

ertotropid system
eructation
erudite
erudition

erythromania
ES
ego strength
electroshock
elopement status
emergency service
environmental stimulation
epileptic syndrome
experimental study
ESB
electric stimulation of the brain
escala inteligencia Wechsler para adultes (EIWA)
escalating conflict
escalation
dose e.
escapade
sexual e.
escape
e. artist
e. behavior
e. conditioning
e. drinking
e. from the ego
e. from freedom
e. from reality
e. into illness
e. learning
e. mechanism
e. phenomenon
e. reaction
e. training
escapism
escapist
eschatology
Escherich sign
eschew
eschrolalia
escort
escutcheon
ESEP
extreme somatosensory evoked potential
Eshmun complex
ESL
English as a second language
ESN
educationally subnormal
esophageal
e. neurosis
e. voice
esophagus psychogenic disorder
esophoria

esoteric
ESP
extrasensory perception
especial
espial
espousal
espouse
esprit
bel e.
e. de corps conditioning
essay
essence
essential
e. alcoholism
e. anosmia
e. convulsion
e. epilepsy
e. feature
e. headache
e. hypertension
e. psychopharmacology
e. seizure
e. tremor (ET)
e. vertigo
essentialism
EST, est
electroshock therapy
electroshock threshold
electroshock treatment
established delusion
establishment
establish predictability
estate guardianship
esteem
e. need
esteem-enhancing
esthematology
esthesia
esthesic
esthesiodic system
esthesiogenesis
esthesiogenic
esthesiography
esthesiology
esthesiomania
esthesiometer
esthesiometry
esthesioscopy
esthesodic
esthetic (*var. of* aesthetic)
estimable

E

NOTES

estimated
> e. learning potential (ELP)
> e. length of stay

estimator

estranged partner

estrangement
> feeling of e.
> inner e.
> sense of e.

estrogen replacement therapy

estromania

estrous cycle

estrual

estrus

esurience

esurient

état criblé

eternal suckling

eternity fear

eternize

eternus
> puer e.

ethamivan

ethanol (ETOH, EtOH)
> e. abuse
> e. abuser
> e. dependence
> e. exposure
> e. intoxication
> e. nonuser
> e. treatment
> e. user
> e. volume fraction (EVF)
> e. withdrawal

ether
> e. base
> cyclic e.
> e. dependence
> e. drunkenness
> e. effect

e-therapy

ethereal

etherism

etherize

etheromania

ethic
> case e.
> work e.

ethical
> e. approach
> e. behavior
> e. concern
> e. conflict
> e. deliberation
> e. dilemma
> e. highbrow
> e. imperative
> e. obligation

> e. principle
> e. reasoning
> e. restraint
> e. risk hypothesis
> e. self

ethically permissible

ethics
> achievement e.
> care e.
> code of e.
> consequentialist e.
> medical e.
> normative e.
> professional e.
> e. of psychiatric research
> situation e.
> situational e.
> structured-based e.
> e. violation
> virtue e.
> Western e.

ethinamate

ethnic
> e. background
> e. bias
> e. factor
> e. hate
> e. minority
> e. prejudice
> e. profiling
> e. reference group
> e. relational behavior (ERB)

ethnocentrism scale

ethnographic approach

ethnography

ethnology

ethnopsychiatry

ethnopsychology

ethogram

ethological
> e. models of personal space
> e. study

ethologist

ethology

ethopharmacology

ethos

ethyl
> e. alcohol (ETOH, EtOH)
> e. alcohol addiction

ethylamine

ethylism

etiolate

etiological
> e. agent
> e. association
> e. complexity
> e. factor
> e. heterogeneity

e. neurological condition
e. relationship
e. validity
etiologic role
etiology, pl. **etiologies**
    delirium due to multiple etiologies
    disease e.
    Four-Factor Theory of E.
    general medical e.
    medical e.
    multifactorial e.
    organic e.
    presumed e.
    substance-induced e.
    e. theory
    unclear e.
etiopathogenesis
etiopathogenic
etiopathology
etiotropic
etiquette
ETOH, EtOH
    ethanol
    ethyl alcohol
etomidate
etoperidone
etryptamine
ETS
    electrical transcranial stimulation
    electrosleep therapy
etymology
EU
    emergency unit
    expected utility
eubiotics
eucaine
EUCD
    emotionally unstable character disorder
euchromatopsy
eucodal
eucrasia
eudemonia
euergasia
eugenicist
eugenics
    negative e.
    positive e.
eugenic sterilization law
eugenism
eugnathia
eugnosia
eukinesia

eukinetic
eulogize
eumetria
eunoia
eunuch
eunuchism
    pituitary e.
eunuchoidism
    female e.
eunuchoid voice
euosmia
eupeptic
euphemism
euphenics
euphonia
euphonic
euphoretic
euphoria
    cannabis-induced e.
    event-related e.
    false e.
    giddy e.
    indifferent e.
    postcoital e.
euphoriant
euphoric
    e. affect
    e. apathy
    e. effect
    e. mood
    e. presentation
    e. speech
euphorigenic effect
euphuism
eupnea
eupraxia
Eurasian
eurymorph
eurytopic
eusthenia
eusthenic
eustress
eutelegenesis
euthanasia
    active e.
    passive e.
    voluntary e.
euthenic
eutherapeutics
euthymia
euthymic
    e. memory

E

NOTES

euthymic (*continued*)
    e. mood
    e. state
euthyroid
eutonia sclerotica
eutonic
eutrophia
evacuant
evacuation
evacuator
evade
evaluability
evaluability-assessment data
evaluating clinician
evaluation
    e. of adolescent
    career e.
    clinical e.
    comprehensive e.
    condescending e.
    e. contract
    contract e.
    court-mandated e.
    criterion e.
    e. of criterion
    cross-sectional e.
    dementia e.
    e. dissemination
    employee e.
    event-related potentials e.
    face-to-face e.
    false e.
    family e.
    home e.
    in-house e.
    e. interview
    job e.
    medical care e. (MCE)
    mental capacity e.
    multiaxial e.
    negative e.
    neurological e.
    neuropsychologic e.
    e. and observation (E&O)
    operational e.
    e. period
    poor performance e.
    psychiatric e.
    psychoeducational e.
    psychological e.
    psychometric e.
    psychosocial factor e.
    rehabilitation e.
    e. research
    social e.
    symptom e.
    testing and e. (T&E)
    e. of training

    transactional e.
    unbiased e.
    e. utilization
    vocational e.
evaluative
    e. rating
    e. reasoning
evaluator bias
evanescent
evangelical
evasion
evasive
    e. behavior
    e. tendency
evasiveness
evenhanded
evening
    e. drinker
    e. drinking
    e. headache
    e. primrose
    e. treatment
event
    acute extrapyramidal e.
    adverse e.
    amnesia for sleep terror e.
    antecedent e.
    catastrophic e.
    cathartic e.
    emotional e.
    entrance e.
    enuretic e.
    exit e.
    external e.
    extrapyramidal e.
    genomic e.
    heinous e.
    independent e.
    life e.
    life-threatening e.
    e. memory
    milestone e.
    multifactorial e.
    negative life e.
    neuroleptic-related e.
    parasuicidal e.
    past e.
    personal e.
    place-specific e.
    positive e.
    potential positive e.
    precipitating e.
    psychosocial e.
    e. recall
    e. recall score
    recent life e. (RLE)
    reexperienced traumatic e.
    sequence of e.'s

sleep-terror e.
stressful e.
time-specific e.
totality of possible e.'s
traumatic life e.
treatment-emergent adverse e.
triggering e.
event-related
e.-r. brain potential study
e.-r. desynchronization (ERD)
e.-r. distress
e.-r. euphoria
e.-r. potential (ERP)
e.-r. potentials evaluation
eventuate
eversion theory of aging
every
e. four hours
e. night
e. other day
e. two hours
everyday
e. activities in life
e. function
EVF
ethanol volume fraction
evict
evidence
admissible e.
amnesia e.
e. of amnesia
anatomic e.
anecdotal e.
biologic e.
blocking e.
e. of blocking
circumstantial e.
clear and convincing e.
compelling e.
e. of dissociation disorder
empirical e.
incontrovertible e.
indirect e.
e. of interruption
e. of intrusion of idiosyncratic material
e. of intrusion of private material
new e.
preponderance of the e.
psychiatric e.
rule of e.
supporting e.

evidence-based
e.-b. medicine (EBM)
e.-b. process
e.-b. psychiatry
evidentiary hearing
evil
e. eye
e. force
e. influence
e. manner
e. omen
e. person
e. reputation
e. spirit
e. temper
e. thoughts
evil-minded
evince
eviration
evocation
evoked
e. affect
e. potential (EP)
e. potential response (EPR)
e. response (ER)
e. somatosensory response
evolution
e. of brain
emergent e.
mental e.
saltatory e.
e. theory
evolutionary intervention
evolutionism
evolve
evulsion
ex
ex post facto
ex post facto research
ex vivo
exacerbated symptoms
exacerbation
e. of acting out
acute e.
disease e.
pain e.
psychotic e.
e. rate
schizophrenic e.
symptom e.
exactitude
exact science

E

NOTES

ex-addict
exaggerated
  e. achievement
  e. belief
  e. communication in schizophrenia
  e. defect
  e. depression
  e. expression
  e. feeling
  e. inferential thinking in
    schizophrenia
  e. movement
  e. negative quality
  e. perception
  e. positive quality
  e. startle response
exaggeration
  e. of inferential behavioral
    monitoring
  e. of language and communication
  e. in wit
exaltation
  reactive e.
exalted paranoia
examination
  e. anxiety
  comprehensive e.
  e. dream
  followup e.
  longitudinal mental status e.
  mental e.
  mental status e. (MSE)
  neurological e.
  neuropathologic e.
  objective e.
  peripheral e.
  physical e. (PE)
  psychiatric e.
  psychological e.
  screening e.
  sexological e.
  status e.
  e. stupor
examiner
  medical e.
  trial e.
example
  clinical e.
exasperate
exceptional
  e. child
  e. stress
exception question
Excerpta Medica
excess
  dietary e.
excessive
  e. acting out

  e. admiration
  e. alcohol intake
  e. concern for defect
  e. crying
  e. daytime sleepiness (EDS)
  e. daytime somnolence
  e. discipline
  e. drug use
  e. emotionality
  e. exercise
  e. fatigue
  e. food intake
  e. gambling
  e. gambling behavior
  e. grooming
  e. guilt
  e. laughing
  e. laxative use
  e. motor activity
  e. need
  e. need for care
  e. optimism
  e. pride
  e. responsibility
  e. rigidity
  e. skin scratching
  e. social anxiety
  e. spending
  e. stress
  e. talking
  e. volubility
  e. worry
excessively
  e. impressionistic speech
  e. loud speech
  e. soft speech
  e. upset
exchange
  angry word e.
  fetal-maternal e.
excipient
excitability of neuron
excitable behavior
excitant
excitation
  catatonic e.
  e. and conduction
  equalization of e.
  e. gradient
  psychogenic e.
  e. psychosis
  e. psychotic reaction
  reactive e.
  subliminal e.
excitation-contraction
excitative psychosis
excitative-type nonorganic psychosis

excitatory
- e. agent
- e. amino acid receptor inhibitor
- e. field
- e. impulse
- e. neurotransmitter
- e. postsynaptic potential (EPSP)
- e. stimulus
- e. synapse

excitatory-inhibitory process

excited
- e. behavior
- e. mood
- e. schizoaffective schizophrenia
- e. state

excitement
- anniversary e.
- catatonic e.
- inhibited sexual e. (ISE)
- manic e.
- mental e.
- e. phase
- e. phase of sexual response cycle
- psychomotor e.
- reactive mental e.
- schizophrenic e.
- sexual e.

excitement-seeking tendency

excitomotor

excitomuscular

excitonutrient

excitor

excitotoxicity

exclamation theory

exclusion
- e. criteria
- diagnosis by e.

exclusive
- mutually e.

excogitate

excommunicate

excommunicative

excoriation
- neurotic e.
- psychogenic e.

excrement fear

excrescence

excretory perversion

excruciate

exculpate

excursive

excusatory

execrable

execrate

executant ego function

executive
- e. aphasia
- e. aspect
- e. control
- e. decision-maker
- e. ego function
- e. function deficit
- e. functioning
- e. functioning disturbance
- e. language
- e. organ
- e. process
- e. speech
- e. stress
- e. system dysfunction

exegesis
- analytic e.

exemplar

exemplify

exencephalia

exencephalic

exencephalous

exencephaly

exercise
- e. addict
- e. addiction
- aerobic e.
- compulsive e.
- container e.
- excessive e.
- holding e.
- imagery e.
- intellectual e.
- intergroup e.
- journaling e.
- e. law
- law of e.
- mental e.
- mirror e.
- modeling e.
- patterning e.
- physical e.
- spiritual e.
- therapeutic e.
- e. therapy
- e. treatment
- verbal memory e.

exercise-induced sympathetic discharge

exerciser container

NOTES

E

exert
exertional headache
exhaustion
>combat e.
>e. death
>e. delirium
>e. management
>mental e.
>nervous e.
>e. paralysis
>e. psychosis
>e. senile dementia
>stage of e.
>e. stage
>e. state
>e. syndrome (EPS)

exhaustive
>e. psychosis
>e. stupor

exhibition
>e. dream
>sexual e.
>e. wit

exhibitionism
>e. paraphilia
>shock e.

exhibitionistic behavior
exhibitionist need
exhilarant
exhilarate
exhortation
ex-husband
exigent
existence
>e. need
>e., relatedness, and growth theory
>(ERG)

existential
>e. analysis
>e. anguish
>e. anxiety
>e. crisis
>e. ego function
>e. living
>e. neurosis
>e. phenomenology
>e. psychiatry
>e. psychoanalysis
>e. psychology
>e. psychotherapy
>e. school
>e. vacuum

existential-humanistic
>e.-h. theory
>e.-h. therapy

existentialism

exit
>e. event
>e. interview

exocathection
exocentric construction
exocytosis
exogamy
exogenesis
exogenetic
exogenous
>e. chemical
>e. depression
>e. factor
>e. obesity
>e. psychosis
>e. smile
>e. stimulation
>e. stress
>e. Zeitgeber

exonerative moral reasoning
exophoria
exopsychic
exorbitance
exorcism
exorcist
exosomatic method
exotic
>e. bias
>e. psychosis

exoticism
expanded consciousness
expansion
>consciousness e.
>e. delusion
>e. idea
>e. mood
>perceptual e.

expansiva
>paraphrenia e.

expansive
>e. delusion
>e. idea
>e. mood
>e. solution

expansiveness
>grandiose e.

expatiate
expectancy
>e. chart
>life e.
>lifetime e.
>e. theory

expectant analysis
expectation
>anxious e.
>apprehension e.
>catastrophic e.
>death e.

e. of death
internal world of e.
e. of life
negative e.
e. neurosis
optimistic e.
realistic e.
serial linguistic e.
unrealistic e.

expected
e. death
e. frequency
e. level of achievement
e. utility (EU)
e. weight gain

expenditure
resting energy e.

experience
accidental e.
adverse childhood e.
affective e.
atypical delusional e.
brief delusional e.
bullying e.
charismatic religious e.
childhood e.
clinical e.
collective e.
common e.
confrontational e.
corrective emotional e.
countertransference e.
cultural e.
culturally sanctioned e.
cutaneous e.
dating e.
deficient affective e.
delusional e.
depersonalization e.
depressive e.
developmental e.
dissociative e.
disturbing e.
dream e.
dysphoric subjective e.
emotional e.
external world e.
false sensory e.
fantasized sexual e.
gambling e.
group e.
hallucinatory e.

heterosexual sexual e.
homosexual sexual e.
horrific e.
human therapeutic e.
identity e.
immediate e.
inner e.
intimate e.
job-sample e.
learning e.
life e.
life-changing spiritual e.
loss e.
mother-child e.
mystical e.
narcolepsy e.
near-death e.
online sexual e.
openness to e.
opposite sex sexual e.
out-of-body e. (OBE)
outside the range of normal
  human e.
overrepresented e.
overwhelming childhood e.
overwhelming intimate e.
paradigmatic stress from life e.
past e.
peak e.
perceptual e.
personal e.
personally saddening e.
physical e.
pleasure e.
practice e.
psychic e.
psychologically overwhelming e.
religious e.
repeated painful e.
same-sex sexual e.
sensory e.
sexual e.
social learning e.
spiritual possession e.
split-off and denied e.
stimulating e.
stress from life e. (SFLE)
stressful life e.
subjective e.
success e.
syntaxic mode of e.
terrifying e.

E

NOTES

253

experience *(continued)*
    thought transfer e.
    transient hallucinatory e.
    traumatic e.
    treatment e.
    troubling e.
    e. with criminal activities
experiential
    e. factor
    e. group
    e. psychotherapy
    e. therapy
experiment
    analog e.
    delayed reaction e.
    double blind e.
    double masked e.
    factorial e.
    field e.
experimental
    e. analysis of behavior
    e. bias
    e. condition
    e. control
    e. design
    e. disorder
    e. drug
    e. error
    e. game
    e. group
    e. hypothesis
    e. intervention
    e. marriage
    e. medication
    e. medicine
    e. method
    e. neurasthenia
    e. neurosis
    e. psychiatry
    e. psychology
    e. psychometric setting
    e. realism
    e. series
    e. sexual activities
    e. study (ES)
    e. therapy
    e. treatment
    e. variable
experimentation
    environmental e.
    pharmacological e.
    role e.
    sexual e.
experimenter
    e. bias
    e. effect
experimenter-expectancy effect

expert
    mental health e.
    e. system
    e. testimony
    e. witness
expertise
expiate
expiation
expiatory
    e. punishment
    e. self-punishment
explain away
explanation
    alternative e.
    post hoc e.
    reassuring e.
explanatory
explicable
explicit
    e. behavior
    e. gesture
    e. language
    e. memory
    e. process
    e. role
    e. type
explicitly religious
exploit
exploitation
    e. of children
    gender e.
    interpersonal e.
exploitative
    e. character
    e. orientation
    e. personality
exploitative-manipulative behavior
exploiter
    professional e.
exploiting type
exploration
    diversive e.
    dream e.
    e. drive
    therapeutic e.
exploratory
    e. behavior
    e. drive
    e. insight
    e. insight-oriented psychotherapy
    (EIO)
    e. therapy
explosion readiness
explosive
    e. aggressive behavior
    e. disturbance
    e. neurotic personality disorder
    e. outburst

e. personality
e. personality disorder
e. psychotic state
e. rage
e. speech
e. temper
explosivity
exposition attitude
expostulate
exposure
e. to abuse
anthrax e.
antipsychotic e.
avoidance of e.
biochemical e.
e. to bioterrorism
e. to biowarfare cue
chronic ethanol e.
cold e.
e. to combat
combat stress e.
common precipitant e.
controlled e.
e. to cue
cue e.
e. deafness
e. to death
disease e.
e. to disease
epidemic germ e.
ethanol e.
exteroceptive e.
fetal e.
germ e.
graded e.
e. to grief
habit e.
e. to hate
e. hierarchy
e. to hostility
imaginal e.
indecent e.
interoceptive e.
neuroleptic e.
occupational e.
e. of person
prolonged e.
e. and response prevention (ERP)
self-directed e.
e. to terrorist activity
toxin e.
e. to toxins

e. to trauma
e. to trigger
e. to violence
e. in vivo
in vivo e.
exposure-based
e.-b. cognitive behavior therapy
e.-b. intervention
expound
expressed
e. emotion (EE)
e. motivation
expression
abrupt shift in affective e.
abstract e.
affective e.
akinesia/diminished emotional e.
appropriate facial e.
behavioral e.
e. of bias
blunted emotional e.
e. of caring
diminished emotional e.
discordant facial e.
disorder of written e.
emotional facial e.
exaggerated e.
facial e.
e. of feeling
e. of grief
e. of hospitality
e. of hostility
inappropriate sexual e.
involuntary emotional e.
lines of e.
e. method
nonverbal e.
obscene e.
parenthetical e.
passivity in anger e.
pattern of e.
e. of prejudice
rapid shift in affective e.
repeated shift in affective e.
restricted range of emotional e.
sexual e.
shallow e.
e. of sharing
staring facial e.
unassertive e.
unhappy facial e.
verbal e.

E

NOTES

expression *(continued)*
    e. with feeling
    written e.
expressionism factor
expressive
    e. amimia
    e. amusia
    e. aphasia
    e. delusion
    e. dysphasia
    e. function
    e. gesture
    e. glance
    e. language
    e. language deficit
    e. language development
    e. language development disorder
    e. language quotient
    e. language skill
    e. movement
    e. pattern
    e. therapy
    e. writing development disorder
expressiveness
    lack of e.
expressive-receptive aphasia
expurgate
expurgatory
extemporaneous
extended
    e. care
    e. counseling
    e. family
    e. family therapy (EFT)
    e. jargon paraphasia
    e. play
    e. sick leave
extended-care
    e.-c. facility
    e.-c. insurance
    e.-c. review
extended-stay review
extension semantics
extensor
    e. plantar response
    e. rigidity
    e. tetanus
    e. thrust
extent
    e. of abuse
    e. of damage
    e. prognosis
extenuating circumstance
exterieur
    milieu e.
exteriorization
exteriorize

external
    e. boundary
    e. capsule
    e. chemical messenger (ECM)
    e. cue
    e. demand
    e. entity
    e. event
    e. force
    e. force control
    e. genitalia
    e. incentive motivation
    e. information
    e. inhibition
    internal versus e. (I-E)
    e. locus of control
    e. meningitis
    e. reality
    e. reward
    e. sense
    e. source
    e. speech
    e. speech stimulus
    e. spirit
    e. stigma
    e. stimulation
    e. stressor
    e. structure
    e. support
    e. support system
    e. validity
    e. world
    e. world experience
externalization
externalize blame
externalized anger
externalizing behavior
externally
    e. directed aggression
    e. oriented thinking (EOT)
exteroceptive
    e. conditioning
    e. exposure
exteroceptor
exteropsychic
extinction
    differential e.
    e. of ego
    order of e.
    perceptual e.
    e. ratio
    resistance to e.
    sensory e.
    tactile e.
    visual e.
extinction-type pattern
extinguish
extirpate

extol
extra
    fecundatio ab e.
extracellular contribution
extraception
extrachromosomal
extract
    kava e.
extractive disorder
extrafamilial sexual abuse
extraindividual behavior
extrajection
extramarital
    e. affair
    e. behavior
    e. intercourse
    e. relations
    e. sex
    e. sexuality
extraneous
    e. movement
    e. noise
extrapolate
extrapsychic conflict
extrapunitive
extrapyramidal
    e. disorder
    e. dyskinesia
    e. epilepsy
    e. event
    e. involvement (EPI)
    e. medication side effect
    e. motor system
    e. rigidity
    e. sign
    e. symptom (EPS)
    e. symptom potential
    e. symptom-sparing
    e. syndrome (EPS)
    e. syndrome symptom
    e. system (EPS)
    e. tract
extrasensory
    e. perception (ESP)
    e. thought transference
extraspective perspective
extratransference issue
extravagant
extraversion (var. of extroversion)
extravert (var. of extrovert)
extravisual

extreme
    e. act of violence
    e. agitation
    e. anxiety
    e. level of violence
    e. negativism
    e. range
    e. somatosensory evoked potential
    (ESEP)
    e. stressor
    e. trauma
extremis
    in e.
extremist
extremity
    phantom e.
extricate
extrinsic
    e. constancy
    e. cortex
    e. epilepsy
    e. motivation
    e. reward
extroceptor
extrospection
extroversion, extraversion
extrovert, extravert
extroverted
    e. personality
    e. type
exuberant
exultant
exultation
ex-wife
eye
    e. accessing cue
    black e.
    e. blink
    e. blink conditioning test
    e. contact
    e. contact avoidance
    crossed e.'s
    dancing e.
    defected e.'s
    deflected e.
    e. dominance
    evil e.
    glassy e.'s
    e. gouging
    lusterless e.'s
    e. memory
    mind's e.

E

NOTES

eye *(continued)*
    e. movement
    e. movement abnormality
    e. movement desensitization
    e. movement desensitization and
      reprocessing (EMDR)
    e. movement reprocessing
    e. preference
    e. psychogenic disorder
    puffy e.
    raccoon e.
    e. scan
    e. scanning
    swollen e.
    e. tracking
eyeball-to-eyeball

eye-blink response
eye-closure reflex
eye-hand coordination
eyelash sign
eyelid
    e. conditioning
    drooping e.
    insufficiency of e.
eye-opener
eye-roll sign
eye-to-eye
eye-voice span
Eysenck
    E. and Gray biological theories of
      personality
    E. model

F
    form response
F+
    good form response
F-
    poor form response
f
    frequency
fable
fables test
fabricate
fabrication
fabulation
facade of competence
face
    about f.
    flushed f.
    immobile f.
    poker f.
    save f.
    staring f.
    unfamiliar f.
    f. up
    f. up to
    f. validity
    f. value
faced
face-hand test
face-off
face-saver
face-saving behavior
facete
facetious
face-to-face
    f.-t.-f. advice
    f.-t.-f. evaluation
    f.-t.-f. meeting
facial
    F. Action Coding System (FACS)
    f. affect
    f. agnosia
    f. apraxia
    f. asymmetry
    f. deceit
    f. diplegia
    f. disfigurement
    f. display
    f. expression
    f. expression automatism
    f. expression interpretation
    f. flushing
    f. grimace
    f. hemiatrophy
    f. hemiplegia
    f. identification

    f. nerve
    f. neuralgia
    f. paralysis
    f. paresis
    f. perception
    f. profiling
    f. recognition
    f. responsiveness
    f. sensation
    f. talk
    f. tic
    f. tremor
    f. twitch
facialis phenomenon
facies, pl. **facies**
    f. dolorosa
    elfin f.
    Hutchinson f.
    mask f.
    masked f.
    masklike f.
    myasthenic f.
    myopathic f.
    myotonic f.
facile
facilitating environment
facilitation
    associative f.
    behavioral f.
    f. of communication
    intracortical inhibition and f.
    reproductive f.
    social f.
    Wedensky f.
facilitory
facility
    board-and-care f.
    childcare f.
    correctional f.
    detention f.
    emergency care f.
    extended-care f.
    health-related f.
    inpatient psychiatric treatment f.
    intermediate care f.
    juvenile detention f.
    long-term care f.
    mental health treatment f.
    psychiatric f.
    rehabilitation f.
    residential treatment f.
    shcltcr f.
    short-term care f.
    substance abuse treatment f.
    treatment f.

F

FACS
    Facial Action Coding System
fact
    f. finding
    f. giver
    f. of life
    f. seeker
faction
    time f.
factitial dermatitis
factitious
    f. disorder, combined type
    f. disorder, physical type
    f. disorder by proxy
    f. disorder, psychological type
    f. illness
    f. illness by proxy
    f. interface disorder
factitious-type neurotic hysteric disorder
facto
    de f.
    ex post f.
factor
    activation f.
    adverse background f.
    age-specific risk f.
    aggression f.
    alpha f.
    f. analysis
    antisocial psychopathic Q f.
    arousability f.
    assimilative f.
    attitudinal risk f.
    background f.
    biologic risk f.
    C f.
    causal f.
    cellular immunity f.
    cleverness f.
    cognitive behavioral f.
    cognitive risk f.
    combined f.
    f. comparison
    f. comparison method
    constitutional f.
    Costa-McCrae f.
    cultural f.
    demographic risk f.
    depression f.
    3-f. dimensional model of
      schizophrenia
    disorder due to combined f.'s
    disorganized f.
    DNA transcription f.
    dysfunctional family f.
    dysphoric Q f.
    emotional f.
    endogenous f.

    environmental f.
    erectile disorder due to
      combined f.'s
    erectile disorder due to
      psychological f.'s
    ethnic f.
    etiological f.
    exogenous f.
    experiential f.
    expressionism f.
    familial risk f.
    father f.
    feedback inhibition f. (FIF)
    Frankenstein f.
    Frohman f.
    G f.
    general f.
    genetic risk f.
    geriatric f.
    gestalt f.
    growth hormone-releasing f.
    hedonic-tone f.
    histrionic Q f.
    human f.
    human growth f. (HGF)
    impulsivity f.
    interest f.
    known organic f.
    lethal f.
    lifestyle f.
    f. loading
    f. matrix
    mauve f.
    method f.
    motivation f.
    motivational f.
    negative f.
    neurotic f.
    noise f.
    nonspecific neurotic f.
    obsessional Q f.
    organic f.
    orthogonal depression f.
    pathogenic f.
    perpetuating f.
    personal f.
    pharmacologic f.
    phenotypic f.
    physiological risk f.
    potential predisposing f.
    precipitating f.
    predictive f.
    predisposing f.
    pregenital f.
    preoedipal f.
    pretraumatic risk f.
    primary risk f.
    protection f.

psychiatric risk f.
psychic f.
psychological f.
psychosexual f.
psychosis f.
psychosocial f.
psychotic f.
Q f.
f. reflection
religious orthodoxy f.
risk f.
rotated f.
f. rotation
S f.
f. of safety (FS)
schizoid Q f.
schizophrenic f.
f. score
significant risk f.
social risk f.
spiritual f.
state f.
subjectivism f.
suicide risk f.
susceptibility f.
f. theory
f. theory of personality
thinking disturbance f. (TDF)
trait f.
uncertainty f.
uncertainty-arousal f.
unconscious f.
unspecified psychological f.
V f.
verbal comprehension f.
violence-promoting f.
will f.
within-family environmental f.
factorial
f. design
f. experiment
f. invariance
f. validity
factual
f. knowledge
f. memory
facultative
faculty
fusion f.
f. fusion
intellectual f.
language f.

mental f.
f. psychology
fad
f. activity
f. diet
illicit drug f.
faddish
faddism
food f.
fading
stimulus f.
FAE
fetal alcohol effect
failed suicide attempt
failing grade
fail-safe
failure
academic f.
attentional f.
brain functional f.
f. to comply
f. to develop
f. to develop empathy
f. to develop relatedness
f. of drug trial
empathic f.
employment f.
erectile f.
f. to fulfill
functional f.
f. to gain weight
f. of lateralization
multiple organ f.
f. of problem solving
recall f.
reproductive f.
sense of f.
f. in social adaptation
f. to sustain consistent work
  behavior
f. to sustain a monogamous
  relationship
therapeutic f.
f. to thrive (FTT)
f. through success
f. to warm
f. to warn
failure-to-grow syndrome
failure-to-thrive syndrome
fain
faint
fight, flee, freeze, or f.

F

NOTES

faint-hearted
fair
> f. minded
> f. sex
> f. shake
> f. spoken

faire
> savoir f.

Fairness in Treatment: Drug and Alcohol Addiction Recovery Act of 1999
fair-weather friend
fait
> f. accompli
> déjà f.

faith
> blind f.
> f. conversion problem
> f. cure
> f. in God
> good f.
> f. healing
> keeping f.
> religious f.
> f. in self
> tenets of f.

fakir
fall
> f. away
> f. off
> f. off the wagon
> f. short
> f. through

fallacious
fallacy
> pathologic f.

fallible
falling
> f. out
> f. risk
> f. sickness

false
> f. accusation
> f. arrest
> f. association
> f. attribution
> f. belief
> f. conditioning
> f. euphoria
> f. evaluation
> f. fluency
> f. friend
> f. hearted
> f. hermaphroditism
> f. hope
> f. identity
> f. image
> f. imprisonment

> f. masturbation
> f. memory
> f. memory syndrome
> f. negative
> f. paracusis
> f. perceptions of movement
> f. positive
> f. pregnancy
> f. pretense
> f. promise
> f. role disorder
> f. sense of security
> f. sensory experience
> f. threshold

falsehood
false-negative
> f.-n. case
> f.-n. diagnosis
> f.-n. response

false-positive
> f.-p. diagnosis
> f.-p. response

falsetto voice
falsifiable hypothesis
falsification
> memory f.
> retrospective f.

falsify
falter
familial
> f. aggregation
> f. aggregation problem
> f. bipolar mood disorder
> f. deficiency
> f. dementia
> f. encephalopathy
> f. hormonal disorder
> f. migraine headache
> f. neuropathy
> f. pattern
> f. periodic paralysis
> f. psychosis
> f. pure depressive disease (FPDD)
> f. risk factor
> f. tendency
> f. transmission
> f. transmission of schizophrenia
> f. unconscious

familiar
> f. correlation coefficient
> f. surroundings

familiarity
famille
> folie á f.
> f. nevropathique

family
> adoptive f.
> alcoholic f.

f. ambiance
f. assessment
f. background
bilineal f.
birth f.
blended f.
f. burden
f. care
f. caregiver
close-knit f.
cohesive f.
f. conference (FC)
f. conflict
f. connectedness
f. constellation
f. counseling
f. counselor
f. court
f. disruption
drug f.
f. dynamics
dysfunctional f.
empowered f.
f. evaluation
f. evaluation scale
extended f.
f. fragmentation
f. group intake
f. group therapy
f. health insurance plan (FHIP)
high-conflict f.
f. history (FH)
f. history of mental illness
  (RHMI)
homeless f.
f. honor
f. identity
f. idiocy
f. incubus
f. interaction
f. intervention
f. involvement
Jukes f.
Kallikak f.
f. loyalty
matrilinear f.
matrilocal f.
f. medicine
f. member
f. member therapy
f. method
f. name

f. neglect
neolocal f.
f. neurosis
nuclear f.
f. obligation
occupational f.
patriarchal f.
patrilineal f.
patrilocal f.
f. pattern
f. perception
f. physician
f. planning
f. process
f. psychiatric history
f. psychotherapy
f. pursuit
reconstituted f.
f. relation
f. relationship
rigid f.
f. risk study
f. romance
f. routine
runs in f.
f. sculpting
f. separation
single-parent f.
f. situation
f. sleeping arrangement
f. social work
f. stability
f. stress
f. strife
f. structural balance
f. support
f. support group
f. support network
f. support system
systemic f.
f. and systemic psychotherapy
f. system interview
f. system research orientation
f. systems theory
f. treatment
f. tree
f. turbulence
f. type
f. unit
f. unit therapy
f. violence
zero f.

F

NOTES

fanaticism
fanatic personality
fanciful
fancy free
fan sign
fantasize
fantasized sexual experience
fantasizing
 active f.
fantastica, phantastica
 paraphrenia f.
 pseudologia f.
fantasticate
fantasy, phantasy
 f. absence
 affect f.
 aggressive f.
 anal rape f.
 f. assessment
 attachment f.
 autistic f.
 cannibalistic f.
 f. cathexis
 compensatory f.
 erotic f.
 eroticized f.
 fellatio f.
 f. figure
 flight into f.
 forced f.
 grandiosity in f.
 hero f.
 hetaeral f.
 homoerotic f.
 incest f.
 incestuous f.
 intense sexual f.
 internal world of f.
 king-slave f.
 f. life
 magic f.
 masochistic sexual f.
 masturbation f.
 night f.
 nonpathological sexual f.
 obsessive f.
 online sexual f.
 paraphiliac f.
 pathognomonic f.
 pathologic sexual f.
 f. period
 f. play
 Pompadour f.
 primal f.
 f. process
 rape f.
 rebirth f.
 rejuvenation f.

 rescue f.
 romance f.
 romantic f.
 schizoid f.
 screen f.
 secondary f.
 sexual f.
 sexually arousing f.
 spider f.
 unconscious f.
 violent f.
 voyeuristic sexually arousing f.
 womb f.
 world-destruction f.
fantasy-based elements of the doctor-patient relationship
fantod
FAP
 fixed action pattern
far-field evoked potential
far-flung
far-off
far-out
far-reaching
farseeing
farsightedness
FAS
 fetal alcohol syndrome
fasciculation
fascinating
fascination
 obsessional f.
fascinum
fashion
 cookbook f.
 multiaxial f.
 nonaxial f.
 probabilistic f.
 ritualistic f.
 singsong f.
 f. statement
fast
 f. activity
 anorexic f.
 f. gradient recalled spectroscopic imaging technique
 f. speech
 f. track
 f. track program
fast-acting agent
fastidious
fastidium
 f. cibi
 f. potus
fastigial pressor response (FPR)
fasting
 religious f.

self-imposed f.
starvation f.
fast-talk
fat
body f.
f. body
f. depot
fatal
f. accident
f. attraction
f. complications of illicit drug use
f. consequence
f. hypothermia
f. mistake
f. overdose
fatale
femme f.
fatalism
fatalistic attitude
fatality
fata morgana
fate
f. analysis
law of common f.
f. neurosis
fated
father
abusive f.
adopted f.
adoptive f.
alleged f. (AF)
biologic f.
birth f.
f. complex
f. confessor
dysfunctional f.
f. factor
f. figure
f. fixation
foster f.
f. hypnosis
f. ideal
f. image
primal f.
f. substitute
surrogate f.
f. surrogate
teenage f.
vaginal f.
father-child bond
father-daughter incest
fatherly

fatidic
fatigue
auditory f.
battle f.
chronic f.
cognitive f.
combat f.
daytime f.
f. disease
disease-related f.
ease of f.
easy f.
emotional f.
excessive f.
mental f.
nervous f.
f. neurosis
operational f.
overwhelming f.
pseudocombat f.
psychogenic f.
sense of f.
f. state
stimulation f.
f. strength
f. stress
sustained f.
f. symptom
f. syndrome
unusual f.
fatiguing vigil
fatness stimulus
fatuity
fatuous
fatuus
ignis f.
faucial
f. paralysis
faugh
fault
find f.
to a f.
faulty judgment
fausse reconnaissance
faut
comme il f.
faute de mieux
faux pas
favor
sexual f.
favorable
favorite son

NOTES

favoritism
faze
FC
    family conference
    formed response of colored area
    foster care
    frontal cortex
    functional capacity
Fc
    shading response to black areas
    shading response to gray areas
FDA
    Food and Drug Administration
      FDA Modernization Act of 1997
FDE
    first episode of depression
fealty
FEAR
    feeling frightened; expecting bad things
    to happen; attitudes and actions that
    help; results and reward
fear
    f. appeal
    f. association
    bad-people f.
    f. of bioterrorism
    building f.
    castration f.
    childhood f.
    cold f.
    combat f.
    f. conditioning
    confinement f.
    contamination f.
    crowd f.
    desire to instill f.
    f. drive
    eating f.
    emptiness f.
    epidemic of f.
    epilepsy f.
    eternity f.
    excrement f.
    free-floating f.
    f. hypnosis
    image eliciting f.
    impregnation f.
    impulse f.
    incapacitating f.
    intense f.
    interoceptive f.
    irrational f.
    lack of f.
    life f.
    lingering f.
    marriage f.
    masking f.
    maturity f.

mirror f.
moisture f.
monster f.
morbid f.
motion f.
mouse f.
night f.
obligations f.
obsessive f.
odor f.
overwork f.
paranoid f.
penis f.
performance f.
pleasure f.
point f.
pregnancy f.
f. reaction
realistic f.
reasonable f.
rejection f.
f. response
scratch f.
semen f.
sermon f.
sex f.
sexual f.
shock f.
sitting f.
skin disease f.
skin injury f.
skyscraper f.
sleep f.
snow f.
sound f.
sourness f.
star f.
story f.
strangeness f.
stranger f.
street f.
subjective f.
sudden f.
suffocation f.
sunlight f.
sunrise f.
talking f.
tapeworm f.
taste f.
f. of terrorism
f. thermometer
thinking f.
thought f.
time f.
tooth f.
train f.
unreasonable f.
vehicle f.

virgin f.
void f.
vomiting f.
weakness f.
wind f.
writing f.

feared
f. disease
f. object
f. single performance situation
f. words

FearFighter computer program tailored for specific fear therapy
fearful C cluster
fearfulness
f. disorder of adolescence
f. disorder of childhood
fear-induced
fear-related
f.-r. belief
f.-r. thought
fearsome
feasible alternative treatment
feat
feature
age-related f.
age-specific f.
agitative f.
f. analysis
antisocial f.
associated descriptive f.
atypical f.
avoidant f.
borderline personality disorder with histrionic f.
catatonic f.
characteristic f.
clinical f.
common shared f.
f. contrasts process
culture-related f.
culture-specific f.
delusional f.
demographic f.
dependent f.
depression with psychotic f.
descriptive f.
diagnostic f.
dominant f.
dysautonomic f.
essential f.
gender f.

gender-specific f.
gross pathological f.
hysteroid f.
insomnia f.
inward expression of anger with ruminative f.
manic f.
melancholic f.
mixed f.
mood-congruent psychotic f.
mood disorder with atypical f.'s
mood disorder with catatonic f.'s
mood disorder with melancholic f.'s
mood-incongruent psychotic f.
narcissistic f.
neurobehavioral f.
neuropsychiatric f.
neurotic f.
nondistinctive f.
obsessional f.
obsessive-compulsive f.
outward expression of anger with impulsive f.
paranoid f.
passive-aggressive f.
pathological f.
personality f.
phenomenological f.
predominant f.
prosodic f.
psychological f.
psychotic f.
schizoid f.
shared phenomenological f.
sociodemographic f.
specific culture, age, and gender f.
specific gender f.
suicidal f.
trait-like f.

febrifacient
febrile
f. delirium
f. psychosis
f. seizure
fecal
f. continence
f. incontinence
feces
feces-child-penis concept
feckless
fecundate

F

NOTES

267

fecundatio ab extra
fecundation
    artificial f.
fecundity
federal
    F. Bureau of Prisons
    f. statute
fed up
feeble-mindedness
    affective f.-m.
    primary f.-m.
feed
    force f.
feedback
    acoustic f.
    afferent f.
    alpha f.
    altered auditory f. (AAF)
    auditory f.
    constructive f.
    control f.
    f. control
    corrective f.
    delayed auditory f.
    efferent f.
    haptic f.
    information f.
    f. inhibition factor (FIF)
    inverse f.
    kinesthetic f.
    f. mechanism
    negative f.
    f. noise
    physiological f.
    positive f.
    proprioceptive f.
    f. sensitivity
    f. system
    tactile f.
    video f.
feeding
    f. behavior
    breast f.
    f. and eating disorder
    fictitious f.
    forced f.
    f. habits
    intravenous f.
    parenteral f.
    f. problem
    f. psychogenic disorder
    sham f.
    f. system
    f. technique
feel-good molecule
feeling
    f. of abandonment
    absence of f.

affected by f.
ambivalent f.
f. analysis
anti-government f.
f. of anxiety
f. apperception
ataxic f.
f. of attachment
f. of being detached from one's body
f. of being detached from one's mental process
f. of being an outside observer of one's life
f. of boredom
community f.
compassionate f.
conflicted f.
f. of control
covert f.
dammed-up f.
f. of despair
f. of detachment
difficulty describing f. (DDF)
difficulty identifying f. (DIF)
f. of dirtiness
f. of disgust
f. of disloyalty
disturbing f.
f. of dominance
f. of doom
f. of dread
f. of electricity
f. of emptiness
f. of estrangement
exaggerated f.
expression of f.
expression with f.
fellow f.
f. frightened; expecting bad things to happen; attitudes and actions that help; results and reward (FEAR)
f. of frustration
f. of grief
group f.
guilt f.
f. of hate
f. of helplessness
f. of hopelessness
inferiority f.
inner f.
f. of insecurity
intensified f.
f. of isolation
lack of f.
loving f.
maladaptive f.

negative f.
f. numb
f. of numbness
obsessive f.
oceanic f.
painful f.
positive f.
premonitory f.
premorbid inferiority f. (PIF)
f. of rage
rageful f.
range of f.
reflection of f.
f. of rejection
f. of remorse
repressed f.
f. of responsibility
f. sensation
sexual f.
f. of shame
sinful f.
sinking f.
subjective emotional f.
substituting f.
superiority f.
f. that self is not real
f. that things are not real
f. tone
tone of f.
transference f.
tridimensional theory of f.
unacceptable f.
f. of unreality
f. of unworthiness
ventilation of f.
verbalization of f.
f. of worthlessness
wounded f.

feeling-talk
FEF
   frontal eye field
Feighner criteria for alcoholism
feign
feigned
   f. bereavement
   f. symptom
feigning
   death f.
Feingold diet
feint
feisty
felicific

felicitate
felicitous
felicity
fellatio fantasy
fellation
fellator
fellatorism
fellatrice, fellatrix
fellow
   f. feeling
   f. man
fellowship
felo-de-se, pl. **felones-de-se**
felon
felonious
felony behavior
felt need
female
   f. biological status
   f. castration
   f. circumcision
   f. climacteric
   f. conditioning
   f. dyspareunia
   f. ejaculation
   f. eunuchoidism
   f. fantasy figure
   f. gender identity
   f. genitalia
   f. homosexuality
   f. hypoactive sexual desire disorder
   f. impersonator
   f. intersex
   marasmic f.
   f. menopause
   f. orgasm
   f. orgasmic disorder
   f. patient
   f. sexual arousal disorder
   f. suffrage
   f. system research orientation
   f. therapist
   f. victim
femaleness
female-to-male transgendered identity
feminine
   f. attitude
   f. identification
   f. identity
   f. mannerism
   f. masochism

NOTES

F

feminine *(continued)*
    f. social role
    f. traits in male
femininity complex
feminism
feminist
feminization
feminize
feminizing
feminizing-testes syndrome
femme fatale
femora
    coitus inter f.
fenestra
    f. ovalis
    f. rotunda
fenestration
feral children
Fere phenomenon
ferocious
ferocity
ferox
    delirium f.
ferrugination
fertility
fertilization
fervent
fervid
fervor
FES
    functional electrical stimulation
    FES figure-drawing test
fester
festinant
festinating gait
festination
fetal
    f. alcohol effect (FAE)
    f. alcohol syndrome (FAS)
    f. death
    f. development
    f. exposure
    f. hydantoin syndrome
    f. injury
    f. movement
    f. screening
fetalism
fetal-maternal exchange
fetation
fetched
feticide
fetish
    f. object
    shoe f.
fetishism
    beast f.
    f. paraphilia
    transvestic f. (TF)

fetishist
fetter
feud
fever
    cabin f.
    high f.
    low f.
    stir f.
feverish
few friends
fey
FH
    family history
FHIP
    family health insurance plan
FI
    fixed interval
fiasco
fibrillary
    f. chorea
    f. myoclonia
    f. tremor
fibrositic headache
fibrous
fickle
fiction
fictitious
    f. feeding
    f. name
fiddle
    second f.
fide
    bona f.
fidelity
fidget
fidgetiness
fidgeting behavior
field
    absolute f.
    abuse f.
    behavior f.
    f. of consciousness
    f. data
    f. defect
    f. dependence
    f. dependence-independence
    electric f.
    excitatory f.
    f. experiment
    f. of fixation
    f. force
    frontal eye f. (FEF)
    f. independence
    minimal audible f. (MAF)
    perceptual f.
    phenomenal f.
    play the f.
    f. property

psychological f.
f. of regard
f. research
f. structure
terminal neuronal f.
f. theory
f. of vision
visual f.
f. work

field-cognition mode
field-tested criterion
FIF
feedback inhibition factor
fight
domestic f.
f., flee, freeze, or faint
f. or flight reaction
gang f.
physical f.
f. for rights
fighting, injuries, sex, threats, self-defense (FISTS)
fight-or-flight
f.-o.-f. stress
Figueira syndrome
figural
f. aftereffect
f. cohesion
f. memory
figurative
f. blind spot
f. knowledge
f. meaning
figure
ambiguous f.
attachment f.
authority f.
childhood f.
empiric-risk f.
fantasy f.
father f.
female fantasy f.
fortification f.
frightening attachment f.
f. and ground
identification f.
inability to trust authority f.
major attachment f.
mother f.
noise f.
simple f.

f. of speech
violent f.
figure-ground
f.-g. distortion
f.-g. perception
figurehead
file
computer f.
encrypted f.
patient f.
protected f.
rank and f.
f. server
filial
f. generation
f. imprinting
f. piety
f. therapy
filiate
filioparental
filter
active f.
band-pass f.
perceptual f.
FIM
functional independence measure
finagle
final
f. analysis
f. diagnosis
f. tendency
finality
financial
f. crisis
f. support
find fault
finding
associated laboratory f.
associated physical examination f.
case f.
clinical f.
comparable f.
empirical f.
equivocal f.
fact f.
neurophysiological f.
neuropsychologic f.
object f.
obtained f.
pathological f.
postmortem f.

F

NOTES

finding *(continued)*
    spurious f.
    tentative f.
fine
    f. electric hair
    f. motor
    f. motor activity
    f. motor coordination
    f. motor movement
    f. motor skill
    f. postural tremor
    f. tactile sensation
finesse
finger
    f. agnosia
    f. anomia
    insane f.
    jerk f.
    lock f.
    f. painting
    f. penetration
    f. phenomenon
    f. pointing
    snap f.
    f. spelling
    spring f.
    f. sucking
    trigger f.
finger-biting behavior
finger-paint
fingerpointing
fingerprint
finger-tapping score
fingertip number writing perception
finger-to-finger test
finical
finicky eatr
finite
finitude
fink
Finn
    Mickey F.
Finnish Adoptive Family Study of Schizophrenia
FIQ
    full-scale intelligence quotient
fire
    ball of f.
    baptism by f.
    f. setter (FS)
    f. setting
firearms
firebug
fire-eater
fire-setting
    f.-s. behavior
    deliberate f.-s.
firing an anchor

firmly held belief
first
    f. admission
    f. aid
    f. episode of depression (FDE)
    f. impression
    f. offense
    f. psychotic episode
    f. rank symptoms of delusion
    f. stage of anesthesia
firstborn
first-class
first-degree biological relative
first-episode
    f.-e. patient
    f.-e. psychosis
    f.-e. schizophrenia
firsthand
first-line therapy
first-order elimination kinetics
first-pass effect
first-rank
    f.-r. psychotic symptom
    f.-r. symptom (FRS)
first-rate
first-signal system
fissure
    anal f.
    central f.
    cerebral f.
    rolandic f.
    f. of Rolando
    sylvian f.
fist clenching
fistfight
FISTS
    fighting, injuries, sex, threats, self-defense
fistula, pl. fistulae, fistulas
    craniosinus f.
fit
    f. of anger
    goodness of f.
    f.'s of horrific temptation
    parental f.
    poorness of f.
    postdormital chalastic f.
    psychomotor f.
    pupil-teacher f.
    rum f.
    running f.
    uncinate f.
fitful sleep
fitness
    inclusive f.
    increased sense of physical f.
    maternal f.
    physical f.

fittest
> survival of the f.

fitting

five-axis system

fixate

fixation
> affect f.
> f. of affect
> anxiety f.
> authority figure f.
> cannibalistic f.
> child f.
> child-parent f.
> father f.
> field of f.
> freudian f.
> gaze f.
> f. hysteria
> libido f.
> line of f.
> mother f.
> f. neurosis
> oral f.
> parent f.
> f. pause
> f. point
> f. reaction
> role f.

fixe
> ideé f.

fixed
> f. action pattern (FAP)
> f. belief
> f. delusion
> f. delusional system
> f. distribution
> f. dose stimulation
> f. dosing
> f. dosing arm
> f. idea
> f. income
> f. internal
> f. interval (FI)
> f. marker
> f. model
> f. pupil
> f. ratio (FR)
> f. reinforcement

fixed-ended session

fixed-interval reinforcement schedule

fixed-ratio reinforcement schedule

fix and focus attention

flaccid
> f. paralysis
> f. speech

flaccidity
> curarization-induced f.

flagellantism

flagellation

flagellomania

flagitious

flagrant

flair

flak

flamboyant behavior

flap
> free bone f.
> liver f.
> sickle f.

flappable

flapping
> f. movement
> f. tremor

flare

flash
> hot f.

flashback
> acid f.
> combat f.
> f. hallucinosis
> intrusive f.
> marijuana f.

flashbulb memory

flasher

flashes
> f. of color
> f. of light

flashing pain syndrome

flashy

flat
> f. affect
> f. electroencephalogram
> f. top wave

flatness
> emotional f.

flattening
> affective f.
> emotional f.

flaunt

flavor
> emotional f.

flaw
> character f.

fleer

F

NOTES

fleeringly
fleeting
    f. auditory hallucination
    f. delusion
    f. illusion
    f. pain
    f. visual hallucination
Flesch formula
Flesh-Kincaid method
fletcherism
flexibilitas
    f. cerea
    f. cerea schizophrenia
flexibility
    behavioral f.
    cognitive f.
    waxy f.
flexible neuroleptic dosing
flexor
    f. spasticity
    f. tetanus
flextime
flicker
    chromatic f.
    f. frequency
    f. fusion
flicker-fusion point
flight
    f. of color
    f. or fight response
    f. from reality
    f. of ideas (FOI)
    f. into disease
    f. into fantasy
    f. into health
    f. into illness
flighty
fling
flippancy
flippant
flirtation
flirtatious behavior
flirting and coquetting
flirty
flittering scotoma
floating transference
floccillation
flocculation
flog
flooding
    emotional f.
    imaginal f.
    implosion f.
flopping tremor
florid
    f. episode
    f. psychosis
    f. symptoms

floridly
    f. delusional
    f. paranoid
flounder
Flourens
    F. doctrine
    F. theory
flout
flow
    absolute f.
    adventitious motor f.
    anterior cingulate f.
    brain blood f.
    cerebral blood f. (CBF)
    f. chart
    prefrontal f.
    regional blood f.
    regional cerebral blood f. (rCBF)
    resting anterior cingulate f.
    f. tracer
    whole brain blood f.
fluanisone
flub
flucindole
fluctuant
fluctuating
    f. affect
    f. course
    f. ego state
    f. level of consciousness
    f. mood disturbance
fluctuation
    attention f.
    core temperature f.
    subsyndromal bipolar mood f.
    temperature f.
fluency
    association f.
    associative f.
    basal f.
    cross-modal f.
    f. disorder
    f. disturbance
    false f.
    intermodal f.
    f. shaping therapy
    speech f.
    f. of thought
    verbal f.
    word f.
fluent
    f. aphasia
    f. aphasic seizure
    f. aphasic speech
    f. paraphasic speech
fluid
    f. balance
    body f.

cerebrospinal f. (CSF)
f. coordination
f. disturbance
f. imbalance
f. intake
f. output
f. overload
f. retention
f. retention syndrome (FRS)
fluidity value
fluke
flummox
flunky
fluoroscopic control
fluoxetine
f. intoxication
f. overdose
f. treatment
flush
flushed face
flushing
facial f.
fluster
flutter
alar f.
ocular f.
flyaway
fly-by-night
Flynn-Aird syndrome
FMR1
fragile X syndrome
FOC
frequency of contact
focal
f. ability
f. conflict theory
f. contralateral routing of signals (FOCALCROS)
f. degeneration
f. epilepsy
f. lateralized dysfunction
f. neurological impairment
f. organic psychosyndrome
f. pathology
f. psychotherapy
f. sclerosis
f. seizure
f. suicide
f. twitch
FOCALCROS
focal contralateral routing of signals

focalize
focus, pl. **foci**
f. of anticipated danger
f. of anxiety
attention f.
characteristic paraphiliac f.
f. of clinical attention
f. of delusional system
epileptic f.
epileptogenic f.
f. group
inward f.
Loyola sensate f.
mirror f.
multiple f.
outward f.
paraphiliac f.
principal f.
restricted f.
sensate f.
somatic f.
f. of thought
unilateral f.
focused
f. analysis
f. delirium
f. expressive therapy
focus-execute component of attention
focusing mechanism
foe
fog
brain f.
mental f.
fogy, fogey
FOI
flight of ideas
foible
foist
folie
f. á cinq
f. circulaire
f. communiquee
f. d'action
f. demonomaniaque
f. des persecutions
f. a deux
f. á double forme
f. á douze
f. du doute
f. du pourquoi
f. á famille
f. gemellaire

NOTES

F

folie *(continued)*
  f. hypocondriaque
  f. imitative
  f. imposee
  f. induite
  f. instantee
  f. morale
  f. musculaire
  f. paralytique
  f. penitentiare
  f. a pleusirs
  f. á quatre
  f. raisonnante
  f. raisonnante meloncolique
  f. simulee
  f. simultanee
  f. à trois
  f. vaniteuse
folk
  f. healer
  f. illness
  f. medicine
  f. psychiatry
  f. psychology
  f. soul
folklore
folksy
folkways
follicularis
follicular phase
follower role
following
  f. behavior
  gaze f.
  f. movement
followup
  f. counseling
  f. data
  f. examination
  f. period
  f. study
  systematic f.
  f. visit
folly
fomentation
fomes ventriculi
fondle
fondling
fondness
food
  f. addict
  f. addiction
  f. additives
  comfort f.
  f. consumption pattern
  f. craving
  f. deprivation
  F. and Drug Administration (FDA)

  f. faddism
  f. habit
  hoard f.
  f. intake
  f. intake abnormality
  f. intake disorder
  junk f.
  f. poisoning
  f. preference
  restricted access to f.
  f. satiation
  f. therapy
  tyramine-rich f.
food-related
  f.-r. behavior
  f.-r. obsessive-like symptom
foolery
foolhardy
foolish business investment
foolproof
foot-drop
footing
  war f.
footloose
forage
foray
forbidden
  f. fruit
  f. impulse
force
  anti-instinctual f.
  catabolic f.
  central f.
  electromotive f. (EMF)
  evil f.
  external f.
  f. feed
  field f.
  f. of habit
  labor f.
  f. majeure
  nerve f.
  outside f.
  psychic f.
  societal f.
  unifying f.
  work f.
forced
  f. alimentation
  f. attitude
  f. cheerfulness
  f. choice
  f. cross-dressing
  f. cross-gender
  f. emigration
  f. fantasy
  f. feeding
  f. hyperventilation

f. impulse
f. laughter
f. medication
f. movement
f. relationship
f. sex
f. sexual encounter
f. sleep
f. smile
f. treatment
f. vibration
f. whisper
forced-choice span of apprehension task
forebrain
limbic f.
foreconscious
foredoom
foreign
f. body
f. custom
f. language
f. standard
f. value
forejudge
forensic
f. consultation
f. determination
f. medicine
f. pathology
f. proof
f. psychiatrist
f. psychiatry
f. psychology
f. setting
foreperiod
foreplay
forepleasure
foreshortened future
foresight
foretell
forethought
forewarn
forfeit
forgery
prescription f.
forgetting
intentional f.
motivated f.
forgotten behavior
forked tongue
forlorn

form
consent f.'s
depot f.
f. discrimination
equivalent f.
free f.
major f.
minor f.
f. perception
f.'s of psychodrama
f. response (F)
f.'s of satisfactory relating
signed consent f.
thought f.
formal
f. contract
f. discipline
f. education
f. logic
f. method
f. operation
f. operational development
f. operations period
f. operations stage
f. testing
f. thought disorder
f. universals
formalized contract
formant
format
nonaxial f.
self-report f.
f. treatment
formate
formation
brainstem reticular f.
compromise f.
concept f.
ego f.
friend f.
gender identity f.
habit f.
identity f.
f. of identity
inhibition f.
mesencephalic reticular f.
omen f.
pathologic character f.
personality f.
posttraumatic symptom f.
reaction f.
replacement f.

NOTES

F

formation *(continued)*
    reversal f.
    substitute f.
    symptom f.
formative
formboard
forme
    folie á double f.
    f. fruste
    f. tardive
formed
    f. belief
    f. image
    f. opinion
    f. response of colored area (FC)
    f. visual hallucination
former
    f. boyfriend
    f. foster home
    f. friend
    f. girlfriend
    f. identity
    f. lover
    f. marriage
    f. partner
    f. relationship
    f. treatment
formication
formidable
formula, pl. **formulae, formulas**
    empirical f.
    Flesch f.
formulary
formulate
formulation
    case f.
    clinical f.
    cultural f.
    dynamic f.
    psychodynamic f.
fornicate
fornication
for-profit hospital
forte
forthcoming
forthright
fortification
    f. figure
    f. scotoma
    f. spectrum
fortify
fortitude
fortuitous
fortuity
fortunate
fortune
    f. hunter
    soldier of f.

fortuneteller
forward
    f. masking
foster
    f. care (FC)
    f. care placement
    f. care system
    f. child
    f. father
    f. grandparent
    f. home
    f. mother
    f. parent
    f. parenting
fostering
    cross f.
fosterling
Fothergill neuralgia
fouetteuse
foul-mouthed
foul play
foul-up
foundation
    biologic f.
    psychological f.
    sociocultural f.
foundling
four
    oriented and alert times f.
    f. times a day
Four-Factor Theory of Etiology
Fourier
    F. analysis
    F. law
four-point restraint
four-way session
foveal vision
FPDD
    familial pure depressive disease
FPR
    fastigial pressor response
FR
    fixed ratio
fraction
    ethanol volume f. (EVF)
fractional analysis
fractionation
fractious
fragesucht
fragging
fragile
    f. sense of self
    f. X chromosome
    f. X syndrome (FMR1)
fragment
fragmentary
    f. delusion
    f. dream image

f. hallucination
f. hallucinations in schizophrenia
f. seizure
fragmentation
f. of ego
family f.
f. of thinking
fragmented
f. communication
f. nighttime sleep
f. sense of self
f. social network
f. syndrome
frail elderly patient
frailty
human f.
frame
analytic f.
f. of reference
frame-up
framework
ecologic f.
multidimensional f.
francomania
francophobe
frank
f. catatonic stupor
f. delirium
f. psychotic symptoms
Frankenstein factor
frantic
fraternal
f. twins
f. twins raised together
fraternize
fratricide
fraud
corporate f.
fraudulent
fraught
FRC
functional residual capacity
freak
speed f.
freaked out
freakish
freaky
free
f. access to process
f. association
f. base
f. bone flap

f. and easy
fancy f.
f. field room
f. form
f. living
f. love
f. play
f. radical scavenger
f. recall
f. recall bias
f. rein
f. response
symptom f.
f. thought
f. will
free-access environment
freebase
cocaine f.
freebasing
freeborn
freedom
f. to choose
degree of f.
escape from f.
loss of f.
freedwoman
free-floating
f.-f. anxiety
f.-f. attention
f.-f. fear
free-handed
free-hand ultrasound-guided intervention
free-hearted
freeload
free-running
freethinker
freezing
f. behavior
f. of movement
f. phenomenon
Fregoli
F. phenomenon
F. syndrome
French
F. kiss
F. leave
frenetic
freneticism
Frenkel
F. movement
F. symptom
frenzied psychomotor activity

F

NOTES

frenzy
    en f.
    presence of f.
frequency (f)
    alpha f.
    f. of anxiety
    band f.
    f. combination
    f. of contact (FOC)
    critical flicker f.
    f. curve
    disease f.
    f. distribution
    f. disturbance
    dominant waking f.
    f. of drug use
    drug use f.
    f. encountered association
    expected f.
    flicker f.
    gambling f.
    gene f.
    intercourse f.
    f. jitter
    law of f.
    f. masking
    relative f.
    f. response
    seizure f. (SF)
    sexual f.
    f. of treatment
    f. of violent act
    waking f.
frequent
    f. crying
    f. derailment
    f. physical complaint
    f. relocation
    f. sadness
fretful
Freud
    F. cathartic method
    F. syndrome
    F. theory
    F. view of depressive disorder
freudian
    f. approach
    f. censor
    f. fixation
    f. psychoanalysis
    f. psychotherapy
    f. slip
    f. theory
    f. theory of personality
freudian-free association
fribble
fricative

friction
    interpersonal f.
Friedmann complex
Friedreich
    F. ataxia
    F. disease
friend
    death of close f.
    fair-weather f.
    false f.
    few f.'s
    f. formation
    former f.
    next f.
    no f.'s
friendless
friendliness
    active f.
    attitude of active f.
friendship
    f. model
    platonic f.
frig
fright
    stage f.
frightened
    f. teen
frightening
    f. attachment figure
    f. circumstance
    f. dream
    f. stimulus
frigid
frigidity
    sexual f.
fringe
    f. of consciousness
    radical f.
    subliminal f.
frippery
frisk
fritter
frivolity
frivolous
Frohlich syndrome
Frohman factor
frolicsome
frontal
    f. based cognition
    f. brain region
    f. cortex (FC)
    f. cortical area
    f. cortical dysfunction
    f. cortical function
    f. eye field (FEF)
    f. headache
    f. lobe
    f. lobe dementia

f. lobe dysfunction
f. lobe function
f. lobe interstitial neuron
f. lobe neuronal density
f. lobe syndrome
f. lobe volume
f. metabolism
f. perceptual disorder
f. release sign
f. subcortical brain circuits
f. sulcus
frontal-cerebellar-thalamic circuitry
frontalis
frontocortical aphasia
frontolenticular aphasia
frontosubcortical dementia
frontotemporal
f. brain atrophy
f. hypometabolism
Frostig-Horne training program
frottage
frotteur
frotteurism paraphilia
frozen watchfulness
FRS
first-rank symptom
fluid retention syndrome
frugal
fruit
forbidden f.
fruition
frump
frumpy
fruste
forme f.
frustrate
frustration
control f.
f. dream
feeling of f.
level of f.
f. response
f. tolerance
frustration-aggression hypothesis
FS
factor of safety
fire setter
FSIQ
full-scale intelligence quotient
FTT
failure to thrive
fucosidosis

fuddle
Fuerstner disease
fugitive
fugue
dissociative f.
epileptic f.
hysterical f.
poriomanic f.
psychogenic f.
psychotic f.
f. state
fulfill
failure to f.
fulfilling
fulfillment
asymptotic wish f.
disguised wish f.
wish f.
fulgurating migraine
full
f. affect
f. blood
f. dependence
f. dose
f. psychotic decompensation
f. psychotic episode
f. recovery
f. relapse
f. remission
f. symptom criterion
f. syndrome
f. wakefulness
full-blown
f.-b. delirium
f.-b. depressive episode
f.-b. panic attack
f.-b. psychosis
f.-b. syndrome
full-dose-treated patient
full-fledged
full-mouthed
full-scale
f.-s. intelligence quotient (FIQ, FSIQ)
f.-s. IQ
full-time
fully organized belief
fulminant
fulminate
fulminating anoxia
fulsome

F

NOTES

function

affective f.
altered f.
arousal f.
autonomic f.
autonomous ego f.
axis f.
behavioral f.
biologic windows on CNS f.
brain f.
brainstem f.
caloric stimulation test for
  vestibular f.
card sorting f.
cerebral cortical f.
cognitive f.
communication f.
communicative f.
f. complex
compromised f.
concept of brain f.
conflict-free f.
cortical f.
day-to-day f.
deteriorating f.
differential f.
diffuse f.
disordered personality f.
dream f.
ego f.
f. engram
episodic memory f.
everyday f.
executant ego f.
executive ego f.
existential ego f.
expressive f.
frontal cortical f.
frontal lobe f.
global f.
gnostic f.
higher cortical f.
higher intellectual f. (HIF)
higher level cognitive f.
higher neural f.
immune f.
impaired limbic-diencephalic f.
impaired sexual f.
impairment of cognitive f.
inability to f.
integrated f.
integrity of brain f.
intellectual f.
intrapsychical f.
inverted-U f.
isomeric f.
language f.
level of cognitive f.

localization of f.
localized f.
maintenance f.
mapping of cortical f.
marginal f.
mediated f.
memory f.
mental f.
motor f.
neurobehavioral f.
noradrenergic system f.
occupational f.
performance-intensity f.
personal f.
phasic f.
f. pleasure
premorbid intellectual f.
preoccupation of bodily f.'s
primary autonomous f.
psychophysical f.
receptive f.
recovery of f.
reduced intellectual f.
referential f.
role f.
semantic memory f.
semi-autonomous systems concept
  of brain f.
semiotic f.
sensory f.
seriatim f.
sexual f.
social f.
spiritual f.
splinter f.
subaverage academic f.
symbolic f.
synthetic f.
thermoeffector f.
thermoregulatory f.
vicarious f.
f. word
working memory f.

functional

f. activation
f. activity
f. age
f. aid
f. ailment
f. analysis
f. anosmia
f. aphasia
f. aphonia
f. approach
f. assessment
f. assessment stage
f. asymmetry
f. autonomy

f. blindness
f. bradykinesia
f. brain imaging study
f. budgeting
f. capacity (FC)
f. cognitive impairment
f. component
f. conformance
f. contracture
f. deafness
f. death
f. decline
f. demand
f. deterioration
f. difference
f. disability
f. disease
f. distance
f. dyspareunia
f. dyspareunia psychosexual dysfunction
f. electrical stimulation (FES)
f. encopresis
f. failure
f. gain testing
f. headache
f. hearing impairment
f. illiteracy
f. illiterate
f. illness
f. imaging data
f. imaging study
f. imaging technique
f. impotence
f. incapacity
f. independence measure (FIM)
f. invariant
f. irritation
f. leadership
f. limitation
f. loss
f. movement
f. neuropharmacology
f. neurosis
f. outcome
f. pain
f. pathology
f. plasticity
f. pragmatic procedure
f. psychiatric syndrome
f. psychogenic disorder
f. psychology

f. psychosis
f. relatedness
f. residual capacity (FRC)
f. shift
f. skill
socially f.
f. spasm
f. status
f. superego structure
f. symbolism
f. type
f. unity
f. vaginismus psychosexual dysfunction
f. voice disorder
functionalism
functionally impaired
functioning
adaptive f.
anxiety-induced impaired social f.
attentional f.
baseline cognitive f.
body f.
borderline intellectual f.
f. brain
brain f.
cognitive f.
community f.
competent, optimal relational f.
decline in academic f.
disrupted, dysfunctional relational f.
disruptive family f.
f. disturbance
domain of f.
dysfunctional relational f.
educational f.
emotional f.
end-state f.
executive f.
general verbal intellectual f.
global f.
good f.
grossly impaired f.
healthy f.
hierarchical f.
impaired attentional f.
impaired cognitive f.
impaired social f.
independent f.
index of sexual f.
intellectual subaverage f.
interpersonal f.

F

NOTES

functioning *(continued)*
    level of f.
    f. level
    level of intellectual f.
    major impairment of f.
    marked decline in academic f.
    f. measure
    neurological f.
    neuropsychologic f.
    normal neurological f.
    occupational f.
    optimal relational f.
    overall cognitive f.
    personality f.
    premorbid level of f.
    psychosocial f.
    quality of sexual f.
    receptor f.
    school f.
    sensory f.
    sexual f.
    social f.
    social-emotional f.
    subaverage academic f.
    subaverage intellectual f.
    superior f.
    unequivocal change in f.
    vasculogenic loss of erectile f.
    verbal intellectual f.
    visuospatial f.
    in vivo brain f.
    vocational f.
    voluntary motor f.
    voluntary sensory f.
fund
    f. of information
    f. of information test
    f. of intelligence
    f. of knowledge
fundamental
    f. approach
    f. attribution error
    f. cognitive process
    f. conceptual problem
    f. neural mechanism
    f. predisposition
    f. psychometric problem
    f. response process
    f. rule of psychoanalysis
    f. social impulse

    f. symptom
    f. tone
    f. wish
funiculitis
funk
funky
funnel plot
furious
furlough psychosis
furor
    epileptic f.
    f. epilepticus
furrowed brows
furtherance
furthest
furthest-neighbor analysis
furtive
fuse
    short f.
fusion
    faculty f.
    f. faculty
    flicker f.
    instinctual f.
    f. state
    telencephalic f.
    unity and f.
fusion-defusion cycle
fuss
fussbudget
fustigate
futile
futilitarian
futility
    medical f.
future
    f. danger
    f. depression
    f. episode
    foreshortened f.
    f. pace
    sense of a foreshortened f.
    f. shock
    f. suicidal act
    f. suicidal behavior
    f. suicide attempt
futuristic thinking
futurology
F-zero

G

G factor

GA

Gamblers Anonymous

GABA

gamma-aminobutyric acid
GABA receptor complex

GAD

generalized anxiety disorder

GAD-specific intervention

gag reflex

GAI

guided affective imagery

gain

antipsychotic-induced weight g.
desire for personal g.
drug-associated weight g.
epinosic g.
expected weight g.
material g.
paranosic g.
peak acoustic g.
primary g.
secondary g.
tertiary g.
weight g.

gainfully employed

gain-loss theory of attraction

gait

abnormal g.
g. abnormality
g. analysis
antalgic g.
g. apraxia
ataxic g.
cerebellar g.
g. disorder
g. disturbance
equine g.
festinating g.
halting g.
helicopod g.
hemiplegic g.
high steppage g.
hysterical g.
narrow-based g.
g. problem
retropulsion of g.
scissor g.
shuffling g.
slowed g.
spastic g.
staggering g.
steady g.
steppage g.

stuttering g.
swaying g.
uncoordinated g.
unsteady g.
waddling g.
wide-based g.

gallery

rogue's g.
shooting g.

gallivant

gallomania

gallows humor

Galton law of regression

galvanic

g. skin reaction
g. skin reflex
g. skin resistance
g. skin response (GSR)
g. skin response biofeedback
g. vertigo

galvanometer

galvanotropism

GamAnon

gamble

g. to escape from depression
lottery g.
urge to g.

gambler

adolescent g.
G.'s Anonymous (GA)
binge g.
compulsive g.
occasional g.
pathologic g.
problem g.
professional g.
recreational g.
regular g.

gambling

g. activity
g. addict
g. addiction
g. attitude
g. behavior
card-game g.
casino g.
g. cessation
compulsive g.
convenience g.
g. cue
g. debt
g. disorder
dog track g.
excessive g.
g. experience

gambling *(continued)*
    g. frequency
    horse race g.
    illegal g.
    g. impulse
    Indian casino g.
    g. industry
    Internet g.
    g. involvement
    legal g.
    legalized g.
    g. need
    g. opportunity
    pathological g. (PG)
    personal skills g.
    g. preoccupation
    g. prevalence
    professional g.
    g. reduction
    riverboat g.
    g. screen
    slot machine g.
    social g.
    sports betting g.
    g. strategy
    g. thought
    underage g.
    g. urge
    video lottery terminal g.
    youth g.
gambling-related difficulty
game
    computer g.
    experimental g.
    graphically violent video g.
    hallucinatory g.
    hate video g.
    language g.
    middle g.
    mixed motive g.
    model g.
    g.'s people play
    g. plan
    play the g.
    g. player
    g. playing
    point-and-shoot video g.
    psychological g.
    g. theory
    video g.
gamine
gamma
    g. alcoholism
    g. movement
    g. wave
gamma-aminobutyric acid (GABA)
gammacism
gamomania

gamy
gang
    g. attack
    g. banger
    g. behavior
    g. colors
    g. encounter
    g. fight
    g. initiation
    g. involvement
    g. member
    g. rape
    street g.
    g. up
    g. war
    g. warfare
ganja
Ganser syndrome
GAP
    Group for the Advancement of Psychiatry
    growth-associated protein
gap
    gender g.
    generation g.
    g. junction
    memory g.
    treatment g.
gargoylism
garish
garnish
garnishment
garrote
garrulity
garrulous affect
GAS
    general adaptation syndrome
gas
    g. chamber
    nerve g.
    g. poisoning
    tear g.
    war g.
gasoline intoxication
gastric
    g. bypass
    g. bypass surgery
    g. lavage
    g. neurasthenia
    g. psychogenic disorder
gastrin
gastrin-inhibiting peptide
gastritis
    alcoholic g.
    nervous g.
gastrointestinal
    g. functional psychogenic
    g. functional psychogenic disorder

g. symptom grouping
g. upset
gastroparalysis
gastroparesis
gastropath
gastroplasty
GAT
group adjustment therapy
gate
g. control theory of pain
g. theory
gate-control
g.-c. hypothesis
g.-c. theory
gatekeeper
gateway drug
gathering
injustice g.
g. of intelligence
rave g.
gating
g. mechanism
g. theory
gauche
Gaucher disease
gaudy
Gault decision
gaunt
gauntlet anesthesia
gaussian
g. curve
g. distribution
gavage
gay
g. bashing
g. liberation
g. rights
gayness
gaze
conjugate g.
consensual g.
g. deficit
g. fixation
g. following
g. impairment
g. paralysis
ping-pong g.
spasticity of conjugate g.
tense g.
gazing
crystal ball g.

GC
gonococcus
G-D syndrome
geisha
gelasmus
gelastic epilepsy
Gelineau syndrome
gemellaire
folie g.
gemistocyte
gemistocytic reaction
gender
g. ambiguity psychosis
appropriate in g.
g. bias
boundaries and g.
g. difference
g. difference psychiatric syndrome
g. differences in anxiety
g. discrimination
g. dysphoria
g. dysphoria syndrome
g. exploitation
g. feature
g. gap
g. identification
g. identity
g. identity board
g. identity confusion
g. identity disorder (GID)
g. identity disorder in adolescence
g. identity disorder of adulthood
g. identity disorder in adults
g. identity disorder of childhood
g. identity disorder in children
g. identity formation
g. identity psychosexual
development
multiple personalities and g.
g. neutrality
g. orientation
personality and g.
g. reassignment
g. role
g. role persistent discomfort
gender-based
g.-b. attitude
g.-b. mental health differences
gender-linked attitude
gender-sensitive psychopharmacology
gender-specific feature

G

NOTES

gene

aberrant g.
autosomal dominant g.
dominant g.
enzyme g.
g. frequency
homeotic g.
g. marker
g. mutation
g. pool
recessive g.
structural g.

genealogy

genera (*pl. of* genus)

general

g. adaptation reaction
g. adaptation syndrome (GAS)
g. adult psychopathology
g. anesthesia
g. anger disorder with aggression
g. anger disorder without aggression
g. clinical interview
g. cognitive status
g. component
g. factor
g. image
g. inquiry (GI)
g. knowledge
g. knowledge score
g. language disability
g. learning ability
g. medical condition (GMC)
g. medical doctor
g. medical etiology
g. medical impairment
g. medical physician
g. medical provider
g. medical treatment
g. medical use
g. memory index
g. mood state
g. paralysis
g. paralysis of the insane (GPI)
g. paresis
g. personality assessment
g. population
g. psychiatric practitioner
g. psychological distress
g. psychology
g. psychopathology
g. relaxation training
g. semantics
g. stress sensitivity
g. symptom
g. systems theory
g. transfer
g. verbal intellectual functioning
g. will

generalise

delire de negation g.

generalist

generality

glittering g.'s

generalization

g. gradient
g. response
stimulus g.
transfer by g.
verbal g.

generalized

g. amnesia
g. anxiety
g. anxiety disorder (GAD)
g. anxiety neurosis
g. auditory agnosia
g. flexion epilepsy
g. headache
g. hyperreflexia
g. intellectual impairment
g. neurotic anxiety state
g. pruritus
g. sexual dysfunction
g. tonic-clonic epilepsy
g. tonic-clonic seizure

generalized-type dyspareunia

generate

generation

g. of affect
baby-boom g.
baby-bust g.
beat g.
filial g.
g. gap
hypothesis g.
me g.
next g.
sandwich g.
second g.
silent g.
g. X
g. Y
g. Z

generational responsibility

generative

g. empathy
g. intervention
g. semantics

generativity versus stagnation

generic

g. negative symptom
g. question
g. skill

generosity

generous

genesial cycle
genesis
genetic

  g. alcoholism
  g. basis
  behavior g.'s
  behavioral g.'s
  g. block
  g. code
  g. component
  g. counseling
  g. counselor
  g. defect
  g. difference
  g. directive
  g. disease
  g. disorder
  g. drift
  g. effect
  g. endowment
  g. engineering
  g. equilibrium
  g. error
  g. heterogenicity
  g. history
  g. influence
  g. involvement
  g. linkage study
  g. loading
  g. makeup
  g. map
  g. marker
  g. material
  g. memory
  g. method
  molecular g.'s
  political g.'s
  population g.'s
  g. predisposition
  psychiatric g.'s
  g. psychology
  g. redundancy
  g. relationship
  g. research
  g. risk factor
  g. screening
  g. sequence
  g. strategy
  g. susceptibility
  g. susceptibility to mental illness
  g. technology
  g. theory

  g. tool
  g. transmission
  g. typing
  g. viewpoint
  g. vulnerability
genetic-dynamic psychiatry
genetic-epidemiologic
geneticism
geneticist
genetotrophic disease
genetous idiocy
genial
geniculate
genidentic
genital

  g. character
  g. erotism
  g. herpes
  g. intercourse
  g. love
  g. maturity
  g. mutilation
  g. organ
  g. pain
  g. phase
  g. primacy
  g. response
  g. sexual contact
  g. stage
  g. stimulation
  g. touching
  g. zone
genitalia
  ambiguous g.
  external g.
  female g.
  male g.
genitalis
  herpes g.
genitality
genitalization
genitourinary psychogenic disorder
genius
genocide
genocopy
genogram
genome
genomic event
genotropism
genotype
  dominant g.

G

NOTES

genotype *(continued)*
    e4/e4 g.
    schizophrenic g.
genotypical
genotypic programming
genteel
gentility
gentle assumption
genu, pl. **genua**
genuine epilepsy
genus, pl. **genera**
geographic
    g. displacement
    g. mobility
geography
geometric
    g. design
    g. hallucination
    g. mean
geophagia
geophagy
geophasia
gephyromania
Gerhardt-Semon law
geriatric
    g. abuse
    g. delinquency
    g. depression
    g. depressive disorder
    g. diagnosis
    g. factor
    g. health care setting
    g. health outcome
    g. medicine
    g. need
    g. neuropsychiatry
    g. patient
    g. population
    g. psychiatrist
    g. psychiatry
    g. psychiatry inpatient service
    g. psychologist
    g. psychology
    g. psychopharmacology
    g. rehabilitation
geriopsychosis
germane
germanomania
germanophile
germ exposure
germinally affected
gerocomia
gerocomy
geromorphism
gerontological psychiatry
gerontologic psychiatry
gerontology
gerontophilia

gerophilia
geropsychiatry
geropsychology
Gesell developmental model
gesellschaft
gestalt
    autochthonous g.
    g. factor
    g. phenomenon
    g. psychiatry
    g. psychology
    g. psychotherapy
    g. theory
    g. therapy
    G. therapy marathon
gestalten
gestaltism
gestaltist
gestate
gestational
    g. diestrus
    g. epilepsy
    g. psychosis
gesticulate
gesticulation
gestural
    g. automatism
    g. communication
gestural-postural language
gesture
    g. of affection
    bizarre g.
    body g.
    clumsy g.
    explicit g.
    expressive g.
    g. of good will
    kinesic g.
    g. language
    obscene g.
    overt g.
    paucity of expressive g.'s
    subtle g.
    suicidal g.
    suicide g.
gesturing communication pattern
GH
    growth hormone
ghastly
Gheel colony
ghetto
    ghetto g.
    psychiatric g.
ghettoize
ghost
    Bidwell g.
    g. image
    g. sickness

ghostlike
GI
    general inquiry
giantism
gibberish aphasia
GID
    gender identity disorder
giddy euphoria
gifted child
gigans
gigantea
gigantism
giggle
giggling
    nervous g.
Gilles de la Tourette syndrome
ginger paralysis
Gingko biloba
ginseng
    Chinese g.
    Panax g.
    Siberian g.
girdle
    g. anesthesia
    g. pain
    g. sensation
girl
    B g.
    call g.
    phallus g.
girlfriend
girlish
given name
giver
    fact g.
giving
    transgenerational role of g.
Gjessing syndrome
glabellar tap
gladden
glance
    expressive g.
glans
    g. clitoridis
    g. penis
glare of light
glasses
    rose-colored g.
glassy eyes
glazed look
glean
glib

glibness
Glick effect
glide
    after g.
    off g.
glissando technique
glitch
glittering generalities
glitz
gloat
global
    g. amnesia
    g. aphasia
    g. attractor state
    g. brain lactate
    g. change
    g. clinical impression score
    g. clinician-rated scale
    g. clinician rating
    g. cognitive deficit
    g. course
    g. delay
    g. dementia
    g. deterioration
    g. distress index
    g. function
    g. functioning
    g. index of distress
    g. loss of language
    g. measure
    g. measure of impairment
    g. metabolism
    g. outcome
    g. paralysis
    g. psychopathology
    g. sociocultural trend
    g. well-being
globi (*pl. of* globus)
globosa
    dysphagia g.
globulin
globus, pl. globi
    g. hystericus
    g. pallidus
gloomy
    habitually g.
glorified self
glorify
glossokinetic potential
glossolalia
glossolysis

NOTES

G

glossopharyngeal
    g. neuralgia
    g. tic
glossoplegia
glossoptosis
glossospasm
glossosteresis
glossosynthesis
gloss over
glossy skin
glottal attack
glottidospasm
glove anesthesia
glucose metabolism
glue
    g. ear
    g. sniffer's rash
    g. sniffing
glue-sniffing habit
glutethimide intoxication
glutton
gluttonous
gluttony
GMA
    gross motor activity
GMC
    general medical condition
gnash
gnashing
gnosia
gnostic function
gnosticism
goal
    g. attainment
    common g.
    gradient g.
    g. gradient
    latent g.
    life g.
    manifest g.
    g. orientation
    g. setting
    short-term g. (STG)
    social g.
    therapeutic g.
    therapy g.
    unattained g.
goal-directed
    g.-d. activity
    g.-d. behavior
goal-limited adjustment therapy
goal-oriented process
goal-setting
go-around
God
    act of G.
    belief in G.
    G. complex

    faith in G.
    relationship with G.
godfather
godless
godlike
godly
godsend
go-getter
going
    easy g.
golden-ager
golden handshake
Goliath syndrome
gonadal
    g. agenesis
    g. cycle
    g. dysgenesis
    g. hormone
gonadocentric
gonads
gonococcal
gonococcus (GC)
gonorrhea
good
    bill of g.'s
    g. faith
    g. form response (F+)
    g. functioning
    g. impression
    g. kid violence
    g. object
    g. old boy
    g. shape
    g. sleep efficiency
good-enough
    g.-e. mother
    g.-e. mothering
good-for-nothing
good-looking
Goodman Lock box
good-natured
goodness of fit
good-tempered
goodwill
goody-goody
goon
Gordon
    G. sign
    G. symptom
gorger-vomiter
Gorlin sign
gormandize
gormless
gory
gospeler
gossip
gossipy
gotu kola

gouge
gouging
    eye g.
gourmand
governess psychosis
Gowers
    G. syndrome
    vasovagal attack of G.
GPI
    general paralysis of the insane
grabby
graceful
graceless
gracious
gradation method
grade
    g. equivalent
    failing g.
    g. norm
    g. rating
    g. scale
    g. skipping
graded
    g. activity
    g. exposure
    g. potential
gradient
    approach g.
    avoidance g.
    axial g.
    effect g.
    excitation g.
    generalization g.
    goal g.
    g. goal
    g. slope
gradual topic shift
graduate
    college g.
graffiti tagger
graft
    cable g.
    nerve g.
    sleeve g.
grammar
    g. development stage
    g. formation stage
    shared g.
grammatical
    g. analysis
    g. equivalent
gramophone symptom

grand
    g. mal
    g. mal epilepsy
    g. mal seizure
    g. mal status
    g. rounds
grande attaque hysterique
grandeur
    delusion of g.
    g. delusion
grandfather complex
grandiloquence
grandiose
    g. concept
    g. content
    g. delirium
    g. delusion
    g. delusion of exceptional talent
    g. expansiveness
    g. idea
    g. ideation
    g. self
    g. subtype
    g. theme
    g. type
    g. type of paranoid disorder
grandiose-type schizophrenia
grandiosity in fantasy
grandma rule
grandparent
    foster g.
grandstand
granted
    take for g.
granulated opium
granulatum
    opium g.
granulocytopenia
granulomatous
grapes
    sour g.
grapevine
graphanesthesia
graphesthesia
graphic
    g. aphasia
    g. description
    g. disorientation
    g. impairment
    g. rating scale
    g. violence

G

NOTES

graphica
    asemasia g.
graphically violent video game
graphic-arts therapy
graphology
graphomania
graphometry
graphomotor
    g. aphasia
    g. technique
graphopathology
graphorrhea
graphospasm
grapple
Grashey aphasia
grasp
    g. and reach
    g. reflex
grasping and groping reflex
Grasset
    G. law
Grasset-Gaussel phenomenon
grata
    persona non g.
grate on the nerves
gratification
    delayed g.
    g. of dependent wishes
    immediate g.
    inability to delay g.
    material g.
    oral g.
    reduced g.
    sexual g.
gratified
    sexually g.
gratify
gratifying work
gratitude
    priori expectation of g.
grave
    delirium g.
    g. delirium
gravel voice
graven image
gravis
    dementia paranoides g.
    neurasthenia g.
    oneirodynia g.
    paranoia dementia g.
gravitate
gravity perception
gray
    g. matter
    g. matter area
    g. matter lactate
    g. matter lactate level

    g. matter region
    g. matter tissue
gray-out
    g.-o. episode
    g.-o. syndrome
gray-white matter difference
greed
greedy
gregarious
gregariousness
grief
    anticipatory g.
    constellation of g.
    g. counselor
    delayed g.
    denied g.
    distorted g.
    exposure to g.
    expression of g.
    feeling of g.
    impacted g.
    inhibited g.
    g. management
    mutual g.
    prolonged g.
    g. reaction
    g. support group
    g. therapy
    traumatic g.
    unresolved g.
    g. work
grief-based attachment
grievance-seeker
grieve
grieving
    inhibited g.
    pathologic g.
grievous
    g. assault
    g. bodily harm
grimace
    facial g.
    tic-like facial g.
grimacing
    prominent g.
grimly adhered-to routine
grimness
grim reaper
grin
    sardonic g.
grinding
    jaw g.
    tooth g.
gripe
grip-strength test
Griselda complex
grisette
grisi siknis

gristly
gritty
groomed
    neatly g.
    poorly g.
    well g.
grooming
    g. deterioration
    excessive g.
groove
grope
groping
gross
    g. impairment
    g. impairment of reality testing
    g. insensitivity
    g. medical error
    g. motor
    g. motor activity (GMA)
    g. motor deficit
    g. motor skill
    g. negligence
    g. neurologic deficit
    g. pathological feature
    g. sensory deficit
    g. stress reaction
grossly
    g. disorganized behavior
    g. impaired functioning
    g. pathogenic care
grotesque
grouchy
ground
    figure and g.
    middle g.
    g. rule
grounded
group
    g. acceptance
    action g.
    g. activity
    g. adjustment therapy (GAT)
    adolescent support g.
    G. for the Advancement of
      Psychiatry (GAP)
    aftercare g.
    age g.
    all-women g.
    amygdala nucleus g.
    g. analysis
    g. analytic psychotherapy
    aspirational g.

attitudinal g.
g. behavior
bereavement support g.
blood g.
g. boundary
buzz g.
g. centered
g. climate
closed g.
CNS disease g.
cognitive behavioral coping skills
  training g.
g. cohesion
community action g.
g. composition
g. consciousness
continuous g.
g. contract
control g.
g. counseling
g. counselor
couple skills g.
crisis g.
criterion g.
cultural reference g.
g. delinquency
g. delinquent reaction
diagnosis-related g.
diagnostic g.
g. difference
g. dimension
diverse g.
g. diversity
g. dynamics
encounter g.
equivalent g.
ethnic reference g.
g. experience
experiential g.
experimental g.
family support g.
g. feeling
focus g.
grief support g.
g. harmony
hate g.
heterogeneous g.
high-risk g.
g. home
horizontal g.
human relations g.
g. identification

NOTES

G

group *(continued)*
 intake diagnostic g.
 intake-orientation g.
 integrity g.
 interact g.
 interest g.
 g. interview
 laissez-faire g.
 leaderless g.
 g. living
 mandated self-help g.
 g. marriage
 matched g.
 g. medicine
 militia g.
 g. mind
 minority g.
 g. morale
 multifamily skills g.
 mutual aid g.
 natural g.
 g. norm
 nurse support g.
 online support g.
 open g.
 g. participation
 peer g.
 personal growth g.
 g. phase
 g. play
 political g.
 g. practice
 g. pressure
 primary support g.
 g. problem-solving
 g. process
 psychoanalytic g.
 psychoeducational g.
 g. psychosis
 g. psychotherapy
 g. psychotherapy session
 rap g.
 reference g.
 regressive-inspirational g.
 g. relations theory
 g. rule
 self-help g.
 sensitivity g.
 sensitivity-training g.
 g. setting
 social reference g.
 socioeconomic g.
 spiritual focus g.
 splinter g.
 g. stage
 g. stress reaction
 g. structure
 structured interactional g.
 study g.
 substance g.
 g. superego
 support g.
 symptom g.
 T g.
 task-oriented g.
 g. test
 thematically related g.'s
 therapeutic g.
 therapeutic play g. (TPG)
 g. therapist
 g. therapy
 training g.
 transient g.
 g. treatment
 work g.
 g. work
groupie
grouping
 clinical g.
 gastrointestinal symptom g.
 heterogenous g.
 homogeneous g.
 homogenous g.
 pain symptom g.
 sexual symptom g.
 symptom g.
groupthink
group-type conduct disorder
grovel
growing
 g. pain
growth
 cognitive g.
 continuous g.
 g. hormone (GH)
 g. hormone-releasing factor
 g. hormone-releasing hormone
 mental g.
 g. period
 personal g.
 surgent g.
 tumultuous g.
 zero population g. (ZPG)
growth-associated protein (GAP)
GROW The Marriage Enrichment Program
grubelsucht
grudge bearing
grueling
gruesome
grumble
grumbling mania
grumpy
Grund symptom
grunge look
grungy

grunt
GSR
  galvanic skin response
GSW
  gunshot wound
GSWH
  gunshot wound to the head
guaiac
  g. negative
  g. positive
guard
  off g.
  old g.
guarded manner
guardedness
  adolescent g.
guardian
  g. ad litem
  court-appointed g.
  legal g.
guardianship
  estate g.
  individual g.
  legal g.
  required g.
guerrilla
  g. tactics
  g. warfare
guess
  second g.
guidance
  anticipatory g.
  g. center
  child g.
  g. clinic
  conscious g.
  g. counselor
  spiritual g.
  vocational g.
guidance-cooperation model
guide
  action g.
  g. dog
  medication g.
  parental failure to g.
  spiritual g.
guided
  g. affective imagery (GAI)
  g. meditation
  g. mourning
guideline
  practice g.

guidepost
guile
guileless
Guillain-Barré syndrome
guilt
  g. by association
  confession of g.
  g. displacement
  excessive g.
  g. feeling
  initiative versus g.
  lack of g.
  misattribution of g.
  neurotic g.
  g. obsession
  pathologic g.
  pathological g.
  pervasive proneness to g.
  preoccupation with g.
  realistic g.
  self-attribution of g.
  self-reported g.
  survivor g.
  g. theme
  unconscious g.
guiltless
guilty
  g. rumination
  g. verdict
Guinon
  tic de G.
guise
Gulf War syndrome
gull-wing pattern
gum
  nicotine g.
  g. opium
gumma
gumopium
gumption
gun
  access to g.'s
  assault g.
  carries a g.
  g. control
  hired g.
  riot g.
  stun g.
  submachine g.
  tommy g.
gunfight
gunfire

NOTES

G

gunman
gunned down
gunnery sergeant
gunrunner
gunshot
    g. wound (GSW)
    g. wound to the head (GSWH)
gurney
guru
gushy
gustation
gustatism
gustatory
    g. anesthesia
    g. audition
    g. aura
    g. hallucination
    g. hyperesthesia
    g. nerve
    g. seizure
gustatory-sudorific reflex

gusto
gutless
gutsy
gwa sha
Gwathmey anesthesia
gymnastics
gymnomania
gynander
gynandrism
gynandroid
gynandromorph
gynatresia
gynecic
gynomonoecism
gyrate
gyration
gyri (*pl. of* gyrus)
gyrosa
gyrospasm
gyrus, pl. **gyri**

h
    human response
HA
    harm avoidance
    high anxiety
habeas corpus
habilitation
habit
    acculturation problem with expression of h.'s
    alcohol h.
    benign h.
    h. cessation
    h. chorea
    cocaine h.
    h. cough
    h. deterioration
    dietary h.
    h. disorder
    h. disturbance
    drug h.
    eating h.
    h. exposure
    feeding h.'s
    food h.
    force of h.
    h. formation
    glue-sniffing h.
    h. hierarchy
    inattention to proper dietary h.
    h. interference
    kick the h.
    laxative h.
    motor h.
    narcotic h.
    nicotine h.
    opium h.
    h. pattern
    poor eating h.
    responsible eating h.
    h. reversal
    h. reversal training (HRT)
    h. spasm
    h. strength
    temporary h.
    h. tic
    h. training
    h. treatment
habitability
habit-forming
habit-training
habitual
    h. act
    h. complaint
    h. criminal

    h. offender
    h. runaway
habitually gloomy
habituate
habituation
    caffeine h.
    cocaine h.
    electrical h.
habitude
habitué
habitus phthisicus
hack
hacker
    computer h.
hackle
HACS
    hyperactive child syndrome
Haeckel biogenic law
haggard appearance
hagiotherapy
hair
    h. denuding
    eating h.
    fine electric h.
    h. plucking
    h. pulling
    spiked h.
hair-pulling behavior
hair-raising
hairsplitting
half-brother
half-hearted attempt at suicide
half-life
    drug h.-l.
half-show
half-sister
half-truth
halfway
    h. children
    h. house
    meet h.
halitosis
hallmark
Halloween effect
hallucinate
hallucinated voice
hallucinating patient
hallucination
    accusatory h.
    affective h.
    alcohol h.
    alcoholic h.
    alcohol-induced h.
    alcohol-induced psychotic disorder with h.'s

H

hallucination *(continued)*
    amphetamine-induced psychotic
      disorder with h.'s
    angel-of-death h.
    anxiolytic-induced psychotic disorder
      with h.'s
    auditory h.
    blank h.
    body-image h.
    cannabis-induced psychotic disorder
      with h.'s
    cenesthesic h.
    cocaine-induced psychotic disorder
      with h.'s
    command auditory h.
    complex h.
    h. of conception
    content of h.
    daytime h.
    depressive auditory h.
    depressive olfactory h.
    depressive visual h.
    dreamlike h.
    drug-induced h.
    elementary h.
    fleeting auditory h.
    fleeting visual h.
    formed visual h.
    fragmentary h.
    geometric h.
    gustatory h.
    hallucinogen-induced psychotic
      disorder with h.'s
    haptic h.
    hypnagogic h.
    hypnopompic h.
    hypnotic-induced psychotic disorder
      with h.'s
    induced h.
    inhalant-induced psychotic disorder
      with h.'s
    kaleidoscope h.
    kinesthesia h.
    kinesthetic h.
    lilliputian h.
    memory h.
    microptic h.
    mood-congruent h.
    mood-incongruent h.
    nocturnal h.
    nonaffective h.
    nonpsychotic h.
    olfactory h.
    organic h.
    overt h.
    h. of perception
    phencyclidine-induced psychotic
      disorder with h.'s

    posttraumatic h.
    prominent h.
    psychotic disorder with h.'s
    reflex h.
    running commentary h.
    sedative-induced psychotic disorder
      with h.'s
    self-destructive h.
    simple h.
    sleep-related h.
    somatic h.
    speech h.
    structured h.
    stump h.
    tactile h.
    tactual h.
    teleologic h.
    temporal h.
    third-person auditory h.
    threatening h.
    transient auditory h.
    transient tactile h.
    transient visual h.
    unformed auditory h.
    unformed visual h.
    unpleasant h.
    vestibular h.
    violent command h.
    visual h.
    vivid h.
hallucinatoria
    paranoia h.
hallucinatory
    h. behavior
    h. dementia
    h. drug
    h. epilepsy
    h. experience
    h. game
    h. image
    h. mania
    h. neuralgia
    h. paranoia
    h. state
    h. state drug psychosis
    h. transient organic
    h. transient organic psychosis
    h. transient organic syndrome
    h. verbigeration
**hallucinatory-type psychoorganic
  syndrome**
hallucinogen
    h. abuse
    h. dependence
    designer h.
    h. hallucinosis
    h. intoxication delirium
    h. persisting perception disorder

sedative h.
h. toxic effect
h. use disorder

hallucinogen-affective disorder
hallucinogen-delusional disorder
hallucinogenesis
hallucinogenic
h. drug
h. drug dependence
h. hallucinosis
h. intoxication
h. overdose

hallucinogen-induced
h.-i. delirium and anxiety disorder
h.-i. psychotic disorder with
delusions
h.-i. psychotic disorder with
hallucinations

hallucinogen-related disorder, not
otherwise specified
hallucinosis
acute h.
alcohol h.
alcoholic h.
h. alcoholic psychosis
alcohol withdrawal h.
bromide h.
drug-induced h.
flashback h.
hallucinogen h.
hallucinogenic h.
organic h.
h. peduncular
peduncular h.
psychoactive substance h.
withdrawal h.

halo
h. effect
h. of light
object h.'s

halogenated inhalational anesthesia
haloperidol condition
haloxazolam
HALT
heroin antagonist and learning therapy
halting
h. gait
h. manner
h. movement
h. speech

haltlose-type personality
hamartomania

hammered
hamper
hand
accoucheur's h.
black h.
dead h.
dominant h.
laying on of h.'s
nondominant h.
h. preference
h. shaking
show one's h.
h. test (HT)
h. tremor
upper h.
h. waving
writing h.

handedness
left h.
handful
handgun
.22-caliber h.
.38-caliber h.
.44-caliber h.
concealed h.
h. control
licensed h.
9 mm h.
h. possession
unlicensed h.

hand-holding
handicap
emotional h. (EH)
severe emotional h. (SEH)
handicapped
educationally mentally h. (EMH)
emotionally h.
mentally h.
perceptually h.
trainable mentally h. (TMH)
handshake
golden h.
hand-to-mouth
h.-t.-m. reaction
hand-washing
h.-w. obsession
handwashing
repeated h.
h. ritual
handwringing
handwrite
handwriting analysis

NOTES

H

hang
> h. around
> h. back
> h. on
> h. out
> h. together
> h. tough

hanged

hanger-on

hanging
> accidental h.
> h. arousal
> h. attempt
> erotized h.
> suicide by h.

hangout

hangover
> daytime sleep h.
> h. effect
> h. headache

hang-up

hanky-panky

hapax legomenon

haphalgesia

haphazard

hapless

haplology

happiness measure

happy-go-lucky

happy puppet syndrome

haptic
> h. feedback
> h. hallucination
> h. perception
> h. system

haptodysphoria

haptometer

haptophonia

harangue

harass

harassment
> email h.
> quid pro quo h.
> same-sex h.
> sexual h. (SH)

harbinger

hard
> h. chancre
> h. line
> h. rock

hard-boiled

harden

hardheaded

hardiness

hard-line

hardness

hard-of-hearing

hardy

Hardy-Weinberg equilibrium

harm
> alcohol-related h.
> h. avoidance (HA)
> grievous bodily h.
> physical h.

harmaline

harm-avoidance need

harm-avoidant trait

harmful
> h. consequence
> h. sexual relationship
> socially h.

harmine

harming
> h. others
> h. self

harmless wit

harmonic
> h. analysis
> h. mean

harmonious interaction

harmonizer

harmony
> group h.
> h. process
> social h.

HARP
> Harvard-Brown Anxiety Disorders
> Research Project

harria

harried

Harris migraine

Harrison Antinarcotic Act

harsh discipline

Hartel technique

Hartnup
> H. disorder

**Harvard-Brown Anxiety Disorders
Research Project (HARP)**

has-been

hashish

hassle

haste

hasten

hastened death

hatchet
> h. job
> h. man

hate
> h. crime
> ethnic h.
> exposure to h.
> feeling of h.
> h. group
> h. video game

hateful

Hatha yoga

hatred
haughty behavior
haunt
haut
    h. mal
    h. mal epilepsy
hauteur
haven
havoc
hawk
Hawthorn effect
hazard
    environmental h.
    moral h.
    occupational h.
hazardous treatment
haze
hazy
HBS
    hyperkinetic behavior syndrome
HCA
    heterocyclic antidepressant
HCD
    higher cerebral dysfunction
HCl
    hydrochloride
        chlorphentermine HCl
        diacetylmorphine HCl
HCR
    hysterical conversion reaction
HDH
    hostility and direction of hostility
HE
    hepatic encephalopathy
head
    h. banging
    h. bobbing
    h. consciousness
    gunshot wound to the h. (GSWH)
    h. of household
    h. injury
    h. jerking
    h. knocking
    h. and neck tremor
    perception of sound inside the h.
    perception of sound outside the h.
    h. rolling
    h. shadow effect
    sound inside the h.
    sound outside the h.
    H. Start program
    swelled h.

    swimming in the h.
    h. tetanus
    h. tilt
    h. trauma
    h. turn technique
    voice inside h.
    voice outside h.
    h. weaving
    H. zone
headache
    acute confusional migraine h.
    aphasic migraine h.
    band-like h.
    benign exertional h.
    bifrontal h.
    bilious h.
    bioccipital h.
    blind h.
    cataclysmic h.
    chronic h.
    circumstantial migraine h.
    classical migraine h.
    cluster h.
    coital h.
    combination h.
    common migraine h.
    complicated migraine h.
    confusional migraine h.
    cyclic h.
    disabling h.
    essential h.
    evening h.
    exertional h.
    familial migraine h.
    fibrositic h.
    frontal h.
    functional h.
    generalized h.
    hangover h.
    hemiparesthetic migraine h.
    histaminic h.
    Horton h.
    ipsilateral h.
    late-life migraine h.
    migraine h.
    Monday morning h.
    muscle contraction h.
    nitrite h.
    nonpulsating h.
    ocular migraine h.
    organic h.
    paroxysmal migraine h.

NOTES

H

headache *(continued)*
    phobia-induced migraine h.
    postcoital h.
    postconcussion h.
    posttraumatic h.
    psychogenic h.
    pulsating h.
    recurrent migraine h.
    reflex h.
    seasonal migraine h.
    sick h.
    sleep-related cluster h.
    suboccipital h.
    sudden-onset h.
    symptomatic h.
    h. syndrome
    temporal h.
    tension migraine h.
    tension-vascular h.
    traumatic h.
    unilateral migraine h.
    vacuum h.
    vascular h.
    vasomotor h.
    weekend h.
head-banging behavior
head-bobbing doll syndrome
head-dropping test
headlong
headquarters
headshrinker
HEADSS
    home life, education level, activities,
    drug use, sexual activity, suicide
    ideation/attempts
headstrong
head-to-head clinical trial
heady
heal
healer
    folk h.
    religious h.
healing
    concept of spiritual h.
    faith h.
    holistic h.
    mental h.
    h. prayer
    h. process
    h. ritual
    spiritual h.
health
    h. behavior
    behavioral h.
    bill of h.
    h. care
    h. care informatics
    change in h.

    community mental h.
    delusion of ill h.
    H., Education, and Welfare (HEW)
    emotional h.
    flight into h.
    H. and Human Services (HHS)
    H. Information Portability and
      Accountability Act of 1996
      (HIPAA)
    h. insurance
    h. issue
    h. law
    h. literacy skills
    h. maintenance organization (HMO)
    mental h.
    National Institute of Mental H.
      (NIMH)
    h. outcome
    H. Plan Employer Data and
      Information Set
    h. policy
    h. professional
    psychological h.
    h. psychology
    public h.
    h. risk
    h. risks from smoking
    h. status
    h. systems agency (HSA)
    h. viewpoint
healthcare
    h. bias
    h. proxy
healthful
health-related
    h.-r. consequence
    h.-r. facility
    h.-r. psychology
    h.-r. variable
healthy
    h. adolescent behavior
    h. aggression
    h. approach
    h. functioning
    h. identification
    h. individual
    h. lifestyle
    h. patient
    h. religious life
hearing
    color h.
    evidentiary h.
    h. impairment
    Riese h.
    speech and h. (S&H)
    h. theory
    thought h.

visual h.
h. voices
hearsay
heart
    bleeding h.
    broken h.
    change of h.
    irritable h.
    pounding h.
    h. psychogenic disorder
    purple h.
    soldier's h.
    take h.
heartache
heartbreak
heartbroken
hearted
    false h.
heartless
heartrending
heartsick
heartstring
heart-to-heart
heat
    h. defense
    h. dissipation
    h. effector
heat-defense response
heated discussion
heat-induced asthenia
heat-loss
    h.-l. apparatus
    h.-l. mechanism
    h.-l. pathway
heaviness
heavy
    h. metal intoxication
    h. metal music
    h. metal screen
    h. smoker
heavy-duty
heavy-handed
heavy-hearted
hebbian
    h. modification
    h. property
Hebb rule
hebephilia
hebephrenia
    manic h.

hebephrenic
    h. dementia
    h. schizophrenia
hebetic
hebetude
heboid
    h. paranoia
    h. praecox
heboidophrenia
Hebrew
heckle
hectic
hector
hedge
hedonic
    h. capacity
    h. drive
    h. level
    h. psychoactive effect
    h. response
    h. volition
hedonic-tone factor
hedonism
hedonistic
    h. activity
    h. orientation
    h. utilitarianism
hedonomania
heed
heedless
heel
    Achilles h.
    h. tap
heel-tap
    h.-t. reaction
    h.-t. test
heel-to-knee test
heightened
    h. anxiety
    h. attention
    h. attention state
    h. awareness
    h. awareness state
    h. sensory perception
height vertigo
Heinis constant
heinous
    h. act
    h. crime
    h. event
heir of the Oedipus complex
helicat

NOTES

H

helicopod gait
helicopodia
heliencephalitis
helienologomania
heliomania
hell
    raise h.
hell-bent
hellcat
hellenologomania
Heller
    H. dementia
    H. syndrome
hellion
hellish
helmet
    neurasthenic h.
help
    cry for h.
    pastoral h.
    plea for h.
    professional h.
    psychiatric h.
    h. seeking
helper
    magic h.
    h. role
    h. therapy
helping
    h. behavior
    h. model
    h. relationship
helpless
helplessness
    feeling of h.
    learned h.
    psychic h.
    self-reported h.
helpmate
help-rejecting complainer
help-seeking behavior
hemeraphonia
hemiacrosomia
hemianalgesia
hemianesthesia
    alternate h.
    crossed h.
hemiapraxia
hemiasynergia
hemiataxia
hemiathetosis
hemiatrophy
    facial h.
    progressive lingual h.
hemiballismic movement
hemiballismus, hemiballism
hemifacial spasm
hemifield of vision

hemihyperesthesia
hemihypertonia
hemihypotonia
hemiopalgia
hemiparesthesia
hemiparesthetic migraine headache
hemiplegia
    contralateral h.
    crossed h.
    double h.
    facial h.
    hysterical h.
    infantile h.
    h. migraine
    nocturnal h.
    spastic h.
hemiplegic
    h. gait
hemisensory loss
hemispasm
hemispatial arousal neglect
hemisphere
    cerebral h.
    dominant h.
    language-dominant h.
    left h.
    right h.
hemispheric
    h. dynamics
    h. lateralization
    h. reliance
hemispherical dysfunction
hemithermoanesthesia
hemitonia
hemitremor
hemizygous
hemlock
    poison h.
    H. Society
hemodynamic system
hemothymia
hemp
henbane
Henmon-Nelson
henpeck
hepatic
    h. coma
    h. encephalopathy (HE)
    h. encephalopathy tremor
    h. injury
    h. porphyria
    h. steatosis
hepatitis
    alcoholic h. (AH)
    infectious h.
hepatolenticular disease
hepatorenal syndrome
hepatosplenomegaly

hepatotoxicity
herbal
    h. medicine
    h. preparation
    h. remedy
herbalism
herbalist
herbiceuticals
herbivorous
herd instinct
hereafter
here-and-now approach
hereditaria
    adynamia episodica h.
    alopecia h.
hereditarian
hereditary
    h. deficiency
    h. disorder
heredity
    environment and h. (E&H)
heredoataxia
heredofamilial
    h. psychosis
    h. tremor
heredo-familial essential microsomia
heredopathia atactica polyneuritiformis
heresiarch
heresy
heretic
heritability
    broad h.
heritable
    h. basis
    h. component
    h. influence
    h. nature
hermaphoditism
hermaphrodism
hermaphrodite
hermaphroditism
    bilateral h.
    false h.
    transverse h.
    true h.
    unilateral h.
hermeticism
hermetic medicine
hermit
hermitage
hero
    h. daydream

    h. fantasy
    intellectual h.
    negative h.
    h. worship
heroin
    h. addiction
    h. antagonist and learning therapy (HALT)
    black tar h.
    cannabis and h.
    cannabis, cocaine and h.
    cocaine and h.
    high-grade h.
    h. injection
    intranasal h.
    liquefied h.
    low-grade h.
    mainlining h.
    h. mixed with powdered milk
    h. overdose
    h. user
    h. withdrawal
hero-worshiper
herpes
    genital h.
    h. genitalis
    h. simplex virus
    h. zoster
    h. zoster meningitis
herpetic
    h. meningoencephalitis
Herrmann syndrome
hersage
hesitancy
    patient h.
hesitant
    h. communication
    h. speech
hesitation phenomenon
hetaeral fantasy
heteresthesia
heterocentric
heteroclite
heterocyclic
    h. agent
    h. antidepressant (HCA)
    h. antidepressant drug
heterodimer
heteroeroticism
heteroerotism
heterogeneity
    clinical h.

NOTES

H

heterogeneity *(continued)*
    etiological h.
    neurophysiological h.
heterogeneous
    h. clinical presentation
    h. condition
    h. group
    h. nuclear RNA
heterogenicity
    genetic h.
    locus h.
heterogenous
    h. disorder
    h. grouping
heterohypnosis
heterokinesia
heterokinesis
heterolalia
heteroliteral
heterologous stimulus
heteromorphic
heteronomous
    h. psychotherapy
    h. stage
    h. superego
heteronomy
heteronymous
heteropathy
heterophasia
heterophemia, heterophemy
heterophonia
heterophoria
heteropsychologic
heteroreceptor
heterorexia
heterosexual
    h. anxiety
    h. behavior
    h. incest
    h. lover
    h. marriage
    h. orientation
    h. pedophile
    h. pedophilia
    h. rape
    h. relationship
heterosexuality
heterosexual sexual experience
heterosome
heterosuggestibility
heterosuggestion
heterotopia
heterotopic pain
heterotopy
heterotrimeric
    h. G protein
    h. postreceptor
heterozygote

heterozygous individual
heuristic
heutoscopy
HEW
    Health, Education, and Welfare
hex, pl. **hexes**
    h. doctor
hexing
    illness ascribed to h.
HFA
    high-functioning autism
HGF
    human growth factor
HHS
    Health and Human Services
HI
    hypoglycemic index
5-HIAA
    5-hydroxyindoleacetic acid
hibernation
hiccup, hiccough
    psychogenic h.
hidden
    h. agenda
    h. meaning
    h. message
    h. observer
    h. observer phenomenon
    h. rage
    h. self
hiding behavior
hidrosis
HIE
    hypoxic-ischemic encephalopathy
hierarchical
    h. functioning
    h. organization
    h. regression analysis
    h. structure
    h. theory of instinct
hierarchy
    anxiety h.
    h. construction
    corporate h.
    dominance h.
    exposure h.
    habit h.
    lifetime h.
    Maslow h.
    motivational h.
    h. of motives
    h. of need
    occupational h.
    response h.
    social h.
hieromania
hierotherapy

HIF
    higher intellectual function
high
    h. adaptive level
    h. affectivity ratio
    h. alpha coefficient
    h. anxiety (HA)
    h. arousal
    h. degree of competency
    drug-induced h.
    h. energy level
    h. fever
    h. frequency deafness
    h. impulsiveness high anxiety
      (HIHA)
    h. impulsiveness low anxiety
      (HILA)
    h. profile
    h. profile crime
    h. profile criminal
    h. quality education
    h. quality parenting
    h. risk
    h. roller
    h. school adolescent
    h. sensitivity
    h. steppage gait
    h. tolerance potential
    h. utilizer
high-alcoholic elixir
high-altitude illness
high-anger individual
highbrow
    ethical h.
high-calorie diet
high-conflict family
high-dose drug
high-emotion scene
high-energy
    h.-e. bond
    h.-e. cellular store
higher
    h. being
    h. brain center
    h. cerebral dysfunction (HCD)
    h. cortical dysfunction
    h. cortical function
    h. dementia
    h. echelon
    h. integrative language processing
    h. intellectual function (HIF)
    h. level cognitive function

    h. level of consciousness
    h. level skill
    h. mental process
    h. neural function
    h. order conditioning
    h. order interaction
    h. power
    h. state of consciousness
    h. status
higher-order emotion-related meaning
highest-ranking item
high-fat diet
high-fiber diet
high-functioning
    h.-f. autism (HFA)
    h.-f. patient
high-grade
    h.-g. defect
    h.-g. heroin
high-intensity transition
high-level perceptual disturbance
high-pitched voice
high-profile
    h.-p. case
    h.-p. patient
high-protein diet
high-resolution MRI
high-risk
    h.-r. activity
    h.-r. approach
    h.-r. behavior
    h.-r. gambling situation
    h.-r. group
    h.-r. lifestyle
    h.-r. patient
    h.-r. population
    h.-r. study
high-spirited buoyancy
high-strung
high-volume hospital
highway hypnosis
HIHA
    high impulsiveness high anxiety
hijacker
HILA
    high impulsiveness low anxiety
Hilgard neo-dissociation theory
Hilton method
HIPAA
    Health Information Portability and
      Accountability Act of 1996
hip-hop culture

NOTES

H

309

hippie culture
hippocampal
    h. activation
    h. amnesia
    h. complex
    h. damage
    h. epilepsy
    h. formation subdivision
    h. raw volume
    h. sclerosis
    h. sprouting
    h. synaptic plasticity
    h. volumetric loss
Hippocratic oath
hippomania
hipster
hipsterism
hired gun
hirsutism
histaminic
    h. cephalalgia
    h. headache
historian
    poor h.
historical
    h. context
    h. data
    h. method
    h. presentation
historicize
history
    h. of abuse
    h. of abusing animals
    alcohol-positive h. (APH)
    biopsychosocial h.
    case h.
    childhood mistreatment h.
    clinical h.
    criminal h.
    h. of cult affiliation
    cyclic h.
    depression h.
    detailed h.
    drinking h.
    drug use h.
    educational h.
    family h. (FH)
    family psychiatric h.
    genetic h.
    life h.
    lifetime h.
    marijuana use h.
    marital h. (MH)
    media h.
    medical h.
    military h.
    h. of mistreatment
    mistreatment h.

    multigenerational h.
    h. of neglect
    no previous h. (NPH)
    occupational h. (OH)
    oral h.
    pain h.
    past h. (PH)
    past personal h.
    personal h. (PH)
    personal psychiatric h.
    personal and social h. (P&SH)
    h. and physical (H&P)
    post relevant h. (PRH)
    premorbid psychiatric h.
    prenatal h.
    h. of present illness (HPI)
    previous h.
    psychiatric family h.
    psychosexual h.
    psychosocial h.
    relationship h.
    reliable h.
    school h.
    seizure h.
    h. of self-mutilation
    sexual abuse h.
    smoking h.
    social h. (SH)
    h. of suicide attempt
    suicide attempt h.
    h. of tobacco use
history-taking
histrionic
    h. character
    h. composite description
    h. diagnostic category
    h. neurotic personality disorder
    h. paralysis
    h. patient
    h. personality
    h. personality disorder score
    h. presentation
    h. Q factor
    h. quality
    h. scale
    h. situation
    h. spasm
histrionism
hit
    h. list
    h. man
hit-and-run
hitting own body
HIV
    human immunodeficiency virus
    HIV illness stage
    HIV risk behavior
HIV-based dementia

hives
HMO
    health maintenance organization
hoard
    h. food
    weapons h.
hoarding
    h. character
    h. and clutter
    compulsive h.
    h. orientation
    h. personality
hoarseness
hoax
hockey-stick strategy
hodomania
Hoffmann
    H. phenomenon
    H. sign
hold
    24-hour h.
holding
    h. environment
    h. exercise
holergasia
holiday
    caffeine h.
    h. depression
    drug h.
    Roman h.
    h. syndrome
    therapeutic drug h.
holier-than-thou attitude
holism
holistic
    h. analysis
    h. approach
    h. healing
    h. medicine
    h. psychology
    h. regimen
    h. treatment
holocaust survivor
holography
holophrase
homage
homatropine
home
    adult foster h.
    h. assessment
    board-and-care h.
    boarding h.

broken h.
    h. care
    h. confinement
    detention h.
    domiciliary care h.
    h. environment
    h. evaluation
    former foster h.
    foster h.
    group h.
    h. invasion victim
    h. language
    h. life, education level, activities,
      drug use, sexual activity, suicide
      ideation/attempts (HEADSS)
    nursing h.
    personal care h.
    h. placement
    rest h.
    returning to h.
    h. schooling
    h. setting
    sheltered h.
    single-parent h.
    h. visit
home-based family management
homebody
homebound
home-health aide
homeland
homeless
    h. child
    h. family
    h. patient
    h. person
    h. shelter
    spiritually h.
homely
homemade
    h. drug paraphernalia
    h. pipe bomb
homemaking responsibility
homeopathic principle
homeopathy
homeostasis
homeostatic
    h. balance
    h. equilibrium
    h. model
    h. principle
homeothermy
homeotic gene

NOTES

H

home-service agency
homesick
homicidal
    h. behavior
    h. ideation
    h. intent
    h. plan
    h. preoccupation
    h. rumination
    h. state
    h. thought
homicide
    justifiable h.
homicide-suicide
    h.-s. pact
    h.-s. protection contract
    h.-s. rate
homicidomania
hominem
    ad h.
homing
homochronous
homoclite
homoerotic
    h. behavior
    h. fantasy
homoeroticism, homoerotism
homoerotism
homogamy
homogenate technique
homogeneity
    cross-cultural h.
homogeneous
    h. grouping
    h. reinforcement
homogenic love
homogenitality
homogenous
    h. grouping
    h. reinforcement
    h. scintillating scotoma
homogeny
homograph
homolateral
homologous stimulus
homonomy drive
homophile
homophobe
homophobia
    internalized h.
    pathological h.
homophobic cult
homorganic
homosexual
    h. behavior
    closet h.
    h. community
    h. complex

    h. conflict disorder
    effeminate h.
    h. incest
    h. lover
    h. marriage
    h. neurosis
    h. orientation
    h. panic
    h. pedophile
    h. pedophilia
    h. relationship
    h. sexual experience
homosexuality
    ego dystonic h.
    female h.
    iatrogenic h.
    latent h.
    male h.
    masked h.
    overt h.
    situational h.
    unconscious h.
homotopic pain
homozygous individual
homunculus
honeymoon period
honor
    court of h.
    family h.
    h. financial obligation
    personal h.
    point of h.
    h. system
honorable discharge
hood
    clitoral h.
hoodwink
hooker
hope
    false h.
    misplaced h.
hopeful
hopelessness
    degree of h.
    feeling of h.
hops
horizon
    closed h.
    open h.
horizontal
    h. conflict
    h. group
    h. mobility
    h. nystagmus
    h. vertigo
hormism
hormonal
    h. difference

h. level
h. maturation
h. sex reassignment
h. sexual reassignment
hormone
antidiuretic h. (ADH)
corticotropin-releasing h.
gonadal h.
growth h. (GH)
growth hormone-releasing h.
h. ingestion
luteinizing h. (LH)
luteinizing hormone-releasing h.
(LHRH)
h. replacement
resistance to thyroid h. (RTH)
sex h.
thyroid-stimulating h. (TSH)
thyrotropin-releasing h. (TRH)
thyrotropin-stimulating h. (TSH)
h. treatment
horrific
h. experience
h. impulse
h. mental imagery
h. temptation
horrify
horror story
hors de combat
horse race gambling
Horton headache
hospice
h. care
h. movement
hospital
h. addiction syndrome
h. admission
h. chaplain
h. and community psychiatry
day h.
for-profit h.
high-volume h.
maximum-security forensic
psychiatric h.
mental h.
h. mortality rate
night h.
not-for-profit h.
open h.
open-door h.
private psychiatric h.
psychiatric h.

h. record
state h. (SH)
state mental h. (SMH)
teaching h.
weekend h.
hospital-based psychiatry
hospitalism
hospitalitis
hospitality
expression of h.
hospitalization
involuntary h.
long-term h.
partial h.
psychiatric h.
short-term h.
voluntary h.
weekend h.
hospitalize
hospitalized setting
host
h. culture
h. mother
hostage
hostile
h. aggression
h. behavior
h. challenge
h. identity
h. mania
h. motive
h. personality
h. response
h. tone
h. transference
h. work environment
hostility
aggressive h.
covert h.
h. and direction of hostility (HDH)
exposure to h.
expression of h.
open h.
paranoid h.
penalty, frustration, anxiety,
guilt, h. (PFAGH)
hot
h. flash
h. line
h. temper
hot-blooded
hotheaded

NOTES

H

313

hotline
>abused-child h.
>abused-wife h.
>crisis h.
>runaway h.
>suicide h.

hot-seat technique

24-hour
>24-h. hold
>24-h. telephone help line

hours
>every four h.
>every two h.

house
>h. arrest
>cooperative urban h.
>halfway h.
>h. husband
>h. physician
>quarter-way h.
>h. rule
>transitional halfway h.

housebound

household
>h. dysfunction
>head of h.
>h. product inhalant
>h. responsibility

housemate

housewife
>h. neurosis
>h. psychosis
>h. syndrome

housing
>satellite h.

hovel

hover

howitzer

howler

HP
>hyperphoria

H&P
>history and physical

HPA
>hypothalamic-pituitary-adrenal

HPI
>history of present illness

HRT
>habit reversal training

HSA
>health systems agency

HT
>hand test
>hypertension

5-HT
>5-HT agonist
>5-HT releasing agent
>5-HT reuptake inhibitor

huang
>ma h.

hubris

hue
>h. and cry
>primary h.

human
>h. companionship
>h. complexity
>h. engineering
>h. factor
>h. factor psychology
>h. figure parts response
>h. frailty
>H. Genome Project
>h. growth factor (HGF)
>h. immunodeficiency virus (HIV)
>h. movement response
>h. nature
>h. potential
>h. prion disease
>h. problem
>h. relation
>h. relations group
>h. relationship
>h. relations training
>h. resources
>h. response (h)
>h. right
>h. sexuality
>h. strength
>h. therapeutic experience

humane treatment

humanism

humanistic
>h. concept
>h. conscience
>h. perspective
>h. philosophy
>h. psychology
>h. school
>h. theory
>h. therapy

humanitarian

humanity
>crime against h.

humanize

humankind

human-motivation theory

human-pet bonding

human-potential
>h.-p. model
>h.-p. movement

humble

humidity effect

humiliate

humiliation

humility

humor
> anal h.
> bitter h.
> cynical h.
> gallows h.
> sense of h.

humoral
> h. immunity
> h. theory

humored

humorless

hunger
> affect h.
> air h.
> h. drive
> drug h.
> h. edema
> narcotic h.
> h. pain
> h. pang
> psychogenic air h.
> social h.
> h. strike

hunter
> fortune h.

hunting behavior

Huntington chorea organic psychosis

hurdle

hurtful

husband
> house h.

husband-to-wife aggression

hustler
> bar h.

Hutchinson
> H. facies
> H. mask
> H. pupil

HV
> hyperventilation

HVS
> hyperventilation syndrome

hwa-byung
> wool h.-b.

hyalophagia

hybrid

hybridization

hydrargyromania

hydration

hydride

hydrocephalus ex vacuo

hydrodipsomania

hydrophobica
> agriothymia h.

hydrophorograph

hydrotherapy

5-hydroxyindoleacetic acid (5-HIAA)

hygieiolatry

hygiene
> criminal h.
> h. deterioration
> inadequate sleep h.
> inappropriate h.
> industrial h.
> mental h.
> minimal personal h.
> personal h.
> poor h.
> sleep h.

hygienic inducement

hymen
> imperforate h.

hymenal membrane

hyofrontality hypothesis in schizophrenia

hypacusic

hypacusis, hypoacusis

hypalgesia, hypoalgesia

hypalgia

hypapoplexia

hyperactive
> h. affect
> h. behavior
> h. child syndrome (HACS)
> h. disorder
> h. sexual arousal
> h. sexual desire
> h. sympathetic response

hyperactive-impulse attention-deficit disorder

hyperactive-impulsive behavior

hyperactivity
> attention deficit disorder with h. (ADD-HA)
> attention deficit disorder without h.
> autonomic h.
> developmental h.
> h. disorder
> dopaminergic h.
> impulsive h.
> h. index
> motoric h.
> prefrontal h.
> h. problem

NOTES

H

hyperactivity *(continued)*
    sympathoadrenal h.
    tactile h.
hyperactivity-impulsivity dimension
hyperacusis, hyperacusia
hyperadrenal constitution
hyperadrenalism
hyperadrenergic state
hyperadrenocorticism
hyperaesthetic
    h. personality
    h. variant of schizoid temperament
hyperageusia
hyperaggressivity
hyperalert
hyperalgesia
    auditory h.
hyperalgia
hyperamnesia
hyperaphia
hyperarousal
    autonomic h.
    physiological h.
    h. symptom
hyperattentiveness to voice tone
hyperbaric medicine
hyperbulia
hypercathexis
hypercompensatory
hypercritical
hyperdynamia
hyperechema
hyperemotional
hyperenergetic behavior
hyperepithymia
hyperergasia
hypereridic state
hyperesthesia
    auditory h.
    cerebral h.
    gustatory h.
    muscular h.
    olfactory h.
    tactile h.
hyperesthetic
    h. memory
    h. zone
hyperevolutism
hyperexcitability
hyperfunction
hypergargalesthesia
hypergasia
hypergenitalism
hypergeusia
hypergnosis
hypergraphia
hyperhedonia
hyperhidrosis

Hypericum perforatum
hyperindependence
hyperingestion
hyperintensity
    h. change
    deep white matter h.
    MRI signal h.
    periventricular h.
    h. rating
    h. severity
    signal h.
    subcortical gray matter h.
    white matter h.
hyperirritability
hyperkinesis, hyperkinesia
    axial h.
    developmental disorder associated
    with h.
    h. index
hyperkinetic
    h. behavior syndrome (HBS)
    h. conduct disorder
    h. conversion reaction
    h. disturbance
    h. dysphonia
    h. encephalopathy
    h. impulse disorder
    h. reaction of childhood
    h. speech
    h. syndrome
    h. syndrome of childhood
hyperlexia
hyperlogia
hypermania
hypermanic
hypermetabolic effect
hypermetabolism
    prefrontal h.
hypermetamorphosis
hypermetria
hypermimia
hypermnesia
hypermyesthesia
hypermyotonia
hypernatremia
hypernatremic encephalopathy
hypernoia
hypernomia
hypernomic
hyperobesity
hyperontomorph
hyperorality
hyperorexia
hyperosmia
hyperpathia
hyperphagia
hyperphagic obesity
hyperphoria (HP)

hyperphrasia
hyperphrenia
hyperphrenic
hyperpipecolatemia
hyperplasia
    adrenal h.
    cerebral h.
    congenital adrenal h.
hyperplastic
hyperpolarization
hyperpolarize
hyperponesis
hyperpragia
hyperpragic
hyperpraxia
hyperprosexia
hyperprosody
hyperpsychosis
hyperpyrexia
hyperquantivalent idea
hyperreflexia
    autonomic h.
    generalized h.
hypersalivation
hyperselaphesia
hypersensibility
hypersensitive
hypersensitivity syndrome
hypersensitization
hypersexual complex
hypersexuality
hypersomnia
    h. associated with depression
    h. disorder
    idiopathic h.
    persistent h.
    primary h.
    transient h.
hypersomnia-type sleep disorder
hypersomnic depression
hypersomnolence disorder
hypertension (HT)
    essential h.
    idiopathic h.
    orthostatic h.
hypertensive
    h. crisis
    h. encephalopathy
hyperthermalgesia
hyperthermia
    ectasy-associated malignant h.
    rebound h.

hyperthermoesthesia
hyperthymia
hyperthymic
    h. personality disorder
    h. temperament
hypertonia
    sympathetic h.
    treatment-emergent h.
hypertonic absence
hypertrophic
    h. cervical pachymeningitis
    h. interstitial neuropathy
hypertychia
hyperventilation (HV)
    autonomic h.
    central neurogenic h.
    forced h.
    neurogenic h.
    psychogenic h.
    h. syndrome (HVS)
    h. test
    h. tetany
hyperverbal
hypervigilance
hypervigilant
hypesthesia, hypoesthesia
    olfactory h.
    vaginal h.
hyphedonia
hypnagogic
    h. hallucination
    h. hallucination image
    h. hallucination imagery
    h. intoxication
    h. perception
    h. reverie
    h. state
    h. vision
hypnagogue
hypnapagogic
hypnic
hypnoanalysis
hypnoanalytic
hypnoanesthesia
hypnocatharsis
hypnogenesis
hypnogenic
    h. spot
    h. zone
hypnogenous
hypnograph
hypnoid state

NOTES

H

hypnologist
hypnology
hypnonarcosis
hypnopompic
    h. hallucination
    h. image
    h. perception
    h. state
hypnosis
    diagnostic use of h.
    direct suggestion under h. (DSUH)
    father h.
    fear h.
    highway h.
    lethargic h.
    major h.
    minor h.
    mother h.
    questioning under h.
    suggestion under h.
    symptom relief through h.
    waking h.
hypnosophy
hypnotherapy
hypnotic
    h. abreaction
    h. abuse
    h. action
    h. activity
    h. agent
    h. amnesia
    h. anesthesia
    h. capacity
    h. delirium
    h. dependence
    h. drug
    h. induction
    h. interview
    h. intoxication
    h. patient
    h. psychotherapy
    h. relationship
    h. relaxation technique training
    h. response
    sedative h.
    h. sleep
    h. state
    h. suggestion
    h. trance
    h. use disorder
    h. withdrawal
    h. withdrawal symptom
hypnotic-dependent
    h.-d. patient
    h.-d. sleep disorder
hypnotic-induced
    h.-i. anxiety
    h.-i. disorder

    h.-i. persisting dementia
    h.-i. psychotic disorder with
      delusions
    h.-i. psychotic disorder with
      hallucinations
    h.-i. sexual dysfunction
hypnotic-sedative drug
hypnotism
hypnotist
hypnotizability
hypnotization
    collective h.
hypnotize
hypoactive
    h. affect
    h. limbic structure
    h. sexual arousal
    h. sexual desire
    h. sexual desire disorder
hypoactivity
hypoacusis (*var. of* hypacusis)
hypoalgesia (*var. of* hypalgesia)
hypocathexis
hypochondria
hypochondriac
    h. language
    h. melancholia
    h. neurosis
    h. paranoia
    h. psychoneurosis
    h. psychoneurotic reaction
hypochondriaca
    melancholia h.
hypochondriacal
    h. complaint
    h. melancholia
    h. neurosis
    h. paranoia
    h. preoccupation
    h. psychogenic disorder
    h. psychoneurosis
    h. psychoneurotic reaction
    h. psychosis
    h. symptom
hypochondriasis
    monosymptomatic h.
    h. neurotic disorder
    h. scale
    h. with poor insight type
hypochoresis
hypocondriaque
    folie h.
hypocrisy
hypocrite
hypodermic
    h. injection
    intracutaneous h.
    intramuscular h.

intravenous h.
h. needle
hypodopaminergic state
hypoesthesia (*var. of* hypesthesia)
hypoesthetic
hypoevolutism
hypofrontality phenomenon
hypofunction
prefrontal h.
testicular h.
hypogeusia
idiopathic h.
hypoglycemia
hypoglycemic
h. delirium
h. encephalopathy
h. index (HI)
hypogonadism with anosmia
hypokinesia, hypokinesis
treatment-emergent h.
hypokinetic
h. anoxia
h. speech
h. syndrome
hypokrisia
hypolepsiomnia
hypologia
hypomania
h. scale
treatment-emergent h.
hypomanic
bipolar I disorder, most recent
episode h.
h. disorder
h. manic-depressive reaction
h. mood episode
h. personality
h. phase
h. psychosis
h. quality
h. scale
h. tendency
hypomanic-depressive reaction
hypomelancholia
hypometabolism
frontotemporal h.
striatal h.
hypometria
hypomnesia
hypomotility
hyponatremia

hyponoia
hyponoic
hyponomic
hypoperfusion
bitemporal h.
cerebellar h.
parietooccipital h.
posterior frontal h.
hypophonia
hypophonic aphasia
hypophoria
hypophrasia
hypophrenic
hypophrenosis
hypophyseopriva
hypophysial, hypophyseal
hypophysiopriva
cachexia h.
hypophysis
catecholamine h.
hypoplasia
cerebral h.
hypoplasticus
status h.
hypopraxia
hypoprosessis
hypoprosody
hypopsychosis
hyporeflexia
hyposensitive
hyposexuality
hyposmia
hyposomnia
h. associated with anxiety
h. associated with depression
h. associated with psychosis
hyposomniac
hyposphresia
hyposthenia
hypostheniant
hyposthenic
hypotaxia
hypotaxis
hypotension
intracranial h.
orthostatic h.
postural h.
hypothalamic
h. area
h. dysfunction
h. nucleus

NOTES

H

hypothalamic *(continued)*
    h. obesity
    h. regulatory input
hypothalamic-pituitary-adrenal (HPA)
hypothalamic-pituitary-adrenocortical
    h.-p.-a. system
hypothalamic-pituitary axis dysfunction
hypothalamus
    anterior h.
    lateral h.
    medial h.
    posterior h.
    ventromedial h.
hypothermia
    accidental h.
    fatal h.
hypothermic disorder
hypothesis, pl. **hypotheses**
    adaptive h.
    alpha, beta, gamma hypotheses
    anniversary h.
    apertural h.
    as-if h.
    beta h.
    biogenic amine h.
    disconnection h.
    dopamine h.
    drift h.
    ethical risk h.
    experimental h.
    falsifiable h.
    frustration-aggression h.
    gate-control h.
    h. generation
    intergroup-contact h.
    matching h.
    maturation h.
    mediumistic h.
    mnemenic h.
    monoamine h.
    neurohumoral h.
    null h.
    quantal h.
    segregation h.
    serotonergic deficiency h.
    specificity h.
    h. testing
    topographic h.
    up-regulation/downregulation h.
hypothesize
hypothetical
    h. continuum
    h. deductive thinking
    h. reasoning
hypothetical-deductive reasoning
hypothymia
hypothymic personality disorder
hypothymism

hypothyroidism
hypovigility
hypoxia
    relative h.
    short-term h.
    toxic h.
hypoxic-ischemic encephalopathy (HIE)
hypoxyphilia
hypoxyphilia-caused death
hysteria
    anxiety h.
    Arctic h.
    canine h.
    Charcot grand h.
    collective h.
    combat h.
    communicable h.
    conversion h.
    defense h.
    dissociative h.
    dissociative-type neurotic h.
    epidemic h.
    fixation h.
    major h.
    mass h.
    minor h.
    h. neurotic disorder
    h. psychoneurosis
    h. psychosis
    h. scale
    St. Louis h.
    studies on h.
    h. study
hysteric
    h. amaurosis
    h. amblyopia
    h. coma-like state
    h. lethargy
    h. paralysis
hysterica
    aura h.
    megalopia h.
    suffocation h.
hysterical
    h. abasia
    h. amnesia
    h. anesthesia
    h. aphonia
    h. ataxia
    h. aura
    h. behavior
    h. blindness
    h. character
    h. character defense
    h. chorea
    h. conversion reaction (HCR)
    h. convulsion
    h. deafness

h. delirium
h. delirium depression
h. dysphoria hysterophilia
h. epilepsy
h. fugue
h. fugue state
h. gait
h. gait disorder
h. hearing impairment
h. hemiplegia
h. insanity
h. joint
h. laughter
h. lithiasis
h. mania
h. movement disorder
h. mutism
h. myodynia
h. neurosis
h. paralysis
h. personality
h. personality disorder
h. polydipsia
h. pregnancy
h. pseudodementia
h. psychogenic disorder
h. psychomotor disorder
h. psychoneurotic reaction
h. psychosis
h. puerilism
h. seizure
h. stuttering
h. syncope

h. torticollis
h. trance
h. tremor
h. vertigo
h. visual loss
h. voices
hysterics
aura h.
megalopia h.
suffocation h.
hystericum
delirium h.
hystericus
clavus h.
globus h.
hysteriform
hysterique
grande attaque h.
hysterocatalepsy
hysteroepilepsy
hysterofrenatory
hysterofrenic
hysterogenic, hysterogenous
h. zone
hysteroid
h. defense
h. dysphoria
h. feature
h. personality
hysterophilia
hysterical dysphoria h.
hysterosyntonic

NOTES

H

I
> I marker
> I tracing

IA
> inactive alcoholic

IACPO
> Inter-American Council of Psychiatric Organizations

iamatology
iambic stress
iatric
iatrogenesis
iatrogenic
> i. addiction
> i. disorder
> i. effect
> i. homosexuality
> i. illness
> i. induction
> i. instability
> i. psychosis
> i. schizophrenia
> i. seizure

iatrogeny
iatrology
iatrophysics
IB
> index of body build

ibogaine
I-boundary
IBS
> irritable bowel syndrome

IBW
> ideal body weight

ICD
> impulse control disorder
> International Classification of Diseases

ICD-9
> International Classification of Diseases, ed. 9
>> ICD-9 code
>> ICD-9 diagnostic codes for Medicare reimbursement

ICD-10
> International Classification of Diseases, ed. 10
>> ICD-10 psychiatric diagnosis

ICD-9CM
> International Classification of Diseases, Clinical Modification, ed. 9

iceberg
> tip of the i.

iceblock theory
Iceland disease
ichnogram

ichthyohemotoxism
ichthyophagia
ichthyosarcotoxin
ichthyotoxin
I-complex
icon
> corporate i.

iconic
> i. memory
> i. sign
> i. storage

iconicity
iconoclasm
iconoclast
iconology
iconomania
ICP
> intracranial pressure

ICPS
> interpersonal cognitive problem solving

ICS
> intracranial stimulation

ICSD
> International Classification of Sleep Disorders: Diagnostic and Coding Manual

ICSW
> International Committee on Social Welfare

ictal
> i. amnesia
> i. automatism
> i. confusional seizure
> i. depression
> i. depression phase of seizure
> i. emotion
> i. period

icteric
icterogenic
icterohepatitis
icteroid
icterus
icthyomania
ictus
> i. epilepticus
> i. paralyticus

ICU
> intensive care unit
>> ICU psychosis

ID
> identification

id
> id anxiety
> id ego
> id interpretation

id *(continued)*
    id psychology
    id resistance
    id sadism
    id wish
idea
    abstract i.
    associated i.
    i. association
    autochthonous i.
    bizarre i.
    complex of i.'s
    compulsive i.
    delusion-like i.
    disconnected i.
    dominant i.
    expansion i.
    expansive i.
    fixed i.
    flight of i.'s (FOI)
    grandiose i.
    hyperquantivalent i.
    imperative i.
    inappropriate i.
    i. of influence
    intruding i.
    intrusive distressing i.
    morbid i.
    obliquely related i.
    obsessional i.
    obtrusive i.
    overcharged i.
    overvalued i.
    permanent dominant i.
    persecutory i.
    persistent inappropriate i.
    persistent intrusive i.
    poverty of i.
    pressure of i.'s
    psychotic-like i.
    recurring i.
    i.'s of reference
    referential i.
    repetitive i.
    ruminative i.
    strongly held i.
    i. of unreality
    unreasonable i.
    unwarranted i.
idea-chase
ideal
    i. beau
    body i.
    i. body weight (IBW)
    i. ego
    ego i.
    father i.
    i. masochism

    narcissistic ego i.
    i. personality
    transient ego i.
idealism
idealist
idealistic notion
idealization
    i. defense mechanism
    primitive i.
idealize
idealized
    i. image
    i. parental imago
    i. self
    i. value
idealizing transference
ideation
    adolescent sexual i.
    elopement i.
    grandiose i.
    homicidal i.
    incoherent i.
    overvalued i. (OVI)
    paranoid i.
    persecution i.
    recurrent suicidal i.
    stress-related paranoid i.
    suicidal i.
    suspicious i.
    transient stress-related paranoid i.
ideational
    i. agnosia
    i. apraxia
    i. shield
    i. style of coping
ideatory apraxia
ideé fixe
id-ego
idem
identical
    i. element
    i. twins
identifiable
    i. antecedent
    i. stress
    i. stressor
identification (ID)
    anthropometric i.
    cause of i.
    cosmic i.
    cross-gender i.
    deep trance i.
    i. defense mechanism
    empathic i.
    facial i.
    feminine i.
    i. figure
    gender i.

I

group i.
healthy i.
letter-word i.
multiple i.
object i.
i. phenomenon
phenomenon i.
primary i.
i. process
projective i.
secondary i.
social i.
i. test
i. transference
trial i.
i. with the aggressor
i. with the dead
identified trait
identifier
identify
identifying
i. data
i. with aggression
identity
adolescent personal i.
adolescent sexual i.
alteration in i.
i. alteration
alternate i.
assumption of new i.
belief about i.
body i.
controlling i.
i. crisis
cultural i.
i. diffusion
i. disorder
i. disorder of adolescence
i. disorder of childhood
i. disturbance
ego i.
i. experience
i. experience integer
false i.
family i.
female gender i.
female-to-male transgendered i.
feminine i.
formation of i.
i. formation
former i.
gender i.

hostile i.
inflated i.
intrapsychic i.
loss of i.
male gender i.
male-to-female transgender i.
masculine i.
multiple distinct i.'s
i. need
new i.
personal i.
place i.
primary i.
i. problem
protector i.
psychosexual i.
sense of i.
sexual i.
social i.
i. state
i. theme
i. versus role diffusion
vocational i.
i. vs. role confusion
identity-disordered children
ideodynamism
ideogenetic
ideogenous
ideogram
ideographic
ideokinetic
i. apraxia
i. praxis
ideological
i. commitment
i. orientation
ideology
ideometabolic
ideometabolism
ideomotion
ideomotor
i. aphasia
i. apraxia
i. signal
ideomotorapraxia
ideophrenia
ideosynchysia
idiocrasy
idiocy
amaurotic axonal i.
amaurotic familial i. (AFI)
axonal i.

NOTES

idiocy *(continued)*
    Aztec i.
    Bielschowsky i.
    cretinoid i.
    developmental i.
    diplegic i.
    epileptic i.
    erethismic i.
    family i.
    genetous i.
    infantile i.
    intrasocial i.
    Kalmuk i.
    microcephalic i.
    moral i.
    paralytic i.
    plagiocephalic i.
    profound i.
    scaphocephalic i.
    sensorial i.
    spastic amaurotic axonal i.
    torpid i.
    traumatic i.
    Vogt-Spielmeyer i.
idiodynamic control
idiogenesis
idioglossia
idiogram
idiographic approach
idiohypnotism
idiolalia
idiologism
idiom
    personal i.
idiomatic usage
idioneurosis
idiopathic
    i. dystonia
    i. encephalopathy
    i. epilepsy
    i. hypersomnia
    i. hypertension
    i. hypogeusia
    i. insomnia
    i. language retardation
    i. neuralgia
    i. psychosis
idiopathy
idiophonia
idiophrenic
    i. insanity
    i. psychosis
idiopsychologic
idioreflex
idiospasm
idiosyncrasy
idiosyncratic
    i. alcohol intoxication

    i. behavior
    i. material
    i. meaning
    i. process
    i. reaction
    i. reasoning
    i. side effect
    i. thinking
    i. topic shifting
idiot
    erethismic i.
    oxycephalic i.
    pithecoid i.
    i. savant
    superficial i.
    torpid i.
idiotic prodigy
idiot-prodigy
idiotrophic
idiotropic type
idiovariation
idle
idol
idolatrous
idolatry
idolism
idolize
idolomania
IDT
    interdisciplinary team
I-E
    internal versus external
        I-E scale
IER
    Institute of Educational Research
IES
    introversion-extroversion scale
IFROS
    ipsilateral frontal routing of signals
ignipedites
ignis fatuus
ignoble
ignominious
ignominy
ignorant
ignore
IHS
    Indian Health Service
I-it relationship
ikota
I-labeled cocaine analog
ill
    i. at ease
    chronically mentally i.
    mentally i.
    object i.
    terminally i.
    i. will

ill-advised
ill-bred
illegal
    i. drug
    i. drug sales
    i. drug synthesis
    i. drug use
    i. gambling
illegible
illegitimate
ill-fated
ill-humored
illicit
    i. drug abuse
    i. drug distribution
    i. drug fad
    i. drug synthesis
    i. drug use
    i. lover
    i. opiate use
    i. opioid
    i. psychoactive drug
    i. psychoactive substance
illimitable
illiteracy
    functional i.
    i. screening
    technological i.
illiterate
    functional i.
ill-mannered
ill-natured
illness
    advantage by i.
    affective i.
    i. ascribed to hexing
    i. as self-punishment
    autoimmune i.
    i. behavior
    bipolar i. (BPI)
    brain i.
    catastrophic i.
    chronic factitious i.
    chronic mental i.
    chronic psychotic i.
    course of i.
    cyclic i.
    debilitating i.
    dementing i.
    disabling mental i.
    dysautonomic i.
    early-onset mental i.

    emotional i.
    escape into i.
    factitious i.
    family history of mental i.
     (RHMI)
    flight into i.
    folk i.
    functional i.
    genetic susceptibility to mental i.
    high-altitude i.
    history of present i. (HPI)
    iatrogenic i.
    Kraepelin classification of mental i.
    legitimate i.
    length of i.
    life-threatening i.
    major mental i.
    manic depressive i.
    mass psychogenic i.
    mass sociogenic i.
    medical i.
    mental i.
    model of i.
    neurological i.
    new-onset mental i.
    no mental i. (NMI)
    nonschizophrenic i.
    objective severity of i.
    outcome of i.
    petition of mental i. (PMI)
    i. phase
    preexisting i.
    present i. (PI)
    progressive dementing i.
    psychiatric i.
    psychogenic i.
    psychosomatic i.
    psychotic i.
    refractory mental i.
    schizophrenic i.
    social class and mental i.
    stress-related i.
    underlying medical i.
    untreated psychiatric i.
    usual childhood i.
illogical
    i. attitude
    i. communication
    i. reasoning
    i. thinking
illogicality
ill-tempered

NOTES

ill-treat
illumination condition
illuminism
ill-use
illusion
- bodily i.
- i. des sosies
- i. of doubles
- dream i.
- fleeting i.
- memory i.
- movement i.
- i. of omnipotence
- optic i.
- optical i.
- i. of orientation
- Poggendorf i.
- i. of power
- i. of power over others
- recurrent i.
- tactile i.
- temporal lobe i.
- transient auditory i.
- transient tactile i.
- transient visual i.
- visual i.
- windmill i.
- Zollner i.

illusional
illusionary misconception
illustrate
illustration
- pornographic i.

IM
- intramuscular

image
- accidental i.
- i. agglutination
- body i.
- changed body i.
- cohesive i.
- concrete i.
- i. control
- dangerous i.
- depersonalized i.
- direct i.
- distorted body i.
- disturbed body i.
- eidetic i.
- i. eliciting disgust
- i. eliciting fear
- i. eliciting neutral emotion
- erotic i.
- false i.
- father i.
- formed i.
- fragmentary dream i.
- general i.

- ghost i.
- graven i.
- hallucinatory i.
- hypnagogic hallucination i.
- hypnopompic i.
- idealized i.
- imperfect i.
- inappropriate i.
- incidental i.
- i. intensifier
- intrusive obsessional i.
- inverted i.
- memory i.
- mental i.
- mirror i.
- mother i.
- motor i.
- negative body i.
- neutral i.
- nurturant i.
- obsessional mental i.
- parent i.
- percept i.
- perception of body i.
- peripheral field i.
- persistent inappropriate i.
- persistent intrusive i.
- personal i.
- poor body i.
- positive i.
- primary mental i.
- i. pseudohallucination
- public i.
- real i.
- i. registration
- sensory i.
- tactile i.
- trailing i.
- transient i.
- unformed i.
- visual i.
- vivid dream i.

image-distorting level
imageless thought
imagery
- affective i.
- auditory i.
- i. code
- eidetic i.
- emotive i.
- i. exercise
- guided affective i. (GAI)
- horrific mental i.
- hypnagogic hallucination i.
- mental i.
- paraphiliac i.
- pictorial i.
- smell i.

tactile i.
taste i.
i. therapy
visual i. (VI)
imaginable process
imaginal
    i. desensitization
    i. exposure
    i. flooding
    i. process
imaginary
    i. companion
    i. language
    i. relationship
imagination
    creative i.
imaginative play
imagine
imagined
    i. abandonment
    i. appearance defect
    i. loss
    i. ugliness
imagines (*pl. of* imago)
imaging
    brain i.
    cerebral dynamic i.
    in vivo i.
    magnetic resonance i. (MRI)
    i. method
    i. modularity
    neuroreceptor i.
    structural brain i.
    structural magnetic resonance i.
    i. study
    two-dimensional proton echo-planar
      spectroscopic i.
imagining
    active i.
    involuntary active i.
    voluntary active i.
imago, pl. **imagines**
    idealized parental i.
imbalance
    autonomic i.
    biochemical i.
    central language i.
    developmental i.
    effort-reward i.
    electrolyte i.
    fluid i.
    intellectual i.

language i.
sympathetic i.
vasomotor i.
imbecile
    moral i.
imbecility
    old-age i.
    senile i.
imbibe
imbibition
imbroglio
IMC
    information memory concentration
imitation
    elicited i.
    morbid i.
    repetition by i.
    spontaneous i.
imitative
    i. behavior
    folie i.
    i. speech
    i. tetanus
immaculate
immanence theory
immature
    i. coping mechanism
    i. defense
    i. personality
    i. personality disorder
immaturity
    emotional i.
    emotionally unstable i.
    perceptual i.
    i. reaction
    social i.
immediacy behavior
immediate
    i. allergy
    i. anxiety
    i. control
    i. echolalia
    i. ejaculation
    i. environment
    i. experience
    i. gratification
    i. memory
    i. memory test
    i. posttraumatic
    i. posttraumatic automatism
    i. posttraumatic convulsion
immediately

NOTES

immedicable
immerge
immersion
immigrant status
imminent justice
immissio penis
immobile
    i. face
    i. state
immobility
    motor i.
    motoric i.
immobilization paralysis
immobilize
immodest
immoral imperative
immoralist
immortalize
immovable
immune
    i. body
    i. deficiency
    i. deficiency syndrome
    i. disorder
    i. function
    i. response
    i. system
    i. system regulation
immunity
    active i.
    humoral i.
    passive i.
    stress i.
immunoblot analysis
immunocompromised
immunodeficiency
    sexually acquired i. (SAID)
immunofluorescence assay
immunogen
    behavioral i.
immunologic
    i. abnormality
    i. aspect
    i. dysfunction
immunological paralysis
immunology
    clinical i.
immunomodulatory
immunosorbent assay
immunosuppression
immunosuppressive effect
immure
immutable
impact
    i. analysis
    developmental i.
    disruptive i.
    pharmacologic i.

    potential i.
    psychological i.
    systemic i.
impacted grief
impair
impaired
    i. affect
    i. affect modulation
    i. arousal
    i. attention
    i. attentional functioning
    i. balance
    i. cognitive functioning
    communicatively i.
    i. concentration
    i. concentration ability
    i. connectedness
    i. consciousness
    i. development
    i. effective communication
    emotionally i.
    functionally i.
    i. impulse control
    i. insight
    i. language
    learning i.
    i. limbic-diencephalic function
    i. memory
    mentally i.
    i. migration of brain neurons
    i. orgasm satisfaction
    i. orientation
    i. performance
    i. relationship
    i. self-care
    i. self-image
    i. self-soothing
    severely mentally i. (SMI)
    i. sexual desire
    i. sexual function
    i. sexual performance
    i. social functioning
    i. social interaction
    i. social judgment
    speech and language i. (SLI)
    i. thinking ability
    i. vision
impairment
    age-associated memory i. (AAMI)
    aphasic phonological i.
    attention i.
    attentional i.
    basic i.
    cerebral i.
    clinically significant i.
    cognitive i.
    i. of cognitive function
    communication i.

i. of consciousness
i. criterion
degree of i.
i. of dementia
disproportionate i.
early speech i.
emotional i.
focal neurological i.
functional cognitive i.
functional hearing i.
gaze i.
generalized intellectual i.
general medical i.
global measure of i.
graphic i.
gross i.
hearing i.
hysterical hearing i.
i. index
initial spoken language i.
intellectual i.
interpersonal i.
language i.
level of i.
life i.
major i.
marked i.
measurable i.
medical i.
memory i.
mental i.
motivation i.
motor i.
narrative speech perception i.
neurocognitive i.
neurologic i.
neuropsychologic i.
nonlanguage cognitive i.
occupational i.
organic i.
perceptual-motor i.
permanent residual i.
phonologic assembly i.
physical i.
psychogenic hearing i.
reading comprehension i.
residual i.
reversible memory i.
school functioning i.
sensory i.
serious i.
severe i.

significant i.
sleep-induced respiratory i.
social functioning i.
speech i.
speech processing i.
spiritual i.
spoken language i.
i. symptom
verbal memory i.
visual memory i.
visual-motor i.
volitional i.

impartial
impasse
    therapeutic i.
impassible
impassion
impassive
impassivity
impatience
impatient
impedance
    i. matching
    i. method
impel
impend
impending
    i. death
    i. decompensation
    i. doom
    i. relapse
impenetrable
imperative
    categorical i.
    i. conception
    ethical i.
    i. idea
    immoral i.
    i. mood
imperceptible
imperception
imperfect
    i. image
    i. image registration
imperfection
imperforate hymen
imperious act
impersistence
impersonal
    i. factual knowledge
    i. projection

NOTES

impersonal *(continued)*
    i. relationship
    i. unconscious
impersonation
impersonator
    female i.
impertinent
imperturbable
impervious
impetuous
impetus
imping
impious
implant
    breast i.
    silicone i.
implausible phenomenon
implement
implementation
    standards i.
implication
    clinical i.
    policy i.
    societal i.
    theoretical i.
implicit
    i. behavior
    i. language
    i. memory
    i. personality theory
    i. process
    i. response
    i. role
implied criticism
implore
implosion
    i. flooding
    i. therapy
implosive therapy
impolite
import
    personal i.
importance
    clinical i.
    diagnostic i.
important
importune
impose
imposee
    folie i.
impostor
    juvenile i.
    i. psychotic manifestation
    i. syndrome
impotence, impotency
    anal i.
    anatomic i.
    atonic i.

    ejaculatory i.
    erectile i.
    functional i.
    organic i.
    orgastic i.
    paretic i.
    penile i.
    primary i.
    psychic i.
    psychogenic i.
    relative i.
    secondary i.
    sexual i.
    symptomatic i.
impotent
impotentia
    i. coeundi
    i. erigendi
impoverished
    i. community
    i. early environment
    i. fantasy life
    i. speech
    i. thought
impoverishment
    intellectual i.
    personality i.
    i. in thinking
impractical
imprecate
imprecise
impregnation fear
impress
impressible
impression
    absolute i.
    clinical i.
    diagnostic i.
    erroneous i.
    first i.
    good i.
    i. management
    mental i.
    i. method
    sensory i.
impressionable
impressive aphasia
imprint
imprinting
    filial i.
imprison
imprisonment
    false i.
improbable
improper
    i. diet
    i. dose
impropriety

I

improved communication skills
improvement
    clinical i.
    cognitive i.
    life-changing i.
    OCD i.
    plateau in i.
    practice-based learning and i.
    pronounced i.
    self-rated i.
    spontaneous i.
    statistically significant i.
    i. training
    transference i.
improvisation
imprudent
impuberism
impudent
impudicity
impugn
impuissant
impulse
    aggressive i.
    base i.
    i. control
    i. control conduct disorder
    i. control disorder (ICD)
    i. control problem
    cruel i.
    excitatory i.
    i. fear
    forbidden i.
    forced i.
    fundamental social i.
    gambling i.
    horrific i.
    inappropriate i.
    inhibitory i.
    intrusive i.
    irresistible i.
    libidinal i.
    i. life
    maladaptive i.
    morbid i.
    nervous i.
    i. neurosis
    nociceptive i.
    obsessional i.
    obsessive i.
    oral i.
    persistent inappropriate i.
    persistent intrusive i.

    i. regulation
    repressed i.
    self-destructive i.
    stealing i.
    unacceptable i.
    unconscious i.
    voluntary i.
    wandering i.
impulse-control
    i.-c. disorder NOS
impulsion
impulsive
    i. act
    i. activity
    i. aggression
    i. behavior
    i. character
    i. dyscontrol
    i. hyperactivity
    i. insanity
    i. madness
    i. neurosis
    i. obsession
    i. outburst
    i. petit mal epilepsy
    i. raptus
    i. spectrum
    i. suicide
    i. tendency
impulsive-aggressive trait
impulsive-compulsive psychopathology
impulsiveness
    low i.
impulsivity
    counteracting i.
    i. factor
    lifetime i.
    i. scale
    self-damaging i.
impunity
impurity
imputability
impute
in
    in absentia
    acting in
    in ano
    in articulo mortis
    being locked in
    in character
    in charge
    in control

NOTES

in *(continued)*
    in extremis
    in loco parentis
    in persona
    in propria persona
    run in
    shut in
    sit in
    turn in
    in vivo
    in vivo brain functioning
    in vivo exposure
    in vivo imaging
    in vivo observation
inability
    i. to concentrate
    i. to cry
    i. to delay gratification
    i. to ejaculate
    i. to enjoy interests
    i. to experience emotion
    i. to finish work
    i. to function
    i. to function independently
    i. to trust authority figure
inaccessibility
inaccessible
inaccurate
inaction
inactive alcoholic (IA)
inactivity
    alert i.
    behavioral i.
inadequacy
    intellectual i.
    personal i.
inadequate
    i. discipline
    i. impulse control
    i. information
    i. literacy
    i. parenting
    i. personality
    i. personality disorder
    i. rapport
    i. response
    i. school environment
    i. sleep hygiene
    i. stimulus
    i. therapy
    i. treatment
inadmissible
inadvertent
inadvisable
inalterable
inamorata
inane
inanimate learning device

inanition
inappetence
inappropriate
    i. affect
    i. appearance
    i. attitude
    i. behavior
    i. circumstance
    i. clothing
    i. crying
    i. dependent care
    i. disrobing
    i. handling of objects
    i. hygiene
    i. idea
    i. image
    i. impulse
    i. laughing
    i. laughter
    i. posture
    i. quality of obsession
    i. relationship
    i. religious training
    i. response
    i. sexual expression
    i. sexuality
    i. social relatedness
    i. thought
    i. urge
    i. verbalizing
    i. voiding
inappropriateness
    sexual i.
    social i.
inarticulate
inassimilable
inattention
    i. dimension
    i. to proper dietary habit
    selective i.
    sensory i.
    visual i.
inattentive behavior
inattentive-type attention deficit hyperactivity disorder
inaudible
in-between
inborn
    i. errors of metabolism
    i. reflex
inbred
inbreeding
    coefficient of i.
incalculable
incapacitate
incapacitating
    i. drowsiness
    i. fear

incapacity
    functional i.
    i. to sustain social bonds
incarcerate
incarcerated
    i. patient
    i. youth
incarceration
    drug-related i.
incarnata
    Passiflora i.
incendiare
    monomanie i.
incendiarism
incendiary arsonist
incense
incentive
    aversive i.
    i. learning
    i. motivation
    positive i.
    i. system
    i. theory
inception
incertitude
incessant speech
incest
    i. barrier
    i. fantasy
    father-daughter i.
    heterosexual i.
    homosexual i.
    mother-daughter i.
    mother-son i.
    i. taboo
incestuous
    i. desire
    i. fantasy
    i. relationship
    i. ties
incidence
    i. rate
    suicide i.
incident
    i. case
    original i.
    parasuicidal i.
    sexual i.
incidental
    i. image
    i. learning
    i. learning language

    i. learning language retardation
    i. memory
    i. stimulus
incipient
    i. schizophrenia
    i. schizophrenia psychosis
    i. schizophrenic psychosis
incisive
incite
incitement premium
incivility
inclement
inclination
    philosophical i.
inclusion
    class i.
inclusive fitness
incoercible
incogitant
incognito
incognizant
incoherence
incoherent
    i. behavior
    i. ideation
    i. patient
    i. speech
income
    fixed i.
    low i.
incommunicado
incomparable
incompatibility
incompatible
    i. behavior
    i. response
incompetence
    ejaculatory i.
    level of i. (LOI)
incompetency
    certificate of i.
    i. proceeding
incompetent
    mentally i.
incomplete
    i. alexia
    i. neurofibromatosis
incomprehensible
    i. speech
    i. thinking
    i. thought
incomputable

NOTES

inconceivable
inconclusive
incongruity
    insensitivity to i.
incongruous affect
inconscient
inconsequential
inconsiderate
    i. behavior
inconsistent
    i. manner
    i. parental discipline
    i. recall
    i. response
inconsolable
inconsonance
inconspicuous
inconstancy
inconstant
incontestable
incontinence
    active i.
    affective i.
    bowel i.
    emotional i.
    fecal i.
    overflow i.
    paradoxical i.
    passive i.
    reflex i.
    urge i.
    urinary i.
incontinent
incontinentia
incontrovertible
    i. evidence
    i. proof
inconvenient
inconvincible
incoordinate
incoordination
incorporation defense mechanism
incorrect
    i. diagnosis
    i. inference
    politically i.
incorrigible
incorruptible
increase
    differential i.
    metabolic i.
    i. speed of thought
increased
    i. arousal
    i. dependence
    i. energy
    i. interpersonal conflict
    i. mortality

    i. responsibility
    i. sense of physical fitness
    i. sexual desire
    i. sexual interest
    i. signal
    i. speech
    i. speed of thought
incredible
incredulous
increment
    sensation i.
increscent
incriminate
incrimination
incrustation
incubation of avoidance
incubus
    family i.
inculcate
inculpable
incult
incurable problem drinker (IPD)
incurious
incursion
IND
    investigational new drug
indagation
indebted
indecency
indecent
    i. assault
    i. exposure
indecision
indecisive
indecisiveness
    parental i.
indecorous
indefatigable
indefensible
indefinable
indefinite
indelible
indelicate
indemnify
indentire
independence
    field i.
    loss of i.
    moral i.
    physical i.
independent
    i. action
    i. event
    i. functioning
    i. group experimental study design
    i. interviewer
    i. living
    i. physical reality

i. play
i. predictor
i. relationship
i. variable
independently
inability to function i.
indescribable
indestructible
indeterminate
i. sex
i. sleep
index, pl. **indices, indexes**
active hostility i. (AHI)
air pollution i.
allergy i. (AI)
alpha i.
ambulation i.
anterior horn i. (AHI)
anxiety i. (AI)
anxiety status i. (ASI)
articulation i.
beta i.
i. of body build (IB)
body mass i. (BMI)
i. case
case i.
cephalic i.
cerebrospinal i.
composite i.
delayed recall i.
delta i.
deterioration i. (DI)
i. of discrimination
empathic i.
i. episode
i. episode of sexual abuse
i. of forecasting efficiency
general memory i.
global distress i.
hyperactivity i.
hyperkinesis i.
hypoglycemic i. (HI)
impairment i.
maturation i.
memory i.
multi-item i.
neurocognitive i.
overall risk i.
perceptual organizational i.
physiological sleepiness i.
pressure-volume i.
putative i.

referential i.
i. of reliability
response i.
schizophrenia i.
i. of sexual functioning
i. of sexuality (IS)
sexuality i.
shift referential i.
spouse abuse i.
status i.
stimulation i. (SI)
switch referential i.
tabular i.
therapeutic i.
theta i.
total response i. (TRI)
i. variable
verbal comprehension i.
indexical
i. communication
i. sign
Indian
I. casino gambling
I. Health Service (IHS)
I. medicine
indicant
indicate
indicatio
i. causalis
i. curativa
i. symptomatica
indication
causal i.
off label i.
symptomatic i.
indicative mood
indicator
risk i.
skill i.'s (SKI)
status i.'s
type i.
indicental
indices (*pl. of* index)
indicis
indict
indictment
bill of i.
indifference
la belle i.
maternal i.
i. to pain syndrome
parental i.

NOTES

indifference *(continued)*
    paternal i.
    i. point
    sexual i.
indifferent
    i. euphoria
    i. to surroundings
indigenous
    i. family culture
    i. worker
indigent
indigestion
    nervous i.
indignant
indignation
    sense of righteous i.
indignity
indirect
    i. aggression
    i. association
    i. evidence
    i. genetic transmission
    i. mechanism
    i. method of therapy
    i. motor system
    i. object
    i. probe
    i. self-destructive behavior (ISDB)
    i. striatopallidal pathway
    i. wit
indiscernible
indisciplinable
indiscreat
indiscreet
indiscretion
    sexual i.
indiscriminate sexual encounter
indisposed
indisposition
indisputable
indistinct
indistinguishable
individual
    affected i.
    age-matched i.
    alcohol-dependent i.
    i. analysis
    androgynous i.
    caffeine-intolerant i.
    caffeine-sensitive i.
    i. care
    cocaine-dependent i.
    i. comprehensive assessment
    i. counseling
    i. counselor
    i. depressive symptom
    i. differences
    drug-dependent i.

    i. guardianship
    healthy i.
    heterozygous i.
    high-anger i.
    homozygous i.
    low-anger i.
    i. marital therapy
    normal i.
    predisposed i.
    i. program
    i. psychology
    i. psychotherapy
    i. psychotherapy session
    i. response
    i. response-specificity
    i. responsibility
    schizophrenia-prone i.
    i. subsystem
    susceptible i.
    i. test
    i. therapist
    i. therapy (IT)
    i. treatment
    i. with schizophrenia
individualist
individualistic
    i. motive
    i. reward structure
individuality
individualized
    i. contract
    i. education program
    i. instruction
individual-specific environment
individuation stage
indoctrination while captive
indole derivative
indolence
indolent
indomitable
indubitable
induced
    i. abortion
    i. association
    i. delusional disorder
    i. factitious symptom
    i. hallucination
    i. insanity
    i. lethargy
    i. paranoid disorder
    i. psychosis
    i. psychotic disorder
    i. sadness
    i. schizophrenia
    i. trance
inducement
    hygienic i.
inductance

induction
- i. coil
- dream i.
- emotion i.
- enzyme i.
- hypnotic i.
- iatrogenic i.
- i. loop
- mood i.
- negative mood i.
- perceptual i.
- positive i.

inductive
- i. problem solving
- i. reactance
- i. reasoning

inductor

induite
- folie i.

indulgence
- plenary i.

indulgent

indurate

industrial
- i. hygiene
- i. organizational psychologist
- i. psychiatry
- i. psychology
- i. psychopath
- i. rehabilitation counselor
- i. sociology
- i. therapy

industrialized culture

industrious

industriousness

industry
- gambling i.
- i. versus inferiority

inebriant

inebriate

inebriation

inebriety

ineducable

ineffable

ineffective
- i. anger
- i. communication pattern
- i. decision making
- i. stimulus
- i. treatment

ineffectively treated

ineffectual parent

inefficient

inelasticity of thought

ineligible

inenarrable

ineptness
- social i.

inept parenting

inequality

inequity

inertia
- motor i.
- principle of i.
- psychic i.
- i. time

inescapable pain

inevitability
- sensation of ejaculatory i.

inevitable

inexorable

inexperience

inexplainable

inexplicable

inexpressible

inexpressive

inexpugnable

inexpungible

infallible

infamous

infamy

infancy
- adjustment reaction of i.
- anal phase of i.
- attachment in i.
- attachment disorder of i.
- bonding in i.
- i. developmental stage
- i. and early childhood disturbance
- reactive attachment disorder of i.
- i. research
- rumination disorder of i.

infant
- i. at risk
- i. behavior record
- i. mortality
- i. narcotic withdrawal
- i. and preschool test
- i. psychiatry
- psychological birth of the human i.
- i. stimulation program

infanticide

NOTES

infantile
    i. affect
    i. amnesia
    i. aphasia
    i. articulation
    i. autism
    i. behavior
    i. convulsion
    i. dementia
    i. diplegia
    i. dynamics
    i. Gaucher disease
    i. hemiplegia
    i. idiocy
    i. masturbation
    i. paresis
    i. perseveration
    i. psychosis
    i. sadism
    i. seduction
    i. seizure
    i. sexuality
    i. spasm
    i. spastic paraplegia
    i. speech
    i. tetany

infantilis
    dementia i.
    mania phantastica i.

infantilism
    Brissaud i.
    cachectic i.
    regressive i.
    sex i.
    sexual i.
    static i.

infantilistic

infantilize

infantum
    autismus i.

infarct
    cerebral i.
    lacunar i.

infarction
    nonhemorrhagic cerebral i.
    silent cerebral i.
    watershed i.

infatuation

infectation

infection
    cerebral i.
    i. organic psychosis
    pediatric autoimmune
     neuropsychiatric disorders
     associated with streptococcal i.
     (PANDAS)

infection-exhaustion psychosis

infection-triggered OCD

infectious
    i. hepatitis
    i. insanity

infectious-exhaustive
    i.-e. psychosis
    i.-e. syndrome

infective psychosis

infecundity

infelicitous

infelicity

infer

inference
    clinical i.
    incorrect i.
    logical i.
    statistical i.
    i. strategy

inferential
    i. behavioral monitoring
    i. behavioral monitoring distortion
    i. perception
    i. perception distortion
    i. statistics
    i. thinking

inferior
    i. frontal sulcus
    i. orbitofrontal complex
    i. parietal region
    i. prefrontal cortex
    i. sibling lifestyle
    i. temporal cortex (ITC)
    i. temporal sulcus

inferiority
    i. complex
    constitutional psychopathic i.
    i. feeling
    industry versus i.
    organ i.
    psychopathic i.

infernal

inferred
    i. conflict
    i. delusional conviction
    i. self-concept scale

infertile

infertility

infestation delusion

infibulation

infidel

infidelity
    delusion of i.
    i. delusion
    marital i.

infighting

infiltration
    i. anesthesia
    paraneural i.
    perineural i.

infinity neurosis
infirmity
inflammatory
inflated
    i. appraisal
    i. identity
    i. knowledge
    i. power
    i. self-esteem
    i. worth
    i. worth theme
inflection
    speech i.
inflexibility
    enduring pattern of i.
inflexible
    i. attitude
    i. pattern
    i. personality trait
inflict
influence
    additive environmental i.
    additive genetic i.
    contextual i.
    delusion of i.
    i. delusion
    developmental i.
    direct genetic i.
    driving under the i. (DUI)
    environmental i.
    evil i.
    genetic i.
    heritable i.
    idea of i.
    media i.
    mystical i.
    outside i.
    passive i.
    putative i.
    i. of religion
    religious i.
influenced psychosis
influential
informal
    i. admission
    i. contract
    i. method
    i. retention
informant report
informatics
    health care i.

information
    afferent thermosensory i.
    assimilating i.
    i. assimilation
    autobiographical i.
    biochemical i.
    i. collection
    contradictory i.
    drug i. (DI)
    educational i.
    emotionally arousing i.
    external i.
    i. feedback
    fund of i.
    inadequate i.
    i. input process
    job i.
    kinetic i.
    learning i.
    i. memory concentration (IMC)
    neurocognitive i.
    nonverbal i.
    i. optimization position
    i. overload
    personal i.
    phonetic i.
    privileged i.
    i. processing
    i. processing bias
    i. processing deficit
    rapidity of analyzing i.
    rapidity of assimilating i.
    release of i.
    i. retrieval
    sensory i.
    structured verbal i.
    i. subtest
    i. technology
    i. theory
    thermosensory i.
    thirdhand i.
    unbiased i.
    i. underload
    unstructured verbal i.
    valid i.
    verbal i.
informational support
informed
    i. consent
    i. decision
informer
infraclass

NOTES

infradian rhythm
infrapsychic
infrequency scale
infrequent interpersonal conflict
infringe
infuriate
infusion
    continuous i.
    lactate i.
ingenious
ingenuity
ingestion
    acute i.
    caffeine i.
    caustic i.
    drug i.
    hormone i.
ingrain
ingrate
ingratiate
ingratiating behavior
ingratiation
ingratitude
ingredient
    psychoactive i.
    toxic i.
in-group
inhabit
inhalant
    absorption of i.
    i. abuse
    i. addiction
    aerosol i.
    amyl nitrate i.
    i. dependence
    household product i.
    i. intoxication
    i. intoxication delirium
    nitrate i.
    nitrite i.
    i. sniffing
    i. use disorder
inhalant-induced
    i.-i. delirium
    i.-i. disorder
    i.-i. persisting dementia
    i.-i. psychotic disorder with
      delusions
    i.-i. psychotic disorder with
      hallucinations
inhalant-related disorder
inhalation
    CO_2 i.
    i. convulsive treatment
    i. of drug
    xenon i.
inhaled anesthesia

inhaler
    amphetamine i.
    nasal i.
    nicotine i.
inharmonious
inherent
inheritability
    disorder i.
inheritable
inheritance
    archaic i.
    autosomal dominant i.
    mendelian rules of i.
    mode of i.
    multifactorial i.
    polygenic i.
inherited
    i. abnormality
    i. releasing mechanism (IRM)
inhibit
inhibited
    i. communication
    emotionally i.
    i. female orgasm
    i. female orgasm psychosexual
      dysfunction
    i. grief
    i. grieving
    i. male orgasm
    i. male orgasm psychosexual
      dysfunction
    i. mania
    i. sexual arousal
    i. sexual desire
    i. sexual desire psychosexual
      dysfunction
    i. sexual excitement (ISE)
    i. sexual excitement psychosexual
      dysfunction
    i. sexual response
inhibited-type
    i.-t. reactive attachment disorder
    i.-t. reactive attachment disorder of
      infancy or early childhood
inhibition
    academic i.
    aim i.
    antidepressant i.
    associative i.
    central i.
    chronic antidepressant i.
    conditioned i.
    i. of delay
    dopaminergic i.
    emotional i.
    i. epilepsy
    external i.
    i. formation

internal i.
i. mechanism
motor i.
occupational i.
pervasive i.
proactive i. (PI)
i. profile
reactive i.
reciprocal i.
retroactive i. (RI)
sexual i.
social i.
specific academic or work i.
work i.
inhibition-action balance
inhibitor
carbonic anhydrase i.
excitatory amino acid receptor i.
5-HT reuptake i.
MAO i.
monoamine oxidase i. (MAOI)
nonselective phosphodiesterase i.
physiological hyaluronidase i. (PHI)
reuptake i.
reversible cholinesterase i.
selective norepinephrine reuptake i.
selective serotonin reuptake i.
(SSRI)
serotonin-norepinephrine reuptake i.
serotonin reuptake i. (SRI)
inhibitory
i. effect
i. epilepsy
i. impulse
i. obsession
i. postsynaptic potential (IPSP)
i. regulatory input
i. tone
in-home crisis stabilization
inhospitable
in-house evaluation
inhuman
inhumane
inhumanity
inimical
iniquity
initial
bystander dominates i.
i. disinhibition
i. interview
i. lag
i. masking

i. onset
i. phase of insomnia
i. spoken language impairment
i. spurt
i. stage
i. stress reaction
i. teaching alphabet
initiate relationship
initiating
i. insomnia
i. structure
initiation
gang i.
i. of goal-directed behavior
treatment i.
i. of treatment
initiative
lack of i.
research i.
i. versus guilt
initiator
initio
ab i.
injectable medication
injected
injection
cerebral i.
death by lethal i.
depot medication i.
heroin i.
hypodermic i.
intracutaneous i.
intradermal i.
intramuscular i.
intrathecal i.
intravascular i.
intravenous i.
lethal i.
long-acting i.
subcutaneous i.
injector
injunction
paradoxical i.
injure
injury
accidental i.
birth i.
brain i.
closed head i. (CHI)
current of i.
deceleration i.
dementia due to traumatic brain i.

NOTES

343

injury *(continued)*
    fetal i.
    head i.
    hepatic i.
    open head i.
    past head i.
    physical i.
    i. potential
    self-induced i.
    self-inflicted bodily i.
    self-inflicted chemical i.
    self-inflicted physical i.
    self-inflicted thermal i.
    toxic i.
    traumatic brain i. (TBI)
    i. of war
    whiplash i.
injustice
    i. collecting
    i. gathering
inkling
inmate
    i. personality
    prison i.
innate
    i. behavior
    i. drive
    i. reflex
    i. releasing mechanism
    i. response system
innateness theory
inner
    i. barrenness
    i. battery cluster
    i. belief
    i. child issue
    i. city community
    i. conflict
    i. control
    i. directed
    i. estrangement
    i. experience
    i. feeling
    i. language
    i. life
    i. need
    i. self-helper
    i. slight
    i. space
    i. tension
    i. thought
    i. vision
    i. world
inner-city adolescent
inner-directed person
innermost
innervate

innervation
    i. apraxia
    motor i.
innocence
    childlike i.
innocent act
innocuous environmental cue
innominata
    substantia i.
innovative
innoxious
innuendo
innutrition
inoculation
    emotional i.
    stress i.
inoperable
inopportune
inordinate
inotropic component
inpatient
    acute psychotic i.
    aggressive psychotic i.
    i. care
    i. drug treatment
    psychiatric i.
    i. psychiatric institution
    i. psychiatric setting
    i. psychiatric treatment facility
    psychotic i.
    schizophrenic i.
    i. service
    i. stay
    i. unit
input
    acoustic i.
    afferent i.
    behavioral i.
    cortical i.
    emotional i.
    hypothalamic regulatory i.
    inhibitory regulatory i.
    phonetic i.
    regulatory i.
input-output mechanism
inquest
inquire
inquiry
    character education i. (CEI)
    general i. (GI)
    systematic i. (SI)
inquisition
inquisitive
inquisitor
inroad
insalubrious
insane
    criminally i.

i. delusion
i. finger
general paralysis of the i. (GPI)
paralysis of the i.
insania lupina
insanity
acute confusional i.
adolescent i.
affective i.
alcoholic i.
alternating i.
American Law Institute Formulation
of I.
basedowian i.
choreic i.
circular i.
climacteric i.
communicated i.
compulsive i.
confusional i.
consecutive i.
constitutional i.
criminal i.
cyclic i.
i. defense
degenerative i.
delusional i.
double i.
doubting i.
dread of i.
drug i.
emotional i.
hysterical i.
idiophrenic i.
impulsive i.
induced i.
infectious i.
intermittent i.
interpretation i.
interpretational i.
manic-depressive i.
moral i.
i. of negation
not guilty by reason of i. (NGI,
NGRI)
partial i.
periodic i.
plea of i.
religious i.
senile i.
simultaneous i.
subacute confusional i.

toxic i.
triple i.
insatiable appetite
insecticide
insecure attachment
insecurity
feeling of i.
social i.
insemination
artificial i.
insenescence
insensate
insensible thirst
insensitive
insensitivity
gross i.
i. to incongruity
insentient
inseparability
linear i.
inseparable
insert
insertion
thought i.
insertion-deletion polymorphism
inside density
insidious onset
insight
absence of i.
analytic i.
emotional i.
exploratory i.
impaired i.
intellectual i.
judgment and i.
lack of i.
i. learning
myopic i.
poor i.
sudden i.
therapeutic i.
i. therapy
true i.
insightful
psychologically i.
insight-oriented
i.-o. approach
i.-o. psychotherapy
i.-o. treatment
insignificant
insinuate
insipid

NOTES

insistent
insolation
insolent
insomnia
    alcohol-related i.
    i. associated with anxiety
    i. associated with depression
    i. associated with psychosis
    bout of i.
    childhood-onset i.
    chronic i.
    drug-dependent i.
    drug-related i.
    i. due to nonorganic origin
    i. feature
    idiopathic i.
    initial phase of i.
    initiating i.
    intermittent i.
    long-term i.
    maintenance i.
    middle i.
    midwinter i.
    nonorganic origin i.
    persistent i.
    i. phase
    primary i.
    psychophysiological i.
    rebound i.
    i. related to another mental
      disorder
    short-term i.
    situational i.
    sleep disorder i.
    sleep-onset i.
    stimulant-induced i.
    i. symptom
    terminal i.
    transient i.
    withdrawal i.
insomniac
insomnia-type
    i.-t. sleep disorder due to general
      medical condition
    i.-t. substance-induced sleep
      disorder
insouciance
inspersion
inspirate
inspiration
inspirational
    i. appeal
    i. group therapy
instability
    affective i.
    autonomic i.
    emotional i.
    iatrogenic i.

    i. in interpersonal relationship
    job i.
    marital i.
    postural i.
    vasomotor i.
    vertebral cervical i.
instantaneous power
instantee
    folie i.
instigate
instigation therapy
instigator
instill
instillation
instillator
instinct
    acquisitive i.
    aggressive i.
    complementary i.
    death i.
    destructive i.
    ego i.
    erotic i.
    herd i.
    hierarchical theory of i.
    life i.
    mother i.
    i. need
    part i.
    partial i.
    i. representative
    i. ridden
    sexual i.
    social i.
instinctive behavior
instinct-training interlocking
instinctual
    i. aim
    i. anxiety
    i. dyscontrol
    i. fusion
    i. renunciation
    i. tension
    i. vicissitude
Institute
    I. of Educational Research (IER)
    I. of Medicine
    I. of Personality and Research
      (IPAR)
institution
    inpatient psychiatric i.
    mental i.
    religious i.
    state psychiatric i.
institutional
    i. care
    i. commitment
    i. environment

i. peonage
i. review board
i. setting
i. transference
institutionalize
instruct
instruction
competency-based i.
individualized i.
unable to follow i.
instructional objective
instrument
action i.
assessment i.
axis I, II i.
personality disorder i.
rating i.
WHO i.
instrumental
i. ADL measurement
i. affair
i. aggression
i. avoidance act
i. conditioning
i. dependence
i. need
i. response
i. support
i. task
instrumentalism
instrumental-relativist orientation
insubordinate
insuccation
insufferable
insufficiency
adrenocortical i.
corticoadrenal i.
i. of eyelid
mental i.
muscular i.
role i.
vertebrobasilar i.
insufficient
i. nocturnal sleep
i. stimulation
insufflation anesthesia
insular
i. cortex tissue
i. sclerosis
insularity
insulate

insulation
i. anesthesia
emotional i.
insulator
insulin
i. abnormality
i. coma treatment
i. shock
i. shock treatment
insult
nutritional i.
putative i.
verbal i.
insuperable
insupportable
insurable
insurance
i. carrier
disability i.
extended-care i.
health i.
liability i.
malpractice i.
short-term i.
unemployment i.
insured patient
insurgent
insurmountable
insusceptibility
intact
cognitively i.
judgment, orientation, memory, abstraction and calculation i. (JOMACI)
naming i.
intake
caffeine i.
caloric i.
cocaine i.
i. diagnostic group
excessive alcohol i.
excessive food i.
family group i.
fluid i.
food i.
intranasal drug i.
i. worker
intake-orientation group
intangible
integer
identity experience i.
integral role

NOTES

integrate
integrated
    i. community
    i. ECT system
    i. function
    i. psychological therapy
integration
    biosocial i.
    cerebral i.
    ego i.
    message i.
    personality i.
    primary i.
    secondary i.
    sensory i.
    social i.
    structural i.
integrative
    i. approach
    i. aspect
    i. learning
integrity
    i. of brain function
    ego i.
    i. group
    physical i.
    i. versus despair
intellect
    ambivalence of the i.
    structure of i. (SI)
intellection
intellectual
    i. ability
    i. activity
    i. agony
    i. aphasia
    i. aura
    i. capacity
    i. deterioration
    i. development
    i. exercise
    i. faculty
    i. function
    i. function deficit
    i. functioning level
    i. hero
    i. imbalance
    i. impairment
    i. impoverishment
    i. inadequacy
    i. insight
    i. maturity
    i. monomania
    i. resource
    i. rigidity
    i. skill
    i. subaverage functioning
    i. superiority

intellectualism
intellectualization communication pattern
intellectualize
intellectualized terms
intellectually sharp
intelligence
    above-average i.
    abstract i.
    aura i.
    biologic i.
    coefficient of i. (CI)
    concrete i.
    crystallized i.
    i. disorder
    fund of i.
    gathering of i.
    low i.
    marginal i.
    measured i.
    mechanical i.
    psychomotor i.
    representative i.
    i. scale
    i. score
    social i.
    superior i.
    i. test
    verbal i.
intelligibility
    i. threshold
intelligible
intemperance
intend
intended victim
intense
    i, affect
    i. affiliation
    i. anger
    i. anxiety
    i. apprehension
    i. autonomic arousal
    i. desire
    i. energy
    i. episodic dysphoria
    i. fear
    i. interpersonal relationship
    i. intoxication
    i. longing
    i. psychological distress
    i. sexual behavior
    i. sexual fantasy
    i. sexual urge
    i. wish
intensification
intensified
    i. action
    i. feeling

intensifier
  image i.
intensity
  affective i.
  delusional i.
  i. of mood
  pain i.
  i. of reaction
  i., severity, and discharge (ISD)
  i. of trauma
  treatment i.
intensive
  i. care community residence
  i. care syndrome
  i. care unit (ICU)
  i. case management
  i. day treatment program
  i. habit pattern
  i. psychotherapy
  i. treatment unit (ITU)
intent
  criminal i.
  homicidal i.
  i. rating
  severity of i.
  suicidal i.
  suicide i.
intention
  i. to deceive
  paradoxical i. (PI)
  i. spasm
  i. tremor
intentional
  i. death
  i. fire setting
  i. forgetting
  i. involuntary behavior
  i. stereotyped movement
  i. tremor
intentionality
intentionally produced symptom
intent-to-treat analysis
interact group
interacting cognitive subsystem
interaction
  accelerated i.
  affective i.
  afferent stimulus i.
  alcohol-methadone i.
  amygdala-prefrontal cortex-locus
    ceruleus i.
  communicative i.

complementarity of i.
complex social i.
demanding i.
differential i.
drug i. (DI)
i. effect
family i.
harmonious i.
higher order i.
impaired social i.
interpersonal i.
mother-infant i.
negative peer i.
neurochemical i.
occupational i.
peer i.
person-environment i.
reciprocal social i.
sexual i.
social i.
state-trait i.
i. term
i. territory
treatment intensity-by-time i.
interactional
  i. childhood psychosis
  i. contract
  i. group psychotherapy
  i. theory of personality
interaction-oriented group therapy
interaction-process analysis
interactive
  i. effect
  i. measurement
  i. phenomenon
  i. voice response system
**Inter-American Council of Psychiatric
  Organizations (IACPO)**
interbody
interbreed
intercalation
intercede
intercept
intercession
interchange
intercommunicate
interconnect
interconnected cerebral region
interconnection
intercostal neuralgia
intercourse
  age at first i.

NOTES

intercourse *(continued)*
    anal i.
    i. anxiety
    buccal i.
    extramarital i.
    i. frequency
    genital i.
    painful i.
    puritanical aversion to i.
    sexual i.
    unprotected i.
intercurrent anxiety
interdependence
interdependent
interdigitate
interdisciplinary
    i. approach
    i. environment
    i. environmental design
    i. team (IDT)
interest
    i. blank
    conflict of i.
    cross-gender i.
    decreased i.
    diminished sexual i.
    i. factor
    i. group
    inability to enjoy i.'s
    increased sexual i.
    interpersonal i.
    i. inventory
    lack of i.
    loss of i.
    low sexual i.
    precocious sexual i.
    range of i.'s
    religious i.
    restricted i.
    i. scale
    i. schedule
    sex i.
    sexual i.
    social i.
    stereotyped i.
interface
    acoustic i.
    emotion-cognition i.
    motor i.
    sensory i.
interfamily
interfere
interference
    anterograde memory i.
    background i.
    habit i.
    i. modification
    i. pattern of discharge

    retrograde memory i.
    sleep i.
    theme i.
    i. theory
    treatment i.
intergang
intergenerational
    i. relation
    i. transmission
    i. trauma
intergradation
intergrade
intergroup-contact hypothesis
intergroup exercise
interhemispheric
    i. asymmetry
    i. transfer
interictal
    i. behavior
    i. behavior syndrome
    i. period
    i. psychosis
interieur
    milieu i.
interindividual variation
interject
interjudge reliability
interleaved learning
interlocking
    instinct-training i.
interlocutor
interlude
intermarriage
intermediary
intermediate
    i. brain syndrome
    i. brain syndrome due to alcohol
    i. care facility
    i. hemispheric dynamics
    i. sex
    i. structure
intermenstrual
intermenstruum
intermetamorphosis
intermingle
intermission
intermittent
    i. aphonia
    i. emotional conflicts or reaction
    i. explosive behavior
    i. explosive disorder
    i. explosive disturbance
    i. insanity
    i. insomnia
    i. melancholia
    i. pain
    i. psychosis
    i. reinforcement

i. reinforcement schedule
i. wakefulness
intermodal fluency
intermorbid
internal
i. architecture neuronal size
i. conflict
i. consistency
i. cue
i. decompression
i. demand
i. drive
fixed i.
i. inhibition
i. locus of control
i. model
i. representation
i. respiration
i. second messenger system
i. selection
i. sensations of anxiety
i. state
i. stimulus
i. stressor
i. validity
i. value
i. versus external (I-E)
i. versus external scale
i. world of belief
i. world of expectation
i. world of fantasy
i. world of perception
internal-external control
internalization
internalize
internalized
i. anger
i. homophobia
i. sense
i. speech
i. validity
internalized-state rating
internalizing
international
I. Association of Group Psychotherapy
i. child pornography ring
I. Classification of Diseases (ICD)
I. Classification of Diseases, Clinical Modification, ed. 9 (ICD-9CM)

I. Classification of Diseases, ed. 9 (ICD-9)
I. Classification of Diseases, ed. 10 (ICD-10)
I. Classification of Sleep Disorders: Diagnostic and Coding Manual (ICSD)
I. Committee on Social Welfare (ICSW)
I. Psychoanalytical Association (IPAA)
I. Society for Adolescent Psychiatry
I. Society for Mental Health Online (ISMHO)
I. Society for the Psychological Treatments of Schizophrenics
I. Society for Sexually Transmitted Disease Research
I. Society for Traumatic Stress Studies
I. Statistical Classification of Diseases and Related Health Problems
I. Transactional Analysis Association (ITAA)
internecine
Internet
I. addiction
I. addiction disorder
I. child pornography
I. counseling
I. gambling
I. psychotherapy
I. relationship
I. sex
I. suicide chat room
interneuronal connection
internship
internuncial
interobserver reliability
interoception
interoceptive
i. awareness
i. cue
i. exposure
i. fear
interoceptor
interpersonal
i. accommodation
i. behavior
i. cognitive problem

NOTES

interpersonal *(continued)*
    i. cognitive problem solving (ICPS)
    i. concern
    i. conflict
    i. consequence
    i. control
    i. crisis
    i. dependence
    i. difficulty
    i. distrust
    i. dysfunction
    i. effectiveness skill
    i. exploitation
    i. friction
    i. functioning
    i. impairment
    i. interaction
    i. interest
    i. issue
    i. loss
    i. morality
    i. network
    i. pathology
    i. personality trait
    i. process
    i. psychiatry
    i. psychotherapy (IPT)
    i. radar
    i. rapport
    i. realm
    i. rejection
    i. relation
    i. relationship
    i. relationship deficit
    i. research orientation
    i. responsibility
    i. role
    i. sensitivity
    i. spacing communication pattern
    i. strain
    i. style
    i. theory
    i. therapy (IPT)
    i. trust
    i. withdrawal
interplay
interpose
interpret
interpretation
    abstract i.
    action i.
    anagogic i.
    analytic i.
    aura i.
    defense i.
    i. delusion
    distortion of i.
    dream i.

    facial expression i.
    id i.
    i. insanity
    mutative i.
    personalized i.
    psychoanalytic i.
    psychodynamic i.
    test i.
    i. test
interpretational insanity
interpreter role
interpretive
    i. leap
    i. therapy
interracial marriage
interrater reliability
interrelate
interrelationship
interrogate
interrupt
interrupted tracing
interrupter device
interruption
    evidence of i.
    repeated REM sleep i.'s
    i. of thought
interruptus
    coitus i.
intersensory
    i. disorder
    i. transfer
intersex
    i. condition
    female i.
    male i.
    true i.
intersexual disorder
intersexuality
intersociety
interstimulation
interstitial
    i. neuritis
    i. neurosyphilis
intersubjective
intertwine
interval
    class i.
    confidence i. (CI)
    fixed i. (FI)
    lucid i.
    i. psychosis
    i. reinforcement
    i. scale
    time i.
    variable i. (VI)
intervene
intervening
    i. act

i. validity
i. variable
intervention
active i.
alternative i.
associated i.
barrier to i.
behavioral i.
biologic i.
clinical facilitated i.
cognitive-behavioral i.
community i.
crisis i.
culture-specific i.
drug i.
early pharmacological i.
early psychotherapeutic i.
educational i.
educative i.
emergency i.
evolutionary i.
experimental i.
exposure-based i.
family i.
free-hand ultrasound-guided i.
GAD-specific i.
generative i.
medical i.
optimal therapeutic i.
outpatient i.
paradoxical i.
pharmacologic i.
pharmacotherapeutic i.
postdisaster psychosocial i.
preventive i.
psychiatric i.
psychological i.
psychopharmaceutical i.
psychopharmacologic i.
psychosocial i.
psychotherapeutic i.
religious i.
remedial i.
i. research
school-based i.
selective preventive i.
spiritual i.
stop, look and listen i.
strategic i.
targeted i.
therapeutic i.
verbal i.

interview
adolescent-parent i.
amobarbital i.
Amytal i.
axis I, II i.
barbiturate-facilitated i.
clinical i.
confidential i.
conjoint i.
counseling i.
diagnostic i.
direct i.
drug-facilitated i.
employment i.
evaluation i.
exit i.
family system i.
general clinical i.
group i.
i. group psychotherapy
hypnotic i.
initial i.
job i.
i. method
nonconfrontational i.
open-ended i.
patient i.
patterned i.
pilot i.
psychiatric i.
psychodynamic i.
psychological i.
research i.
semistructured diagnostic i.
stress i.
structured clinical i.
i. technique
i. therapy
unstructured i.
Zarit burden i.
interviewer
i. effect
independent i.
i. training
interviewing technique
interview-related
i.-r. item
i.-r. parental environment item
inter vivos
intestinal psychogenic disorder
intimacy
delusional belief in i.

NOTES

intimacy *(continued)*
   i. principle
   rejection of i.
   sense of i.
   sexual i.
   i. versus isolation
   i. versus self-absorption
intimate
   i. experience
   i. human relation
   i. relationship
   sexually i.
   i. zone
intimidate
intimidating
   i. behavior
   i. others
intolerable
   i. behavior
   i. inner conflict
   i. side effect
intolerance
   alcohol i.
   caffeine i.
   drug i.
intonation
   voice i.
intoxicant
intoxicate
intoxicated
   driving while i. (DWI)
   legally i.
intoxication
   acute alcohol i.
   alcohol i.
   alcohol pathological i.
   amphetamine i.
   anticonvulsant i.
   anxiolytic i.
   anylcyclohexylamine i.
   barbiturate i.
   bromide i.
   Burundanga i.
   caffeine i.
   cannabis i.
   carbon dioxide i.
   carbon disulfide i.
   carbon monoxide i.
   chronic i.
   cocaine i.
   i. delirium
   drug i.
   drug pathological i.
   i. episode
   ethanol i.
   fluoxetine i.
   gasoline i.

   glutethimide i.
   hallucinogenic i.
   heavy metal i.
   hypnagogic i.
   hypnotic i.
   idiosyncratic alcohol i.
   inhalant i.
   intense i.
   i. level
   marijuana i.
   metal i.
   narcotic chemical i.
   nicotine i.
   opioid i.
   i. organic psychosis
   organic psychosis drug i.
   pathological i.
   pathologic alcohol i.
   pathologic drug i.
   phencyclidine i.
   physiological i.
   psychoactive substance i.
   reversible i.
   sedative i.
   severe i.
   sign of alcohol i.
   substance i.
   substance-induced i.
   sympathomimetic i.
   i. syndrome
   water i.
intoxication-type organic psychosis
intracellular
   i. contribution
   i. energy metabolism
   i. metabolic process
   i. second messenger
   i. second messenger system
intraception
intraceptive signaling
intracisternal
intraclass correlation
intraconscious personality
intracortical inhibition and facilitation
intracranial
   i. brain volume
   i. disorder
   i. hypotension
   i. infection organic psychosis
   i. pressure (ICP)
   i. raw volume
   i. stimulation (ICS)
intracrine
intractable
   i. grand mal epilepsy
   i. pain
intractive pain

intracutaneous
>i. hypodermic
>i. injection

intradermal injection
intrafamilial
>i. conflict
>i. relationship
>i. sexual abuse

intramedullary canal
intramuscular (IM)
>i. absorption
>i. administration
>i. hypodermic
>i. injection

intranasal
>i. drug intake
>i. heroin

intraneuronal argentophilic Pick inclusion body
intransigent
intrapersonal conflict
intrapopulation
intrapsychic
>i. ataxia
>i. change
>i. conflict
>i. distortion
>i. distress
>i. identity
>i. origin
>i. personality trait
>i. style
>i. world

intrapsychical function
intrapsychology
intrasocial idiocy
intrathecal injection
intravaginal
intravascular injection
intravenous (I.V.)
>i. cocaine
>i. drug use
>i. drug user
>i. feeding
>i. hypodermic
>i. injection
>i. medication
>i. treatment

intra vitam
intrepid
intricate

intrigue
>romantic i.
>sexual i.

intriguing
intrinsic
>i. asthma
>i. behavior
>i. capacity
>i. constancy
>i. damage
>i. motivation
>i. reflex
>i. relationship
>i. reward

introduce
introject
introjection
>i. defense mechanism

introjective-projective cycle
intropunitive response
introspect
introspection
>phenomenalistic i.

introspectionism
introspective method
introtensive
>i. personality style
>i. problem-solving style

introversion
>passive i.
>social i. (SI)

introversion-extroversion
>i.-e. continuum
>i.-e. scale (IES)

introversive
>i. problem-solving style
>i. tendency
>i. trait

introvert
introverted
>i. disorder of adolescence
>i. disorder of childhood
>i. personality disorder
>i. schizoid personality
>i. schizothymia
>i. type

intrude
intruding idea
intrusion
>ego-dystonic i.
>i. score

NOTES

intrusive
    i. behavior
    i. distressing idea
    i. flashback
    i. impulse
    i. memory
    i. obsessional image
    i. recollection
    i. sexual disorder
    i. symptom
    i. thought
    i. treatment
    i. urge
intubation
intuition
intuitive
    i. encounter
    i. judgment
    i. stage
    i. type
inure
invade
invalid
invalidating environment
invalidism
invaluable behavior
invariable behavior
invariance
    factorial i.
invariant
    functional i.
invasion
    aggressive i.
    personal space i.
    i. of privacy
invasive
    i. treatment
invective
inveigh
inveigle
inventory
    academic i.
    adaptive behavior i.
    adjustment i.
    i. adjustment
    adolescent i.
    anxiety i.
    anxiety status i. (ASI)
    aptitude i.
    assessment i.
    attitude i.
    behavior i.
    career i.
    child abuse i.
    child depression i.
    child development i.
    clinical i.
    coping i.

    counseling i.
    cultural i.
    depression i.
    development i.
    diagnostic i.
    employment i.
    environmental i.
    interest i.
    leadership i.
    learning i.
    i. of loss
    management i.
    motivational i.
    obsessive-compulsive i. (OCI)
    orientation i. (OI)
    parent i.
    perception i.
    personality i.
    picture i.
    psychological i.
    psychosomatic i. (PSI)
    readiness i.
    relationship i.
    risk i.
    satisfaction i.
    self-report personalities i.
    self-report psychological i.
    sex i. (SI)
    skill i.
    social stress and functionability i. (SSFI)
    social stress and functionality i.
    stress and functionability i.
    task i.
    teacher i.
    teacher attitude i.
    i. test
    Test Anxiety I. (TAI)
    values i.
inversal
    language i.
inverse
    i. agonist
    i. feedback
    i. relationship
inversion
    absolute i.
    affect i.
    amphigenic i.
    occasional i.
    i. relationship
    sex role i.
    sexual i.
    sleep i.
invert
inverted
    i. image

i. Oedipus
i. radial reflex
inverted-U function
invested
emotionally i.
investigate
investigation
drug under i.
eating disorder i. (EDI)
postmortem i.
principal i.
psychoanalytic i.
investigational
i. drug
i. new drug (IND)
investment
emotional i.
foolish business i.
inveterate drinking
invidious
invincible
inviolable
inviolacy motive
invisible college
inviting
invocational psychosis
invoke
involuntary
i. active imagining
i. admission
i. behavior
i. civil commitment
i. discharge
i. ECT
i. emotional expression
i. hospitalization
i. manslaughter
i. medication
i. motion
i. motor movement
i. outpatient commitment
i. pauses in speech
i. premonitory urge
i. response
i. retention
i. state of trance
i. time-out
i. treatment
i. twitch
i. vocalization
i. whispering

involution
senile i.
involutional
i. depression
i. melancholia
i. paranoia
i. paranoid psychosis
i. paranoid reaction
i. paranoid state
i. paraphrenia
i. period
i. psychotic reaction
involve
involved
sexually i.
involvement
brain i.
ego i.
emotional i.
extrapyramidal i. (EPI)
family i.
gambling i.
gang i.
genetic i.
lack of i.
personal i.
subcortical brain i.
invulnerable
inward
i. aggression
i. expression of anger with ruminative feature
i. focus
i. picture
inwardly directed anger
iotacism
IPAA
International Psychoanalytical Association
IPAR
Institute of Personality and Research
IPD
incurable problem drinker
I-persona
ipsation
ipsilateral
i. cerebellar ataxia
i. deficit
i. frontal routing of signals (IFROS)
i. headache

NOTES

ipsilateral *(continued)*
    i. loss
    i. reflex
IPSP
    inhibitory postsynaptic potential
IPT
    interpersonal psychotherapy
    interpersonal therapy
IQ
    full-scale IQ
    IQ test
irascible
irate
ire
irk
irksome
IRM
    inherited releasing mechanism
ironclad
ironic aspect
irony
irradiation-induced mental deterioration
irrational
    i. action
    i. anger
    i. argument
    i. behavior
    i. desire
    i. fear
    i. type
irrationality
irreality level
irreconcilable
irrecoverable
irrecusable
irredeemable
irreformable
irrefragable
irrefutable
irregular
    i. movement
    i. sleep pattern
    i. sleep-wake pattern
irregularity
irrelevant
    i. answer
    i. external stimuli
    i. language
    i. pair
irreminiscence
irreparable
irrepressible
irreproachable
irresistibility
irresistible
    i. apprehension
    i. impulse
    i. sleep

irresoluble
irresolute
irresponsibility
    consistent i.
    criminal i.
irresponsible
    i. acting out
    i. parenting
    i. work behavior
irresponsive
irretrievable
irreverence
irreverent communication
irreversibility
irreversible
    i. coma
    i. shock
irritability
    acoustic i.
    electric i.
    marked i.
irritable
    i. bowel
    i. bowel syndrome (IBS)
    i. heart
    i. mania
    i. mood
    i. morosity
    i. syndrome
    i. testis
irritant
irritate
irritation
    cerebral i.
    functional i.
    i. therapy
irrumation
irruption
I-R specificity
IRT
    item response theory
IS
    index of sexuality
Isakower phenomenon
ischemia organic psychosis
ischemic pathology
ISD
    intensity, severity, and discharge
ISDB
    indirect self-destructive behavior
ISE
    inhibited sexual excitement
island
    i. of control
    social i.
Islander
    Pacific I.
islet of precocity

I

Isle of Wight Study
ISMHO
International Society for Mental Health
Online
isocaloric
isochronal
isochronism
law of i.
isodynamic
isoeffect
isolate
social i.
isolated
i. delusion
emotionally i.
i. explosive disorder
i. explosive disturbance
isolation
i. of affect
alcoholism in i.
i. amentia
i. aphasia
autistic i.
i. effect
feeling of i.
intimacy versus i.
social i.
i. syndrome
isolative behavior
isomeric function
isomorphism
isopathic principle
isophilic
isosexual
isotypical
issue
aging i.
biologic i.
boundary i.
cosmetic i.
end-of-life i.
extratransference i.
health i.
inner child i.
interpersonal i.
late-life substance abuse i.
legal i.
lifestyle i.
nature-nurture i.
personal i.
preexisting underlying emotional i.
process i.

psychological i.
psychosocial i.
public health i.
reality i.
recovery i.
rehabilitative i.
reimbursement i.
skirt the i.
spiritual i.
take i.
termination i.
theologic i.
treatment i.
treatment-relevant i.
underlying emotional i.
weight i.
IT
individual therapy
ITAA
International Transactional Analysis
Association
ITC
inferior temporal cortex
itching
item
i. analysis
axis I, II i.
cultural i.
i. difficulty
i. discrimination parameter
highest-ranking i.
interview-related i.
interview-related parental
environment i.
jargon-free i.
parental environment i.
personality-descriptive i.
i. response theory (IRT)
scale i.
i. scaling
i. selection
SWAP-200 i.
i. validity
i. weighting
item-total correlation
iterate
I-thou relationship
itinerate
ITU
intensive treatment unit
I.V.
intravenous

NOTES

I.V. *(continued)*
  I.V. drug abuse
  I.V. drug use

ivory tower

jabber
jacket
jackknife seizure
jack-of-all-trades
Jackson
    J. epilepsy
    J. law
    J. rule
    J. sign
jacksonian
    j. convulsion
    j. epilepsy
    j. seizure
Jacobson
    J. view of depressive disorder
jactatio
    j. capitis nocturna
    j. capitis nocturnus
jactitation, jactation
    periodic j.
jaded
jag
    arousal j.
    crying j.
    j. drinker
    j. drinking
jail
    j. cell
    j. days per year
    j. diversion program
    j. sentence
jailbait
jail-based treatment program
JaK
    Janus kinase
Jakob-Creutzfeldt disease organic psychosis
Jamaica ginger paralysis
jamais
    j. phenomenon
    j. vu
    j. vu aura
James-Lange-Sutherland theory
James-Lange theory of emotion
Janet
    J. disease
Janus-faced
janusian thinking
Janus kinase (JaK)
jape
jargon
    j. agraphia
    j. aphasia
    organ j.
    organic j.

    j. paraphasia
    semantic j.
jargon-free item
jargonistic
jaundice
    nuclear j.
jaunty
jaw
    j. grinding
    j. jerk
    j. reflex
jaw-winking
jaw-working reflex
JCAHO
    Joint Commission on Accreditation of Healthcare Organizations
JCHIH
    Joint Commission on Mental Illness and Health
jealous
    j. rage
    j. subtype
    j. type
    j. type of paranoid disorder
jealousness
jealous-type
    j.-t. delusion
    j.-t. schizophrenia
jealousy
    alcoholic j.
    j. delusion
    delusional j.
    morbid j.
    projected j.
    retrospective ruminative j.
    sibling j.
jeer
Jekyll and Hyde personality
Jenny Craig diet
jeopardize
jerk
    Achilles j.
    ankle j.
    chin j.
    crossed adductor j.
    crossed knee j.
    j. finger
    jaw j.
    knee j.
    supinator j.
jerking
    head j.
    j. movement
jest
jester

J

jet
- j. lag phenomenon
- j. lag sleep disorder
- j. lag-type dyssomnia
- j. set

jetsetter
Jewish
Jezebel
jilt
jinx
jitter
- frequency j.

jittery
jive
JLO
- judgment of line orientation

JND
- just noticeable difference

job
- j. analysis
- j. change
- j. characteristics model
- j. component method
- j. design
- j. dimensions
- j. enrichment
- j. evaluation
- hatchet j.
- j. information
- j. instability
- j. interview
- j. loss
- j. performance
- j. placement
- j. pressure
- j. reinstatement
- j. retirement
- j. satisfaction
- snow j.
- j. specification
- j. stability
- j. stress
- j. tenure

job-hopping
jobless
job-related stress
job-sample experience
job-specific test
Jocasta complex
jock
jocose
jocosity
jocular
Joffroy
- J. sign

joiner

joint
- J. Commission on Accreditation of Healthcare Organizations (JCAHO)
- J. Commission on Mental Illness and Health (JCHIH)
- j. custody
- hysterical j.
- neuropathic j.
- j. play
- j. psychogenic disorder
- j. sense

joker
joking mania
Jolly reaction
jolt
JOMACI
- judgment, orientation, memory, abstraction and calculation intact

Jonah words
Joubert syndrome
joule
journal
- J. of the Addictions
- J. of Consulting and Clinical Psychology
- J. of Psychiatric Research

journaling exercise
journalize
journey
jovial
joyless
joyous
Juanism
- Don J.

jubilation
Judaism
judge
judgmatic
judgment
- automatic j.
- clinical j.
- comparative j.
- critical j.
- diagnostic j.
- faulty j.
- impaired social j.
- j. and insight
- intuitive j.
- j. of line orientation (JLO)
- moral j.
- negative j.
- j., orientation, memory, abstraction and calculation intact (JOMACI)
- personal j.
- poor j.
- qualitative j.
- quantitative j.

social j.
value j.
judgmental
judicature
judicial process
judicious
juggle
jugglery
Jukes family
jumble
jumbo
mumbo j.
jumper disease of Maine
jumpers
jumping
j. Frenchmen of Maine syndrome
jumpy
junctim
junction
gap j.
juncture
closed j.
open j.
Jung
J. method
J. theory
jungian
j. psychoanalysis
j. psychology
j. theory
junk food
juramentado
jurisdiction
jurisprudence
dental j.
medical j.
jury
special j.
traverse j.
trial j.
jus primae noctis
justice
imminent j.

juvenile j.
J. in Mental Health Organization
social j.
j. system
justifiable
j. homicide
j. reaction
justified
therapeutically j.
justify
just noticeable difference (JND)
juvantibus
diagnosis ex j.
juvenescence
juvenile
j. aggression
antisocial j.
j. chorea
j. competence
j. court
j. court consultant
j. criminal
j. delinquency
j. delinquent
j. detention facility
j. era
j. impostor
j. justice
j. justice system
j. myoclonic epilepsy
j. nonneuropathic Niemann-Pick
disease
j. offender
j. officer
j. paralytic dementia
j. paresis
j. psychosis
j. tabes
j. violence
juvenilis
dementia paralytica j. (DPJ)
juvenilism
juvenility

J

NOTES

KAB
    knowledge, attitude, behavior
kahuna
kainomania
kakergasia
kakosmia
kakotrophy
kaleidoscope hallucination
Kallikak family
Kallmann syndrome
Kalmuk idiocy
Kanner syndrome
kappa
    k. coefficient
    k. opiate receptor
    k. opioid
karma
katagogic tendency
katasexuality
kathisomania
katzenjammer
kava
    k. extract
    kava k.
kavain
kavalactones
kavapyrones
Kayser-Fleischer ring
K complex
Keeler polygraph
keenly aware
keep
    recognize, empathize, think, hear,
       integrate, notice, k. (RETHINK)
keeping faith
keirospasm
Kempf disease
kempt
Kendell classification
kernel complex
Kernig sign
ketanserin
ketazolam
ketoacidosis
    alcoholic k. (AKA)
    diabetic k.
ketoaciduria
ketogenic diet
ketosteroid
key
    k. concept
    k. question
    k. symptom
keying
    empirical-criterion k.

khat
kick
    k. around
    k. the habit
    k. out
kicky
kiddie porn
kidnapper
killer
    k. cult
    detection of adolescent k.'s
    serial k.
    teen k.
    time k.
killing
    mercy k.
killjoy
kilogram
kilounit
kilovolt (kV)
kilovoltage peak (kVp)
kimilue
kin
    next of k.
kinanesthesia, cinanesthesia
kinase
    Janus k. (JaK)
    protein k. C (PKC)
kindergarten
kindhearted
kindling
    k. effect
    K. pattern
kindly
kindness
kinephantom
kinesalgia
kinesiatrics
kinesic
    k. behavior
    k. gesture
kinesigenic ataxia
kinesiology
kinesioneurosis
kinesiotherapy
kinesipathy
kinesis
kinesomania
kinesthesia hallucination
kinesthesiometer
kinesthesis
kinesthetic
    k. analysis
    k. apraxia
    k. aura

K

kinesthetic *(continued)*
   k. cue
   k. feedback
   k. hallucination
   k. method
   k. perception
   k. sensation
   k. sense
   k. technique
kinetic
   k. analysis
   k. ataxia
   chemical k.'s
   k. drive
   k. energy
   first-order elimination k.'s
   k. information
   k. model
   k. modeling
   k. tremor
   zero-order elimination k.'s
kinetism
kinetogenic
kinetosis
kinetotherapy
king-slave fantasy
kinky-hair disease
kinship
   k. network
   k. system
KIPS
   knowledge information processing system
kiss
   French k.
   k. off
   tongue k.
kissing
   k. behavior
kit
kitchen
   soup k.
kitten
   sex k.
klazomania
Klein
   K. death wish
   K. suffocation alarm theory
   K. view of depressive disorder
Kleine-Levin syndrome
kleptolagnia
kleptomania
kleptomaniac
kleptomanic behavior
Klinefelter syndrome
Klippel-Feil syndrome
klismaphilia
klutz
Klüver-Bucy syndrome

knavery
knee
   k. jerk
   k. phenomenon
kneippism
knight move
knismogenic
knismolagnia
knock
   k. off
   k. over
   k. up
knocked up
knocking
   head k.
knockout drops
knot
   love k.
   lover's k.
knotty
know-how
know-it-all
knowledge
   acquired k.
   k., attitude, behavior (KAB)
   carnal k.
   competence k.
   factual k.
   figurative k.
   fund of k.
   general k.
   impersonal factual k.
   inflated k.
   k. information processing system
    (KIPS)
   lack of k.
   sources of sexual k.
   k. structure
   k. test
   k. theme
knowledgeable
known
   k. group validity
   k. organic factor
know-nothing
knuckle under
Kohlberg developmental model
kohlbergian theory of moral reasoning
   development
Kohnstamm phenomenon
kola
   gotu k.
kolyphrenia
kolytic
Korean War
koro
   k. psychosis
   k. syndrome

Korsakoff
    K. alcoholic psychosis
    K. amnesia
    K. disease
    K. nonalcoholic psychosis
    K. syndrome
Kosovo
Krabbe syndrome
Kraepelin
    K. classification of mental illness
    K. diagnostic system
    K. disease
    K. schema
kraepelinian
    k. subtype
    k. view of psychosis
Kraepelin-Morel disease

krauomania
Kretschmer type
kudos
kudzu
kuru
Kussmaul
    K. aphasia
    K. coma
Kussmaul-Landry paralysis
kV
    kilovolt
kVp
    kilovoltage peak
kymatism
kymogram
kymograph
Kyofusho

NOTES

K

LA
> low anxiety

lab

label
> designer l.

labeling theory

la belle indifference

labialism

labial paralysis

labile
> l. emotionality
> l. mood
> l. personality disorder
> l. range of affect

lability
> affective l.
> emotional l.
> mood l.

labiochoreic stuttering

labiorum
> morsicatio l.

labor
> l. camp
> l. force

laboratory
> l. abnormality
> basement l.
> clinical l.
> l. data
> l. diagnosis
> diagnostic l.
> NIDA-certified forensic
>   toxicology l.
> personal growth l.
> l. study
> l. training

laboratory-method model

laborer
> manual l.

labyrinthine
> l. disorder
> l. righting reflex
> l. sense
> l. speech

lachrymose

lacing agent

lack
> l. of academic success
> l. of confidence
> l. of control
> l. of courage
> l. of efficacy
> l. of empathy
> l. of energy
> l. of expressiveness
> l. of family support
> l. of fear
> l. of feeling
> l. of future planning
> l. of guilt
> l. of initiative
> l. of insight
> l. of interest
> l. of interoceptive awareness
> l. of involvement
> l. of knowledge
> l. of mature defense
> l. of memory
> l. of motivation
> l. of patience
> l. of penetrance
> l. of performing to potential
> l. of reactivity
> l. of remorse
> l. of restraint
> l. of self-confidence
> l. of self-discipline
> l. of speech
> l. of structure
> l. of vocational success
> l. of will

laconic speech

laconism

lactate
> brain l.
> global brain l.
> gray matter l.
> l. infusion
> regional brain l.
> white matter l.

lactation

lactational diestrus

lactic acidosis

lactoovovegetarian diet

lactotrophic

lactovegetarian diet

lacuna, pl. **lacunae, lacunas**
> l. cerebri
> superego l.

lacunaire

lacunar
> l. amnesia
> l. dementia
> l. infarct
> l. state
> l. stroke
> l. syndrome

lacunaris
> status l.

lacunas (*pl. of* lacuna)

L

LAD
>language acquisition device

ladder
>abstraction l.
>counseling l.

lady
>bag l.

Laennec cirrhosis

Lafayette pegboard

lag
>circadian rhythm sleep disorder, jet l.
>cultural l.
>initial l.
>maturational l.
>terminal l.

laid back

laissez-faire
>l.-f. group
>l.-f. leader
>l.-f. leadership pattern

laliatry

lallation

lalling

lalochezia

lalognosis

lalomania

laloneurosis

lalopathology

lalopathy

laloplegia

lalorrhea

L-alpha-acetylmethadol

lambaste

lambdacism

lambitus

lame

lament

lancinating

Landau-Kleffner syndrome

landmark
>developmental l.

Landry-Guillain-Barré syndrome

Landry paralysis

lane of childhood

language
>l. ability
>l. acquisition device (LAD)
>l. area
>artificial l.
>l. arts
>l. assessment
>l. associated cortex
>automatic l.
>l. barrier
>behavior l.
>l. behavior
>body l.

l. boundary
l. center
l. change
l. and communication
l. and communication distortion
communication in sign l.
l. comprehension
l. comprehension and production
l. content
daughter l.
l. deficit
delayed l.
l. development
l. developmental delay disorder
deviant l.
l. difficulty
l. disability
l. disorder in dementia
l. disturbance
dominant l.
l. dysfunction
egocentric l.
emotive l.
English as a second l. (ESL)
l. enrichment therapy (LET)
erotic l.
executive l.
l. experience approach (LEA)
explicit l.
expressive l.
l. faculty
foreign l.
l. function
l. function deterioration
l. game
gestural-postural l.
gesture l.
global loss of l.
home l.
hypochondriac l.
imaginary l.
l. imbalance
impaired l.
l. impairment
implicit l.
incidental learning l.
inner l.
l. inversal
irrelevant l.
l. lateralization
legal l.
l. localization
loss of l.
l. manipulation
metaphoric l.
mixed receptive-expressive l.
negotiating l.
nonspecific l.

nonverbal l.
obscene l.
oral l.
organic l.
l. origin
l. pathology
primitive psychosomatic l.
l. problem
l. processing
l. purist
l. quotient
l. recovery
religious l.
l. scale
scatological l.
school l.
l. screening
sign l.
l. skills learning retardation
l. and speech disorder
spoken l.
subcultural l.
syntaxic l.
target l.
l. theory
l. therapist
l. therapy
twin l.
unknown l.
vulgar l.
written l.
l. zone
language-dominant hemisphere
language-processing
languid
languish
languor
languorous
lanugo
Laotian
laparotomaphilia
lapse
l. of awareness
memory l.
lapsus
l. calami
l. lingua
l. memoriae
larcenist
larcenous
larceny

large
at l.
larval
l. epilepsy
l. sadism
l. schizophrenia
larvated epilepsy
laryngeal
l. anesthesia
l. chorea
l. crisis
l. epilepsy
l. paresthesia
l. psychophysiologic reaction
l. syncope
l. vertigo
laryngoparalysis
LAS
laxative abuse syndrome
lascivia
lasciviency forced laughter
lascivious
l. hysterical laughter
lashing
lassitude
last
l. chance
l. ditch
l. straw
l. word
latah, lata, lattah
l. syndrome
latchkey
l. child
l. children
late
l. adolescence
l. adulthood
l. life
l. life developmental stage
l. luteal phase dysphoric disorder
l. paraphrenia
l. reaction
l. speech development
l. traumatic epilepsy
late-age trauma
late-emerging medical side effect
late-life
l.-l. migraine
l.-l. migraine headache
l.-l. schizophrenia
l.-l. substance abuse issue

L

NOTES

latency
> Erickson theory of l.
> mean sleep l.
> l. period (LP)
> l. period psychosexual development
> l. phase
> prolonged sleep l.
> rapid eye movement l.
> reduced rapid eye movement l.
> reflex l.
> l. of reply
> l. of response
> short REM l.
> short sleep l.
> sleep l.
> l. stage

latency-age children
late-night activity
latent
> l. class analysis
> l. content
> l. epilepsy
> l. goal
> l. homosexuality
> l. learning
> l. meaning
> l. period
> l. psychosis
> l. reflex
> l. response
> l. schizophrenia
> l. schizophrenic reaction
> l. tetany
> l. thought
> l. zone

late-onset
> l.-o. category
> l.-o. schizophrenia

later
> l. life
> l. reading disorder

lateral
> l. dominance
> l. geniculate nucleus (LGN)
> l. hemispheric dynamics
> l. hypothalamus
> l. orbitofrontal cortex
> l. rostral supplementary motor area
> l. ventricle
> l. vertigo

laterality
> crossed l.
> dominant l.
> mixed l.

lateralization
> cortical l.
> failure of l.

> hemispheric l.
> language l.

lateralized
> l. dysfunction
> l. rapid activating task

lateralizing abnormality
lateriflora
> Scutellaria l.

later-life depression
lateropulsion
lathyrism
Latino
lattah (*var. of* latah)
laudable
laudanum
laugh
> nervous l.
> l. off
> sardonic l.

laughing
> l. disease
> excessive l.
> inappropriate l.
> l. sickness

laughter
> compulsive l.
> drawn l.
> forced l.
> hysterical l.
> inappropriate l.
> lasciviency forced l.
> lascivious hysterical l.
> obsessive l.
> pathological l.
> l. reflex
> spasmodic l.
> spontaneous l.
> uncontrollable l.
> uncontrolled l.

Laurence-Biedl syndrome
Laurence-Moon-Bardet-Biedl syndrome
Laurence-Moon-Biedl syndrome
Laurence-Moon syndrome
lavage
> gastric l.

law
> l. abiding
> l. of advantage
> American Academy of Psychiatry and L. (AAPL)
> assimilation l.
> l. of assimilation
> l.'s of association
> autonomic affective l.
> l. of avalanche
> l. of average localization
> biogenetic mental l.
> l. breaker

Briggs l.
Charpentier l.
l. of closure
l. of coercion to the biosocial
  mean
l. of cohesion
l. of combination
command l.
l.'s of commitment
l. of common fate
l. of constancy
l. of contiguity
l. of contrast
court of l.
cyberstalking l.'s
Dale l.
l. of denervation
l. of diminishing return
l. of effect
effect l.
empirical l.
l. enforcement agency
l. of equality
equality l.
equipotentiality l.
eugenic sterilization l.
l. of exercise
exercise l.
Fourier l.
l. of frequency
Gerhardt-Semon l.
Grasset l.
Haeckel biogenic l.
health l.
l. of isochronism
Jackson l.
Leyden l.
martial l.
Megan L.
mendelian l.
mental health l.
Merkel l.
Müller l.
Murphy's l.
natural l.
Ohm l.
parallel l.
Pitres l.
poor l.
l. of precision
l. of referred pain
l. of relativity

restraint l.
l. of retrogenesis
Ribot l.
Ritter l.
Rosenbach l.
seclusion l.
Semon l.
Semon-Rosenbach l.
stalking l.'s
talion l.
three strikes l.
van der Kolk l.
Weber-Fechner l.
Yerkes-Dodson l.
law-abiding citizen
law-and-order orientation
lawbreaker
lawful behavior
lawless
lawsuit
lawyer
  trial l.
laxative
  l. abuse
  l. abuse syndrome (LAS)
  l. addiction
  l. of choice (LOC)
  l. dependence
  l. habit
  l. misuse
lay analysis
layer
  arachnoid l.
  tangential l.
laying on of hands
layman
lazy listening
LCU
  life change unit
LD
  learning disability
  lethal dose
LEA
  language experience approach
LEAD
  longitudinal expert evaluation using all
    available data
lead
  l. encephalopathy
  l. neuropathy
  l. palsy
  l. paralysis

L

NOTES

lead *(continued)*
    l. pipe contraction
    l. poisoning
leaden paralysis
leader
    authoritarian l.
    laissez-faire l.
    l. match
    l. role
    team l. (TL)
leaderless
    l. group
    l. group discussion (LGD)
    l. group therapy
leadership
    l. behavior
    dual l.
    functional l.
    l. inventory
    l. potential
    l. power struggle
    l. role
    spiritual l.
    l. theory
    l. training
lead-pipe rigidity
leaf, pl. **leaves**
    cassina l.
    coca l.
leak
leakage
    verbal l.
leap
    interpretive l.
Lear complex
learned
    l. autonomic control
    l. drive
    l. dysfunctional behavior
    l. helplessness
    material previously l.
learner
    auditory l.
    slow l.
learning
    l. ability
    l. aptitude
    associate l.
    association l.
    associative l.
    attachment l.
    avoidance and escape l.
    cognitive theory of l.
    concept l.
    conceptual l.
    l. cue
    l. curve
    l. defect

l. development
l. development disorder
l. difficulty
l. disabilities specialist
l. disability (LD)
l. disabled
discrimination l.
dissociated l.
dissociation of l.
l. by doing
emotional l.
escape l.
l. experience
l. impaired
incentive l.
incidental l.
l. information
insight l.
integrative l.
interleaved l.
l. inventory
latent l.
l. material
l. mechanism
l. model
l. new information disturbance
observational l.
operant l.
paired-associates l.
l. paradigm
passive l.
passive-avoidance l.
perceptual l.
perceptual-motor l.
probability l.
l. problem
problem-based l.
l. psychogenic disorder
l. retardation
reversal l.
rote verbal l.
self-directed l. (SDL)
sensate focus l.
serial list l.
l. session
l. set
sexual l.
state-dependent l.
l. strategy
stress effect on l.
subliminal l.
systems-based l.
l. task
l. theory
Thorndike trial-and-error l.
transfer of l.
trial-and-error l.
verbal l.

vicarious l.
visceral l.

least
l. noticeable
l. preferred
l. resistance
l. restrictive alternative

least-effort principle
leather restraint
leave
l. of absence (LOA)
absent without l. (AWOL)
authorized l.
extended sick l.
French l.
medical l.
l. on pass (LOP)
sick l.
unauthorized l. (UL)

leaves (*pl. of* leaf)
leaving
Leboyer method
lecanomancy
lecher
lecherous
lechery
lecheur
left
l. handedness
l. hemisphere
l. hemisphere dominance
l. parietal association metabolism

left-hand dominant
left-handedness
left-out sibling profile
leftward asymmetry
leg
cold mottled insensate l.
l. phenomenon

legal
l. age
l. approach
l. blindness
l. capacity
l. commitment
l. consequence
l. contract
l. counselor
l. criteria for competency
l. decision
l. deliberation
l. determination

l. dilemma
l. divorce
l. drug
l. gambling
l. guardian
l. guardianship
l. issue
l. language
l. medicine
l. opioid
l. psychiatry
l. psychology
l. repercussion of violent behavior
l. responsibility
l. sanction
l. separation
l. standard

legality
legalized gambling
legally
l. committed
l. drunk
l. intoxicated
l. separated (LS)

legasthenia
legendary
Legendre sign
legislation
mental health l.

legitimacy
legitimate illness
legitimize
legomenon
hapax l.

Leichtenstern
L. phenomenon
L. sign

leipolalia
leisure
l. activity
l. awareness
l. skill
l. time

length
cycle l.
l. of episode
l. of illness
l. of patient stay (LOPS)
l. of stay (LOS)

lengthened off-time (LOT)
lengthening reaction
leniency

L

NOTES

lenient
lenticular aphasia
leprosy
> dry l.

leprotica
> alopecia l.

leptin
> l. level
> l. secretion
> l. signal

leptophonia, leptophonic
Leri sign
lesbian
lesbianism
Lesch-Nyhan syndrome
lesion
> self-inflicted l.

less
> l. pervasive disorder
> l. than maximal effect

lesson
> object l.
> trial l.

LET
> language enrichment therapy

let down
lethal
> l. blow
> l. catatonia
> l. dose (LD)
> l. factor
> l. injection
> l. overdose

lethality
> l. rating
> l. scale
> severity of l.
> suicide l.

lethargic
> l. hypnosis
> l. patient
> l. stupor

lethargy
> hysteric l.
> induced l.
> lucid l.

letheomania
lethica aphasia
lethologica
letter
> l. blindness
> Dear John l.
> scarlet l.

letter-number sequencing
letter-word identification
lettuce opium
levallorphan
levamphetamine

level
> l. of abstraction
> action l.
> activity l.
> aggression l.
> agitation l.
> alcohol l.
> l. of alertness
> alertness l.
> alpha l.
> androgen l.
> annoyance l. (AL)
> anxiety l.
> l. of anxiety
> l. of arousal
> aspiration l.
> automatic phrase l.
> basal resistance l.
> below detectable l.'s (BDL)
> beta l.
> blood l.
> blood alcohol l. (BAL)
> l. of care
> circulating leptin l.
> cognitive awareness l.
> l. of cognitive function
> cognitive impairment l.
> cohesiveness l.
> l. of cohesiveness
> comfort l.
> confidence l.
> l. of confidence
> conflict l.
> l. of conflict
> l. of consciousness (LOC)
> criterion l.
> current defense l.
> defense l.
> defensive dysregulation l.
> l. of defensive dysregulation
> delta l.
> denervation l.
> l. of depression
> desire l.
> l. of development
> developmental l.
> difficulty l.
> disability l.
> disavowal l.
> discomfort l.
> l. of disruption
> dissociation l.
> l. of disturbance
> drug l.
> l. of education
> educational l.
> effective l.
> effort l.

endurance l.
energy l.
engagement l.
l. of expressed emotion
l. of frustration
functioning l.
l. of functioning
gray matter lactate l.
hedonic l.
high adaptive l.
high energy l.
hormonal l.
image-distorting l.
l. of impairment
l. of incompetence (LOI)
intellectual functioning l.
l. of intellectual functioning
intoxication l.
irreality l.
leptin l.
l. of liability
lithium l.
low educational l.
low energy l.
maintenance l.
major image-distorting l.
medication l.
mental inhibition l.
minor image-distorting l.
occupational l.
operant l.
l. of pain tolerance
pathological l.
peak and trough l.
perceptual l.
performance l.
phallic l.
plasma leptin l.
posttest l.
pragmatic l.
predominant current defense l.
preoedipal l.
primitive emotional l.
l. of psychological pain
psychopathology l.
l. of psychosocial stress
reduced aggression l.
reference zero l.
l. of resistance
resistance l.
l. of response
l. of risk

risk l.
sensory l.
serotonin l.
serum l.
significance l.
social functioning l.
society l.
symptom l.
therapeutic blood l.
theta l.
tolerance l. (TL)
toxic l.
uncertainty l.
vegetative l.
white matter lactate l.
leveling
leveling-sharpening
level-of-care criterion
levirate
levitation
levity
lewd
lewdness
Lewy body variant of Alzheimer disease
lexica concept
lexical
l. agraphia
l. ambiguity
l. processing
lex talionis
Leyden
L. ataxia
L. law
L. neuritis
LGD
leaderless group discussion
LGN
lateral geniculate nucleus
LH
luteinizing hormone
LHRH
luteinizing hormone-releasing hormone
liability
l. abuse
l. insurance
level of l.
vicarious l.
weight l.
liaison
l. nursing

L

NOTES

liaison *(continued)*
  l. psychiatrist
  l. psychiatry
liar
  pathologic l.
  pathological l.
lib
  ad l.
libation
liberal
  l. cutoff score
liberate
liberation
  gay l.
  women's l.
liberomotor
libidinal
  l. development
  l. drive
  l. energy
  l. impulse
  l. object constancy
  l. phase
  l. transference
  l. type
libidinal-cathexis
libidinization
libidinous
libido
  l. analog
  l. binding
  bisexual l.
  change in l.
  dammed-up l.
  decreased l.
  diminished l.
  displaceability of l.
  ego l.
  l. fixation
  loss of l.
  mobility of l.
  normal l. (NL)
  object l.
  organ l.
  l. organization
  plasticity of l.
  primal l.
  l. quantum
  sexual l.
  l. stasis
  l. theory
  traumatization of the l.
  viscosity of l.
  l. wish
libido-binding
license
  revocation of driver's l.

licensed
  l. handgun
  l. marriage and family therapist
  l. practical nurse (LPN)
  l. professional counselor (LPC)
  l. psychologist
  l. vocational nurse (LVN)
licentious
Lichtheim
  L. aphasia
  L. sign
licit psychoactive drug
Liddle psychomotor poverty
lid tic
lie
  bald-faced l.
  l. detection
  l. detector
  life l.
  l. scale
  white l.
liebestod
Liepmann apraxia
lieutenant
life, pl. **lives**
  adaptation to l.
  adjustment reaction of later l.
  adult l.
  appetite for l.
  change of l.
  l. change unit (LCU)
  l. circumstance problem
  l. course
  l. crisis
  l. cycle
  l. cycle change
  l. cycle theory
  dating l.
  deprived early l.
  l. difficulty
  direct threat to l.
  l. energy
  l. event
  everyday activities in l.
  l. expectancy
  expectation of l.
  l. experience
  fact of l.
  fantasy l.
  l. fear
  feeling of being an outside
    observer of one's l.
  l. goal
  healthy religious l.
  l. history
  l. impairment
  impoverished fantasy l.
  impulse l.

inner l.
l. instinct
late l.
later l.
l. lie
love l.
mental l.
noon of l.
l. organization
overstimulated home l.
phase of l.
philosophy of l.
l. plan
prayerful l.
prime of l.
purpose in l. (PIL)
quality of l.
reading activities in l.
real l.
religious l.
right to l.
l. script
l. sentence
sexual l.
sheltered l.
l. space
l. span
l. span development
l. stage
l. stress
l. stressor
l. support system
sustenance of l.
l. table
threat to l.
tumultuous l.
vegetative l.
vicissitudes of l.
l. years

life-changing
l.-c. improvement
l.-c. spiritual experience
life-cycle
l.-c. adjustment
l.-c. transition
life-event stress theory
lifeless
lifeline
lifelong
l. affiliation
l. obesity
l. personality disorder
l. sexual dysfunction

lifelong-type
l.-t. dyspareunia
l.-t. vaginismus
life span development
lifestyle
alternative l.
antisocial l.
balanced l.
l. change
disciplined l.
l. factor
healthy l.
high-risk l.
inferior sibling l.
l. issue
l. modification
nomadic l.
nontraditional l.
l. prejudice
sedentary l.
traditional l.
unstable l.
life-threatening
l.-t. behavior (LTB)
l.-t. condition
l.-t. danger
l.-t. disease
l.-t. event
l.-t. illness
lifetime
l. aggression
l. anxiety disorder
l. behavior
l. depression criterion
l. episode
l. expectancy
l. hierarchy
l. history
l. impulsivity
l. personality
l. prevalence
l. risk
life years
lifter
weight l.
ligand selection
light
l. diet
l. drinking
flashes of l.
glare of l.
halo of l.

L

NOTES

light *(continued)*
    l. sleep (LS)
    l. therapy
    l. touch sensation
    l. trance
    l. treatment
    l. treatment for winter depression
lighter fluid dependence
lightheaded
lightning
    white l.
light-therapy-induced mood disorder
likability
    peer l.
likable
likelihood of recurrence
lilliputian hallucination
limb
    abnormal position of distal l.'s
    phantom l.
    l. psychogenic disorder
limbi (*pl. of* limbus)
limbic
    l. activation
    l. brain region
    l. circuit
    l. circuitry
    l. dopamine receptor
    l. dysregulation
    l. effect
    l. epilepsy
    l. forebrain
    l. leucotomy for treatment of OCD
    l. lobe
    l. structure
    l. system
    l. system disorder
    l. zone
limbic-related region
limb-kinetic apraxia
limbus, pl. **limbi**
limen, pl. **limina**
    difference l.
liminal stimulus
liminometer
limit
    class l.
    medication l.
    method of l.'s
    normal l.'s
    off l.'s
    physiological l.
    l. setting
    within normal l.'s (WNL)
limitation
    conceptual l.
    empirical l.
    functional l.

    l. of movement (LOM)
    sex l.
    technical l.
    technological l.
limited
    l. activity
    l. diet
    l. effect
    l. responsibility
    l. support
    l. symptom attack
    l. war
limited-capacity retrieval
limiting decision
limit-setting
    l.-s. for adolescent
    l.-s. parenting
limit-testing behavior
limophoitas
limophthisis
limosis
limotherapy
limp-wristed
line
    developmental l.'s
    l. of duty
    l.'s of expression
    l. of fixation
    hard l.
    hot l.
    24-hour telephone help l.
    pure l.
    soft l.
    Ullmann l.
lineage
linear
    l. inseparability
    l. perspective
    l. thought process
    l. type
linen
    dirty l.
liner
lingering fear
lingua, pl. **linguae**
    lapsus l.
lingual
    l. delirium
linguistic
    l. approach
    l. content of task
    l. determinism
    l. disorganization
    l. disturbance
    l. savant
    l. style
linguistic-kinesic method

linguistics
    anthropological l.
lining
    silver l.
link
    causal l.
    pathophysiological l.
linkage
    associative l.
    l. object
    sex l.
    l. worker
lip
    l. biting
    l. erotism
    l. pursing
    l. reading
    l. reflex
    l. smacking
lipolytic enzyme
lipophilic
liquefied heroin
liquidation
    l. of attachment
liquid diet
liquor
    malt l.
lisping
Lissauer dementia paralytica
Lissauer-type paresis
lissencephalia, lissencephaly
list
    hit l.
    l.'s preoccupation
listen
    unable to l.
listening
    l. attitude
    diotic l.
    l. language quotient
    lazy l.
    passive l.
    l. with the third ear
listless
litem
    guardian ad l.
literacy
    l. deficiency
    inadequate l.
    patient l.
    l. test
    visual l.

literal
    l. agraphia
    l. alexia
    l. meaning
    l. paraphasia
    l. paraphrasia
literalis
    paralalia l.
literate
    computer l.
literature
    clinical l.
    l. review
lithiasis
    hysterical l.
lithium
    l. action on first messenger
    l. action on membranes
    l. action on second messenger
    l. dose
    l. level
litigious
    l. delusional state
    l. environment
    l. paranoia
litigiousness
littering
live
    l. birth
    l. on welfare
    l. in the project
    l. together
    will to l.
live-in relationship
liver
    l. cirrhosis
    cirrhotic l.
    l. damage
    l. disease
    l. disease organic psychosis
    l. flap
    l. function test
    palpable l.
    l. span
livid
living
    activities of daily l. (ADL)
    ambivalence about l.
    l. arrangement
    capacity for independent l.
    daily l.
    existential l.

L

NOTES

living *(continued)*
    free l.
    group l.
    independent l.
    reasons for l.
    simulated activities of daily l.
      (SADL, SADLs)
    l. situation
    standard of l.
    l. standard
    task of independent l.
    vicarious l.
    l. wage
    l. will
lizard
    lounge l.
LOA
    leave of absence
    loosening of association
load
    case l.
    sensory l.
loading
    factor l.
    genetic l.
    salient l.
    l. strategy
loafer
loaner
    psychological l.
loath, loth
loathe
loathsome
lobar
    l. dysfunction
    l. sclerosis
lobata
    Pueraria l.
lobe
    contralateral parietal l.
    l. dysfunction
    frontal l.
    limbic l.
    occipital l.
    parietal l.
    posterodorsal temporal l.
    prefrontal l.
    temporal l.
lobectomy
    temporal l.
    transorbital l.
lobotomy
    prefrontal l.
    l. syndrome
    transorbital l.
LOC
    laxative of choice
    level of consciousness

    locus of control
    loss of consciousness
local
    l. convulsion
    l. epilepsy
    l. excitatory state
    l. potential
    l. response
    l. sign
    l. syncope
    l. tic
    l. vasoconstrictive action
localis paracusis
locality attachment
locality-specific pattern of aberrant
    behavior
localization
    l. agnosia
    auditory l.
    l. of behavior
    cerebral l.
    l. of function
    language l.
    law of average l.
    point l.
    l. of symptoms
localized
    l. amnesia
    l. epilepsy
    l. function
    l. weakness
location
    action l.
    brain l.
    cerebral l.
    l. constancy
LOC-C
    locus of control-chance
LOC-E
    locus of control-external
LOC-I
    locus of control-internal
loci (*pl. of* locus)
lock
    l. finger
    scalp l.
locked
    l. cell
    l. door seclusion
    l. hospital unit
    l. room
    l. in state
    l. ward
locking
    phase l.
loco
    l. plant
    l. weed

locoism
locomotion
locomotive
locomotor
    l. activity
    l. arrest
    l. ataxia
locomotor-genital stage
locomotorium
LOC-PO
    locus of control-powerful others
locum tenens
locura
locus, pl. **loci**
    l. ceruleus neuron
    chromosomal loci
    l. of control (LOC)
    l. of control-chance (LOC-C)
    l. of control-external (LOC-E)
    l. of control-internal (LOC-I)
    l. of control-powerful others (LOC-PO)
    l. heterogenicity
    l. minoris resistentiae
    quantitative trait loci (QTL)
locution
LOD
    logarithm of odds
log
    activity l.
    drug information l. (DIL)
logagnosia
logagraphia
logamnesia
logaphasia
logarithm
    l. of odds (LOD)
    l. of the odds score
logasthenia
logic
    formal l.
    perverted l.
    trance l.
logical
    l. analysis of automatic thought
    l. inference
    l. memory
    l. memory subtest score
    l. memory test
    l. operation
    l. positivism

logistic
    l. curve
    l. regression
    l. regression equation
logoclonia
logographic
logokophosis
logomachy
logomania
logoneurosis
logopathy
logoplegia
logorrhea
logospasm
logotherapy
LOI
    level of incompetence
loiterer
Lolita
lolling
LOM
    limitation of movement
    loss of movement
loneliness
lonely
loner
    psychological l.
lonesome
long
    l. latency response
long-acting
    l.-a. barbiturate
    l.-a. injectable medication
    l.-a. injection
long-circuiting
longevity
    marital l.
long-half-life anxiolytic substance
long-hot-summer effect
longing
    intense l.
    passive-receptive l.
longitudinal
    l. assessment
    l. course
    l. course specifier
    l. data
    l. experimental study design
    l. expert evaluation using all available data (LEAD)
    l. mental status examination
    l. method

L

NOTES

longitudinal *(continued)*
    l. observation
    l. scan
    l. study
long-lasting drug effect
long-lived
long-stay ward
long-suffering
long-term
    l.-t. abstinence
    l.-t. associative memory
    l.-t. care
    l.-t. care facility
    l.-t. commitment
    l.-t. consequence
    l.-t. course
    l.-t. course of abuse
    l.-t. data
    l.-t. declarative memory
    l.-t. dependence
    l.-t. detoxification program
    l.-t. disability (LTD)
    l.-t. disease
    l.-t. effect
    l.-t. effectiveness
    l.-t. effects of trauma
    l.-t. heavy use
    l.-t. hospitalization
    l.-t. insomnia
    l.-t. maintenance treatment
    l.-t. management
    l.-t. memory (LTM)
    l.-t. mental health program
    l.-t. mortality rate
    l.-t. naturalistic study
    l.-t. outcome
    l.-t. pattern
    l.-t. potentiation (LTP)
    l.-t. psychotherapy
    l.-t. risk
    l.-t. storage
    l.-t. storage of memory
    l.-t. therapy
look
    glazed l.
    grunge l.
    paranoid l.
look-alike
    amphetamine l.-a.
looking-glass self
loop
    basal ganglia-cingulate gyrus-frontal
      lobe l.
    calibrated l.
    induction l.
loopy
loosening of association (LOA)

LOP
    leave on pass
LOPS
    length of patient stay
loquacious
loquaciousness
loquacity
LOS
    length of stay
loser
losing
    l. control
    l. time
loss
    age-related hearing l.
    amygdala volumetric l.
    l. of appetite
    appetite l.
    approval l.
    autonomy l.
    l. of autonomy
    l. of belief
    l. of biographical memory
    l. of boundaries of ego
    l. of breadwinner
    central sensory l.
    cognitive l.
    l. of consciousness (LOC)
    l. of control
    cortical sensory l.
    dense sensory l.
    l. discrimination
    dissociated sensory l.
    l. of effect
    ego boundary l.
    l. of ego boundary
    l. of energy
    l. experience
    l. of freedom
    functional l.
    hemisensory l.
    hippocampal volumetric l.
    hysterical visual l.
    l. of identity
    imagined l.
    l. of independence
    l. of interest
    l. of interest in usual activity
    interpersonal l.
    inventory of l.
    ipsilateral l.
    job l.
    l. of language
    l. of libido
    l. of loved one
    major l.
    mechanical functional l.
    memory l.

monocular visual l.
l. of motivation
motor l.
l. of movement (LOM)
multiple l.
nerve l.
neuronal l.
nonnormative hair l.
object l.
l. of orientation
parental l.
past l.
perceived l.
peripheral sensory l.
personal l.
l. of pleasure
postsurgical l.
pregnancy l.
psychogenic hearing l.
real l.
recent l.
l. of relationship
l. of response
self-induced hair l.
semen l.
l. of semen
l. of sensation
l. of sensitivity
significant l.
sleep l.
soul l.
spousal l.
stocking-and-glove sensory l.
symbolic l.
threat of job l.
unresolved l.
volumetric l.
weight l.
l. of zest

lost
l. privileges (LP)
l. in thought
LOT
lengthened off-time
loth (*var. of* loath)
lottery gamble
loud
l. music
l. speech
Louis-Bar syndrome

lounge
l. lizard
l. music
loup-garou
louse, pl. **lice**
love
l. affair
anal-sadistic l.
capacity to l.
l. child
deficiency l.
Dorian l.
free l.
genital l.
homogenic l.
l. knot
l. life
make l.
monkey l.
mother l.
l. need
object l.
l. object
passive object l.
phallic l.
platonic l.
Polybus l.
pregenital l.
productive l.
puppy l.
l. relationship
sexual l.
smother l.
tough l.
transference l.
loveboat
loved
love-hate relationship
loveless
lovely
lovemaking
lover
distraught former l.
former l.
heterosexual l.
homosexual l.
illicit l.
l.'s knot
lovesick
loving
delusional l.

NOTES

L

loving *(continued)*
> l. feeling
> l. parenting

low
> l. alpha coefficient
> l. anger threshold
> l. anxiety (LA)
> l. back pain psychogenic disorder
> l. delirium
> l. dose
> l. education
> l. educational level
> l. energy
> l. energy level
> l. fever
> l. frustration tolerance
> l. impulsiveness
> l. income
> l. intelligence
> l. profile
> l. self-confidence
> l. sensory environment
> l. sexual desire
> l. sexual interest
> l. social desirability
> l. stimulation environment
> l. threshold of competency
> l. tolerance potential

low-activity situation
low-anger individual
low-calorie diet
low-complexity movement
low-dose
> l.-d. strategy
> l.-d. treatment

lowered mood
lower-intensity treatment
low-fat diet
low-grade
> l.-g. heroin
> l.-g. thought disorder

low-key response
lowlife
low-magnitude stressor subscale
low-minded
low-salt diet
low-spirited
low-stimulation
> l.-s. situation

low-tyramine diet
loxia
loyalty
> doubts of l.
> family l.
> unjustified doubt of l.

Loyola sensate focus

LP
> latency period
> lost privileges

LPC
> licensed professional counselor

LPN
> licensed practical nurse

LS
> legally separated
> light sleep

LSD
> lysergic acid diethylamide
> LSD dependence
> LSD reaction

LSD-type perception
LTB
> life-threatening behavior

LTD
> long-term disability

LTM
> long-term memory

LTP
> long-term potentiation

lubricant
lubricious
lucid
> l. interval
> l. lethargy

lucidification
lucidity
lucrative
lucubrate
ludic
ludicrous
lues
luetic curve
lugubrious
lumbarization
luminescence of object
lump in the throat
lunacy
lunatic
lupina
> insania l.

lupus
lure
Luria technique
lurid
lush
lust
> l. dynamism
> l. murder

lusterless eyes
lustful
luteal
> l. phase
> l. phase assessment

luteinizing
    l. hormone (LH)
    l. hormone-releasing hormone
      (LHRH)
luxuriate
LVN
    licensed vocational nurse
lycanthropy
lycomania
lycorexia
lygophilia
lying
    pathologic l.

    pathological l.
    repetitive l.
lymphatic psychogenic disorder
lynch
lysatotherapy
lysergic
    l. acid
    l. acid amide
lyssa
lytic cocktail
lz R
    total response

NOTES

L

MA
mental age
migraine with aura
M/A
mood and/or affect
MAB
management of assaultive behavior
MAC
maximum allowable cost
macabre
mace
macerate
maceration
Macewen
M. sign
M. symptom
machiavellian
machiavellianism
machinate
machination
machinator
machinery
machismo
macho manner
macrobiotic diet
macrocranium
macroencephalon
macroesthesia
macrographia, macrography
macrogyria
macromania
macromaniacal delirium
macropsia
macrostereognosis
maculocerebral
Madame Butterfly syndrome
madcap
MADD
mixed anxiety depression disorder
madden
maddening
made-to-order dream
Mad Hatter syndrome
madhouse
madly
madman
madness
impulsive m.
raving m.
Madonna complex
Madonna-prostitute complex
madwoman
MAF
minimal audible field

magazines
sexually charged m.
magdalen
Magenblase syndrome
magic
black m.
m. bone
communication m.
compulsive m.
cursing m.
m. fantasy
m. helper
m. mushroom
m. omnipotence
m. phase
m. thinking
magical thinking
magicked
magisterial
magna
cisterna m.
Magnan
M. sign
M. trombone movement
magnanimity
magnet
m. reaction
m. reflex
magnetic
m. apraxia
m. attraction
m. crisis
m. personality
m. resonance imaging (MRI)
m. resonance spectroscopy (MRS)
m. seizure therapy
magnetism
animal m.
magnetometer
magnific
magnification
magnificent
magnify
magniloquence
magniloquent
magnitude
perturbation m.
magusucht
mahatma
ma huang
maid
old m.
maidenhair tree
maiden name

M

maidica
    psychoneurosis m.
maim
main
    m. d'accoucheur
    m. effect
    m. en crochet
    M. syndrome
    m. treatment modality
mainline
mainlining heroin
mainstream
maintenance
    m. dose
    drug m.
    m. drug
    m. drug therapy
    m. function
    m. insomnia
    m. level
    m. medication
    methadone m.
    m. minimum
    minimum m.
    perceptual m.
    physiological m.
    short-term m.
    m. striving
    m. treatment
    m. treatment program
    weight loss m.
maitre de plaiser
majeure
    force m.
major
    m. affective disorder
    m. attachment figure
    m. break
    chorea m.
    m. depression
    m. depressive affective psychosis
    m. depressive disorder (MDD)
    m. depressive disorder, recurrent
    m. depressive episode (MDE)
    m. epilepsy
    m. form
    m. hypnosis
    m. hysteria
    m. image-distorting level
    m. impairment
    m. impairment of functioning
    m. life activity
    m. life change
    m. life stress
    m. loss
    m. mental illness
    m. mood disorder
    m. motor aphasia

    m. motor seizure
    m. psychiatric disorder
    m. psychiatric syndrome
    m. risk period
    m. role obligation
    m. role therapy (MRT)
    m. solution
    m. tranquilizer
majority society
make
    m. believe
    m. love
    m. out
    m. sense
make-believe
    m.-b. play
    m.-b. world
makeup
    genetic m.
    mental m.
making
    career decision m.
    m. change test
    clinical decision m.
    competent decision m.
    decision m.
    end-of-life decision m.
    ineffective decision m.
    real-life decision m.
    tyrannical decision m.
mal
    cerebral m.
    comitial m.
    m. de la rosa
    m. de ojo
    m. de pelea
    m. d'orient
    grand m.
    haut m.
    petit m.
    m. puesto
    m. rosso
malabsorption
maladaptation
maladaption
maladaptive
    m. behavioral change
    m. coping
    m. coping mechanism
    m. defense mechanism
    m. feeling
    m. impulse
    m. pattern of behavior
    m. pattern of emotion
    m. pattern of motivation
    m. pattern of substance abuse
    m. pattern of thought
    m. personality

m. personality pattern
m. personality trait
m. problem-solving strategy
m. psychological change
m. reaction
m. reaction to a stressor
m. response
m. thought
m. way
maladaptively aggressive youth
maladie
m. des tics
m. du doute
m. du pays
maladjusted
sexually m.
maladjustment
sexual m.
social m.
vocational m.
malady
malaise
postexertional m.
malapert
malaria
cerebral m.
therapeutic m.
malcontent
maldevelopment
male
m. alcoholism subtype
m. biological status
m. bond
m. castration
m. circumcision
m. climacteric
m. climacteric syndrome
m. dyspareunia
m. dyspareunia male erectile disorder
m. erectile disorder
m. erectile dysfunction
feminine traits in m.
m. gender identity
m. genitalia
m. homosexuality
m. hypoactive sexual desire disorder
m. intersex
m. menopause
m. orgasm
m. patient

m. pattern alopecia
m. rape
m. therapist
m. victim
maledict
malediction
malefaction
malefactor
maleficence
maleficent
maleness
male-to-female transgender identity
malevolence
malevolent
m. behavior
m. concern
m. distrust
m. thought system
malfeasance
malfunction
malice
malicious mischief
malign
malignancy
malignant
m. brain neoplasm
m. neurosis
m. psychosis
m. stupor
m. trend
malinger
malingerer
malingering disorder
malleability
malleable
malleation
mallet
anger m.
mall treatment concept
malnourished
m. child
malnutrition
malodorous
malpractice
m. insurance
malternative drink
malt liquor
maltreat
maltreatment
child m.
childhood m.
elder m.

M

NOTES

malvaria
malversation
mammalian
    m. teratology
    m. tissue
mammalingus
mammonist
man
    drug-using m.
    eight stages of m.
    enlisted m.
    Erikson eight stages of m.
    fellow m.
    hatchet m.
    hit m.
    medicine m.
    non-drug-using m.
    personal m.
    wise old m.
manacle
manage
    difficult to m.
manageable
managed
    m. care
    M. Care Appropriateness Protocol
    m. care environment
management
    adolescent anger m.
    anger m.
    anxiety m.
    m. of assaultive behavior (MAB)
    behavioral m.
    clinical m.
    conflict m.
    conservative m.
    contingency m.
    crisis m.
    diet m.
    drug m.
    exhaustion m.
    grief m.
    home-based family m.
    impression m.
    intensive case m.
    m. inventory
    long-term m.
    medication m.
    multidimensional pain m.
    obesity m.
    pain m.
    participative m.
    pharmacological m.
    psychological m.
    psychosocial m.
    reflux m.
    seizure m.
    stress m.

    style of leadership and m.
    weight m.
manager style appraisal
MANCOVA
    multivariate analysis of covariance
mandate
mandated self-help group
mandatory treatment
maneuver
    body concept-exploration m.
    body contact-exploration m.
    passive-aggressive m.
    tactical m.
manganese mask
manhandle
manhood
manhunt
mania
    absorbed m.
    acute alcoholic m.
    acute hallucinatory m.
    adolescent m.
    akinetic m.
    alcoholic m.
    anxious m.
    atypical m.
    biting m.
    chronic alcoholic m.
    classic euphoric m.
    collecting m.
    compulsive m.
    copying m.
    dancing m.
    delirious m.
    depressed m.
    doubting m.
    drug-induced m.
    dysphoric m.
    ephemeral m.
    epileptic m.
    grumbling m.
    hallucinatory m.
    hostile m.
    hysterical m.
    inhibited m.
    irritable m.
    joking m.
    peracute m.
    periodic m.
    periodical m.
    m. phantastica infantilis
    political m.
    pornographic m.
    postpartum m.
    m. a potu
    prepubertal m.
    process m.
    puerperal m.

pure m.
m. rating score
reactive m.
reasoning m.
recommencement m.
recurrent episode chronic m.
religious m.
seaman m.
m. secandi
secondary m.
senile m.
single-episode chronic m.
squander m.
stage 3 m.
stupor m.
transitory m.
unipolar m.
unproductive m.
m. with rapid cycling
maniacal grief reaction
maniac catatonia
manic
m. agitation
m. bipolar disorder
m. child
m. delirium
m. depression
m. depressive
m. depressive illness
m. excitement
m. feature
m. hebephrenia
m. mood
m. mood episode
m. mood theme
m. patient
m. phase
m. psychosis
m. reaction
schizoaffective disorder, m.
m. speech
m. stare
m. state
m. stupor
m. symptom
m. syndrome
m. temperament
manic-depressive
m.-d. affective psychosis
m.-d. disorder
m.-d. insanity
perplexed-type m.-d.

m.-d. reaction
m.-d. syndrome
manicky
manic-like episode
manie
m. de perfection
m. de rumination
m. a potu
manifest
m. anxiety
m. content
m. destiny
m. dream
m. goal
m. symptom
m. tetany
manifestation
behavioral m.
characteristic m.
clinical m.
m. of depression
m. of emotion
impostor psychotic m.
neuroimaging m.
neuropsychiatric m.
neuropsychologic m.
neurotic m.
objective m.
physiological m.
psychiatric m.
psychogenic physiological m.
psychophysiologic m.
psychotic m.
m. of resistance
subjective m.
underlying psychological m.
m. of violence
manifested disability
manifestly observable symptom
manifold
manipulability
manipulable
manipulanda
manipulate
manipulation
m. communication pattern
emotional m.
environmental m.
language m.
m. stage
manipulative
m. behavior

NOTES

manipulative *(continued)*
    m. device
    m. drive
    m. pseudohallucination
    m. technique
manipulatory task
mankind
manliness
manly
man-machine system
manner
    allosteric m.
    authoritative m.
    bedside m.
    bellicose m.
    condescending m.
    detached m.
    m.'s deterioration
    devious m.
    elementary m.
    evil m.
    guarded m.
    halting m.
    inconsistent m.
    macho m.
    part-object m.
    patronizing m.
    secretive m.
    superior m.
    sustained m.
    unkempt m.
    unusual m.
mannered
mannerism
    childlike m.
    feminine m.
    speech m.
mannish
Mannkopf sign
mannosidosis
MANOVA
    multivariate analysis of variance
manslaughter
    involuntary m.
manslayer
mansuetude
mantic
mantle sclerosis
mantra
manual
    m. communication
    Crime Classification M. (CCM)
    m. dexterity
    diagnostic m.
    Diagnostic and Statistical M. (DSM)
    Diagnostic and Statistical M., Revision IV (DSM-IV)

    m. dominance
    International Classification of Sleep Disorders: Diagnostic and Coding M. (ICSD)
    m. laborer
    m. sadism
    self-help m.
    m. stimulation
manual-based interpersonal psychotherapy
manumit
many-sided
many things
many-valued
MAO
    monoamine oxidase
    MAO inhibitor
MAOI
    monoamine oxidase inhibitor
MAOI-serotonergic agent
MAOI-tricyclic agent
map
    brain electrical activity m.
    cognitive m.
    genetic m.
    personal skills m.
    z score m.
maple sugar syrup urine disease
maplike skull
mapping
    behavior m.
    brain m.
    brain electrical activity m. (BEAM)
    cognitive m.
    cortical m.
    m. of cortical function
    speech and motor m.
    topographic m.
mar
marasmic
    m. female
    m. state
marasmus
    nutritional m.
Marateaux-Lamy disease
marathon
    drug-fueled music m.
    Gestalt therapy m.
    m. group psychotherapy
    m. session
marauder
Marcé study
Marchant zone
Marchiafava-Bignami disease
mareos
margin
marginal
    m. consciousness

m. function
m. intelligence
m. thinking
m. transvestite
marginalis
alopecia m.
marginalization
marginalized
marginally therapeutic dose
Marie ataxia
Marie-Robinson syndrome
marijuana, marihuana
m. delirium
m. delusional disorder
m. dependence
m. flashback
m. intoxication
m. preparation
m. psychosis
m. use history
mariposia
marital
m. adjustment
m. conflict
m. counseling
m. counselor
m. couples group therapy
m. discord
m. disharmony
m. disruption
m. dissatisfaction
m. history (MH)
m. infidelity
m. instability
m. longevity
m. problem
m. satisfaction
m. schism
m. skew
m. stability
m. status
m. stress
m. turbulence
mark
easy m.
marked
m. anger
m. anxiety
m. decline in academic functioning
m. depression
m. impairment
m. irritability

m. motor agitation
m. tension
marker
biochemical phenotypic m.
circadian m.
fixed m.
gene m.
genetic m.
I m.
phenotypic m.
psychological m.
m. X syndrome
marketing personality
marking
analog m.
marksman
markswoman
marriage
arranged m.
civil m.
cluster m.
common law m.
companionate m.
compassionate m.
consanguineous m.
m. contract
m. of convenience
m. counseling
m. counselor
m. encounter
experimental m.
m. fear
former m.
group m.
heterosexual m.
homosexual m.
interracial m.
mixed m.
nonconsanguineous m.
open m.
open-end m. (OEM)
pluralism m.
m. response
m. ritual
same-sex m.
sandbox m.
shotgun m.
stability of m.
starter m.
symbiotic m.
synergic m.
m. therapy

M

NOTES

marriage *(continued)*
    traditional m.
    trial m.
    troubled m.
    unconsummated m.
    m. vows
marshal
    sky m.
martial
    m. arts
    m. law
Martin-Bell syndrome
martyr complex
martyrdom
marvel
marvelous
marxism
marxist
masculation
masculine
    m. attitude
    m. attitude in female neurotic
    m. identity
    m. protest
    m. social role
masculinity
masculinity-femininity scale
masculinization
masculinize
masher
mask
    death m.
    m. facies
    Hutchinson m.
    manganese m.
masked
    m. affection
    m. anxiety
    m. depression
    m. deprivation
    m. epilepsy
    m. facies
    m. homosexuality
    m. obsession
masking
    background m.
    backward visual m.
    behavioral m.
    central m.
    effective m.
    m. efficiency
    m. fear
    forward m.
    frequency m.
    initial m.
    maximum m.
    m. pain
    perceptual m.

    peripheral m.
    m. stimulus
    upward m.
masklike facies
Maslow hierarchy
masochism
    erotogenic m.
    feminine m.
    ideal m.
    mental m.
    moral m.
    sexual m.
    social m.
    verbal m.
masochist
masochistic
    m. behavior
    m. character
    m. character defense
    m. component
    m. personality
    m. personality disorder
    m. ritual
    m. sabotage
    m. sexual activity
    m. sexual fantasy
    m. sexual urge
    m. wish
    m. wish dream
masquerade
mass
    m. action theory
    m. behavior
    black m.
    m. hysteria
    m. media
    m. method
    m. movement
    m. murderer
    m. polarization
    m. psychogenic illness
    m. psychology
    m. reflex
    m. sociogenic illness
    m. terrorism
    m. therapy
    thermogenic tissue m.
massacre
massacrer
massage
    electrovibratory m.
    nerve-point m.
    m. parlor
    tremolo m.
    vibratory m.
massager
masse
    en m.

massed negative practice
masseur
masseuse
massive
    m. seizure
massotherapy
master
    m. of avoidance
    M. of Science in Nursing (MSN)
    M. of Social Work (MSW)
masterful
mastermind
Masters and Johnson studies
mastery
    motive m.
    m. motive
masticatoria
    monoplegia m.
masticatory
    m. diplegia
    m. spasm
Mast syndrome
masturbate
masturbation
    anal m.
    m. behavior
    compulsive m.
    m. equivalent
    false m.
    m. fantasy
    infantile m.
    mutual m.
    psychic m.
    public m.
    symbolic m.
masturbator
masturbatory
    m. activity
    m. pain
match
    leader m.
    perceptual-motor m.
matchbox sign
matched group
matching
    m. hypothesis
    impedance m.
    prototype m.
    m. test
matchmaker
mate
    soul m.

materfamilias
material
    clinical m.
    emotional m.
    evidence of intrusion of
      idiosyncratic m.
    evidence of intrusion of private m.
    m. gain
    genetic m.
    m. gratification
    idiosyncratic m.
    learning m.
    neutral m.
    m. previously learned
    m. symbolism
    unstructured verbal m.
    verbal m.
materialism
materialistic
materialization
materialize
maternal
    m. abuse
    m. attachment
    m. attitude
    m. behavior
    m. competency
    m. depression
    m. deprivation
    m. deprivation syndrome
    m. desertion
    m. drive
    m. dysfunction
    m. fitness
    m. indifference
    m. neglect
    m. overprotection
    m. problem-solving strategy
    m. rejection
    m. relationship
    m. role
    m. stress
maternity blues
math achievement
mathematical
    m. ability
    m. skill
    m. symbol
mathematics
    assessment in m.
    m. disorder

NOTES

M

mating
    assortative m.
    assortive m.
    m. behavior
    nonrandom m.
    random m.
matriarch
matriarchy
Matricaria recutita
matrices (*pl. of* matrix)
matricide
matrilinear family
matrilocal family
matrimony
matrix, pl. **matrices**
    dural graft m.
    factor m.
    therapeutic m.
matroclinous
matrocliny
matron
matronism
matter
    central gray m. (CGM)
    cortical gray m.
    deep white m.
    dorsal gray m.
    gray m.
    midbrain m.
    parahippocampal white m.
    periventricular white m.
    sclerosis of white m.
    subcortical gray m.
    subcortical white m.
    theologic m.'s
    white m.
matter-of-fact
mattoid
maturate
maturation
    cognitive m.
    emotional m.
    hormonal m.
    m. hypothesis
    m. index
    mitosis, migration and m.
    neurological m.
    principle of anticipatory m.
    psychological m.
    m. rate
    retarded m.
maturational
    m. change
    m. crisis
    m. lag
mature
    m. defense
    m. minor rule

maturity
    biologic m.
    cognitive m.
    emotional m.
    m. fear
    genital m.
    intellectual m.
    mental m.
    motor m.
    psychological m.
    m. rating
    m. scale
matutinal epilepsy
maudlin drunkenness
maul
mau-mau
maunder
mauve factor
maven, mavin
maverick
mawkish
maximal
    m. contrast
    m. effect
    m. electroshock
    m. electroshock seizure (MES)
    m. stimulus
maximation
    ego m.
maximum
    m. acoustic output
    m. allowable cost (MAC)
    m. intensity projection
    m. intent rating
    m. lethality rating
    m. masking
    m. permissible dose
    m. recommended human dose
    (MRHD)
    m. security
    m. security unit
    m. tolerable amount
maximum-security
    m.-s. forensic psychiatric hospital
    m.-s. prison
Mayberg limbic-cortical dysregulation model
mayhem
maze
    m. behavior
MBD
    minimal brain dysfunction
McCullough-Pitts
    M.-P. model
    M.-P. neuron
MCE
    medical care evaluation

MCR
mother-child relationship
MD
mentally deficient
MDD
major depressive disorder
MDE
major depressive episode
MDSO
mentally disordered sex offender
meager
meals
after m.
before m. (a.c.)
skip m.
mealy-mouthed
mean
m.'s for anxiety
arithmetic m.
assumed m.
m. deviation
geometric m.
harmonic m.
m. intracranial raw volume
law of coercion to the
biosocial m.
m. normalized whole brain volume
m. sleep latency
standard error of the m. (SEM)
statistical m.
m. total weighted sum score
meaning
affect-related m.
double m.
effort after m.
emotion-related m.
figurative m.
hidden m.
higher-order emotion-related m.
idiosyncratic m.
latent m.
literal m.
psychological m.
m. reframing
sliding of m.'s
subtle m.
symbolic m.
transferred m.
unknown m.
will to m.

meaningful
m. conversation
m. interpersonal relationship
meaningless
meanness
measurable impairment
measure
abuse m.
achievement identification m.
adjustment m.
affect intensity m.
assessment m.
attentional m.
avoidance m.
m. of balance
baseline m.
behavioral assessment m.
biologic m.
central tendency m.
m. of central tendency
cognitive m.
m. of competence
course of illness m.
diagnostic m.
dissociation m.
functional independence m. (FIM)
functioning m.
global m.
happiness m.
neglect m.
neurocognitive m.
neuropsychologic m.
number-recency m.
objective m.
outcome m.
overall cognitive m.
phenomenological m.
physiological m.
pretreatment m.
psychometric m.
psychopathology m.
psychotherapeutic m.
quality of life m.
quantitative m.
reactive m.
Schutz m.
self-report m.
sensitive m.
social adjustment m.
sociodemographic m.
state-dependent m.
symptom m.

M

NOTES

measure *(continued)*
    therapeutic m.
    unambiguous m.
    unobtrusive m.
measured
    m. capacity
    m. dose
    m. intelligence
measurement
    absolute m.
    educational m.
    EEG activity m.
    m. effect
    m. error
    error of m.
    instrumental ADL m.
    interactive m.
    mental m.
    psychomotor m.
MEC
    minimum effective concentration
mecca
mechanical
    m. anosmia
    m. aptitude
    m. functional loss
    m. intelligence
    m. vertigo
mechanics
    body m.
mechanism
    abnormalities in sleep-wake
      timing m.
    acting out defense m.
    adaptation m.
    adaptive defense m.
    adjustment m.
    alerting m.
    analogous brain m.
    arousal boost m.
    arousal reduction m.
    association m.
    attentional m.
    balance m.
    basic brain m.
    brain metabolic m.
    causal m.
    causative m.
    cognitive m.
    compensation defense m.
    compensatory m.
    conversion defense m.
    coping m.
    cross-correlation m.
    defense m.
    denial defense m.
    direct causative
      pathophysiological m.

displacement defense m.
dissociation defense m.
ego defense m.
emotional m.
endogenous brain m.
escape m.
feedback m.
focusing m.
fundamental neural m.
gating m.
heat-loss m.
idealization defense m.
identification defense m.
immature coping m.
incorporation defense m.
indirect m.
inherited releasing m. (IRM)
inhibition m.
innate releasing m.
input-output m.
introjection defense m.
learning m.
maladaptive coping m.
maladaptive defense m.
mediating m.
mental m.
metabolic m.
neural m.
neurobiological m.
neutralizing m.
outgoing m.
pain m.
pathophysiological m.
perceptual cognitive m.
pharmacological m.
physiological m.
plastic compensatory m.
Pollyanna m.
postsynaptic compensatory m.
primary m.
projection defense m.
rationalization defense m.
reaction formation defense m.
regression defense m.
relapse m.
sex arousal m. (SAM)
shared m.
sleep m.
sour-grapes m.
specific pathophysiological m.
sublimation defense m.
substitution defense m.
sweet-lemon m.
symbolization defense m.
thermogenic m.
triggering m.
undoing defense m.
mechanistic approach

mechanize
mechanology
mechanoreflex
mechanotherapy
mechanothermy
meconism
meddle
meddlesome behavior
meddling
Medea complex
medial
    m. frontal cortex
    m. frontal lobe syndrome
    m. hemispheric dynamics
    m. hypothalamus
    m. orbitofrontal cortex
    m. prefrontal cortex
    m. rostral supplementary motor area
    m. temporal memory system
    m. temporal structure
median
    center m.
    m. sagittal plane
    statistical m.
mediate
mediated
    m. function
    m. response
mediating
    m. effect
    m. mechanism
mediation
    cognitive m.
    conflict m.
    peer m.
    verbal m.
mediator
Medica
    Excerpta M.
medicable
Medicaid
medical
    m. advice
    m. anthropology
    m. assistance
    m. attention
    m. audit
    m. care
    m. care evaluation (MCE)
    m. center
    m. comorbidity

    m. complications of obesity
    m. condition
    m. consultant
    m. contraindication
    m. deliberation
    m. discharge
    m. doctor
    m. effect
    m. emergency
    m. ethics
    m. etiology
    m. examiner
    m. futility
    m. history
    m. identification tag
    m. illness
    m. impairment
    m. intervention
    m. jurisprudence
    m. leave
    m. model
    m. morbidity
    m. necessity
    M. Outcomes Study (MOS)
    m. power of attorney
    m. problem
    m. profession
    m. professional
    m. provider
    m. psychoanalyst
    m. psychology
    m. psychotherapy
    m. reason
    m. record
    m. review
    m. sociology
    m. staff
    m. staff member
    m. stress
    m. symptom
    m. syndrome
    m. treatment
    m. use
    m. utilization
    m. value system
medicament
medicamentosa
    alopecia m.
Medicare
medicaster
medicate
medicated patient

M

NOTES

medication
m. abuse
active antidepressant m.
adjunctive m.
agonist m.
antagonist m.
antianxiety m.
anticholinergic m.
antidepressant m.
antiepileptic m.
antihypertensive m.
antipsychotic m.
antiretroviral m.
antiseizure m.
anxiolytic m.
attitude to m. (AM)
beta adrenergic m.
blackmarket m.
m. change
cheeking m.
conservative m.
continuous antipsychotic m.
continuous maintenance m.
m. contraindication
conventional antipsychotic m.
cyclic m.
depot m.
m. dosage
experimental m.
forced m.
m. guide
injectable m.
intravenous m.
involuntary m.
m. level
m. limit
long-acting injectable m.
maintenance m.
m. management
neuroleptic m.
m. noncompliance
over-the-counter m.
patient guide to m.
peripherally acting
  anticholinergic m.
poor response to m.
prescription m.
psychiatric m.
psychoactive m.
psychotropic m.
m. reduction
m. refractoriness
m. refusal
m. regimen
m. side effect
m. stigma
sublingual m.
substitutive m.

supportive m.
m. tapering
m. taper schedule
targeted m.
m. treatment
m. trial
unnecessary m.
up-to-date m.
weight-neutral psychotic m.
medication-induced
m.-i. movement
m.-i. movement disorder
m.-i. parkinsonism
m.-i. postural tremor
m.-i. tardive dyskinesia
medication-resistant schizophrenia
medication-taking behavior
medicinal
patent m.'s
medicine
Academy of Psychosomatic M.
  (APM)
alternative m.
American Academy of Pain M.
  (AAPM)
American Academy of Sleep M.
  (AASM)
American Society of Addiction M.
  (ASAM)
artificial intelligence in m. (AIM)
aviation m.
Band-Aid m.
behavioral m.
clinical m.
comparative m.
complementary m.
compound m.
m. concept
constitutional m.
diploma in psychological m.
  (DPM)
domestic m.
dosimetric m.
emergency m.
environmental m.
evidence-based m. (EBM)
experimental m.
family m.
folk m.
forensic m.
geriatric m.
group m.
herbal m.
hermetic m.
holistic m.
hyperbaric m.
Indian m.
Institute of M.

legal m.
m. man
mental m.
modern Western m.
neo-hippocratic m.
nutritional m.
Office of Alternative M. (OAM)
patent m.
physical m.
preclinical m.
prescription-only m. (POM)
preventive m.
psychologic m.
psychosomatic m. (PSMed)
rational m.
social m.
socialized m.
suggestive m.
Western m.
m. woman
medicolegal
medicomechanical
medicopsychological
medicopsychology
medicosocial
medievalism
mediocrity
meditate
meditatio mortis
meditation
guided m.
mindfulness m.
principle of Buddhist m.
Qi Gong movement-based m.
transcendental m. (TM)
meditation-based stress reduction
meditative tradition
medium, pl. **media**
media history
media influence
mass media
spiritual m.
m. trance
media violence
violent media
mediumistic hypothesis
medley
chance m.
medulla, pl. **medullae**
m. oblongata
medullary
m. canal

m. narcosis
m. syndrome
medullovasculosa
zona m.
meek
meemies
screaming m.
meet halfway
meeting
face-to-face m.
12-step m.'s
megacephalic
megacephalous
megacolon
psychogenic m.
megalgia
megaloencephalic
megaloencephalon
megaloencephaly
megalographia, megalography
megalomania
megalomanic, megalomaniac
megalopia, megalopsia
m. hysterica
m. hysterics
Megan Law
megavitamin therapy
me generation
megrim
meiosis
melancholia
acute m.
affective m.
m. affective psychosis
agitated m.
m. attonita
chronic m.
climacteric m.
convulsive m.
hypochondriac m.
m. hypochondriaca
hypochondriacal m.
intermittent m.
involutional m.
menopausal m.
panphobic m.
paranoid m.
paretic m.
puberty m.
puerperal m.
reactive m.
recurrent m.

M

NOTES

melancholia (*continued*)
   m. religiosa
   senile m.
   sexual m.
   m. simplex
   m. stuporosa
   stuporous m.
   suicidal m.
   m. vera
   m. with delirium
   m. zoanthropy
melancholic, melancholiac
   m. constitutional type
   m. depression
   m. feature
   m. involutional reaction
   m. mood
   m. personality
melancholicus
   raptus m.
melancholium
   omego m.
melancholy
melatonin
melee
meliorism
melioristic
Melissa officinalis
melitracen
Mellanby effect
mellow
mellowness
melodramatic
melodramatize
melomania
meloncolique
   folie raisonnante m.
meltdown
member
   adolescent gang m.
   couple m.
   m. of a coven
   cult m.
   family m.
   gang m.
   medical staff m.
   neo-Nazi gang m.
   skinhead gang m.
   staff m.
   surviving family m.
   team m. (TM)
membrane
   hymenal m.
   lithium action on m.'s
   neuronal m.
   m. phenotype
memento mori
memoir

memorabilia
memorable
memoration
   amnesic m.
memoriae
   lapsus m.
memorial
memorialist
memorialize
memorize
memory
   m. ability
   accuracy of m.
   affect m.
   m. afterimage
   amnesia loss of m.
   m. amplification
   anterograde loss of m.
   associative m.
   auditory m.
   autobiographic m.
   automatic m.
   behavioral m.
   m. bias
   biographical m.
   body m.
   Bower model of mood-
     congruent m.
   m. buffer
   buffer m.
   childhood m.
   childhood trauma m.
   coast m.
   conscious m.
   m. consolidation
   constructive m.
   declarative m.
   decreased m.
   m. defect
   delayed m.
   m. for design (MFD)
   m. deterioration
   m. difficulty
   digit-symbol and incidental m.
   m. disability
   m. disorder
   m. distortion
   distributed m.
   m. disturbance
   disturbance of m.
   echoic m.
   m. by emotion
   emotional m.
   emotionally loaded event m.
   m. encoding
   episodic m.
   euthymic m.
   event m.

explicit m.
eye m.
factual m.
false m.
m. falsification
figural m.
flashbulb m.
m. function
m. function deficit
m. gap
genetic m.
m. hallucination
hyperesthetic m.
iconic m.
m. illusion
m. image
immediate m.
impaired m.
m. impairment
implicit m.
incidental m.
m. index
intrusive m.
lack of m.
m. lapse
logical m.
long-term m. (LTM)
long-term associative m.
long-term declarative m.
long-term storage of m.
m. loss
loss of biographical m.
minute m.
nondeclarative m.
m. organization
overconsolidation of m.
painful m.
panoramic m.
m. paradigm
m. passage
m. performance
permanent m.
personal m.
photographic m.
physiological m.
pleasant m.
primary m.
priming m.
m. process
m. processing
prospective m.
m. questionnaire

m. quotient (MQ)
racial m.
recall m.
m. recall
recent past m.
recognition m.
recovered m.
recursive autoassociative m.
m. reference
remote m.
replacement m.
m. retention
m. retrieval strategy
retrograde loss of m.
retrospective gaps in m.
m. romance
rote m.
m. scale
m. score
m. screen
screen m.
secondary verbal m.
selective m.
semantic m.
senile m.
sequence m.
sequential m.
short-term m. (STM)
short-term declarative m.
m. skill
somatic m.
m. span
state-dependent m.
m. storage
stress effect on m.
subconscious m.
m. symbol
m. for symbolic unit (MSU)
m. system
m. task
m. test
m. theory
top-down organization of m.
m. trace
m. training
m. transfer
unconscious m.
unhappy m.
verbal working m.
visual spatial m.
visuospatial m.
working m.

M

NOTES

memory-continuous performance
MEMPHIS
> Memphis Educational Model Providing Handicapped Infant Services

Memphis Educational Model Providing Handicapped Infant Services (MEMPHIS)
menace
menacing
ménage à trois
menarche
mendacious
mendacity
Mendel
> M. instep reflex

mendelian
> m. law
> m. rules of inheritance

mendelism
mendicancy
> pathologic m.
> pathological m.

mendicant
menerik
menial
meningeal neurosyphilis
meningis
meningism
meningismus psychosis
meningitis, pl. **meningitides**
> external m.
> herpes zoster m.
> occlusive m.
> syphilitic m.

meningoencephalitis
> herpetic m.
> syphilitic m.

meningomyelitis
meningovascular syphilis
meninx
Menninger Clinic Treatment Intervention Project
menopausal
> m. depression
> m. distress
> m. melancholia
> m. paranoid psychosis
> m. paranoid reaction
> m. paranoid state
> m. paraphrenia
> m. status

menopause
> adjustment reaction of m.
> female m.
> male m.
> m. neurosis

Mensa
mens rea

menstrual
> m. cramp
> m. psychogenic disorder

menstruation
> psychogenic painful m.

mensuration
mental
> m. aberration
> m. ability
> m. abnormality
> m. abuse
> m. act
> m. activity
> m. age (MA)
> m. agitation
> m. agraphia
> m. alertness
> m. anesthesia
> m. apparatus
> m. arousal
> m. asthenia
> m. asymmetry
> m. ataxia
> m. audition
> m. blind spot
> m. block
> m. capacity
> m. capacity evaluation
> m. chemistry
> m. chronometry
> m. competence
> m. competency
> m. concept
> m. confusion
> m. control
> m. data
> m. defect
> m. deficiency
> m. deficit
> m. depression
> m. derangement
> m. deterioration
> m. deterioration battery
> m. development
> m. disability
> m. discipline
> m. disease
> m. disorder
> m. disorder due to alcoholism
> m. disorder due to a general medical condition
> m. disorganization
> m. distress
> m. disturbance
> m. dynamism
> m. eclipse
> m. ego
> m. energy

m. evolution
m. examination
m. excitement
m. exercise
m. exhaustion
m. faculty
m. fatigue
m. fog
m. function
m. growth
m. healing
m. health
m. health advocate
M. Health Association (MHA)
m. health care
m. health care professional
m. health clinic (MHC)
m. health community
m. health counseling
m. health counselor
m. health court
M. Health Early Intervention, Treatment, and Prevention Act of 2000
M. Health Equitable Treatment Act of 2001
m. health expert
m. health law
m. health legislation
M. Health Parity Act of 1998
m. health practitioner
m. health professional
m. health provider
m. health reform
m. health resource
m. health service
m. health specialist
m. health system
m. health treatment
m. health treatment facility
m. health worker
m. hospital
m. hygiene
m. hygiene clinic
m. illness
m. image
m. imagery
m. impairment
m. impression
m. inhibition level
m. institution
m. insufficiency

m. life
m. makeup
m. masochism
m. maturity
m. measurement
m. mechanism
m. medicine
m. metabolism
m. model
m. obtundation
m. pain
m. patient organization
m. patient sterilization
m. patient warehousing
m. phenomenon
m. process
m. psychoneurotic disorder
m. retardation (MR)
m. retardation, severity unspecified
m. scale
m. scotoma
m. set
m. shock
m. skills
m. speed
m. stability
m. state
m. status
m. status change
m. status cognitive task
m. status examination (MSE)
m. status examination record
m. status examination report (MSER)
m. status schedule (MSS)
m. status test
m. stress
m. structure
m. subnormality
m. subnormality disorder
m. suffering
m. symptom
m. tension
m. testing
The M. Health Association of Michigan
m. topography
m. upset
m. workload
mentalis
mentalism
mentalist

M

NOTES

mentalistic
mentality
  dominant m.
mentally
  m. competent
  m. defective
  m. deficient (MD)
  m. deranged
  m. disabled
  disordered m.
  m. disordered offender
  m. disordered sex offender
    (MDSO)
  m. handicapped
  m. ill
  m. impaired
  m. incompetent
  m. obtunded
  m. retarded
  m. retarded child
  m. retarded persons' rights
mentation
  altered m.
  change in m.
  normal m.
  m. rate
  subjective m.
menticide
mentionable
mentis
  abalienatio m.
  alienatio m.
  compos m.
  non compos m.
mentor
mentoring program
mentulomania
MEP
  motor evoked potential
  multimodality evoked potential
meperidine
  analog of m.
mephenesin
mercenary
merciful
merciless
mercuralis
  erethism m.
mercurial
  m. behavior
  m. tremor
mercury encephalopathy
mercy killing
mere-exposure effect
merergasia
merergastic
meretricious

mergent
  partial m.
  total m.
merger state
merit
  m. ranking
  m. rating
meritocracy
meritorious
Merkel law
merosmia
merycism
MES
  maximal electroshock seizure
mescal button
mescalism
mesencephalic reticular formation
mesencephalitis
mesencephalon
mesial
  m. prefrontal cortex
  m. prefrontal cortical area
mesmeric crisis
mesmerism
mesmerize
mesmeromania
mesoblastic sensibility
mesocortical
  m. dopamine pathway
mesolimbic
  m. dopamine
  m. dopamine pathway
  m. selectivity
mesolimbic-mesocortical tract
mesomorph
mesomorphic constitutional type
mesoneuritis
mesontomorph
mesopsychic
message
  conflicting m.
  covert m.
  cryptic m.
  dichotic m.
  diotic m.
  hidden m.
  m. integration
  mixed m.
  overt m.
  subliminal m.
  threatening m.
  two-sided m.
messenger
  chemical m.
  external chemical m. (ECM)
  intracellular second m.
  lithium action on first m.
  lithium action on second m.

m. RNA
second m.
messiah complex
messianic
messianism
mesylate
meta-analysis
metabolic
    m. abnormality
    m. acidosis
    m. activation
    m. activity
    m. alkalosis
    m. anomaly
    m. anoxia
    m. asymmetry
    m. capability
    m. change
    m. coma
    m. conversion
    m. defect
    m. derangement
    m. difference
    m. disease organic psychosis
    m. disorder
    m. disturbance
    m. dysperception
    m. effect
    m. encephalopathy
    m. energy
    m. increase
    m. mechanism
    m. nutritional model
    m. process
    m. rate
    m. response
    m. tolerance
    m. tremor
    m. variability
    m. volume depletion
metabolism
    abnormal m.
    alcohol m.
    m. at rest
    basal m.
    brain m.
    brain glucose m.
    caffeine m.
    carbohydrate m.
    cerebellar m.
    cerebral glucose m.
    cortical m.

cytochrome P450 m.
dopamine m.
energy m.
frontal m.
global m.
glucose m.
inborn errors of m.
intracellular energy m.
left parietal association m.
mental m.
methadone m.
mineral m.
myelin m.
neuronal m.
parallel pathways of m.
prefrontal m.
psychotropic m.
purine m.
pyrimidine m.
regional brain glucose m.
striatal m.
striatus-orbitofrontal m.
metabolite
    active m.
    dopamine m.
    neurotransmitter m.
metachlorophenylpiperazine
metaclazepam
metacognitive capacity
metacommunication
metaerotism
metaethics
metaevaluation
metagenesis
metagnosis
metakinesis
metal
    m. intoxication
    m. object
metalanguage
metalinguistic
metallic tremor
metamemory
metamorphic paralogia
metamorphopsia
metamorphose
metamorphosis
    behavioral m.
    m. sexualis paranoica
metamotivation
metaneeds
metapathology

M

NOTES

metapelet
metaphase
metaphor
    religious m.
metaphoric
    m. language
    m. paralogia
    m. symbolism
metaphrenia
metaphysics
metapramine
metapsyche
metapsychiatry
metapsychics
metapsychological profile
metapsychology
metasyncrisis
metatabi
metatarsalgia
metatrophia
metatrophy
metatropism
metempirical
metempsychosis
met-enkephalin
meter
    biofeedback m.
methadone
    m. addiction
    m. block
    m. center
    m. dependence
    m. maintenance
    m. maintenance treatment (MMT)
    m. maintenance treatment program
    m. metabolism
methamphetamine
    m. abuse
    m. addiction
    m. dependence
methilepsia
method
    adjustment m.
    m. of administration
    adoptee family m.
    alternative m.
    m.'s analysis
    analytic m.
    anecdotal m.
    approximation m.
    m. of approximation
    aristotelian m.
    m. of ascertainment
    assessment m.
    behavior m.
    biofeedback m.
    biographical m.
    bisensory m.

brain imaging m.
Brasdor m.
case m.
cathartic m.
chewing m.
classification m.
clinical m.
cognitive m.
complete-learning m.
confluence m.
m. of constant stimuli
Cooper m.
correlation m.
cross-sectional m.
m. of defining criterion
m. of delivery
diagnostic m.
dose reduction m.
Dubois m.
equal-and-unequal-cases m.
equal-appearing-intervals m.
equivalent m.
exosomatic m.
experimental m.
expression m.
m. factor
factor comparison m.
family m.
Flesh-Kincaid m.
formal m.
Freud cathartic m.
genetic m.
gradation m.
Hilton m.
historical m.
imaging m.
impedance m.
impression m.
informal m.
interview m.
introspective m.
job component m.
Jung m.
kinesthetic m.
Leboyer m.
m. of limits
linguistic-kinesic m.
longitudinal m.
mass m.
metric m.
Milligan annihilation m.
minimal-change m.
minimum separable m.
Montessori m.
Moore m.
need-press m.
nonpurging m.
numerical cipher m.

observational m.
obstruction m.
operant m.
optimal m.
part-learning m.
Pavlov m.
pedigree m.
plateau m.
preferred m.
proband m.
purging m.
Purmann m.
Q m.
Q-Sort m.
rating m.
recall m.
reconstruction m.
relearning m.
review m.
rhythm m.
Rochester m.
Scarpa m.
scientific m.
m. of self-injury
sibship m.
steady-state m.
structured clinical interview m.
suicide m.
swallow-belch m.
synthetic m.
systematic m.
Tadoma m.
Taylor series linearization m.
Trager m.
Wardrop m.
Xe clearance m.
methodical chorea
methodologic
methodology
   Q m.
methomania
methylated spirit addiction
methyldopa
   alpha m.
methylphenidate
   m. administration
   m. challenge test
methylphenidate-induced change
metiapine
meticulous
metonymic distortion
metonymy

metopoplasty
Metrazol
   M. shock therapy
   M. shock treatment
metric method
metromania
metronoscope
mettle
mettlesome
Metz
   Bad Wildungen M. (BWM)
Meyer theory
MF
   multifactorial model
MFD
   memory for design
MH
   marital history
MHA
   Mental Health Association
MHC
   mental health clinic
MIA
   missing in action
mianserin
miasma theory
mice
Mickey Finn
micosis
   spastic m.
micrencephalia, micrencephaly
micrencephalous
microcephalic idiocy
microcephalus
microcephaly
   schizencephalic m.
microcheilia
microcosm of words
microdysgenesia
microelectrode technique
microencephaly
microgeny
microglia
microgliomatosis
microgliosis
micrography
microgyria
microinjection
micromania
micromaniacal delirium
micromelia
microphonia

M

NOTES

micropsia
micropsy
micropsychophysiology
micropsychosis
micropsychotic
    m. dimension
    m. episode
microptic
    m. delirium
    m. hallucination
microsomia
    heredo-familial essential m.
microsurgery
microsuture
microtia
micturate
micturition
    m. psychogenic disorder
    m. syncope
Midas punishment
midbrain
    m. deafness
    m. dysfunction
    m. matter
mid childhood
middle
    m. adolescence
    m. adulthood
    m. age
    m. age pedophilia
    m. class
    m. class community
    m. frontal sulcus
    m. game
    m. ground
    m. insomnia
    play both ends against the m.
    m. school
    m. school adolescent
middle-aged
middlebrow
middle-class youth
middleman
midfrontal
midlife crisis
midline nuclei
midpontine wakefulness
Midtown Manhattan Study
midwinter insomnia
mien
mieux
    faute de m.
Mignon delusion
migraine
    abdominal m.
    acute confusional m.
    aphasic m.
    circumstantial m.

    classic m.
    cluster m.
    common m.
    fulgurating m.
    Harris m.
    m. headache
    hemiplegia m.
    late-life m.
    ocular m.
    ophthalmic m.
    ophthalmoplegic m.
    paroxysmal m.
    m. personality
    seasonal m.
    tension m.
    unilateral m.
    vestibular m.
    m. with aura (MA)
migraineur
migrainoid
migrainous neuralgia
migrant
migrate
migration
    m. adaptation
    adjustment following m.
    cultural adjustment following m.
    m. psychosis
migratory
mild
    anxiety reaction, m. (ARM)
    m. ataxia
    m. delusion
    m. depression
    m. disability
    m. eccentricity in demeanor
    m. neurocognitive disorder
milenperone
milestone
    developmental m.
    m. event
milieu
    m. environment
    m. exterieur
    m. interieur
    sociocultural m.
    structured m.
    therapeutic m.
    m. therapy
milipertine
militant
militaristic
militarize
military
    m. chaplain
    m. forensic psychiatry
    m. history

m. neurosis
m. psychology
militate
militia group
militiaman
milk
heroin mixed with powdered m.
milk-ejection reflex
Millard-Gubler syndrome
Milles syndrome
Milligan annihilation method
milling crowd
Milton model
mime
mimesis
mimetic
m. chorea
m. paralysis
m. seizure
mimic
m. convulsion
m. seizure
m. spasm
m. speech
m. tic
mimica
asemasia m.
mimicked
mimicry
mimmation
minaprine
minatory
mince
mind
m. blindness
m. control
disharmonious state of m.
m.'s eye
group m.
miniature m.
mortal m.
one-track m.
open m.
m. pain
m. power
prelogical m.
m. reader
m. reading
m. set
state of m.
subconscious m.

theory of m.
wandering m.
mind-altering
m.-a. drug
m.-a. substance
mind-bending
mind-blowing
mind-body
m.-b. dualism
m.-b. problem
mind-boggling
minded
absent m.
fair m.
small m.
social m.
tender m.
mindedness
psychological m.
small m.
mind-expanding
mindful
mindfulness
m. meditation
m. skills
mindfulness-based stress reduction
mindless
mindset
mineral metabolism
miner's cramp
mingy
miniature
m. mind
m. system
minimal
m. audible field (MAF)
m. audible pressure
m. brain damage
m. brain dysfunction (MBD)
m. cue
m. personal hygiene
m. provocation
m. residual symptom
m. risk
minimal-change method
minimalist
minimization of emotional detail
minimize
minimizes responsibility
minimizing stimulation
minimum
m. dose

M

NOTES

minimum *(continued)*
    m. duration
    m. effective concentration (MEC)
    m. intensity projection
    maintenance m.
    m. maintenance
    m. separable method
minimum-change therapy
minion
minister
ministry
minor
    m. analysis
    chorea m.
    m. depressive disorder
    emancipated m.
    m. epilepsy
    m. form
    m. hypnosis
    m. hysteria
    m. image-distorting level
    m. penalty
    m. stimulus
    m. tranquilizer
minority
    m. community
    m. discrimination
    ethnic m.
    m. group
    m. group psychiatry
    racial m.
    underrepresented m.
minute
    m. memory
    m. object
miosis
    paralytic m.
    spastic m.
miracle
miraculous
mirage
mirror
    m. drawing
    m. exercise
    m. fear
    m. focus
    m. image
    one-way m.
    m. sign
    m. speech
    m. technique
    m. transference
    m. writing
mirroring
    crossover m.
    m. the transference
mirror-writing
mirth

miryachit, myriachit
misaction
misala
misalignment
misalliance
misandry
misanthropia
misanthropy
misapplication
misattribution of guilt
misbehave
misbehaving child
misbehavior
    sexual m.
misbelief
miscalculate
miscarriage
miscast
miscegenation
mischance
mischief
    malicious m.
mischievous behavior
misclassify
miscode
miscommunication
misconception
    illusionary m.
misconduct
    sexual m.
misconstrue
miscreant
misdemeanor
misdiagnose
misdiagnosis
misdirection phenomenon
miser
miserable
miserliness
miserly
miserotia
misery
    emotional m.
misfit
misfortune
misgiving
mishandle
mishap
misidentification
misinformation effect
misinterpret
misjudge
mislead
mismatch
misnomer
misocainia
misogamy
misogynist

misogynistic
misogyny
misologia
misology
misoneism
misopedia, misopedy
misperception
    sleep state m.
misplace
misplaced
    m. hope
    m. objects test
misprision
mispronounce
misquote
misrepresent
missed
    m. abortion
    m. diagnosis
    m. dose
    m. school
missexual
missiles
missing in action (MIA)
mistake
    basic m.
    category m.
    fatal m.
mistreat
mistreatment
    history of m.
    m. history
mistress
mistrust
    basic m.
    trust vs. m.
misty-eyed
misuse
    alcohol m.
    diuretic m.
    laxative m.
mitamachen
Mitchell treatment
mite
    delirium m.
mitgehen
mitigate
mitigated echolalia
mitis
    catatonia m.
    dementia paranoides m.
    epilepsia m.

mitissima
mitochondria
mitochondrial
Mitofsky-Aaksberg random digit dialing
  procedure
mitosis
    m., migration and maturation
mitten pattern
mix
    case m.
mixed
    m. anxiety depression disorder
    (MADD)
    m. aphasia
    m. bag
    m. bipolar affective psychosis
    bipolar I disorder, most recent
    episode m.
    m. bipolar state
    bipolar type m.
    m. cerebral dominance
    m. chancre
    m. compulsive states psychasthenia
    m. design
    m. development developmental
    delay disorder
    m. disturbance stress reaction
    m. drink
    m. feature
    m. foot dominant
    m. laterality
    m. mania episode
    m. manic-depressive psychosis
    m. marriage
    m. message
    m. model
    m. mood episode
    m. mood state
    m. motive game
    m. neurosis
    m. paralysis
    m. paralytic conversion reaction
    paranoid-affective organic
    psychosis, m.
    m. personality disorder
    m. presentation
    m. psychoneurosis
    m. psychoneurotic disorder
    m. psychopathic personality
    m. receptive-expressive language
    m. reinforcement
    m. schizophrenia

M

NOTES

mixed (*continued*)
    m. schizophrenic-affective psychosis
    m. specific developmental disorder
    m. substance abuse
    m. symptom picture with
      perceptual disturbance
    m. type
    m. up
mixed-sex group composition
mixed-type
    m.-t. delusion
    m.-t. epilepsy
    m.-t. psychopathic
    m.-t. psychopathic personality
    m.-t. schizophrenia
mixoscopia bestialis
mixoscopy
mixture
    m. approach
    color m.
    m. theory
mix-up
MMECT
    multimonitored electroconvulsive
    treatment
9mm handgun
MMPI
    MMPI Code Type
MMT
    methadone maintenance treatment
MMUS
    multiple medically unexplained symptom
M'Naghten
    M. rule
    M. test
mneme
    phylogenetic m.
mnemenic, mnemic
    m. hypothesis
    m. theory
mnemism
    theory of m.
    m. theory
mnemonic
    m. strategy
    m. system
    m. trace
mob
    m. behavior
    m. psychology
mobile
    m. crisis outreach team
    m. spasm
    upwardly m.
mobility
    m. disability
    geographic m.
    horizontal m.

    m. of libido
    upward m.
    vertical m.
mobilization reaction
mobilize
mobocracy
mock
mockery
modal
    m. adaptive task
    m. dose
modality
    main treatment m.
    sensory m.
    suboptimal treatment m.
    tactile sensory m.
    therapeutic m.
    treatment m.
    visual sensory m.
modality-specific
mode
    enactive m.
    field-cognition m.
    m. of inheritance
    parataxic m.
    protaxic m.
    prototaxic m.
    quiet wakefulness m.
    syntaxic m.
model
    active-passive m.
    adversary m.
    affective schematic mental m.
    affect-related schematic mental m.
    affect trauma m.
    awareness training m.
    behavioral m.
    biomedical m.
    biopsychosocial m.
    Blos developmental m.
    Bowen m.
    Bowlby developmental m.
    brain m.
    categorical m.
    cognitive m.
    contingency m.
    cost-reward m.
    developmental-vulnerability m.
    dimensional m.
    dual-arousal m.
    ecological systems m.
    educational-socialization m.
    ego m.
    Erickson developmental m.
    Eysenck m.
    fixed m.
    friendship m.
    m. game

Gesell developmental m.
guidance-cooperation m.
helping m.
homeostatic m.
human-potential m.
m. of illness
internal m.
job characteristics m.
kinetic m.
Kohlberg developmental m.
laboratory-method m.
learning m.
Mayberg limbic-cortical
   dysregulation m.
McCullough-Pitts m.
medical m.
mental m.
metabolic nutritional m.
Milton m.
mixed m.
multifactorial m. (MF)
multimodal treatment m.
Munich cooperative m.
mutual participation m.
nonaffective schematic mental m.
parent-child m.
m. penal code
PLISSIT M.
psychodynamic-experiential m.
psychological m.
m. psychosis
public health m.
random m.
role m.
schematic mental m.
single-major-locus m.
SML m.
social integration-disintegration m.
socially intimate m.
standard kinetic m.
stress-diathesis m.
subcortical dysfunction m.
teacher-student m.
treatment m.
modeled behavior
modeling
abstract m.
behavioral m.
covert m.
m. exercise
kinetic m.
participant m.

moderate
m. ataxia
m. depression
m. difficulty
m. mental retardation
m. mental subnormality
moderate-to-severe depression
moderator variable
modern
m. psychiatry
m. Western medicine
modernize
modest
modesty
modification
active m.
behavior m.
body m.
carbonyl m.
dietary m.
environment m.
environmental m.
hebbian m.
interference m.
lifestyle m.
modified
m. ECT therapy
m. Stroop effect
modularity
imaging m.
modulated affect
modulating
modulation
affect m.
amplitude m. (AM)
dopaminergic m.
emotional m.
impaired affect m.
modulator
module
modus operandi
mogiarthria
mogigraphia
mogilalia
mogiphonia
mogul
moieties
moil
moisture
m. fear
m. fear-molar approach

M

NOTES

MOJAC
    mood, orientation, judgment, affect,
    content
molar approach
mold
molecular
    m. genetics
    m. neuropathology
    m. psychiatry
molecule
    feel-good m.
molest
molestation
    child m.
molester
    child m.
    serial child m.
molilalia
molimen, pl. **molimina**
    m. climactericum virile
moll
mollify
molluscum, pl. **mollusca**
mollycoddle
Molotov cocktail
mom
    deadbeat m.
moment
    m. of aggression
    m. of truth
momentarily
momentary tearfulness
momentous
moment-to-moment mood change
momentum
momism
monandry
monarchical
monastic
monathetosis
Monday morning headache
monde
    beau m.
monesthetic
monestrous
money
    ability to manage m.
    m. management ability
    old m.
monism
monistic
monition
monitor
    body m.
monitoring
    baseline m.
    behavioral m.
    clinical m.

    close clinical m.
    distortion of inferential
     behavioral m.
    electronic m.
    exaggeration of inferential
     behavioral m.
    inferential behavioral m.
    seizure m.
    m. technique
monk
monkey
    m. love
    m. therapist
monoamine
    m. hypothesis
    m. oxidase (MAO)
    m. oxidase inhibitor (MAOI)
monochorea
monocular visual loss
monocyclic antidepressant
monoecious
monoecism
monogamist
monogamous relationship
monogamy
monogynous
monogyny
monoideic somnambulism
monoideism
monolithic adult block
monologue
    collective m.
monomania
    affective m.
    emotional m.
    intellectual m.
monomaniac
monomanie
    m. du vol
    m. erotique
    m. incendiare
monomoria
monomyoplegia
mononeuralgia
mononeuritis multiplex
mononoea
mononuclear
monoparesis
monoparesthesia
monophagia
monophagic
monophagism
monophasia
monophasic
monoplegia masticatoria
monoplegic psychogenic disorder
monopolar depression
monopolization communication pattern

monopolize
monopsychosis
monorecidive chancre
monoscenism
monosexual
monospasm
monosyllabic speech
monosymptom
monosymptomatic
    m. circumscription
    m. hypochondriacal psychosis
    m. hypochondriasis
    m. neurosis
monotheism
    Moses and m.
monotherapy
monotone
    m. speech
    m. voice
monotonic
monotonous
    m. speech
    m. voice
monotony
monotropic
monoxide
    carbon m.
monozygotic twins (MZ)
monster fear
monstrosity
monstrous
Montessori method
month
    abstinent days per m.
monthly
monumental
mood
    abnormal m.
    absence of depressed m.
    absence of elevated m.
    adjustment disorder with angry m.
    adjustment disorder with
      anxious m.
    adjustment disorder with mixed
      anxiety and depressed m.
    m. and/or affect (M/A)
    anxious m.
    m. brightening
    m. change
    m. chart
    m. cluster score
    m. congruent

consistent m.
dark m.
dejected m.
depressed m.
depth of m.
m. deterioration
m. disorder
m. disorder due to a general
  medical condition
m. disorder patient
m. disorder with atypical features
m. disorder with catatonic features
m. disorder with melancholic
  features
m. disorder with postpartum onset
m. disorder with rapid cycling
m. disorder with seasonal pattern
m. disturbance
duration of m.
dysphoric m.
elated m.
elevated m.
m. elevation
m. elevator
m. episode
erratic m.
euphoric m.
euthymic m.
excited m.
expansion m.
expansive m.
imperative m.
indicative m.
m. induction
intensity of m.
irritable m.
labile m.
m. lability
lowered m.
manic m.
melancholic m.
morbid m.
nondepressed m.
normal m.
normal range of m.
m., orientation, judgment, affect,
  content (MOJAC)
m. profile
prominent irritable m.
public health m.
pure m.
quality of m.

M

NOTES

mood *(continued)*
 m. reactivity
 m. regulator
 m. responsivity
 rhythmic m.
 sad m.
 shift in m.
 m. shift
 somber m.
 m. spectrum disorder
 m. stabilization
 m. stabilizer
 m. stabilizing agent
 m. state
 subjunctive m.
 m. swing
 m. swing affective psychosis
 m. swing syndrome
 m. symptom
 m. symptomatology
 unpleasant m.
 unstable m.
 usual m.
 vascular dementia with
  depressed m.
mood-altering
 m.-a. drug
 m.-a. substance
mood-balance
mood-congruent
 m.-c. delusion
 m.-c. hallucination
 m.-c. psychotic feature
mood-cyclic disorder
mood-elevating drug
mood-incongruent
 m.-i. delusion
 m.-i. hallucination
 m.-i. psychotic feature
moodiness
 developmental m.
moody
Mooney
Moonies
mooning
moon phase
moon-phase study
moonshine
moonstruck
Moore
 M. method
 M. syndrome
moot point
mope
moperone
mora
moral
 m. anxiety

 m. assessment
 m. ataxia
 m. behavior
 m. code
 m. conduct
 m. consistency
 m. deficiency
 m. deficiency personality disorder
 m. development
 m. emotion
 m. hazard
 m. idiocy
 m. imbecile
 m. independence
 m. insanity
 m. judgment
 m. masochism
 m. objection
 m. oligophrenia
 m. outrage
 m. philosophy
 m. pride
 m. principle
 m. realism
 m. relativism
 m. right
 m. theory
 m. thought
 m. treatment
 m. turpitude
 m. value
 m. wrongdoing
morale
 acquired folie m.
 folie m.
 group m.
moralism
moralist
morality
 m. of constraint
 m. of conventional role conformity
 m. of cooperation
 interpersonal m.
 m. of self-accepted moral principle
 sphincter m.
moralize
morally
morass
moratorium
 psychosexual m.
 psychosocial m.
morbid
 m. anxiety
 m. dependence
 m. desire
 m. doubt
 m. fear
 m. idea

m. imitation
m. impulse
m. jealousy
m. mood
m. obesity
m. perplexity
m. response
m. risk
m. rumination
m. thirst
morbidity
medical m.
persistent m.
psychiatric m.
psychosocial m.
morbidostatic
mordancy
mordant
mores
sexual m.
social m.
Morgagni
M. syndrome
morgana
fata m.
mori
memento m.
moria
moribund state
Morita
M. psychotherapy
M. therapy
morning
m. after
m. bright light therapy
m. drinking
m. glory seeds dependence
morning-after pill
moron
moronity
morose
morosity
irritable m.
morpheme
circumfix m.
morphine
m. addiction
m. dependence
m. withdrawal
morphine-like action
morphinism
morphinist

morphinistic
morphinization
morphinomania
morphinomaniac
morphiomania
morphogenetic
morphological
m. deformation
m. difference
m. rule
morphologic teratogenicity
morphology
planum temporale m.
morphometric
m. abnormality
m. analysis
m. technique
morphosynthesis
morsicatio
m. buccarum
m. labiorum
mortal
m. mind
m. sin
mortality
actual m.
drug-associated m.
increased m.
infant m.
prediction of m.
m. rate
reproductive m.
m. risk
risk factor for m.
m. trend
mortally
mort douce
mortification
mortify
mortis
in articulo m.
meditatio m.
mortisemblant
MOS
Medical Outcomes Study
mosaicism
Moses and monotheism
mosque
mother
biologic m.
birth m.
m. card

M

NOTES

mother *(continued)*
>complete m.
>m. complex
>m. confessor
>dysfunctional m.
>m. figure
>m. fixation
>foster m.
>good-enough m.
>host m.
>m. hypnosis
>m. image
>m. instinct
>m. love
>opioid-dependent m.
>phallic m.
>m. substitute
>M. Superior complex
>m. surrogate
>surrogate m.
>working m.

mother-child
>m.-c. attachment
>m.-c. bond
>m.-c. dyad
>m.-c. experience
>m.-c. relationship (MCR)

mother-daughter incest
mother-infant
>m.-i. attachment
>m.-i. bonding
>m.-i. interaction
>m.-i. proximity
>m.-i. relationship

mothering
>good-enough m.
>multiple m.

motherly
mother-son incest
motile
motility
>m. disorder
>m. psychosis

motion
>brownian m.
>m. fear
>involuntary m.
>m. perception
>phenomenal m.
>m. picture violence
>set in m.
>m. sickness
>voluntary m.

motivate
motivated
>m. error
>m. forgetting

motivating operation

motivation
>achievement m.
>adult m.
>m. analysis
>m. analysis testing
>being m.
>characteristic pattern of m.
>childhood m.
>competence m.
>competing theories of m.
>m. for cross-dressing
>decreased m.
>deficiency m.
>m. deterioration
>expressed m.
>external incentive m.
>extrinsic m.
>m. factor
>m. impairment
>incentive m.
>intrinsic m.
>lack of m.
>loss of m.
>maladaptive pattern of m.
>personal m.
>positive m.
>primary m.
>prosocial m.
>psychological m.
>reduced m.
>m. research
>secondary m.
>m. for self-injury
>sexual m.
>suicide m.
>true m.
>unconscious m.
>work m.

motivational
>m. enhancement therapy
>m. factor
>m. hierarchy
>m. inventory
>m. process
>m. selectivity

motive
>abundant m.
>achievement m.
>m. achievement
>aroused m.
>autonomy of m.'s
>competitive m.
>conflicting m.
>cooperative m.
>deficiency m.
>hierarchy of m.'s
>hostile m.
>individualistic m.

inviolacy m.
mastery m.
m. mastery
personal social m.
physiological m.
safety m.
ulterior m.
m. for violent act
motley
motor
m. ability
m. abreaction
m. activity
m. agraphia
m. alexia
m. amusia
m. aphasia
m. apraxia
m. area
m. ataxia
m. aura
m. behavior
m. compliance
m. control of the ego
m. conversion symptom
m. coordination
m. cortex
m. cortical center
m. dapsone neuropathy
m. deficit
m. depressant
m. development
m. disability
m. disinhibition
m. evoked potential (MEP)
fine m.
m. function
gross m.
m. habit
m. image
m. immobility
m. impairment
m. inertia
m. inhibition
m. innervation
m. interface
m. loss
m. maturity
m. movement
m. nerve
m. nerve conduction
m. neurosis

m. passivity
m. performance
m. performance test
m. perseveration
m. persistence
m. phenomenon
m. planning
m. point
m. psychogenic disorder
m. psychosis
m. region
m. response
m. restlessness
m. retardation
m. sign
m. skill
m. skill disturbance
m. skills disorder
m. slowing
m. speed
m. system
m. task
m. theory of thought
m. threshold
m. tic
m. tic disorder
transcortical m.
m. vocalization
m. zone
motoric
m. abnormality
m. hyperactivity
m. immobility
m. reproduction process
motorium
motor-verbal
m.-v. tic
m.-v. tic disorder
motor-vocal tic disorder
moulage
mount
mourn
mourning
guided m.
m. work
mouse, pl. **mice**
CRF knockout mice
m. fear
mouth
downturned corners of the m.
dry m.
nothing by m. (NPO, n.p.o., npo)

NOTES

M

mouth *(continued)*
 poor m.
 twisted m.
mouthing
 object m.
mouthy
movable, moveable
move
 knight m.
 opening m.
movement
 m. abnormality
 active m.
 adventitious m.
 alpha m.
 anomalous m.
 arcuate m.
 associated m.
 automatic m.
 ballistic m.
 beta m.
 bodily m.
 body m.
 brownian m.
 cardinal ocular m.
 choreic m.
 choreiform m.
 clonic m.
 compensatory m.
 complex whole body m.
 constraint of m.
 decomposition of m.
 discordance of m.
 m. disorder
 m. disorder effect
 dyskinetic m.
 dysmetric hand m.
 dyspractic m.
 dysrhythmic m.
 dystonic m.
 encounter m.
 epsilon m.
 exaggerated m.
 expressive m.
 extraneous m.
 eye m.
 false perceptions of m.
 fetal m.
 fine motor m.
 flapping m.
 following m.
 forced m.
 freezing of m.
 Frenkel m.
 functional m.
 gamma m.
 halting m.
 hemiballismic m.

hospice m.
human-potential m.
m. illusion
intentional stereotyped m.
involuntary motor m.
irregular m.
jerking m.
limitation of m. (LOM)
loss of m. (LOM)
low-complexity m.
Magnan trombone m.
mass m.
medication-induced m.
motor m.
myoclonic m.
neurobiotactic m.
nonrapid eye m. (non-REM,
 NREM)
nonrhythmic stereotyped motor m.
passive m.
paucity of m.
perseverative m.
poverty of m.
purposeful m.
purposeless m.
purposive m.
quasi-purposive m.
random m.
rapid alternating m. (RAM)
rapid eye m. (REM)
rapid fine m.
rapid motor m.
rapid repetitive m.
recurrent motor m.
reflex m.
reflexive m.
repetitive imitative m.
rhythmic slow eye m.
roving eye m.
roving ocular m.
saccadic eye m.
m. scale
sleep m.
smooth pursuit eye m. (SPEM)
spontaneous m.
stereotyped body m.
stereotyped motor m.
stereotypic motor m.
sudden motor m.
m. symptom
synkinetic motor m.
m. therapist
m. therapy
tonic-clonic m.
tremulous m.
vermicular m.
vestibular m.
visual pursuit m.

volitional m.
voluntary muscle m.
withdrawal m.
women's liberation m.
movies
sexually charged m.
moving object
moxa
moxibustion
moxie
Moynahan syndrome
Mozart effect
MPD
multiple personality disorder
MPS
mucopolysaccharidosis
MQ
memory quotient
MR
mental retardation
MRHD
maximum recommended human dose
MRI
magnetic resonance imaging
high-resolution MRI
MRI signal hyperintensity
structural MRI
MRI volumetry
MRS
magnetic resonance spectroscopy
MRT
major role therapy
MSE
mental status examination
MSER
mental status examination report
MSIS
multistate information system
MSN
Master of Science in Nursing
MSS
mental status schedule
MST
multisystemic therapy
MSU
memory for symbolic unit
MSW
Master of Social Work
multiple stab wounds
MT
music therapy

MTP
multidisciplinary treatment plan
MTR
Music Therapist, Registered
mucinosa
alopecia m.
muck
muckrake
mucopolysaccharidosis,
pl. **mucopolysaccharidoses (MPS)**
mucosal
muddleheaded
muddle through
muddy
mudslinger
Muenzer-Rosenthal syndrome
muffle
mugged
mugger
mulato
muliebrity
mulish
mull
Müller law
multiaxial
m. classification
m. classification system
m. evaluation
m. fashion
multicomponent
m. behavioral treatment
m. program
multicultural environment
multidetermination
multidimensional
m. assessment
m. assessment of outcome
m. construct
m. family therapy
m. framework
m. pain management
m. scale for rating psychiatric
patients
multidirectional
multidisciplinary
m. group psychiatry
m. treatment plan (MTP)
multidrug
multifacet circumplex
multifaceted nature
multifactorial
m. etiology

M

NOTES

multifactorial *(continued)*
    m. event
    m. inheritance
    m. model (MF)
multifamilial
multifamily skills group
multifarious
multifocal thought
multiforme
multiforme-like
multifunctional
multigenerational history
multi-impulsivity syndrome
multi-infarct
    m.-i. psychosis
multi-item
    m.-i. index
    m.-i. test
multilayered
multimodal
    m. behavior therapy
    m. therapeutic approach
    m. treatment model
multimodality evoked potential (MEP)
multimonitored electroconvulsive treatment (MMECT)
multiorgasmic
multiphase
multiple
    m. analysis
    m. anxiety comorbidity
    m. association
    m. baseline design
    m. birth
    m. cognitive deficits
    m. correlation
    m. delusions
    m. distinct identities
    m. domains of self
    m. ego state
    m. family therapy
    m. focus
    m. identification
    m. life difficulty
    m. loss
    m. medically unexplained symptom (MMUS)
    m. mothering
    m. neuritis
    m. organ failure
    m. personalities and gender
    m. personality
    m. personality crime
    m. personality disorder (MPD)
    m. psychotherapy
    m. regression
    m. regression technique
    m. reinforcement
    m. relationship
    m. role playing
    m. sclerosis-type organic psychosis
    m. sexual partner
    m. spontaneous orgasms
    m. stab wounds (MSW)
    m. tics with coprolalia
    m. victimization
multiple-choice
    m.-c. assessment
    m.-c. testing
multiple-dose regimen
multiple-episode patient
multiple-tracer approach
multiplex
    dysostosis m.
    mononeuritis m.
    myoclonus m.
multiplication
    m. of personality
    m. table test
multiplicity
    target m.
multipolarity
multisensory
multispeaker phonetic noise
multistate
    m. drug distribution ring
    m. information system (MSIS)
multistep task
multisynaptic
multisystemic
    m. therapy (MST)
    m. therapy approach
multitalented
multitude
multitudinous
multivalence
multivariable
multivariate
    m. analysis
    m. analysis of covariance (MANCOVA)
    m. analysis of variance (MANOVA)
    m. study
    m. technique
multiversity
mum
mumble
mumbling automatism
mumbo jumbo
mummery
mummy attitude
Munchausen
    M. disease by proxy
    M. by proxy syndrome
    M. syndrome by proxy

mundane realism
Munich cooperative model
munificent
mu opiate receptor
murder
    lust m.
    m. rampage
    m. suspect
    m. trial
    witness to m.
murderer
    mass m.
    serial m.
murderess
murderous predation behavior
murky
murmur
    brain m.
Murphy's law
muscaria
    Amanita m.
muscarine-agonist-induced
muscarine blockade
muscarinic
    m. cholinergic receptor
    m. receptor blockade
muscle
    buccinator m.
    m. contraction headache
    m. erotism
    m. pleasure
    m. psychogenic disorder
    m. rigidity
    m. spasm
    m. twitch
    vascular m.
muscle-relaxing effect
musculaire
    folie m.
muscular
    m. anesthesia
    m. body
    m. hyperesthesia
    m. insufficiency
    m. reflex
    m. sense
    m. tension
muscular-anal stage
muscularis
musculoskeletal psychogenic disorder
musculospiral paralysis
muse

mushroom
    magic m.
music
    background m.
    bebop m.
    m. blindness
    m. deafness
    heavy metal m.
    loud m.
    lounge m.
    punk m.
    rap m.
    spatial m.
    M. Therapist, Registered (MTR)
    m. therapy (MT)
musical
    m. agraphia
    m. alexia
    m. stimulus
    m. therapy
musician's cramp
musicogenic epilepsy
musicomania
musicotherapy
musomania
mussitans
    delirium m.
mussitation
mustard
    nitrogen m.
mutable
mutacism
mutagenicity
mutation
    gene m.
    m. rate
    testicular feminization m. (TFM)
mutative interpretation
mute
    m. patient
    m. state
muted voices
muteness
mutilate
mutilation
    genital m.
    sadistic m.
mutism
    akinetic m.
    catatonic m.
    elective m.
    hysterical m.

NOTES

M

mutism *(continued)*
  relative elective m.
  selective m.
  traumatic m.
  voluntary m.
mutter
muttering delirium
Mutt and Jeff approach
mutual
  m. affective responsiveness
  m. aid group
  m. consent
  m. grief
  m. masturbation
  m. participation model
  m. pretense awareness
  m. regard
  m. respect
  m. trust
mutual-help services
mutualism
mutuality
mutually exclusive
muzzy
myalgia
myasthenia
myasthenic
  m. facies
  m. reaction
  m. syndrome
mycophagy
mydriasis
  alternating m.
  paralytic m.
  spasmodic m.
  spastic m.
  springing m.
mydriatic rigidity
myelapoplexy
myelatelia
myelauxe
myelin metabolism
myeloplegia
myelosyphilis
Myers-Briggs psychological test
myobradia
myocardiopathy
  alcoholic m.
myocarditis
  toxic m.
myocelialgia
myoclonia
  fibrillary m.
myoclonic
  m. absence
  m. astatic epilepsy
  m. convulsion

  m. movement
  m. seizure
myoclonica
  dementia m.
  dyssynergia cerebellaris m.
myoclonus
  m. epilepsy
  m. multiplex
  nocturnal m.
  stimulus sensitive m.
myodynia
  hysterical m.
myodystony
myofascial pain
myogenic paralysis
myoglobin
myoinositol
myokymia
myoneuralgia
  postural m.
myoneurasthenia
myoneuroma
myopalmus
myoparalysis
myoparesis
myopathic
  m. facies
  m. paralysis
myopathy
  acute alcoholic m.
  alcoholic m.
myopic insight
myorhythmia
myosalgia
myoseism
myotone
myotonia neonatorum
myotonic facies
myotony
myriachit *(var. of* miryachit)
myriad
mysophilia
mysophobic
mystic
  m. paranoia
  m. union
mystica
  unio m.
mystical
  m. experience
  m. influence
mysticism
  purveyor of m.
mystification
mystify
mystifying behavior
mystique
mytacism

myth
    personal m.
    sexual m.
mythical
mythological theme

mythomania
myxedema depression
myxedematous
MZ
    monozygotic twins

NOTES

M

N
numerical aptitude
  N protein
NA
Narcotics Anonymous
n-Ach
achievement need
nadir
nag
nagger
nail
  n. biter
  n. biting
NAIP
National Association of Inpatient
  Physicians
naivete
naive wit
name
  birth n.
  family n.
  fictitious n.
  given n.
  maiden n.
name-calling
name-dropping
naming intact
nance
napalm burn
NAPHS
National Association of Psychiatric
  Health Systems
naphtha
napping phenomenon
NarcAnon
narcissism
  acquired situational n.
  body n.
  ego n.
  primary n.
  primitive n.
  secondary n.
narcissistic
  n. character
  n. character structure
  n. composite
  n. diagnosis
  n. dynamics
  n. ego ideal
  n. equilibrium
  n. feature
  n. neurotic personality disorder
  n. object choice
  n. personality

  n. personality disorder (NPD)
  n. Q score
  n. quality
  n. rage
  n. scale
  n. self-concept
  n. self-peeping
  n. tendency
  n. transference
  n. vulnerability
  n. wounding
narcoanalysis
narcoanesthesia
narcocatharsis
narcohypnia
narcohypnosis
narcolepsy
  n. cataplexy syndrome
  n. experience
  non-REM n.
narcoleptic tetrad
narcomania
narcomatous
narcose
narcosis
  basal n.
  continuous n.
  medullary n.
  nitrogen n.
narcosomania
narcostimulant
narcosuggestion
narcosynthesis
narcotherapy
narcotic
  n. abuse
  n. addict
  n. addiction
  n. agonist drug
  n. antagonist
  n. antagonist drug
  n. blockade
  n. blocking drug
  n. chemical intoxication
  n. drug dependence
  n. habit
  n. hunger
  n. poisoning
  n. withdrawal
Narcotic Addict Treatment Act
Narcotics Anonymous (NA)
narcotism
narcotize

N

narrative
n. account
n. data
n. description
n. speech
n. speech perception
n. speech perception impairment
n. therapy
narrow
straight and n.
narrow-based gait
narrowed attention span
narrow-minded
nasal inhaler
nasality
assimilated n.
nascentium
national
N. Association of Inpatient Physicians (NAIP)
N. Association of Psychiatric Health Systems (NAPHS)
N. Association of Social Workers
N. Association of Veterans Affairs Chiefs of Psychiatry (NAVACP)
N. Center for Health Statistics
n. character
N. Comorbidity Study (NCS)
N. Depressive and Manic-Depressive Association (NDMDA)
n. epithet
N. Guild of Catholic Psychiatrists (NGCP)
N. Institute of Mental Health (NIMH)
N. Institute of Mental Health-Diagnostic Interval Schedule (NIMH-DIS)
N. Institute of Mental Health-Epidemiologic Catchment Area (NIMH-ECA)
N. Institute of Mental Health - Epidemiologic Catchment Area Program
N. Institute of Mental Health-Epidemiologic Catchment Area Program
N. Institute of Neurological and Communicative Disorders and Stroke
N. Mental Health Association (NMHA)
N. Mental Illness Screening Project
N. Psychological Association for Psychoanalysis
N. Rehabilitation Association
N. Resource Center on Domestic Violence

N. Vietnam Veterans Readjustment Study
nativism
nativist theory
natural
n. disaster
n. emotion
n. environment
n. group
n. law
n. selection
n. theology
naturalism
naturalistic
n. design
n. followup study
naturalness
nature
demanding in n.
dilatory n.
heritable n.
human n.
multifaceted n.
negative n.
pathologic n.
pejorative n.
sexual n.
sexually violent n.
n. versus nurture
nature-nurture issue
naturopath
naturopathy
nauseam
ad n.
nauseant
nauseate
nausea and vomiting (N&V)
nauseous
nautomania
NAVACP
National Association of Veterans Affairs Chiefs of Psychiatry
naysayer
nazism, naziism
NCP programming wand
NCS
National Comorbidity Study
ND
nondirective
N-desmethylclozapine
NDMDA
National Depressive and Manic-Depressive Association
near-death experience
neatly groomed
nebbish
nebulous

necessary
    as n.
    n. condition
    n. task
necessitate
necessitous
necessity
    medical n.
neck
    bent-over n.
    buffalo n.
    n. reflex
    stiff n.
    wry n.
necking
necromancy
necromania
necromimesis
necrophagous
necrophile
necrophilia, necrophilism, necrophily
necrophilous
necrosadism
necrosis
    n. negation
    neuronal n.
    occlusal n.
need
    achievement n. (n-Ach)
    n. for admiration
    affective n.
    affiliation n.
    blithely ignored n.
    n. for care
    certificate of n.
    changing n.
    clinical n.
    cognitive n.
    community n.
    n. for constant attention
    n. to control
    diverse n.
    emotional n.
    esteem n.
    excessive n.
    exhibitionist n.
    existence n.
    felt n.
    gambling n.
    geriatric n.
    harm-avoidance n.
    hierarchy of n.

    identity n.
    inner n.
    instinct n.
    instrumental n.
    love n.
    oral n.
    personal n.
    physiological n.
    primary n.
    psychological n.
    n. for punishment
    repressed n.
    seclusion n.
    n. for sleep
    submerged individual n.
    succorance n.
    n. tension
    togetherness n.
    transcendence n.
    unmet dependency n.
needed
    as n. (prn, PRN)
need-fear dilemma
needle
    contaminated n.
    dirty n.
    hypodermic n.
    n. sharing
    n. stick
    n. track
    n. user
needle-related HIV risk behavior
needless repetition
need-press method
nefarious
Neftel disease
negate
negation
    delire de n.
    delirium of n.
    n. delusion
    delusion of n.
    n. of the ego
    insanity of n.
    necrosis n.
negative
    n. affect
    n. attitude
    n. behavior
    n. body image
    n. change
    n. command

N

NOTES

negative *(continued)*
    n. conditioning
    n. conditioning for sleep
    n. correlation
    n. delusion
    n. diagnosis
    n. emotion
    n. emotionality
    n. eugenics
    n. evaluation
    n. expectation
    n. factor
    false n.
    n. feedback
    n. feeling
    guaiac n.
    n. hero
    n. immunosuppressive effect
    n. judgment
    n. life event
    n. mood induction
    n. mood state
    n. nature
    n. Oedipus
    n. outcome
    n. peer interaction
    n. picture-caption pair
    n. practice
    n. predictive power
    n. quality
    n. reinforcement
    n. reinforcer
    n. relation
    n. relationship
    n. response
    n. ruler of the soul
    n. score
    n. scotoma
    n. self-comparison
    n. self-concept
    n. self-image
    n. symptom
    n. symptomatology
    n. symptom dimension
    n. therapeutic reaction
    n. transference
    true n.
    n. utilitarianism
    n. variation
    n. voice
negative-affect alcoholism
negatively
    n. bathmotropic
    n. correlated region
negative-symptom schizophrenia
negativism
    active n.
    adolescent n.

    catatonic n.
    command n.
    extreme n.
    sexual n.
    toddler n.
negativistic
    n. behavior
    n. bias
    n. personality disorder
    n. response
negativity
    endogenous n.
neglect
    adult survivor of n.
    child n.
    n. of child
    n. of duty
    elder adult n.
    emotional n.
    family n.
    hemispatial arousal n.
    history of n.
    maternal n.
    n. measure
    organic n.
    parent n.
    paternal n.
    perceived n.
    problems related to n.
    sensory n.
    spatial n.
    survivor of n.
    n. syndrome
    unilateral organic n.
    unilateral spatial n.
    unilateral visual n.
    visual n.
neglecta
    self-inflicted dermatitis n.
neglected child
neglectful
negligence
    contributory n.
    gross n.
    professional n.
negligent
negligible routine
negotiable
negotiate
negotiating
    n. goals skills
    n. language
    n. routines skills
    n. rules skills
negotiation
    contract n.
    problem-solving n.
negrophile

nemesis
NEO
    neuroticism, extroversion, openness
neoassociationism
neoatavism
neoconnectionism
neocortex
neocortical
    n. association area
    n. region
neofreudian
neographism
neography
neo-hippocratic medicine
neo-kraepelian classification
neolalia
neolallism
neolocal family
neologism
neomimism
neomnesis
neomyerian era
neonatacide
neonatal
neonatorum
    myotonia n.
    tetanus n.
neo-Nazi gang member
neophasia
    polyglot n.
neophilia
neophilism
neophrenia
neophyte
neoplasia
neoplasm
    malignant brain n.
neopsychic
neosleep
neoteny
nepenthe
nepenthic
nepotism
nerd
nerve
    accommodation of n.
    acoustic n.
    auditory n.
    autonomic n.
    n. cell death
    n. cell survival
    n. conduction

    n. conduction study
    n. conduction velocity
    cranial n.
    n. deafness
    efferent n.
    facial n.
    n. force
    n. gas
    n. graft
    grate on the n.'s
    gustatory n.
    n. loss
    motor n.
    n. pain
    n. root
    sensory n.
    trigeminal n.
    vagus n.
    vestibular n.
    war of n.'s
nerveless
nerve-point massage
nerve-racking
nervimotility
nervimotion
nervimotor
nervine
nervios
    ataque de n.
nervosa
    anorexia n. (AN)
    bulimia n.
    chronic anorexia n.
    dysphagia n.
    dysphoria n.
nervosus
    status n.
nervous
    n. asthma
    n. bladder
    n. breakdown
    n. chill
    n. clucking
    n. consumption
    n. debility
    n. depression
    n. disease
    n. exhaustion
    n. fatigue
    n. gastritis
    n. giggling
    n. impulse

N

NOTES

nervous *(continued)*
    n. indigestion
    n. laugh
    n. stomach
    n. system
    n. tension
    n. vomiting
nervousness
nervy
nest
    empty n.
    n. syndrome
network
    artificial neural n.
    Body Awareness Resource N.
      (BARNY)
    communication n.
    cortical n.
    delusional n.
    Drug Abuse Warning N. (DAWN)
    family support n.
    fragmented social n.
    interpersonal n.
    kinship n.
    neural n.
    Practice Research N.
    n. therapy
networking
Neumann syndrome
neural
    n. activation
    n. darwinism
    n. deficit
    n. efficiency
    n. mechanism
    n. network
    n. plasticity
    n. structure
    n. substrate
    n. system
neuralgia
    atypical n.
    epileptiform n.
    facial n.
    n. facialis vera
    Fothergill n.
    glossopharyngeal n.
    hallucinatory n.
    idiopathic n.
    intercostal n.
    migrainous n.
    periodic migrainous n.
    reminiscent n.
    stump n.
    suboccipital n.
    supraorbital n.
    symptomatic n.
    trigeminal n.

neuralgic pain
neuralgiform
neuramebimeter
neuranagenesis
neurapraxia
neurasthenia
    acoustic n.
    aviator's n.
    experimental n.
    gastric n.
    n. gravis
    n. neurotic disorder
    n. praecox
    primary n.
    professional n.
    pulsating n.
    sexual n.
    traumatic n.
neurasthenic
    n. helmet
    n. neurosis
    n. personality
    n. psychoneurosis
    n. psychoneurosis reaction
    n. psychoneurotic reaction
neuremia
neurergic
neurexeresis
neurexin
neuriatria, neuriatry
neurility
neurimotility
neurimotor
neuritic
    n. atrophy
    n. plaque
neuriticum
    atrophoderma n.
neuritis, pl. **neuritides**
    axial n.
    central n.
    descending n.
    Eichhorst n.
    endemic n.
    interstitial n.
    Leyden n.
    multiple n.
    optic n.
    parenchymatous n.
    peripheral n.
    segmental n.
    suboccipital n.
    toxic n.
    traumatic n.
neuroadaptation
neuroallergy
neuroanalysis

neuroanatomic
  n. circuit
  n. connection
neuroanatomy
  behavioral n.
neuroaugmentation
neuroaugmentive
neurobehavioral
  n. consequence
  n. feature
  n. function
  n. readaptation
  n. symptom
  n. syndrome
neurobiochemistry
neurobiological
  n. cause
  n. mechanism
  n. perspective
neurobiology
  behavioral n.
  n. of early childhood development
neurobiotactic movement
neuroborreliosis
neurochemical
  n. change
  n. disequilibrium
  n. interaction
  n. pathway
  n. research
neurochemistry
  behavioral n.
neurocirculatory
  n. asthenia
  n. psychogenic disorder
neurocladism
neurocognition
neurocognitive
  n. alteration
  n. deficit
  n. disorder
  n. impairment
  n. index
  n. information
  n. measure
  n. process
neurocristopathy
neurodegeneration
neurodegenerative
  n. disease
  n. process

neurodevelopmental
  n. disorder
  n. dysfunction
  n. pattern
  n. telencephalic ontogenic process
neurodynia
neuroethology
neurofeedback training (NT)
neurogenic
  n. atrophy
  n. bladder
  n. hyperventilation
  n. reaction
  n. shock
  n. shock syndrome
neurogenous
neurogram
neurography
neurohormone
neurohumor
neurohumoral
  n. hypothesis
  n. transmission
neurohypophysis
neuroimaging
  n. approach
  n. assessment
  n. manifestation
  structural n.
neuroinduction
neurointerventional
neurokym
neuroleptic
  n. adjunct
  n. agent
  n. anesthesia
  conventional n.
  n. dosage
  n. dose
  n. dose-dependent akathisia
  n. dosing
  n. drug
  n. exposure
  n. malignant syndrome (NMS)
  n. medication
  n. responsivity
  traditional n.
  n. treatment
  n. treatment of childhood conduct
    disorder
  typical n.
  n. use

NOTES

N

neuroleptic-free patient
neuroleptic-induced
    n.-i. acute dystonia
    n.-i. acute movement disorder
    n.-i. akathisia
    n.-i. akinesia
    n.-i. dysphoria
    n.-i. parkinsonism
    n.-i. postural tremor
    n.-i. tardive dyskinesia
neuroleptic-naive patient
neuroleptic-related event
neuroleptic-resistant schizophrenic
neuroleptization
    rapid n.
neurolinguistic
    n. assessment
    n. deficit
    n. programming
neurologic
    n. cognition
    n. disorder
    n. impairment
    n. restitution
neurological
    n. amnesia
    n. condition
    n. control
    n. defect
    n. dysfunction
    n. evaluation
    n. examination
    n. functioning
    n. illness
    n. maturation
neurology
    American Board of Forensic
      Psychiatry and N. (ABFPN)
    American Board of Psychiatry
      and N. (ABPN)
    behavioral n.
neurolysis
neuromessenger
neurometric analysis
neurometrics
neuromimesis
neuromodulator
neuromotor
neuromuscular
    n. rehabilitation
neuromyasthenia
neuron
    A9 n.
    bipolar n.
    cholinergic n.
    cold-sensitive n.
    n. doctrine
    excitability of n.

    frontal lobe interstitial n.
    n. II
    impaired migration of brain n.'s
    locus ceruleus n.
    McCullough-Pitts n.
    nonsynaptic n.
    noradrenergic n.
    presynaptic n.
    projection n.
    sensory n.
    serotonergic n.
    upper motor n.
    warm-sensitive n.
neuronal
    n. activation
    n. activity
    n. circuit
    n. damage
    n. loss
    n. membrane
    n. metabolism
    n. necrosis
    n. plasticity
    n. process
    n. size
    n. somata
neuronopathy
    sensory n.
neuronophage
neuronyxis
neuropathic
    n. diathesis
    n. joint
    n. pain
neuropathogenesis
neuropathologic examination
neuropathology
    Alzheimer disease n.
    molecular n.
neuropathy
    alcoholic peripheral n.
    alcohol-induced peripheral n.
    asymmetric motor n.
    autonomic n.
    buffer n.
    diphtheritic n.
    familial n.
    hypertrophic interstitial n.
    lead n.
    motor dapsone n.
    onion bulb n.
    peripheral autonomic n.
    segmental n.
    symmetric distal n.
    vitamin B12 n.
neuropharmacology
    functional n.
neurophilic

neurophonia
neurophthalmology
neurophysin
neurophysiological
    n. assessment
    n. finding
    n. heterogeneity
    n. study
    n. testing
neurophysiology
neuroplegic
neuroprotective
neuropsychiatric
    n. condition
    n. feature
    n. manifestation
    n. movement disorder
    n. psychiatry
    n. test
neuropsychiatrist (NP)
    American College of N.'s
neuropsychiatry (NP)
    geriatric n.
neuropsychic
neuropsychologic, neuropsychological
    n. area
    n. assessment
    n. battery
    n. characteristic
    n. disorder
    n. domain
    n. evaluation
    n. finding
    n. functioning
    n. impairment
    n. manifestation
    n. measure
    n. performance
    n. resource
    n. test
    n. testing
neuropsychologically relevant task
neuropsychology
    clinical n.
    cognitive n.
neuropsychometric test
neuropsychopathic
neuropsychopathy
neuropsychopharmacology
neuropsychophysiological
neuropsychosis
neuroreceptor imaging

neurorecidive
neurorecurrence
neuroregulator
neurorelapse
neuroscience
    behavioral n.
    cognitive n.
    psychotherapeutic n.
neuroscientist
    clinical n.
neurosis, pl. **neuroses**
    accident n.
    actual n.
    acute conditioned n. (ACN)
    acute posttraumatic n.
    analytic n.
    anancastic n.
    anxiety n.
    artificial n.
    association n.
    asthenic n.
    battle n.
    cardiac n.
    cardiovascular n.
    character n.
    chronic posttraumatic n.
    climacteric n.
    collective n.
    combat n.
    compensation n.
    compulsion n.
    compulsive n.
    conversion hysteria n.
    conversion type hysterical n.
    countertransference n.
    craft n.
    death n.
    decompensative n.
    depersonalization n.
    depressive n.
    dissociative-type hysterical n.
    ego n.
    environmental n.
    esophageal n.
    existential n.
    expectation n.
    experimental n.
    family n.
    fate n.
    fatigue n.
    fixation n.
    functional n.

N

NOTES

neurosis *(continued)*
    generalized anxiety n.
    homosexual n.
    housewife n.
    hypochondriac n.
    hypochondriacal n.
    hysterical n.
    impulse n.
    impulsive n.
    infinity n.
    malignant n.
    menopause n.
    military n.
    mixed n.
    monosymptomatic n.
    motor n.
    neurasthenic n.
    noogenic n.
    obsessional n.
    obsessive-compulsive n.
    occlusal n.
    occupational n.
    oedipal n.
    organ n.
    organic n.
    pain-type anxiety n.
    panic-type anxiety n.
    pension n.
    performance n.
    perhaps n.
    phobic-anxiety-depersonalization n.
    phobic obsessional n.
    postconcussion n.
    posttraumatic n.
    prison n.
    professional n.
    progredient n.
    promotion n.
    psychasthenic n.
    psychoanalytic n.
    railroad n.
    regression n.
    regressive transference n.
    retirement n.
    senile n.
    sexual n.
    situation n.
    situational posttraumatic n.
    success n.
    Sunday n.
    suppression n.
    symptom n.
    transference n.
    traumatic n.
    uprooting n.
    vagabond n.
    vegetative n.
    visceral n.

    war n.
    weekend n.
neurospasm
neurosteroid
neurosthenia
neurostimulator
neurosyphilis
    asymptomatic n.
    cerebral n.
    congenital n.
    ectodermogenic n.
    interstitial n.
    meningeal n.
    parenchymatous n.
    vascular n.
neurotension
neurothekeoma
neurotherapeutics, neurotherapy
neurotic
    n. acting out
    alopecia n.
    n. anxiety state
    n. delinquency
    n. depression
    n. depressive state
    n. direction profile
    n. excoriation
    n. factor
    n. feature
    n. guilt
    n. hysteric disorder
    n. manifestation
    masculine attitude in female n.
    n. mental disorder
    passive-aggressive n.
    n. personality
    n. personality disorder
    n. process
    n. reaction
    n. reaction brain syndrome
    n. resignation
    n. rumination
    n. state with depersonalization
    n. state with depersonalization
      episode
    n. style
neurotica
    alopecia n.
neurotic-depressive reaction
neuroticism
neuroticism, extroversion, openness (NEO)
neuroticum
neurotization
neurotize
neurotmesis
neurotogenic
neurotonic

neurotony
neurotoxic
neurotoxin
    therapeutic botulinum n.
neurotransmission
    chemical n.
    dopamine n.
    dysregulated n.
    serotonergic n.
neurotransmitter
    acetylcholine as n.
    biogenic amine n.
    catecholamine n.
    coexistence of n.
    excitatory n.
    n. metabolite
    peptide n.
    putative n.
    n. receptor
    specific n.
    n. synthesizing enzyme
    n. system
neurotrauma
neurotripsy
neurotrophasthenia
neurotrophic
    brain-derived n.
    neurotrophic atrophy
neurotrophy
neurotropic effect
neurotrosis
neurovegetative
    n. sign
    n. symptom
neutral
    n. attitude
    n. image
    n. material
    n. party
    socially n.
    n. spirit
    n. stimulus
neutrality
    gender n.
    therapeutic gender n.
neutralization rule
neutralize
neutralized anxiety
neutralizer
neutralizing mechanism
never-medicated patient
nevoid amentia

nevropathique
    famille n.
new
    n. age
    n. age suicide prevention
    n. evidence
    N. Hampshire rule
    N. Haven study
    n. identity
    n. normal
    n. responsibility
    n. treatment
    n. wave
    N. York Longitudinal Study
    (NYLS)
newborn
    n. abuse
    n. drug withdrawal
Newcastle classification
new-generation
    n.-g. antipsychotic
    n.-g. antipsychotic drug
newly
    n. abstinent alcoholic
    n. diagnosed
    n. emergent categorical change
new-onset
    n.-o. mental illness
    n.-o. seizure
new-work effort
next
    n. friend
    n. generation
    n. of kin
nexus, pl. nexus
NGCP
    National Guild of Catholic Psychiatrists
NGI, NGRI
    not guilty by reason of insanity
niacin deficiency
Nicaragua
niche
    quiet n.
    social n.
nickname
nicotine
    n. abstinence
    n. abuse
    n. addiction
    n. administration
    n. craving
    n. dependence

N

NOTES

nicotine *(continued)*
    n. gum
    n. habit
    n. inhaler
    n. intoxication
    n. nasal spray
    n. organic brain disorder
    n. patch
    n. pharmacology
    n. poisoning
    n. replacement product
    n. replacement therapy
    n. transdermal system
    n. use
    n. use disorder
    n. user
    n. withdrawal
    n. withdrawal symptom
nicotine-induced disorder
nicotine-related
    n.-r. disorder NOS
    n.-r. disorder, not otherwise
    specified
nicotinic
    n. acid deficiency
    n. cholinergic receptor
    n. receptor blockade
nictation
nictitans
    spasmus n.
nictitate
nictitating spasm
nictitation
NIDA-certified forensic toxicology laboratory
Nielsen syndrome
Niemann-Pick disease
niente
niggling
night
    every n.
    n. fantasy
    n. fear
    n. hospital
    n. pain
    n. palsy
    n. residue
    n. rider
    slept all n. (SAN)
    n. terror
    wedding n.
night-eating syndrome
nightly
nightmare
    n. disorder
    recurrent n.
    vivid n.

nightshade
    deadly n.
    n. poisoning
nighttime
    n. activity
    n. agitation
    n. awakening
nigra
    substantia n.
nihilism
    n. theme
    therapeutic n.
nihilistic delusion
NIMH
    National Institute of Mental Health
NIMH-DIS
    National Institute of Mental Health-
    Diagnostic Interval Schedule
NIMH-ECA
    National Institute of Mental Health-
    Epidemiologic Catchment Area
nine-digit task
Ninjitsu
nipping
nirvana principle
nisus
nitpick
nitpicking
nitrate inhalant
nitrite
    n. headache
    n. inhalant
nitrocellulose
nitrogen
    blood urea n. (BUN)
    n. mustard
    n. narcosis
nitrous oxide dependence
NL
    normal libido
    NL CICI
NLC&C
    normal libido, coitus, and climax
NMHA
    National Mental Health Association
NMI
    no mental illness
NMS
    neuroleptic malignant syndrome
N,N-dimethyltryptamine
NO
    nitric oxide
no
    no friends
    no mental illness (NMI)
    no previous history (NPH)
    no response

no sense
no trauma personality disorder
noc
nocere
primum non n.
nociassociation
nociceptive
n. impulse
nociceptor
noci-influence
nociperception
noctambulation
noctambulism
noctimania
noctis
jus primae n.
nocturna
enuresis n.
jactatio capitis n.
nocturnal
n. agitation
n. confusion
n. diarrhea
n. drinking syndrome
n. eating syndrome
n. emission
n. epilepsy
n. hallucination
n. hemiplegia
n. myoclonus
n. panic attack
n. paralysis
n. paroxysmal dystonia
n. penile tumescence (NPT)
n. penile tumescence study
n. penile tumescence test
n. restlessness
n. seizure
n. sleep episode
n. vertigo
nocturnus
jactatio capitis n.
pavor n.
nocuous
nodal behavior
nodding
n. off
n. spasm
node
noematachograph
noematachometer
noematic

noesis
noetic anxiety
no-fault
no-good
no-holds-barred
noire
bete n.
noise
ambient n.
n. analyzer
background n.
complex n.
n. condition
diagnostic n.
extraneous n.
n. factor
feedback n.
n. figure
multispeaker phonetic n.
phonetic n.
pink n.
random n.
white n.
noiseless
noisiness
noisome
noisy
noli me tangere
nolo contendere
nomad
nomadic lifestyle
nomadism
nomenclature
psychiatric n.
standard psychiatric n.
nominal
n. aphasia
nominalism
nominalist
nominalization
nomogram
d'Ocagne n.
nomograph
nomological
nomothetic approach
non
n. compos mentis
n. possumus
n. sequitur
sine qua n.
non-24-hour sleep-wake syndrome

N

NOTES

nonability
    cognitive n.
nonabrasive
nonacceptable
nonadaptive
nonaddicting
nonaffective
    n. hallucination
    n. psychosis
    n. schematic mental model
nonage
nonaggressive
    n. objectionable behavior
nonaggressive-type undersocialized
  conduct disorder
nonalcoholic
nonattentive
nonautistic
nonaxial
    n. fashion
    n. format
nonbarbiturate
nonbelief
    religious n.
nonbeliever
nonbipolar major depression
nonbizarre
    n. delusion
    n. symptom
noncaloric
noncausal possibility
nonchalance
nonchalant
noncharismatic
noncognitive subscale
noncoherent
noncoital stimulation
noncombatant
noncommissioned officer
noncommittal
noncomparable
noncomplementary role
noncompliance
    medication n.
    n. with medical treatment
noncompliant
noncomprehension
nonconclusive
nonconcur
nonconflicting
nonconformance
nonconformist
nonconformity
nonconfrontational
    n. communication skills
    n. interview
nonconfrontive therapy
nonconsanguineous marriage

nonconsenting
    n. adult
    n. partner
    n. patient
noncontrastive distribution
noncontributory
noncontroversial
nonconvulsive status epilepticus
noncooperative
noncued memory pattern
noncustodial parent
nondeclarative memory
nondefense
nondeficit schizophrenia
nondemented
nondependent adult abuse
nondepressed mood
nondescript
nondirective (ND)
    n. approach
    n. psychotherapy
    n. therapy
nondisclosure
nondiscretionary
nondiscriminatory
nondisease
    psychogenic cardiac n.
nondistinctive feature
nondominant hand
nondopaminergic
nondrinker
non-drug-using
    n.-d.-u. man
    n.-d.-u. woman
nonegalitarian
nonentity
nonesuch
nonevent
nonexistence
nonexistent
nonextrapyramidal neurologic sign
nonfatal
nonfattening
nonfearful panic disorder
nonfeasance
nonfluency
nonfluent
    n. aphasia
    n. aphasic seizure
    n. aphasic speech
nonfocal elevation
nonfunctional
nongambling partner
nongeneral phobic
nongeriatric
nonhazardous
nonhemorrhagic cerebral infarction
nonhereditary

nonhero
nonictal
nonidentical
noninvasive
    n. brain imaging study
    n. operation
noninvolvement
nonjudgmental attitude
nonketotic
non-kraepelinian chronic schizophrenia
nonlanguage cognitive impairment
nonlinear
    n. developmental curve
    n. distortion
nonlinguistic
nonmajor depression
nonmaleficence
nonmedical personnel
nonmoral
nonnarcotic analgesic
nonnegative
nonnegotiable
non-neuroleptic-induced tremor
nonneuronal
nonnormative hair loss
nonobjective
no-nonsense
nonopioid
nonorganic
    n. origin
    n. origin insomnia
    psychogenic paranoid n.
    n. psychosis
    n. steep disorder
nonorgasmic
nonorthodox
no-no tremor
nonparametric tests of significance
nonparaphilic compulsive sexual
  behavior
nonparkinsonian tremor
nonparticipant observer
nonparticipatory
nonpartisan
nonpathological
    n. amnesia
    n. anxiety
    n. dissociation
    n. reaction
    n. sexual fantasy
    n. substance use
nonpersistent

nonperson
nonpharmacologically induced tremor
nonphobic anxiety behavior therapy
nonplus
nonplussed
nonpredictive
nonprescription
    n. drug
    n. drug abuse
    n. drug addiction
nonproband
nonproblematic drinking
nonproductive
    n. activity
    n. behavior
nonpsychotic
    n. Alzheimer patient
    n. anxiety
    n. hallucination
    n. mental disorder
    n. onset of symptoms
    n. posttraumatic brain syndrome
    n. psychiatric disorder
    n. severity psychoorganic
    n. severity psychoorganic syndrome
    n. signs and symptom
    n. unipolar depression
    unspecified mental disorder, n.
nonpsychotropic drug
nonpublic residential treatment center
nonpulsating headache
nonpurging method
nonrandom
    n. mating
    n. rating
nonrapid eye movement (non-REM,
  NREM)
nonreactive depression
nonreader
Non-Reading
nonrecall
nonrecognition
    spatial n.
nonrecurrent
nonreduplicated babbling
nonregressive schizophrenia
non-REM
    nonrapid eye movement
      non-REM narcolepsy
nonreporting
nonresidency
nonresistant

N

NOTES

nonrespondent
nonresponder
nonresponsive state
nonrestorative sleep
nonrestraint
nonrestrictive
nonrhythmic
    n. stereotyped motor movement
    n. vocalization
nonrigid
nonschizophrenic illness
nonscientific
nonselective phosphodiesterase inhibitor
nonself source
nonsense
    n. syndrome
    n. in wit
nonsensical
    n. speech
    n. statement
nonsensuous
nonserotonergic
nonsexist
nonsexual boundary violation
nonshivering thermogenesis
nonsignificant
    n. difference
    n. protective effect
    n. trend
nonsmoker (NS)
nonsocial
nonspeaking
nonspecific
    n. abnormality
    n. abnormality on EEG
    n. arousal
    n. benefit
    n. binding
    n. effect
    n. language
    n. neurotic factor
    n. neurotic syndrome (NSN)
    n. research
    n. response rate
    n. stress
    n. syndrome
    n. system
nonstandard
nonstarter
nonstress-induced personality disorder
nonsubstance-induced mental disorder
nonsuffocation panicker
nonsuicidal depressed patient
nonsupport
nonsymbolic
nonsynaptic neuron
nonsystematic schizophrenia
nonsystematized delusion

nontherapeutic
non-tic-related obsessive-compulsive
   disorder
nontoxic
    n. substance
nontraditional lifestyle
nontranssexual cross-gender disorder
nontrivial value
nonturbulence subscale
nonturning against self (NTS)
nonunique
nonuser
    ethanol n.
nonverbal
    n. abstractive ability
    n. behavior
    n. communication
    n. cue
    n. expression
    n. information
    n. intellectual capacity
    n. language
    n. reasoning
    n. synthesizing ability
    n. task
nonviable
nonviolence
nonviolent
    n. behavior
    n. crime
    n. delinquent
    n. stalker
nonvocal communication
noogenic neurosis
nookleptia
noology
noon of life
noopsyche
noose
noothymopsychic ataxia
nootropic
noradrenaline dementia of Alzheimer
   type
noradrenergic
    n. drug
    n. effect
    n. neuron
    n. receptor
    n. synapse
    n. system
    n. system function
norepinephrine
    n. neurotransmitter systems
    peripheral n.
norepinephrine-selective
norm
    age n.
    age-appropriate societal n.

cultural n.
deviation from physiological n.
grade n.
group n.
occupational n.
percentile n.
physiological n.
social n.
societal n.
subculture n.
n. violator
normal
n. affect
n. affective processing
n. aging
n. anxiety
n. autistic phase
n. child
n. childhood development
n. circuitry
n. curve
n. distribution
n. heat defense
n. individual
n. libido (NL)
n. libido, coitus, and climax (NL CICI, NLC&C)
n. limits
n. mentation
n. mood
n. neonatal nursery
n. neurological functioning
new n.
n. personality
n. range
n. range of mood
n. sadness
n. subject
n. thermogenesis
n. thinking
n. transition
n. valence
n. voluntary napping phenomenon
normalcy
normality
normalization principle
normalize
normalized
n. whole brain volume
norm-assertive stance
normative
n. aging process

n. aspect
n. behavior
n. crisis
n. data
n. ethics
normative-referenced
normatologically
normatological research
normatology
normethadone
normothymatic
normotonic
normotype
norms
NOS
not otherwise specified
NOS category
impulse-control disorder NOS
nicotine-related disorder NOS
PDD NOS
personality disorder NOS
phencyclidine-related disorder NOS
noser
nosey (*var. of* nosy)
nosh
nosocomion, nosocomium
nosogenesis
nosogeny
nosological
nosology
psychiatric n.
nosomania
nosophilia
nosotropic
n. drug
n. drug dementia of Alzheimer type
nostalgia
nostalgic
nostalgist
nostomania
nostrum
nosy, nosey
not
n. applicable (N/A)
n. guilty by reason of insanity (NGI, NGRI)
n. otherwise specified (NOS)
n. prisoner of war (NPOW)
n. significant (NS)
n. supportive
n. turning against the self

N

NOTES

notable
notably
notanencephalia
notation
notch
note blindness
noteworthy
not-for-profit hospital
nothing by mouth (NPO, n.p.o., npo)
nothingness
Nothnagel syndrome
noticeable
    least n.
notifiable
notification
notion
    idealistic n.
notoriety
notorious
noumenal
noumenon
nourish
nourishment
nous
nouveau riche
nouvelle vague
novation
novel
    n. antipsychotic
    n. antipsychotic drug
    n. memory task
    n. recall task
    n. stimulus
    n. task performance
novelistic
novelty
    n. seeking
    n. speaking (NS)
novelty-seeking trait
novice
no-win relationship
noxa
noxious
    n. agent
    n. stimulus
NP
    neuropsychiatrist
    neuropsychiatry
NPD
    narcissistic personality disorder
NPH
    no previous history
NPO, n.p.o., npo
    nothing by mouth
NPOW
    not prisoner of war
NPT
    nocturnal penile tumescence

NREM
    nonrapid eye movement
      NREM sleep
NS
    nonsmoker
    not significant
    novelty speaking
NSN
    nonspecific neurotic syndrome
NT
    neurofeedback training
NTS
    nonturning against self
nuance
nubile
nubility
nuchal rigidity
nuclear
    n. depression
    n. family
    n. jaundice
    n. problem
    n. schizophrenia
    n. transsexual
    n. transvestite
    n. war
nuclei (*pl. of* nucleus)
nucleopetal
nucleotide
nucleus, pl. nuclei
    anterior n.
    cell n.
    central tegmental n.
    cerebellar nuclei
    dorsal raphe nuclei
    Edinger-Westphal n.
    ego n.
    hypothalamic n.
    lateral geniculate n. (LGN)
    midline nuclei
    pontine n. (PN)
    pulvinar n.
    reticular thalamic n.
    n. reuniens
    serotonergic raphe nuclei
    spinal trigeminal n.
    subthalamic n.
    superior salivary n. (SSN)
    suprachiasmatic nuclei
    supraoptic n.
nude
nudism
nudist
nudity
nudomania
nugatory
nuisance complaint
nuke

null hypothesis
nullify
numb
    feeling n.
number
    chromosome n.
    Drug Enforcement Administration n.
    (DEA#)
    n. dysgnosia
    n. one
    series of n.'s
    900 n. sex
    n. 3 traced on patient's palm test
number-recency measure
numbing
    emotional n.
    psychic n.
    n. sensation
    sense of n.
    n. symptom
numbness
    emotional n.
    feeling of n.
    psychic n.
    sleep n.
    waking n.
numen
numerical
    n. aptitude (N)
    n. cipher method
    n. reasoning skills
    n. score
    n. thinking
numerologist
numerology
numinous
nunnation
nuptial
nurse
    n. aide
    licensed practical n. (LPN)
    licensed vocational n. (LVN)
    n. practitioner
    psychiatric n.
    registered n. (RN)
    school n.
    n. station
    n. support group
    visiting n.
nursing
    n. home
    n. home placement

    liaison n.
    Master of Science in N. (MSN)
nurturant image
nurture
    nature versus n.
nurturer
nurturing
    n. environment
    n. relationship
nut
    betel n.
nutans
    chorea n.
    epilepsia n.
    spasmus n.
nutation
nutriceutical
    n. data
    n. product
nutrient
nutriment
    emotional n.
Nutri/System diet
nutrition
    American Institute of N. (AIN)
    autotrophic n.
    total parenteral n. (TPN)
    n. treatment
nutritional
    n. adequacy
    n. amblyopia
    n. amenorrhea
    n. change
    n. deficiency
    n. deficiency disorder
    n. edema
    n. insult
    n. marasmus
    n. medicine
    n. polyneuropathy
    n. status
    n. therapy
    n. type cerebellar atrophy
nutritionist
nutritious
nutritive
    n. enema
    n. equilibrium
nutriture
N&V
    nausea and vomiting
nyctalgia

N

NOTES

nyctalopia
nyctaphonia
nyctophilia
nyctophonia
NYLS
New York Longitudinal Study
nymph
nymphet
nympholepsy
nymphomania
active n.
platonic n.

nymphomaniac
nymphomaniacal
nystagmus
downbeat n.
horizontal n.
retraction n.
rotary n.
toxic n.
vertical n.

O-A
  objective-analytic
OA
  object assembly
  Overeaters Anonymous
OAM
  Office of Alternative Medicine
OAP
  occupational ability pattern
oath
  Hippocratic o.
OBD
  organic brain disease
  organic brain disorder
obdormition
obduracy
obdurate
OBE
  out-of-body experience
obedience
  automatic o.
  deferred o.
  destructive o.
obedient behavior
obese
  o. adolescent
  o. body
  o. child
  o. patient
obesity
  adult-onset o.
  alimentary o.
  o. care
  endocrine o.
  endogenous o.
  exogenous o.
  hyperphagic o.
  hypothalamic o.
  lifelong o.
  o. management
  medical complications of o.
  morbid o.
  psychogenic o.
  simple o.
  o. treatment
obesogenous
obfuscate
obfuscation
  terminological o.
obfuscatory
object
  o. addict
  o. addiction
  agent, action, and o.
  o. agnosia

analytic o.
anxiety o.
o. of arousal
o. assembly (OA)
o. attachment
o. attitude
bad o.
o. blindness
o. cathexis
o. choice
o. concept
o. constancy
o. of a delusion
feared o.
fetish o.
o. finding
good o.
o. halos
o. identification
o. ill
inappropriate handling of o.'s
indirect o.
o. lesson
o. libido
linkage o.
o. loss
love o.
o. love
luminescence of o.
metal o.
minute o.
o. mouthing
moving o.
paraphiliac o.
part o.
o. permanence
pointed o.
primary transitional o.
o. relation
o. relationship
o. relations theory
religious o.
o. reversal test
secondary transitional o.
sex o.
o. shadow
sharp o.
substitute o.
o. test (OT)
test o.
transitional o.
twirling of o.
objectifying attitude
objection
  moral o.

O

objectionable behavior
objectivation
objective
    o. anxiety
    o. assessment
    behavioral o.
    o. correlative
    o. criticism
    o. examination
    instructional o.
    o. manifestation
    o. measure
    operational o.
    o. orientation
    o. pain
    performance o.
    principal o.
    o. psychobiology
    o. psychology
    o. psychotherapy
    o. reality
    o. scoring
    o. self-awareness
    o. sensation
    o. severity
    o. severity of illness
    o. sign
    social o.
    o. sociogram
    o. symptom
    o. test (OT)
    o. trauma characteristic
    o. type
    o. vertigo
objective-analytic (O-A)
objectivism
objectivity
object-love
    primary o.-l.
objects
objurgate
obligate
obligation
    ethical o.
    family o.
    honor financial o.
    major role o.
    role o.
    therapist o.
obligations
    o. fear
    patient o.
obligatory
    o. occurrence
    o. perception
    o. relay station
oblige
obliquely related idea

obliquity
obliterate
obliterative
oblivion
obliviousness to social cue
oblivious to surroundings
oblongata
    medulla o.
obloquy
obmutescence
obnoxious
obnubilation
OBS
    organic brain syndrome
obscene
    o. expression
    o. gesture
    o. language
    o. phone call
    o. telephone caller
    o. wit
obscenity
obscenity-purity complex
obscurantism
obscure
obscuring fundamental truth
observable disability
observation
    around-the-clock o.
    behavioral o.
    careful o.
    clinical o.
    clinician o.
    close o.
    o. commitment
    continuous o.
    o. delusion
    delusion of o.
    direct o.
    evaluation and o. (E&O)
    longitudinal o.
    participant o.
    o. period
    preclinical o.
    quantified clinical o.
    random o.
    receptive-expressive o. (REO)
    research o.
    serial o.
    systematic quantitative o.
    o. technique
    unselective o.
    in vivo o.
observational
    o. learning
    o. learning theory
    o. method

observer
> o. drift
> hidden o.
> nonparticipant o.
> participant o.
> o. position

obsession
> aggressive o.
> alien o.
> contamination o.
> counting o.
> ego-dystonic o.
> erotic o.
> guilt o.
> hand-washing o.
> impulsive o.
> inappropriate quality of o.
> inhibitory o.
> masked o.
> o. psychasthenia
> pure o.
> quality of o.
> religious o.
> revenge o.
> rooted o.
> rotted o.
> sexual o.
> somatic o.
> suicidal o.
> symmetry o.
> o. syndrome

obsessional
> o. anxiety
> o. brooding
> o. character
> o. compulsive inventory alpha
> o. fascination
> o. feature
> o. idea
> o. impulse
> o. mental image
> o. neurosis
> o. personality
> o. personality disorder
> o. psychoneurosis
> o. psychoneurotic reaction
> o. Q factor
> o. rehearsal
> o. rumination
> o. slowness
> o. state
> o. syndrome

> o. thinking
> o. thought
> o. type

obsessionalism
obsessionality
obsessive
> o. attack
> o. behavior
> o. doubt
> o. fantasy
> o. fear
> o. feeling
> o. feelings of responsibility
> o. impulse
> o. laughter
> o. neurotic style
> o. personality
> o. personality disorder
> o. preoccupation
> o. psychogenic disorder
> o. psychoneurotic reaction
> o. rumination
> o. thought

obsessive-compulsive
> o.-c. behavior
> o.-c. disorder (OCD)
> o.-c. disorder with poor insight type
> o.-c. feature
> o.-c. inventory (OCI)
> o.-c. neurosis
> o.-c. neurotic disorder
> o.-c. personality
> o.-c. personality disorder (OCPD)
> o.-c. psychoneurosis
> o.-c. reaction
> o.-c. symptom

obsessively bitter
obsessiveness
obsessive-ruminative tension state
obsolescence
> role o.

obstacle sense
obstinate progression
obstipation
obstipatio paradoxa
obstreperous
obstruction
> o. box
> o. drive
> o. method

NOTES

O

obstruction *(continued)*
    thought o.
    visual o.
obstructionism
obstruent
obtained finding
obtrude
obtrusive idea
obtundation
    mental o.
obtunded
    mentally o.
obtundent
obturator
obtuse
obtusion
obvious proof
occasional
    o. gambler
    o. inversion
    o. sexual aversion
occipital
    o. association
    o. association cortical area
    o. cortex
    o. cortex tissue
    o. lobe
    o. sulcus
occipitotemporal cortex
occiput
occlusal
    o. necrosis
    o. neurosis
occlusion
    artery o.
occlusive meningitis
occult
    o. blood
    o. head trauma
occultism
occupancy
    D_2 o.
    preferential o.
    receptor o.
occupation
    British Manual of the Classification
      of O.'s
    sedative o.
    stimulating o.
occupational
    o. ability
    o. ability pattern (OAP)
    o. activity
    o. adjustment
    o. analysis
    o. checklist (OCL)
    o. choice
    o. cramp

    o. crisis
    o. deafness
    o. delirium
    o. disease
    o. drinking
    o. dysfunction
    o. exposure
    o. family
    o. function
    o. functioning
    o. hazard
    o. hierarchy
    o. history (OH)
    o. impairment
    o. inhibition
    o. interaction
    o. inventory
    o. level
    o. neurosis
    o. neurotic disorder
    o. norm
    o. problem
    o. psychiatry
    o. psychogenic disorder
    o. psychoneurosis
    o. rehabilitation
    o. skill training
    o. spasm
    o. stability
    o. stress
    o. test
    o. therapist (OT)
    o. therapy (OT)
    o. tic
occupationally effective
occurrence
    obligatory o.
OCD
    obsessive-compulsive disorder
    anterior capsulotomy for treatment
      of OCD
    anterior cingulotomy for treatment
      of OCD
    augmentation agent overactivity in
      OCD
    behavioral avoidance test for OCD
    bilateral anterior capsule deep brain
      stimulation for OCD
    caudate nucleus overactivity in
      OCD
    cingulate gyrus overactivity in
      OCD
    OCD improvement
    infection-triggered OCD
    limbic leucotomy for treatment of
      OCD
    OCD patient
    OCD responsiveness

ritual injury in OCD
OCD spectrum disorder
thalamus overactivity in OCD
oceanic feeling
ochlomania
OCI
  obsessive-compulsive inventory
OCL
  occupational checklist
ocnophile
O'Connor vs Donaldson
OCPD
  obsessive-compulsive personality
  disorder
ocular
  o. apraxia
  o. bobbing
  o. dominance column
  o. flutter
  o. migraine
  o. migraine headache
  o. paralysis
ocularis
  angor o.
oculomotor
  o. apraxia
  o. disturbance
  o. response
odaxesmus
odaxetic
ODD
  oppositional defiant disorder
odd
  o. behavior
  o. belief
  logarithm of o.'s (LOD)
  o. man out
  o.'s ratio (OR)
  o. speech
odd-eccentric cluster
odd-even method reliability coefficient
oddity
odious
odium
odogenesis
odonterism
odontoneuralgia
odontoprisis
odor
  body o. (BO)
  o. fear
odorant

odoriferous
odorivection
odorous
ODS
  Operation Desert Storm
odynometer
odynophagia
odynophonia
Odysseus pact
odyssey
oedipal
  o. behavior
  o. complex
  o. conflict
  o. neurosis
  o. period
  o. phase
  o. situation
  o. stage
oedipism
Oedipus
  complete O.
  O. complex
  inverted O.
  negative O.
  O. period
OEM
  open-end marriage
oenomania
Oenothera biennis
off
  o. balance
  better o.
  blow o.
  carry o.
  cooling o.
  o. effect
  fall o.
  o. glide
  o. guard
  kiss o.
  knock o.
  o. label indication
  laugh o.
  o. limits
  nodding o.
  pop o.
  o. putting
  rip o.
  shrug o.
  slough o.
  throw o.

NOTES

O

off *(continued)*
    touch o.
    o. the wagon
offbeat
offender
    adolescent sex o.
    habitual o.
    juvenile o.
    mentally disordered o.
    mentally disordered sex o. (MDSO)
    registered sex o.
    repeat sex o.
    sex o. (SO)
    status o.
    Task Force on Sexually
      Dangerous O.'s
    violent o.
offending agent
offense
    alcohol o.
    alcohol-related o.
    capital o.
    first o.
    sex o.
    statutory o.
    violent o.
offensive
    o. chat-room dialogue
office
    O. of Alternative Medicine (OAM)
    O. of Juvenile Justice and
      Delinquency Prevention
    O. of National Drug Control
      Policy
    o. seclusion
officer
    juvenile o.
    noncommissioned o.
    probation o.
officinalis
    Melissa o.
officious
offish
offscouring
offset
offsetting
off-the-cuff
off-the-record
off-the-wall
off-time
    lengthened o.-t. (LOT)
off-track betting
ogle
ogler
ogre
OH
    occupational history

OHIO
    only handle it once
    OHIO rule
Ohm law
OI
    orientation inventory
oikiomania
oikiotropic
oikofugic
oikomania
oinomania
ojo
    mal de o.
olanzapine-associated DKA
old
    o. age
    o. guard
    o. maid
    o. money
old-age
    o.-a. dementia
    o.-a. imbecility
    o.-a. psychiatry
    o.-a. therapy
old-fashioned
old-sergeant syndrome
olfactie, olfacty
olfaction
olfactism
olfactoria
olfactory
    o. amnesia
    o. anesthesia
    o. aura
    o. erotism
    o. hallucination
    o. hyperesthesia
    o. hypesthesia
    o. pathway
    o. psychomotor seizure
    o. reference syndrome
    o. stimulation
olfacty
olfacty *(var. of olfactie)*
oligergasia
oligodendrite
oligodendroblastoma
oligodendrocyte
oligodendroglioma
oligodipsia
oligodontia
oligomania
oligomenorrhea
oligophrenia
    moral o.
    phenylpyruvic o.
    polydystrophic o.
oligophrenic

oligopsychia
oligoria
oligosthenic
oligothymia
oligothymic
oligotrophia
oligotropy
olivopontocerebellar
ombudsman
OMC
> short orientation-memory-concentration test

OMD
> organic mental disorder

Omega sign
omego melancholium
omen
> o. formation

ominous
omission
> o. of duty
> o. in wit

omissive
omnipotence
> illusion of o.
> magic o.
> thought o.
> o. of thought

omnipotency
omnipotent infantile sadism
omnipotently
omnipresent dysphoria
omniscience
omniscient
omnisexual
omnisexuality
omophagia
OMS
> organic mental syndrome

on
> carry on
> cast on
> on edge
> on effect
> hang on
> set eyes on
> set foot on
> on the skin
> on top of the world
> on the wagon

onanism
> buccal o.

onanist
once
> only handle it o. (OHIO)

oncocytoma
oncogene
Ondine curse
one
> day o.
> loss of loved o.
> number o.
> o. own control

one-dimensional
Oneida community
oneiric, oniric
> o. delirium

oneirique
> delire o.

oneirism
oneiroanalysis
oneirocritical
oneirodelirium
oneirodynia
> o. activa
> o. gravis

oneirogenic
oneirogmus
oneirogonorrhea
oneirogonos
oneiroid
> o. schizophrenia
> o. state

oneirology
oneiromancy
oneironanalysis
oneironosus
oneirophrenia
oneiroscopy
one-night stand
one-on-one supervision
onerous
oneself
> play with o.
> will to be o.

one-sided
one-to-one situation
one-track mind
one-upmanship
one-way mirror
ongoing
> o. cognitive process
> o. neuroleptic treatment

oniomania

O

NOTES

onion bulb neuropathy
oniric, oneiric
online
    o. counseling
    o. education
    o. encounter
    International Society for Mental Health O. (ISMHO)
    o. mental health care
    o. pharmacy
    o. pornography
    o. relationship
    o. sexual activity
    o. sexual addiction
    o. sexual experience
    o. sexual fantasy
    o. support community
    o. support group
    o. therapy
only
    o. handle it once (OHIO)
    o. handle it once rule
onology
onomatomania
onomatopoeia
onomatopoiesis
onotoanalysis
onotogenesis
onset
    abrupt o.
    acute o.
    adolescent o.
    age at o.
    o. of agitation
    childhood o.
    dementia of the Alzheimer type, with early o.
    dementia of the Alzheimer type, with late o.
    initial o.
    insidious o.
    mood disorder with postpartum o.
    o. of sleep
    sudden o.
    o. of symptoms
on-task behavior
on-the-job bias
on-the-wagon
ontoanalysis
ontogenesis
ontogenic process
ontogeny
    psychic o.
ontology
onus
onychophagia
onychophagy
onychotillomania

OOB
    out of bed
OOC
    out of control
oophagia
OP
    outpatient
opacity
open
    o. awareness
    o. discussion
    o. group
    o. head injury
    o. horizon
    o. hospital
    o. hostility
    o. juncture
    o. marriage
    o. mind
    o. place
    o. posture
    o. quotient
    o. seclusion restriction
    o. up
    o. ward
open-cue situation
open-door
    o.-d. hospital
    o.-d. policy
open-ended
    o.-e. interview
    o.-e. question
    o.-e. session
open-end marriage (OEM)
opener
opening
    o. move
    o. sound
    o. statement
open-label trial
openness to experience
open-ward status
operandi
    modus o.
operant
    autoclitic o.
    o. behavior
    o. behaviorism
    o. conditioning
    o. learning
    o. level
    o. method
    o. reserve
    o. therapy
operation
    O. Anaconda
    concrete o.
    decompression o.

O. Desert Storm (ODS)
dissectible cognitive o.
effector o.
formal o.
logical o.
motivating o.
noninvasive o.
o.'s research (OR)
security o.
sensor o.

operational
o. definition
o. evaluation
o. fatigue
o. objective
o. planning
o. research
o. sign
o. thought

operative behavior
operatoire
pensee o.
ophidiomania
ophidiophilia
ophryosis
ophthalmia
ophthalmic
o. migraine
ophthalmoplegic migraine
opiate
o. abstinence
o. abstinence syndrome
o. addiction
o. antagonist
o. overdose
o. poisoning
o. receptor

opiate-free urine screen
opiate-induced emergency
opinion
formed o.
personal o.
o. poll
o. questionnaire
second o.
o.'s toward adolescents (OTA)
opinionated
opinionnaire
opioid
o. abuse
o. antagonist
o. dependence

endogenous o.
illicit o.
o. intoxication
o. intoxication delirium
kappa o.
legal o.
o. overdose
o. peptide
o. poisoning
o. receptor
o. substitute
o. tolerance
o. use
o. use disorder
o. withdrawal

opioid-dependent
o.-d. mother
o.-d. patient
opioid-induced
o.-i. delirium
o.-i. psychotic disorder
o.-i. sexual dysfunction
opiomania
opiophagism
opiophagorum
opisthoporeia
opisthotonic
opisthotonoid
opium (O)
o. addiction
belladonna and o. (B&O)
Boston o.
cannabis and o.
crude o.
o. den
o. deodoratum
deodorized o.
o. dependence
granulated o.
o. granulatum
gum o.
o. habit
lettuce o.
o. poisoning
o. poppy
powdered o.
pudding o.
o. pulveratum
o. tincture
o. use
o. wine

opiumism

NOTES

O

opotherapy
Oppenheim
    O. syndrome
opportunist
opportunity
    educational o.
    equal employment o.
    gambling o.
    sexual o.
    social o.
    o. for theft
opposed
    diametrically o.
opposite
    o. affect state
    o. biological sex
    o. phase
    polar o.
    relational o.
    o. sex peer
    o. sex sexual experience
opposition
    o. breathing
    passive o.
    o. respiration
oppositional
    o. attitude
    o. behavior
    o. defiance
    o. defiant disorder (ODD)
    o. disorder
    o. disorder of adolescence
    o. disorder of childhood
    o. thinking
oppress
oppression
oppression-artifact disorder
oppressive
opprobrium
    public o.
opsomania
optative
optesthesia
optic
    o. agnosia
    o. agraphia
    o. aphasia
    o. ataxia
    o. illusion
    o. neuritis
optical
    o. alexia
    o. illusion
    o. projection
Optifast diet
optimal
    o. care
    o. development

    o. diet
    o. group size
    o. interpersonal distance
    o. method
    o. relational functioning
    o. relationship
    o. therapeutic intervention
    o. treatment
    o. treatment strategy
optimal-stimulation principle
optimism
    excessive o.
    oral o.
    period of o.
    therapeutic o.
optimistic
    o. atmosphere
    o. expectation
optimize
optimum dose
option
    activity, interest, o. (AIO)
    therapeutic o.
    treatment o.
opulent
OR
    odds ratio
    operations research
oral
    o. administration
    o. aggressive
    o. anxiety
    o. apraxia
    o. behavior
    o. biting period
    o. character
    o. coitus
    o. communication
    o. contraceptive
    o. crisis
    o. dependence
    o. dose
    o. ego
    o. erotism
    o. fixation
    o. gratification
    o. history
    o. impulse
    o. language
    o. language skill
    o. need
    o. optimism
    o. orientation
    o. personality
    o. pessimism
    o. phase
    o. primacy
    o. route

o. sadism
o. sensory ability
o. sex
o. stage
o. stage psychosexual development
o. state
o. stereotypy
o. stimulation
o. supplementation
o. test
o. triad

oral-aggressive character
oral-eroticism phase
oral-genital contact
oral-incorporative phase
oralism
orality
oral-nasal acoustic ratio
oral-passive character
oral-receptive character
oral-sadistic cathexis
oral-sensory stage
orange

Agent O.

Orbeli effect
orbicularis

sign of the o.
tic o.

orbit
orbital

o. decompression
o. prefrontal cortex

orbitofrontal

o. activity
o. area
o. cortex
o. pathway
o. region

orbitomedial syndrome
orchidomania
order

birth o.
chronological o.
court o.
o. of extinction
outpatient commitment o.
pecking o.
putting affairs in o.
rank o.
restraining o.

ordering and arranging

orderliness

compulsive o.
organic o.
o. preoccupation

orderly behavior
ordinal position
ordinate
ordure
orectic
Oregon Adolescent Depression Project
orexia
orexigenic
oreximania
orexis
organ

auxiliary o.
end o.
o. erotism
executive o.
genital o.
o. inferiority
o. inferiority complex
o. jargon
o. libido
o. neurosis
o. pleasure
o. speech
target o.
o. transplantation

organic

o. affective syndrome
o. amnesia
o. amnestic syndrome
o. anxiety
o. anxiety disorder
o. approach
o. brain disease (OBD)
o. brain disorder (OBD)
o. brain dysfunction
o. brain syndrome (OBS)
o. contracture
o. deafness
o. defect
o. delirium
o. delusion
o. delusional disorder
delusional transient o.
o. dementia
o. dyscontrol
o. epilepsy
o. etiology
o. factor

NOTES

O

organic *(continued)*
    o. hallucination
    hallucinatory transient o.
    o. hallucinosis
    o. hallucinosis syndrome
    o. headache
    o. impairment
    o. impotence
    o. jargon
    o. language
    o. mental disorder (OMD)
    o. mental syndrome (OMS)
    o. mood disorder
    o. mood syndrome
    o. neglect
    o. neurosis
    o. orderliness
    o. pain
    o. persona
    o. personality disorder
    o. pleasure
    o. psychiatric disorder
    o. psychiatry
    psychoactive substance-induced o.
    o. psychosis
    o. psychosis drug intoxication
    o. psychosyndrome
    o. psychotic condition
    o. psychotic state
    o. reaction
    o. repression
    o. speech
    o. therapy
    o. variable
    o. vertigo

organica
    alalia o.

organic-affective syndrome
organic-functional dilemma
organicism
organicist
organicity
    o. screening

organism
    empty o.

organismic
    o. causation
    o. psychology
    o. variable

organization
    action o.
    borderline personality o.
    care o.
    cytoarchitectural o.
    defense o.
    disrupted sleep o.
    health maintenance o. (HMO)
    hierarchical o.

    Inter-American Council of Psychiatric O.'s (IACPO)
    Joint Commission on Accreditation of Healthcare O.'s (JCAHO)
    Justice in Mental Health O.
    libido o.
    life o.
    memory o.
    mental patient o.
    peer review o. (PRO)
    perceptual o.
    personality o.
    preferred provider o.
    pregenital o.
    o. preoccupation
    Professional Standards Review O. (PSRO)
    psychic o.
    religious o.
    sleep o.
    social welfare o.
    spatial o.
    temporal o.
    topographical o.
    trait o.
    welfare o.
    World Health O. (WHO)

organizational
    o. chaos
    o. entry
    o. plan
    o. psychology
    o. skills
    o. structure

organized
    o. activity
    o. care psychiatry
    o. play
    o. religion

organizer
    decision-making o.

organizing principle
organogenesis
organogenetic, organogenic
organoleptic
organotherapy
orgasm
    coital o.
    o. delay
    dry o.
    o. dysfunction
    female o.
    inhibited female o.
    inhibited male o.
    male o.
    multiple spontaneous o.'s
    paradoxical o.
    pharmacogenic o.

premature female o.
premature male o.
o. satisfaction
vaginal o.

orgasmic
o. anhedonia
o. capacity
o. cephalalgia
o. deficiency
o. deficiens
o. disorder
o. dysfunction
o. phase
o. phase of sexual response cycle
o. platform
o. problem
o. reconditioning

orgasmus deficiens
orgastic
o. impotence
o. potency
o. release

orgiastic
orgone therapy
orgy
oriental nightmare-death syndrome
orientation
academic o. (AO)
autopsychic o.
behavioral research o.
biologic research o.
bisexual o.
cognitive research o.
coronal o.
o. cue
delusion of o.
o. disorder
disturbed o.
double o.
ego-dystonic o.
exploitative o.
family system research o.
female system research o.
gender o.
goal o.
hedonistic o.
heterosexual o.
hoarding o.
homosexual o.
ideological o.
illusion of o.
impaired o.

instrumental-relativist o.
interpersonal research o.
o. inventory (OI)
judgment of line o. (JLO)
law-and-order o.
loss of o.
objective o.
oral o.
psychodynamic research o.
reality o. (RO)
receptive o.
religious o.
reverse o.
reversed o.
sagittal o.
same-sex o.
o. session
sexual o.
spatial o.
spiritual o.
subjective o.
temporal o.
theoretical o.
transverse o.
whole focus o.

orientation-memory-concentration test
oriented
alert and o.
alert, cooperative, and o. (ACO)
o. and alert times four
o. and alert times three
o. in all spheres
awake, alert, and o. (AAO)
past o.
o. to person, place, and time
present o.
reality o. (RO)
o. to time and place
well o.

orienting
o. reflex
o. response

orifice
body o.
o. picking

origin
bleeding of undetermined o. (BUO)
bruising of undetermined o. (BUO)
culture of o.
insomnia due to nonorganic o.
intrapsychic o.
language o.

NOTES

O

origin *(continued)*
    nonorganic o.
    psychodynamic o.
    psychogenic o.
    tic disorder of organic o.
    undetermined o. (UO)
    o. of violence
original
    o. incident
    o. response
    o. trauma
originaria
    paranoia o.
ornery
ornithinemia
ornithomania
orofacial dyskinesia
orofaciodigital syndrome
orogenital
    o. activity
    o. sex
orphan
    o. drug
    o. train
    O. Train Heritage Society
orthergasia
orthobiosis
orthodox
orthogenesis
orthogenetic
orthogenic
orthogenics
orthogonal
    o. combination
    o. depression factor
orthograde degeneration
orthographic
orthography
orthomolecular
    o. psychiatry
orthonasia
orthophrenia
orthopsychiatry
orthostasis
orthostatic
    o. hypertension
    o. hypotension
orthosympathetic
orthothaniasia
oscillating tremor
oscillation
    behavioral o.
oscillations of attachment
osmoceptor
osmodysphoria
osmolagnia
osmolality
osmoreceptor

osmotherapy
osphresia
osphresiolagnia
osphresiophilia
osphresis
ossification
ossify
ostentatious
osteoplastic
osteoporosis
    posttraumatic o.
    senile o.
ostracism
    peer o.
ostracize
OT
    objective test
    object test
    occupational therapist
    occupational therapy
OTA
    opinions toward adolescents
OTC
    over the counter
Othello
    O. delusion
    O. syndrome
other
    avoidance of o.'s (AO)
    danger to o.'s
    dangerous to o.'s
    o. directed
    harming o.'s
    illusion of power over o.'s
    o. interpersonal problem
    intimidating o.'s
    locus of control-powerful o.'s
      (LOC-PO)
    relating to o.'s
    significant o.
    o. specified family circumstance
    o. type personality disorder
    o. woman
other-directed person
otiose
otohemineurasthenia
otoneurasthenia
Ouija board
oust
out
    acting o.
    asocial acting o.
    o. of bed (OOB)
    blacking o.
    o. of the blue
    o. of bounds
    o. of character
    chill o.

o. of the closet
o. of control (OOC)
dry o.
exacerbation of acting o.
excessive acting o.
falling o.
freaked o.
hang o.
irresponsible acting o.
kick o.
make o.
neurotic acting o.
odd man o.
passive-aggressive acting o.
read o.
roached o.
rub o.
rule o. (R/O)
sexual acting o.
shut o.
sign o.
sit o.
skip o.
social acting o.
speak o.
spell o.
stand o.
take o.
talk o.
talking it o.
throw o.
time o.
o. of touch
o. of touch with reality
tripped o.
violent acting o.
washed o.
o. of wedlock
wipe o.
working o.

outburst
aggressive o.
o. of anger
anger o.
angry o.
behavioral o.
explosive o.
impulsive o.
tearful o.
temper o.
uncharacteristic o.

verbal o.
violent o.
outcast
social o.
outcome
o. assessment
clinical o.
o. domain
functional o.
geriatric health o.
global o.
health o.
o. of illness
long-term o.
o. measure
multidimensional assessment of o.
negative o.
primary efficacy o.
psychosocial symptom o.
o. study
therapeutic o.
treatment o.
untoward o.
o. variable
well-formed o.
outcome-based therapy
outdoing wit
outer-provider
outframing
outgoing mechanism
outlandish
outlet
creative o.
o. for success
outlier
outlook
pessimistic o.
out-of-body
o.-o.-b. experience (OBE)
o.-o.-b. sensation
out-of-control
o.-o.-c. adolescent
o.-o.-c. behavior
out-of-mind sensation
outpatient (OP)
o. basis
o. care
o. clinic
o. commitment order
o. intervention
o. mental health clinic setting
o. patient population

NOTES

O

outpatient *(continued)*
    o. program
    o. psychiatric help seeking
    o. psychotherapy
    o. treatment
outpatient-based psychiatry
output
    o. disability
    energy o.
    fluid o.
    maximum acoustic o.
    reduced verbal o.
    sympathetic o.
outrage
    moral o.
outrageous
outre
outreach
    assertive o.
    o. program
    o. services
outside
    o. activity
    o. activity avoidance
    o. control
    o. density
    o. force
    o. influence
    o. the range of normal human
      experience
    o. stimulus
outward
    o. expression of anger with
      impulsive feature
    o. focus
ovalis
    fenestra o.
over
    bind o.
    blow o.
    o. the counter (OTC)
    gloss o.
    knock o.
    slough o.
    talk o.
    throw o.
    working o.
overachiever
overact
overactivity
    psychomotor o.
overadequate-inadequate reciprocity
overage
overall
    o. cognitive functioning
    o. cognitive measure
    o. depressive symptom
    o. disability

    o. psychopathology
    o. risk index
overanxious
    o. disorder
    o. disorder of adolescence
    o. disorder of childhood
    o. reaction
overbearance
    phallic o.
overbearing
overbreathing
    voluntary hysterical o.
overburden
overcharged idea
overcome
overcommit
overcommitment
overcompensation
overconcern
overconcrete speech
overconfident
overconscientious personality disorder
overconsciousness
overconsolidation of memory
overcontrolled eating plan
overcorrection
overcrowding
overdependence
    social o.
overdependency
overdependent attitude
overdetermination
overdiagnosis
overdominance
overdominant
overdose
    accidental o.
    amphetamine o.
    barbiturate o.
    benzodiazepine o.
    down from o.
    drug o.
    fatal o.
    fluoxetine o.
    hallucinogenic o.
    heroin o.
    lethal o.
    opiate o.
    opioid o.
    paregoric o.
    sedative o.
    stimulant o.
    talk-down from o.
Overeaters Anonymous (OA)
overeating
over-elaborate speech
overestimation
overexertion

overextension
overflow
    o. encopresis
    o. incontinence
overidentification
overinclusion
overinclusiveness
overindependence
overindulge
overinvolvement
overlap
    DSM disorder o.
    symptom o.
overlapping agitation
overlay
    emotional o.
    psychogenic o.
    supratentorial o.
overlearning
overload
    attention o.
    fluid o.
    information o.
    sensory o.
    stimulus o.
overly stimulating treatment
overmanning
overmedicated
overmedication
overmobilization
overoptimistic
overplay
overpopulation
overpower
overprescribed
overproduction
overprotection
    maternal o.
    parental o.
    o. score
overprotective parent
overreaction
    emotional o.
overreactive disorder
overrepresented
    o. characteristic
    o. experience
overresponse
oversee
oversensitive
oversexed
overshadow

overshadowing
    diagnostic o.
oversimplify
oversleeping
oversoul
overstatement
overstay
overstep
overstimulated home life
overstimulation
overstrain
overstress
overt
    o. agitation
    o. behavior
    o. behavior consequences of divorce
    o. compliance
    o. compliance masking covert resistance
    o. criticism
    o. gesture
    o. hallucination
    o. homosexuality
    o. message
    o. rage
    o. response
    o. sensitization
    o. signs of anger
    o. signs of depression
    o. signs of powerlessness
    o. signs of shame
    o. signs of sorrow
    o. weeping
overtalkative
over-the-counter
    o.-t.-c. drug abuse
    o.-t.-c. drug addiction
    o.-t.-c. drug-related disorder
    o.-t.-c. medication
overthrow
overtone
    psychic o.
overture
overvaluation
overvalued
    o. idea
    o. ideation (OVI)
overventilation
overweight
overwhelm
overwhelmed subjectivity

O

NOTES

overwhelming
>   o. anxiety
>   o. childhood experience
>   o. depression
>   o. fatigue
>   o. intimate experience
>   o. stress

overwork fear

overwrought

OVI
>   overvalued ideation

ownership
>   sense of o.

oxidant

oxidase
>   monoamine o. (MAO)
>   platelet monoamine o.

oxidative

oxyaphia

oxyblepsia

oxycephalia

oxycephalic idiot

oxyesthesia

oxygen
>   o. deficiency
>   o. deprivation
>   o. therapy

oxygen-carrying capacity

oxygen-deprived sexual arousal

oxygen-depriving activities

oxygeusia

oxylalia

oxylate

oxyopia

oxyosmia

oxyosphresia

oxypathia

oxypertine

oxyphonia

oxyphresia

ozoline

PA
> paranoia
> passive-aggressive
> physician's assistant
> psychoanalysis
> psychoanalyst
> psychogenic aspermia
> psychosocial assessment

PAB
> positive attention behavior

pace
>> change of p.
>> future p.

pacemaker
>> cerebral p.
>> endogenous circadian p.

pachygyria
pachyleptomeningitis
pachymeningitis
>> hypertrophic cervical p.
>> pyogenic p.

pacification
Pacific Islander
pacificism
pacifist
pacify
pacing
>> p. behavior
>> ceaseless p.
>> restless p.

package-testing
packer
packet
packs per day (PPD)
pact
>> devil's p.
>> homicide-suicide p.
>> Odysseus p.
>> suicide p.

PAD
> primary affective disorder
> psychoaffective disorder

pad
>> visuospatial scratch p.

padded
>> p. cell
>> p. room

paddled
pagan
paganism
paganize
pagophagia
pain
>> abdominal p.
>> anatomic site of p.

> atypical p.
> p. avoidance
> p. behavior
> burning p.
> central p.
> chest p.
> chronic p.
> p. clinic
> p. complaint
> p. control
> core p.
> degree of p.
> deliberate infliction of p.
> diminished response to p.
> p. disorder, chronic
> p. and distress score
> dream p.
> p. dysfunction syndrome (PDS)
> ecstatic p.
> ejaculatory p.
> endogenous p.
> p. exacerbation
> fleeting p.
> functional p.
> gate control theory of p.
> genital p.
> girdle p.
> growing p.
> heterotopic p.
> p. history
> homotopic p.
> hunger p.
> inescapable p.
> p. intensity
> p. intensity threshold
> intermittent p.
> intractable p.
> intractive p.
> law of referred p.
> level of psychological p.
> p. management
> masking p.
> masturbatory p.
> p. mechanism
> mental p.
> mind p.
> myofascial p.
> nerve p.
> neuralgic p.
> neuropathic p.
> night p.
> objective p.
> organic p.
> pathologic p.
> pelvic p.

P

pain *(continued)*
    p. perception
    phantom limb p.
    physical manifestation of p.
    posttraumatic p.
    pounding p.
    prepsychotic p.
    p. presentation
    p. principle
    psychic p.
    psychogenic chest p.
    psychogenic pelvic p.
    psychogenic penis p.
    psychogenic precordial p.
    psychogenic testicular p.
    psychogenic testis p.
    psychogenic uterus p.
    psychological p.
    psychosocial p.
    pulsating p.
    p. questionnaire
    p. reaction
    recalcitrant p.
    p. receptor
    referred p.
    p. relief
    residual p.
    response to p.
    rest p.
    scrotal p.
    searing p.
    secondary p.
    sexual p.
    shooting p.
    somatoform p.
    p. somatoform disorder
    soul p.
    spiritual p.
    stabbing p.
    p. state
    stinging p.
    p. stricken
    subjective p.
    superficial p.
    p. symptom
    p. symptom grouping
    p. threshold
    p. tolerance
    p., touch and stroke psychiatric syndrome
    unendurable psychological p.
    unexplained p.
    unrelenting p.
    vice-like p.
    wandering p.
painful
    p. affect
    p. anesthesia

    p. consequence
    p. feeling
    p. intercourse
    p. memory
    p. paraplegia
    p. point
    p. ritual
    p. stimulus
    p. symptom
    p. thought
paining
painkiller
pain-pleasure principle
painstaking
painter's encephalopathy
painting
    action p.
    finger p.
paint thinner
pain-type
    p.-t. anxiety
    p.-t. anxiety neurosis
pair
    p. bond
    coherent negative picture-caption p.
    coherent positive picture-caption p.
    control picture-caption p.
    irrelevant p.
    negative picture-caption p.
    picture-caption p.
    positive picture-caption p.
    reference picture-caption p.
pair-bond
paired
    p. associates
    p. dreams
paired-associates learning
palatoplegia
palaver
paleopsychology
paleosensation
palikinesia, palicinesia
palimony
palindrome
palindromia
palindromic encephalopathy
palinesthesia
palingnosticum
palingraphia
palinmnesis
palinopsia
palinphrasia palipraxia
paliopsy
paliphrasia
palipraxia
    palinphrasia p.
pallanesthesia
pallesthesia

pallesthetic
palliate
palliative care
pallid
pallidal
    p. cell
    p. syndrome
pallidectomy
pallidoamygdalotomy
pallidoansotomy
pallidotomy
pallidum
pallidus
    globus p.
pallor
palmar reflex
palmesthesia
palmi
palmic
palmist
palmistry
palmodic
palpable liver
palpitant
palpitate
palpitation
palsy
    craft p.
    creeping p.
    lead p.
    night p.
    posticus p.
    pressure p.
    Saturday night p.
    shaking p.
    supranuclear gaze p.
    trembling p.
    wasting p.
palter
paltry
pamoate
pamper
panacea
Panax ginseng
panchreston
pancreatic
pancreatitis
    alcoholic p.
PANDAS
    pediatric autoimmune neuropsychiatric
      disorders associated with streptococcal
      infection

pandemic epidemiology
pandemonium
pander
pandiculation
pandy
panel
    continuous p.
    personality p.
panendoscopy
panesthesia
panethnic
pang
    hunger p.
pangenesis
panglossia
panhandling
panic
    p. attack
    p. attack neurotic anxiety
    p. attack neurotic anxiety state
    p. button
    p. delirium
    p. diathesis
    p. disorder (PD)
    p. disorder with agoraphobia
    p. disorder without agoraphobia
    homosexual p.
    primordial p.
    situational p.
    p. symptom
    p. symptomatology
panic-agoraphobic spectrum
panic-disordered patient
panic-free state
panicker
    nonsuffocation p.
    suffocation p.
panicky voice
panic-spectrum phenomenon
panic-stricken
panic-type
    p.-t. anxiety
    p.-t. anxiety neurosis
Panism
    Peter P.
panky
panoramic memory
panphobic melancholia
panplegia
pan-potency
panpsychism
pansexualism

NOTES

P

pantalgia
pantheism
panthodic
panting
pantomime
panum phenomenon
PAP
    passive-aggressive personality
Papaver somniferum
paper pica
Papez
    P. circle
    P. circuit
    P. theory of emotion
papilla, pl. **papillae**
papillary
papilledema
papillomatosis
PAR
    PAR Admissions Testing program
paraballism
parablepsia
parabrachial area
parabulia
paracenesthesia
paracentesis
paracentral
    p. gray area
    p. scotoma
parachromatopsia
parachromopsia
parachute reflex
paracinesia, paracinesis
paracousis
paracusis, paracusia
    false p.
    localis p.
parademential
paradigm
    biopsychosocial p.
    p. clash
    cocktail party p.
    diathesis-stress p.
    learning p.
    memory p.
    physiological p.
    risk p.
    p. shift
    transference p.
paradigmatic
    p. response
    p. shift
    p. stress from life experience
paradipsia
paradox
paradoxa
    obstipatio p.

paradoxical
    p. anxiety
    p. cold
    p. combination
    p. depression
    p. incontinence
    p. injunction
    p. intention (PI)
    p. intervention
    p. orgasm
    p. pupil
    p. pupillary phenomenon
    p. reaction
    p. response
    p. sleep
    p. technique
    p. therapy
    p. undressing
    p. warmth
paraequilibrium
paraeroticism, paraerotism
paraesthesia
paraesthetica
    pseudomelia p.
parafunction
paragammacism
paragenital
parageusia
parageusic
paragnomen
paragrammatism
paragraphia
paragraph-meaning test
paragraph recall test
parahippocampal white matter
parahypnosis
parahypophysis
parakinesia, parakinesis
paralalia literalis
paralambdacism
paralanguage
paraldehydism
paraleprosis
paralepsy
paralexia
paralgesia
paralgesic
paralgia
paralimbic region
parallax
parallel
    culturally p.
    p. dream
    p. law
    p. pathways of metabolism
    p. play
    p. processing
    p. subsystem

parallelism
    cultural p.
    psychoneural p.
    psychophysical p.
paralogia
    metamorphic p.
    metaphoric p.
    thematic p.
    themomatic p.
paralogism
paralogistic
paralogy
paralysis, pl. **paralyses**
    acute atrophic p.
    alcoholic p.
    ascending p.
    bilateral abductor p.
    bilateral adductor p.
    catatonic cerebral p.
    central p.
    compression p.
    conjugate p.
    conversion p.
    crossed p.
    exhaustion p.
    facial p.
    familial periodic p.
    faucial p.
    flaccid p.
    gaze p.
    general p.
    ginger p.
    global p.
    histrionic p.
    hysteric p.
    hysterical p.
    immobilization p.
    immunological p.
    p. of the insane
    Jamaica ginger p.
    Kussmaul-Landry p.
    labial p.
    Landry p.
    lead p.
    leaden p.
    mimetic p.
    mixed p.
    musculospiral p.
    myogenic p.
    myopathic p.
    nocturnal p.
    ocular p.

    periodic p.
    postdormital sleep p.
    posticus p.
    predormital sleep p.
    pressure p.
    progressive bulbar p.
    pseudohypertrophic muscular p.
    psychogenic p.
    sensory p.
    sleep p.
    sodium-responsive periodic p.
    spinal p.
    supranuclear p.
    unilateral abductor p.
    unilateral adductor p.
    wasting p.
    work p.
paralytic
    p. abasia
    congenital syphilitic p.
    p. dementia
    p. idiocy
    p. miosis
    p. mydriasis
    p. psychosomatic disorder
paralytica
    p. aphonia
    dementia p.
    Lissauer dementia p.
paralyticus
    ictus p.
paralytique
    folie p.
paralyzant
paralyze
paralyzed
paralyzer
paralyzing
    p. depression
    p. vertigo
paramania
paramedical
parameter
    chance response p.
    item discrimination p.
    pharmacokinetic p.
    psychiatric p.
    treatment intensity p.
parametric
    p. study
    p. test of significance
paramilitary

NOTES

P

paramimia
paramnesia
    reduplicative p.
paramour
paramusia
paramyoclonus
paramyotonia
    congenital p.
    symptomatic p.
paramyotonus
paranalgesia
paranee
paranesthesia
paraneural infiltration
paranoia, pl. **paranoides (PA)**
    acquired p.
    acute hallucinatory p.
    affect-laden p.
    alcoholic p.
    amentia paranoides
    amorous p.
    classical p.
    conjugal p.
    p. and delusions psychiatric
     syndrome
    dementia paranoides
    p. dementia gravis
    dissociative p.
    eccentric p.
    erotic p.
    exalted p.
    p. hallucinatoria
    hallucinatory p.
    heboid p.
    hypochondriac p.
    hypochondriacal p.
    involutional p.
    litigious p.
    mystic p.
    p. originaria
    paranoidal p.
    p. paranoid state
    persecutory p.
    projectional p.
    p. querulans
    p. querulans paranoid state
    querulous p.
    reformatory p.
    rudimentary p.
    Seglas-type p.
    senile p.
    p. senilis
    p. simplex
paranoiac (*var. of* paranoic)
    p. character
    p. psychosis
    reformatory p.

paranoica
    aphonia p.
    aphrasia p.
    metamorphosis sexualis p.
paranoid
    p. behavior
    p. belief system
    p. condition
    p. delusional belief
    p. dementia
    p. erotism
    p. fear
    p. feature
    floridly p.
    p. grandiose delusion
    p. hostility
    p. ideation
    p. involutional reaction
    p. litigious state
    p. look
    p. melancholia
    p. neurotic personality disorder
    p. personality
    p. psychoneurosis
    p. reaction type
    p. scale
    p. schizophrenia
    p. schizophrenic psychosis
    schizophrenic reaction, acute, p.
     (SR/AP)
    schizophrenic reaction, chronic, p.
     (SR/CP)
    sensitive Beziehungswahn p.
    p. tendency
    p. thinking
    p. trait
    p. transient organic psychosis
    p. trend
paranoid-affective organic psychosis,
  mixed
paranoidal paranoia
paranoides (*pl. of* paranoia)
paranoidism
paranoid-schizoid position
paranoid-schizotypal personality disorder
paranoid-type
    p.-t. alcoholic psychosis
    p.-t. arteriosclerotic dementia
    p.-t. arteriosclerotic psychosis
    p.-t. presenile dementia
    p.-t. psycho-organic syndrome
    p.-t. schizophrenia
    p.-t. schizophrenic disorder
    p.-t. senile dementia
    p.-t. senile psychosis
paranomasia
paranomia

paranormal
- p. capacity
- p. cognition
- p. phenomenon

paranosic gain

paranosis

paraparesis

paraparetic

parapathetic proviso

parapathy

paraphasia
- extended jargon p.
- jargon p.
- literal p.
- thematic p.
- verbal p.

paraphasic error

paraphasis

paraphemia

paraphenomenon

paraphernalia
- drug p.
- homemade drug p.
- paraphiliac p.

paraphia

paraphilia
- atypical p.
- exhibitionism p.
- fetishism p.
- frotteurism p.
- pedophilia p.
- transvestism p.
- voyeurism p.

paraphiliac, paraphilic
- p. behavior
- p. coercive disorder
- p. fantasy
- p. focus
- p. imagery
- p. object
- p. paraphernalia
- p. pornography
- p. preference
- p. stimulus

paraphonia

paraphonic state

paraphora

paraphrasia
- literal p.
- thematic p.

paraphrenia
- climacteric p.

- p. confabulans
- p. expansiva
- p. fantastica
- involutional p.
- late p.
- menopausal p.
- p. paranoid state
- presenile p.
- p. systematica

paraphrenic
- p. dementia
- p. schizophrenia

paraphronia

paraphysial, paraphyseal

parapithymia

paraplectic

paraplegia
- alcoholic p.
- congenital spastic p.
- infantile spastic p.
- painful p.
- senile p.
- superior p.
- tetanoid p.

paraplegic

parapoplexy

parapraxia

paraprofessional

parapsia

parapsis

parapsychology

parapsychosis

parareaction

parareflexia

pararhotacism

parasexuality

parasigmatism

parasites of the superego

parasitic
- p. superego
- p. vampirism

parasitosis

parasocial speech

parasomnia

parasomniac
- p. consciousness
- p. conscious state

parasomnia-type substance-induced sleep disorder

paraspasm

parasuicidal
- p. behavior

NOTES

P

parasuicidal *(continued)*
    p. event
    p. incident
parasympathetic
    p. epilepsy
    p. nervous system (PNS)
parasympathicotonia
parasympatholytic
parasympathomimetic drug
parasympathotonia
paratactic distortion
parataxic
    p. distortion
    p. mode
parataxis, parataxia
parateresiomania
parathormone
parathymia
parathyreopriva
    tetania p.
paratonia progressiva
paratrophy
paratypic
paraverbal therapy
parchment crackling
pardon
pardonable
parectropia
paregoric
    p. overdose
    p. poisoning
pareidolia
parencephalia
parencephalous
parenchymatous
    p. neuritis
    p. neurosyphilis
parens patriae
parent
    absent p.
    p. abuse
    abusive p.
    adoptive p.
    alcoholic p.
    P.'s Anonymous
    p. anxiety rating scale
    p.'s at risk
    authoritarian rejecting-neglecting p.
    battered p.
    biologic p.
    p. burnout
    childhood loss of a p.
    controlling p.
    critical p.
    custodial p.
    p. effectiveness training
    p. ego state
    p. fixation

    foster p.
    p. image
    ineffectual p.
    p. inventory
    p. neglect
    noncustodial p.
    overprotective p.
    permissive p.
    p. perplexity
    problem p.
    raging p.
    refrigerator p.
    rejecting p.
    rejecting-neglecting p.
    search for p.
    separation from p.
    strict p.
    substance-abusing p.
    p. subsystem
    surrogate p.
    surviving p.
    p. therapist program
    ungiving p.
    weak p.
    weekend p.
    P.'s Without Partners (PWP)
parent-adult-child (PAC)
parental
    p. abuse
    p. attitudes toward sex
    p. behavior
    p. care
    p. control
    p. control problem
    p. criticism
    p. custody
    p. death
    p. denial
    p. divorce
    p. dysfunction
    p. environment
    p. environment characteristic
    p. environment item
    p. failure to guide
    p. feeding practice
    p. fit
    p. indecisiveness
    p. indifference
    p. loss
    p. marital problem
    p. overprotection
    p. perplexity
    p. rejection
    p. right doctrine
    p. rights
    p. separation
    p. socioeconomic class

p. spontaneity
p. value
parent-child
p.-c. bond
p.-c. conflict
p.-c. conflict counseling
p.-c. dyad
p.-c. group therapy
p.-c. model
p.-c. rapport
p.-c. relational problem
p.-c. relationship
p.-c. transmission
parenteral
p. alimentation
p. drug
p. drug administration
p. feeding
parenthetical expression
parenthood
Planned P.
parent-infant bonding
parenting
p. ability
erratic p.
foster p.
high quality p.
inadequate p.
inept p.
irresponsible p.
limit-setting p.
loving p.
positive p.
reciprocal p.
refrigerator p.
p. skill
p. style
unpredictable p.
parentis
in loco p.
parent-offspring bond
parent-to-child aggression (PTCA)
parepithymia
parerethisis
parergasia
paresis
alcoholic p.
facial p.
general p.
infantile p.
juvenile p.
Lissauer-type p.

paresthesia
laryngeal p.
paresthetica
digitalgia p.
paresthetic conversion reaction
paretic
p. curve
p. dementia
p. impotence
p. melancholia
p. psychosis
pargyline
Parham decision
parietal
p. cortex
p. lobe
p. lobe dysfunction
p. neocortical association area
p. skull bone
temporal, occipital, p. (TOP)
p. tissue
parietooccipital aphasia
parietooccipital hypoperfusion
parietotemporal
p. area
p. perfusion deficit
parlor
massage p.
parmia
parody in wit
parole
condition of p.
p. violation case
parolee
paroneiria salax
paroniria
p. ambulans
p. salax
paronomasia
parorexia
parosmia
parosphresia
parousiamania
paroxysm
paroxysmal
p. activity
p. convulsion
p. drinking
p. dyskinesia
p. dystonia
p. migraine
p. migraine headache

NOTES

P

477

paroxysmal *(continued)*
    p. phenomenon
    psychogenic p.
    p. psychosis
    p. seizure
    p. sleep
    p. trepidant abasia
parricide
parrotlike speech pattern
parry
pars, pl. **partes**
    p. pro toto
parsimony
part
    p. instinct
    p. object
partake
part-brain
partes *(pl. of* pars)
partial
    p. adjustment
    p. agonist
    p. aim
    p. amnesia
    p. complex seizure
    p. correlation
    p. cross-dressing
    p. delirium
    p. delusion
    p. epilepsy
    p. hospitalization
    p. hospital patient population
    p. hospital setting
    p. insanity
    p. instinct
    p. mergent
    p. nominal aphasia
    p. organic psychosyndrome
    p. permanent disability
    p. recovery
    p. regression
    p. reinforcement
    p. remission
    p. sensory seizure
    p. tonic seizure
partialis
    psychopathia p.
partialism
    persistent p.
partiality
partially disabled
partial-reinforcement effect (PRE)
participant
    p. modeling
    p. observation
    p. observer
    self-help p.
participate

participation
    group p.
participative management
particle
particular
    bill of p.'s
    p. complex
    p. task
particularism
particularity
particulate
parting of the ways
parti pris
partisan
partitive
part-learning method
partner
    abusive p.
    bed p.
    compulsive fixation on an
      unobtainable p.
    consenting p.
    distraught former p.
    estranged p.
    former p.
    multiple sexual p.
    nonconsenting p.
    nongambling p.
    Parents Without P.'s (PWP)
    phallic p.
    p. relational problem
    sexual p.
    sleeping p.
    surrogate sexual p.
partner-swapping
part-object manner
parturition
party
    neutral p.
    rave p.
paruresis
parviculata
    alopecia p.
PAS
    personality assessment system
pas
    faux p.
PASO
    primitive aggressive self-organization
pass
    leave on p. (LOP)
    weekend p.
passage
    bird of p.
    p. comprehension
    memory p.
    rite of p.
Passiflora incarnata

passing stranger effect
passion
    crime of p.
passionate attitude
passionelle
    attitude p.
    psychose p.
passive
    p. accommodation
    p. aggression
    p. algolagnia
    p. analysis
    p. avoidance
    p. behavior
    p. castration complex
    p. dependence
    p. euthanasia
    p. immunity
    p. immunization therapy
    p. incontinence
    p. influence
    p. introversion
    p. learning
    p. listening
    p. mode of consciousness
    p. movement
    p. object love
    p. opposition
    p. parasitic psychopathy
    p. personality
    p. reaction
    p. recreation
    p. resistance
    p. therapist
    p. transport
    p. tremor
    p. vocabulary
passive-aggressive (PA)
    p.-a. acting out
    p.-a. behavior
    p.-a. feature
    p.-a. maneuver
    p.-a. neurotic
    p.-a. neurotic personality
    p.-a. neurotic personality disorder
    p.-a. personality (PAP)
    p.-a. reaction
    p.-a. scale
passive-avoidance learning
passive-dependent
    p.-d. personality (PDP)
    p.-d. reaction

passively phrased question
passive-receptive longing
passivism
passivity
    active p.
    p. in anger expression
    delusion of p.
    p. delusion
    motor p.
password
past
    p. alcoholism
    p. behavior
    criminal p.
    p. event
    p. experience
    p. head injury
    p. history (PH)
    p. lifetime disorder
    p. loss
    p. month alcohol use
    p. oriented
    p. personal history
    p. suicidal act
    p. suicide attempt
    p. tic
    violent p.
past-life hypnotic regression
pastoral
    p. care
    p. counseling
    p. counselor
    p. help
    p. psychiatry
past-pointing
patch
    nicotine p.
    transdermal p.
patchy amnesia
patent
    p. medicinals
    p. medicine
    p. medicine abuse
paterfamilias
paternal
    p. abuse
    p. attitude
    p. behavior
    p. care
    p. competency
    p. deprivation
    p. desertion

NOTES

P

paternal (*continued*)
   p. drive
   p. indifference
   p. neglect
   p. rejection
   p. relationship
paternalism
paternity
   p. blues
   proof of p.
   p. suit
   p. test
pathema
pathematic aphasia
pathemia
pathergasia
pathetic
pathetism
pathic
pathoclisis
pathocure
pathodixia
pathoformic
pathogen
   behavioral p.
   p. of violence
pathogenesis
   biologic p.
pathogenic, pathogenetic
   p. care
   p. factor
   p. family pattern
pathogenicity
pathogeny
pathognomic
pathognomonic
   p. fantasy
   p. sign
pathognomy
pathognostic
pathography
   psychoanalytic p.
   psychoanalytical p.
pathohysteria
pathokinesis
patholesia
pathologic
   p. alcohol intoxication
   p. amenorrhea
   p. behavior
   p. care
   p. character formation
   p. communication
   p. condition
   p. diagnosis
   p. drowsiness
   p. drug intoxication
   p. drug intoxication drug psychosis

   p. drunkenness
   p. emotionality
   p. fallacy
   p. gambler
   p. gambling disorder (PGD)
   p. grief reaction
   p. grieving
   p. guilt
   p. intoxication alcoholic psychosis
   p. liar
   p. lying
   p. mendicancy
   p. nature
   p. pain
   p. personality
   p. preoccupation
   p. process
   p. reaction to alcohol
   p. reflex
   p. sexual fantasy
   p. sexuality
   p. sleepiness
   p. substance use
   p. swindler
   p. trait
pathological
   p. change
   p. communication
   p. crying
   p. dissociation
   p. drunkenness
   p. emotionality
   p. feature
   p. finding
   p. gambling (PG)
   p. grief reaction
   p. guilt
   p. homophobia
   p. intoxication
   p. laughter
   p. level
   p. liar
   p. lying
   p. mendicancy
   p. mood state
   p. personality
   p. preoccupation
   p. response
   p. sexuality
   p. sleepiness
   p. study
   p. swindler
pathology
   association deficit p.
   aural p.
   borderline p.
   brain p.
   character p.

cognitive p.
cortical p.
deep white matter p.
focal p.
forensic p.
functional p.
interpersonal p.
ischemic p.
language p.
personality p.
psychosocial p.
structural p.
subcortical p.
white matter p.
pathology-induced memory reconstruction
pathomania
pathomimesis
pathomimia
pathomimicry
pathomiosis
pathomorphism
pathoneurosis
pathophilia
pathophrenesis
pathophysiological
p. basis
p. cascade
p. link
p. mechanism
p. pattern
p. process
p. role
pathophysiologic process
pathophysiology
pathoplasty
pathopsychology
pathopsychosis
pathos
pathosis
attitudinal p.
pathway
anterior cingulate p.
auditory p.
basic brain p.
biochemical p.
brain dopaminergic p.
cerebellar p.
dopamine p.
dopaminergic p.
dorsolateral p.
heat-loss p.
indirect striatopallidal p.

mesocortical dopamine p.
mesolimbic dopamine p.
neurochemical p.
olfactory p.
orbitofrontal p.
pilomotor p.
serotonergic p.
spinoreticulothalamic p.
p. stimulation
ventral amygdala fugal p.
visceromotor p.
patience
lack of p.
patient (pt)
p. abuse
acutely psychotic schizophrenic p.
p. advocate
agitated p.
akinetic p.
American Academy on Physician and P. (AAPP)
amnesic p.
analytic p.
antisocial p.
aphasic p.
at-risk p.
p. authentication
p. autonomy
P.'s Bill of Rights
bipolar p.
borderline p.
catatonic p.
chronically depressed p.
clinic p.
comatose p.
combative p.
community-residing p.
p. compliance
consenting p.
p. contract
dangerous p.
p. data bank
p. delay
delirious p.
demented p.
dementia p.
depressed p.
disheveled p.
disoriented p.
p. disquietude
disruptive psychotic p.
dissociative p.

NOTES

P

481

patient *(continued)*
 drug-free p.
 dual diagnosis p.
 dysphoric p.
 p. education
 elderly depressed p.
 p. and family services (PFS)
 female p.
 p. file
 first-episode p.
 frail elderly p.
 full-dose-treated p.
 geriatric p.
 p. guide to medication
 hallucinating p.
 healthy p.
 p. hesitancy
 high-functioning p.
 high-profile p.
 high-risk p.
 histrionic p.
 homeless p.
 hypnotic p.
 hypnotic-dependent p.
 incarcerated p.
 incoherent p.
 insured p.
 p. interview
 lethargic p.
 p. literacy
 male p.
 manic p.
 medicated p.
 mood disorder p.
 multidimensional scale for rating
  psychiatric p.'s
 multiple-episode p.
 mute p.
 neuroleptic-free p.
 neuroleptic-naive p.
 never-medicated p.
 nonconsenting p.
 nonpsychotic Alzheimer p.
 nonsuicidal depressed p.
 obese p.
 p. obligations
 OCD p.
 opioid-dependent p.
 panic-disordered p.
 peregrinating problem p.
 person in the p.
 p. placement criterion
 posttraumatic p.
 potentially dangerous p.
 problem p.
 psychiatric p.
 psychotic Alzheimer p.
 rapid metabolizer p.'s

 p. resistance
 p. responsibility
 p. rights
 sadistic p.
 p. satisfaction
 schizophrenic p.
 schizophreniform p.
 schizotypal p.
 self-destructive p.
 slow metabolizer p.'s
 stuporous p.
 suicidal depressed p.
 symptomatic p.
 target p.
 treatment-intolerant p.
 treatment-refractory p.
 uninsured p.
 unipolar p.
 unmedicated p.
 unresponsive p.
 violent pediatric p.
 young-old p.
patient-care audit
patient-centered
 p.-c. approach
 p.-c. services
patient-controlled analgesia (PCA)
patient-oriented consultation
patriae
 parens p.
patriarch
patriarchal family
patricide
patrilineal family
patrilocal family
patrimony
patronize
patronizing manner
patronymic
pattern
 action p.
 activation p.
 advanced sleep-phase p.
 affectomotor p.
 p. of aggression
 agreed-on p.
 p. analysis
 anomalous parental vocal p.
 p. of antisocial behavior
 authoritarian leadership p.
 autosomal dominant p.
 avoidance p.
 behavior p.
 beta p.
 binge eating p.
 blame-placing communication p.
 p. of care

change in sleep p.
changing sleep-wake p.
characteristic p.
checkerboard p.
chronic p.
chronically disabling p.
communication p.
p. of conduct
delusional thought p.
democratic leadership p.
destructive family relationship p.
desynchronized discharge p.
p. of detachment
developmental p.
discharge p.
p. discrimination
disturbed sleep p.
enduring p.
erotic-arousal p.
p. of expression
expressive p.
extinction-type p.
familial p.
family p.
fixed action p. (FAP)
food consumption p.
gesturing communication p.
gull-wing p.
habit p.
ineffective communication p.
inflexible p.
intellectualization communication p.
intensive habit p.
interpersonal spacing
  communication p.
irregular sleep p.
irregular sleep-wake p.
Kindling p.
laissez-faire leadership p.
long-term p.
maladaptive personality p.
manipulation communication p.
mitten p.
monopolization communication p.
mood disorder with seasonal p.
neurodevelopmental p.
noncued memory p.
occupational ability p. (OAP)
parrotlike speech p.
pathogenic family p.
pathophysiological p.
persistent p.

personality p.
pervasive p.
p. of pervasive unhappiness
phenomenal p.
positive spike p.
power struggle leadership p.
prototypical course p.
rapid-cycling p.
p. recognition
reflex p.
repeating p.
repetitive p.
p. of repetitive behavior
response p.
role p.
scapegoating communication p.
seasonal p.
p. of self-injury
semantic argument
  communication p.
p. sensitive epilepsy
shared thought p.
silence communication p.
sleep p.
specific dynamic p.
speech p.
stable sleep-wake p.
symptom response p.
syndrome p.
syndromic p.
temporal p.
thought p.
touching communication p.
validation communication p.

patterned interview
pattern-induced epilepsy
patterning
  p. exercise
  p. psychotherapy
  p. vision
paucity
  p. of data
  p. of expressive gestures
  p. of movement
  p. of reports
  p. of speech
  p. of speech content
pauperize
pause
  apneic p.
  fixation p.

NOTES

P

483

pause (*continued*)
    respiratory p.
    p. in speech
Pausinystalia yohimbe
pauvre
    autisme p.
Pavlov
    P. method
    P. theory of schizophrenia
pavlovian conditioning
pavlovianism
pavor
    p. diurnus
    p. nocturnus
    p. scleresis
pay
    take-home p.
payer
Paykel classification
pays
    maladie du p.
PBG
    porphobilinogen
PC
    phrase construction
    picture completion
    PC subtest
PCA
    patient-controlled analgesia
    principal-components analysis
PCP
    phencyclidine
PCP-induced anxiety disorder
PCP-related disorder, not otherwise specified
PD
    panic disorder
    personality disorder
    problem drinker
    psychopathic deviant
    psychotic depression
PDD
    pervasive developmental disorder
    primary degenerative dementia
    PDD NOS
PDDAT
    primary degenerative dementia of Alzheimer type
PDP
    passive-dependent personality
PDR
    Physicians' Desk Reference
PDS
    pain dysfunction syndrome
PE
    physical examination
    probable error

peace
    disturb the p.
    p. pipe
peaceful coexistence
peacemaker role
peacetime
peak
    p. absorption spike
    p. acoustic gain
    p. behavioral effect
    p. clipping
    p. experience
    kilovoltage p. (kVp)
    p. level of drug activity
    p. score
    p. and trough level
Pearson correlation coefficient pedantic
PEC
    politico-economic-conservatism
    PEC scale
peccant
peccavi
pecking order
pectoralgia
pectoris
    angor p.
peculiar
    p. behavior
    p. personality trait
peculiarity
pedagogy
pedantic
    Pearson correlation coefficient p.
pederast
pederasty
pediatric
    p. autoimmune neuropsychiatric disorders associated with streptococcal infection (PANDAS)
    p. growth chart
    p. psychiatry
    p. psychologist
    p. psychology
    p. psychopharmacology
pediatrics
    developmental-behavioral p.
    Society for Developmental and Behavioral P.
pedication
pedigree
    p. method
    p. study
pedionalgia
pedioneuralgia
pedohebephilia
pedologia
pedologist
pedology

pedomorphism
pedophile
    heterosexual p.
    homosexual p.
pedophilia
    adolescent p.
    bisexual p.
    heterosexual p.
    homosexual p.
    middle age p.
    p. paraphilia
    senescent p.
pedophilic
    p. behavior
    p. stimulus
pedotrophy
peduncular
    hallucinosis p.
    p. hallucinosis
pedunculotomy
peeping Tom
peer
    p. abuse
    age p.
    p. anxiety
    p. censure
    conflicts with p.'s
    p. criticism
    p. group
    p. interaction
    p. interactional situation
    p. likability
    p. mediation
    opposite sex p.
    p. ostracism
    p. play
    p. pressure
    p. rating
    rejection by p.'s
    p. relationship
    p. review
    p. review organization (PRO)
    same-sex p.
    sex play with p.'s
    p. support
    p. support for violence
peer-helping service
peer-to-peer conflict resolution
peeve
peevish
pegboard
    Lafayette p.

pejoration
pejorative
    p. delusion
    p. nature
    p. voice
pejorism
pelea
    mal de p.
peliagroid
pellagra
    pellagra sine p.
pellagragenic
pellagral
pellagrin
pellagroid
pellagrous
pellucidum
    septum p.
pelvic
    p. pain
    p. thrusting
penal code
penalize
penalty
    p., frustration, anxiety, guilt, hostility (PFAGH)
    minor p.
penance
penchant
pendulous
pendulum of diagnosis
penectomy
penetrable
penetrance
    lack of p.
penetrate
penetration
    finger p.
    p. response
penile
    p. arousal
    p. impotence
    p. plethysmograph
    p. prosthesis
    p. tumescence
penilingus
penis, pl. **penes**
    artificial p.
    p. captivus
    p. envy
    erector p.
    p. fear

NOTES

P

penis *(continued)*
    glans p.
    immissio p.
    p. pride
    tenesmus p.
    p. wish
penitence
penitent
penitentiare
    folie p.
penitentiary
penniless
penology
pense
    deja p.
pensee
    arriere-p.
    p. operatoire
    tic de p.
penses
    echo des p.
pension neurosis
pentapeptide
pentetrazol
penurious
penury
peonage
    institutional p.
people
    recognition of p.
    p. skills
    street p.
peotillomania
pep
    p. talk
Pepper syndrome
peptide
    beta amyloid p.
    delta sleep-inducing p.
    gastrin-inhibiting p.
    p. neurotransmitter
    opioid p.
    sleep-inducing p.
    tau protein p.
    vasoactive intestinal p. (VIP)
per
    p. anum
    p. capita
    p. day (/d)
    p. rectum
    p. vaginam
peracute mania
perazine
perceived
    p. danger
    p. emotional abandonment
    p. interpersonal rejection
    p. loss

    p. maternal dysfunction
    p. neglect
    p. parental dysfunction
    p. power
    p. reality
    p. sin
    p. trauma characteristic
percentage
percentile
    p. norm
    p. rank
    p. score
percept
    p. analysis
    body p.
    delusional p.
    p. image
perceptible
perception
    aberration of p.
    abnormal p.
    abstract p.
    alteration in time p.
    altered mind-body p.
    altered sensory p.
    altered time p.
    p. analysis
    auditory space p.
    automorphic p.
    binocular p.
    p. of body image
    body-image p.
    clerical p. (Q)
    color p.
    conscious p.
    cross-modality p.
    p. deficit
    depth p.
    p. disorder
    distance p.
    distorted p.
    p. disturbance
    disturbance of p.
    ecological p.
    p. ego
    p. of the environment
    exaggerated p.
    extrasensory p. (ESP)
    facial p.
    family p.
    figure-ground p.
    fingertip number writing p.
    form p.
    gravity p.
    hallucination of p.
    haptic p.
    heightened sensory p.
    hypnagogic p.

hypnopompic p.
inferential p.
internal world of p.
p. inventory
kinesthetic p.
p. localized within the body
LSD-type p.
motion p.
narrative speech p.
obligatory p.
pain p.
person p.
physiognomic p.
posthallucinogen p.
proprioceptive p.
p. of reality
sensory p.
situational p.
size p.
social p.
p. of sound
p. of sound inside the head
p. of sound outside the head
space p.
p. of spatial relations
speech p.
stereognostic p.
subconscious p.
subliminal p.
substance-induced p.
tactile kinesthetic p.
time p.
touch p.
transactional theory of p.
true p.
visual p.
weight p.
perception-hallucination
perceptive
p. deafness
p. epilepsy
perceptivity
perceptorium
perceptual
p. abnormality
p. analysis
p. anchoring
p. aspect
p. closure
p. cognitive mechanism
p. consciousness
p. consistency

p. constancy
p. cue
p. cycle
p. defect
p. defense
p. deficit
p. deprivation
p. disability
p. disorder
p. distortion
p. emotive stimulus
p. error
p. expansion
p. experience
p. extinction
p. field
p. filter
p. immaturity
p. induction
p. learning
p. level
p. maintenance
p. masking
p. motor abilities disturbance
p. motor ability
p. motor dysfunction
p. organization
p. organizational index
p. process
p. psychology
p. restructuring
p. retardation
p. rivalry
p. schema
p. segregation
p. sensitization
p. set
p. skill
p. sociogram
p. speed
p. structure
p. style
p. symptoms
p. synthesis
p. training
p. transformation
p. vigilance
perceptual-identification test
perceptually handicapped
perceptual-motor
p.-m. disability
p.-m. impairment

NOTES

P

perceptual-motor *(continued)*
    p.-m. learning
    p.-m. match
    p.-m. region
    p.-m. skill
perch
percipient
percussion
percutaneous stimulation
perdida del alma
peregrinating problem patient
perencephaly
perennial dream
perfect
    p. negative relationship
    p. performance
    p. positive relationship
perfectible
perfection
    manie de p.
    p. state
perfectionism preoccupation
perfectionist
perfectionistic personality
perfervid
perfidious
perfidy
perforate
perforation
perforator
perforatum
    Hypericum p.
performance
    p. abnormality
    academic p.
    p. anxiety
    as-if p.
    p. assessment
    attentional p.
    automaticity of p.
    p. characteristic
    cognitive p.
    decreased work p.
    p. fear
    impaired p.
    impaired sexual p.
    job p.
    p. level
    memory p.
    memory-continuous p.
    motor p.
    neuropsychologic p.
    p. neurosis
    novel task p.
    p. objective
    perfect p.
    poor school p.
    psychometric p.

    psychomotor p.
    quality of p.
    recall p.
    p. requirement
    school p.
    p. score
    sexual p.
    p. situation
    social p.
    standard of p.
    task p.
    p. task
    p. test
    vocational p.
    work p.
performance-intensity function
performative speech
performer
performing symbolically
perfunctory
perhaps neurosis
periamygdaloid cortex
perianal
periarterial sympathectomy
periblepsis
perichareia
periciazine
pericranitis
periencephalitis
perikaryal
peril
perilous
    p. activity
    p. course
periluteal phase dysphoric disorder
perimeningitis
perineometer
perineural
    p. anesthesia
    p. infiltration
perineuritis
period
    adaptation p.
    apneic p.
    apneustic p.
    child raising p.
    chum p.
    concrete operation p.
    crisis p.
    p.'s of crisis
    critical p.
    depression p.
    developmental p.
    discrete p.
    drug-free p.
    enactive p.
    endogenous circadian p.
    evaluation p.

fantasy p.
followup p.
formal operations p.
growth p.
honeymoon p.
ictal p.
interictal p.
involutional p.
latency p. (LP)
latent p.
major risk p.
observation p.
oedipal p.
Oedipus p.
p. of optimism
oral biting p.
practicing p.
prenatal p.
preoperational thought p.
p. prevalence
prodromal p.
psychological refractory p.
refractory p.
REM p.
p.'s of remission
sadness p.
sensorimotor intelligence p.
silent p.
sleep onset REM p.
storm-and-stress p.
thought p.
treatment p.

periodic
   p. catatonia
   p. drinker
   p. drinking
   p. insanity
   p. jactitation
   p. mania
   p. migrainous neuralgia
   p. paralysis
   p. psychosis of puberty
   p. reinforcement
   p. reinforcement relationship
   p. screening
periodical mania
periodicity theory
periontogenic
perioral tremor
peripatetic
peripheral
   p. anesthesia

p. autonomic neuropathy
p. catecholamine
p. catecholamine receptor
p. cholinergic activity
p. cue test
p. epilepsy
p. examination
p. field image
p. masking
p. nervous system (PNS)
p. neuritis
p. norepinephrine
p. sensation
p. sensory loss
p. sympathomimetic effect
p. tabes
peripheralism
peripheralist psychology
**peripherally acting anticholinergic
  medication**
periphery
periphrastic
peripolar zone
periproctic
perirectal
perirectitis
perish
perispondylitis
peristasis
peritonism
peritraumatic
   p. dissociation
   p. predictor
periurethral
perivaginal
periventricular
   p. gray matter area
   p. gray region
   p. hyperintensity
   p. white matter
perjury
perky
permanence
   p. concept
   object p.
permanent
   p. disability
   p. dominant idea
   p. epilation
   p. memory
   p. planning
   p. residual impairment

NOTES

P

permeable
permeation
permissible
    p. dose
    ethically p.
permission
permissive
    p. environment
    p. hypothesis of affective disorders
    p. parent
permissiveness
permit
permutation
perneoscrotal
perneovaginal
pernicious trend
peroneal phenomenon
peroral
peroration
peroxisomal proliferator receptor
  (PPAR)
perpend
perpetrate
perpetrator of violence
perpetual
perpetuate
perpetuating factor
perpetuator of abuse
perpetuity
perplex
perplexed manic-depressive psychosis
perplexed-type
    p.-t. manic-depressive
    p.-t. manic-depressive psychosis
perplexing behavior
perplexity
    morbid p.
    parent p.
    parental p.
    p. psychosis
    p. state
    vague p.
persecute
persecution
    p. complex
    delirium of p.
    delusion of p.
    p. delusion
    folie des p.'s
    p. ideation
    social p.
    p. syndrome
    p. theme
persecutor
persecutory
    p. anxiety
    p. delusion
    p. delusional disorder

    p. delusional system
    p. idea
    p. paranoia
    p. subtype
    p. type
    p. type of paranoid disorder
persecutory-type schizophrenia
perseverate
perseveration
    p. deficit
    infantile p.
    motor p.
    p. set
    verbal p.
perseverative
    p. error
    p. functional autonomy
    p. movement
    p. response
    p. speech
    p. trace
persevere
Persian Gulf War syndrome
persist
persistence
    motor p.
persistent
    p. anxiety
    p. delusion
    p. discomfort
    p. emotional condition
    p. hypersomnia
    p. inappropriate idea
    p. inappropriate image
    p. inappropriate impulse
    p. insomnia
    p. intrusive idea
    p. intrusive image
    p. intrusive impulse
    p. morbidity
    p. motor activity
    p. partialism
    p. pattern
    p. pattern of conduct
    p. puberism
    p. rumination
    p. thought
    p. tremor
    p. vegetative state (PVS)
    p. vegetative state disorder
persisting
    p. dementia
    p. disorder
person
    aged p.
    composite p.
    p. culture
    p. deixis

displaced p.
disturbed p.
dominant p.
evil p.
exposure of p.
homeless p.
inner-directed p.
p. in need of supervision
other-directed p.
p. in the patient
p. perception
religious p.
significant supporting p.
spectral relationship to famous p.
spiritual p.
street p.
time, place, and p. (TP&P)
p. with AIDS (PWA)

persona
in p.
p. non grata
organic p.
in propria p.
symbolic p.

personable

personal
p. adjustment
p. agenda
p. agony
p. anguish
p. assault
p. attribution
p. audit
p. belief
p. care
p. care home
p. communication
p. construct
p. construct theory
p. control
p. counselor
p. data sheet
p. demoralization
p. development
p. disposition
p. distance zone
p. document analysis
p. dysjunction
p. effects
p. episode
p. equation
p. event

p. experience
p. factor
p. followup data
p. function
p. growth
p. growth group
p. growth laboratory
p. history (PH)
p. history questionnaire
p. honor
p. hygiene
p. identity
p. identity confusion
p. idiom
p. image
p. import
p. inadequacy
p. inadequacy theme
p. information
p. involvement
p. issue
p. judgment
p. locus of control (PLC)
p. loss
p. man
p. memory
p. memory score
p. motivation
p. myth
p. need
p. opinion
p. psychiatric history
p. recovery
p. relationship
p. relevance
p. response
p. responsibility
p. satisfaction
p. skills gambling
p. skills map
p. and social history (P&SH)
p. social motive
p. space
p. space invasion
p. spirituality
p. unconscious
p. value

personalism

personality
abnormal p.
p. abnormality
acromegaloid p.

NOTES

P

personality *(continued)*
  action-oriented p.
  addiction-prone p. (APP)
  addictive p.
  affective p.
  aggressive p.
  alexithymic p.
  allotropic p.
  alternating p.
  altruistic p.
  amoral psychopathic p.
  anal p.
  anal-retentive p.
  anancastic p.
  antisocial p. (ASP)
  antisocial neurotic p.
  antisocial trends psychopathic p.
  as-if p.
  asocial trends psychopathic p.
  p. assessment
  p. assessment system (PAS)
  asthenic p.
  authoritarian p.
  avoidant p.
  basic p.
  borderline p.
  brooding p.
  Cattell factorial theory of p. (CFTP)
  p. change
  p. change disorder
  p. change due to a general medical condition
  p. change due to a general medical condition, aggressive type
  p. change due to a general medical condition, aphasic type
  p. change due to a general medical condition, disinhibited type
  p. change due to a general medical condition, labile type
  p. change due to a general medical condition, paranoid type
  p. characteristic
  charismatic p.
  chronic hypomanic p.
  p. clash
  coarctated p.
  coconscious p.
  codependent p.
  composite p.
  compulsive p.
  p. configuration
  controlling p.
  p. cult
  cult of p.
  cycloid p.

cyclothymic p.
dependent p.
depressive p.
p. deterioration
p. development
p. deviation
diehard p.
p. dimension
p. disintegration
p. disorder (PD)
p. disorder diagnosis
disordered p.
p. disorder instrument
p. disorder NOS
p. disorder profile
p. disorder score
p. disorders scale
p. disorder taxonomy
p. disorder typology
disturbed p.
dominant p.
double p.
dual p.
dynamic p.
p. dynamics
p. dysfunction
dyssocial p.
eccentric p.
emotional p.
emotionally unstable p.
epileptic p.
exploitative p.
explosive p.
extroverted p.
Eysenck and Gray biological theories of p.
factor theory of p.
fanatic p.
p. feature
p. formation
freudian theory of p.
p. functioning
p. and gender
haltlose-type p.
histrionic p.
hoarding p.
hostile p.
hyperaesthetic p.
hypomanic p.
hysterical p.
hysteroid p.
ideal p.
immature p.
p. impoverishment
inadequate p.
inmate p.
p. integration
interactional theory of p.

intraconscious p.
introverted schizoid p.
p. inventory
Jekyll and Hyde p.
lifetime p.
magnetic p.
maladaptive p.
marketing p.
masochistic p.
melancholic p.
migraine p.
mixed psychopathic p.
mixed-type psychopathic p.
multiple p.
multiplication of p.
narcissistic p.
neurasthenic p.
neurotic p.
p. neurotic disorder
normal p.
obsessional p.
obsessive p.
obsessive-compulsive p.
oral p.
p. organization
p. panel
paranoid p.
passive p.
passive-aggressive p. (PAP)
passive-aggressive neurotic p.
passive-dependent p. (PDP)
pathologic p.
pathological p.
p. pathology
p. pattern
p. pattern disturbance
perfectionistic p.
physiological basis of p.
posttraumatic p.
premorbid p.
prepsychotic p.
presenting p.
p. problem
p. process
productive p.
psychoinfantile p.
p. psychologist
p. psychology
p. psychoneurosis
psychoneurotic p.
psychopathic p.
p. questionnaire

p. reaction
receptive p.
repressive p.
p. research
p. researcher
role theory of p.
sadistic p.
schizoid p.
schizophrenic p.
schizothymic p.
schizotypal schizoid p.
Schneider definition of p.
schneiderian criteria for
  depressive p.
seclusive p.
secondary p.
seductive p.
self-defeating p.
shut-in p.
sociopathic p.
p. sphere
split p.
stable p.
stormy p.
p. structure
p. syndrome
syntonic p.
p. test
p. trait disturbance
p. trait stability
p. trait theory
type A, B p.
ulcer p.
unstable p.
unusual p.
viscosity p.
volatile p.
von Zerssen circumplex model of
  premorbid p.
personality-descriptive
  p.-d. item
  p.-d. statement
personalization
personalized interpretation
personally
  p. saddening experience
  p. significant anniversary
personate
person-centered theory
person-environment interaction
personification
  eidetic p.

NOTES

P

personified self
personify
personnel
  p. date
  nonmedical p.
  p. placement
  p. psychology
  p. selection
  p. test
  p. training
personology
perspective
  alternating p.
  alternative p.
  atmospheric p.
  behavioral p.
  biologica p.
  categorical p.
  clinical p.
  developmental p.
  extraspective p.
  humanistic p.
  linear p.
  neurobiological p.
  psychoanalytic p.
  psychosocial p.
  religious p.
  symptomatic p.
  temporal p.
perspective-taking skills
perspicacious
perspiration
perspire
persuade
persuasion
  coercive p.
  p. therapy
persuasive communication
pertinacious
pertinence
pertinent
Pertofrane
perturb
perturbation magnitude
pervasive
  p. affect
  p. anger disorder
  p. anhedonia
  p. anxiety
  childhood-onset p.
  p. desire for death
  p. developmental disorder (PDD)
  p. disinhibited type of
    developmental disorder
  p. distrust
  p. emotion
  p. impairment of development
  p. inhibition

  p. pattern
  p. and persistent maladaptive
    personality traits
  p. pessimism
  p. problem
  p. proneness to guilt
  p. self-criticism
  p. unhappiness
perverse
perversion
  excretory p.
  polymorphous p.
  sex p.
  sexual p.
pervert
  sexual p.
perverted
  p. appetite
  p. logic
  p. sexuality
  p. thinking
pervigilium
PES
  psychiatric emergency service
pessimism
  chronic p.
  oral p.
  pervasive p.
  self-reported p.
  therapeutic p.
pessimist
pessimistic
  p. attitude
  p. outlook
pestilent
PET
  psychiatric emergency team
petechial
Peter
  P. Panism
  P. Principle
pethidine
petit
  p. mal
  p. mal epilepsy
  p. mal status
  p. mal variant seizure
petition of mental illness (PMI)
petrification
pettifog
petting behavior
petty punishment
petulance
petulant
peyote
  p. cactus
  p. dependence
peyotism

PFAGH
  penalty, frustration, anxiety, guilt, hostility
PFAMC
  psychological factors affecting medical condition
pfropfhebephrenia
pfropfschizophrenia
PFS
  patient and family services
  picture frustration study
PG
  pathological gambling
PGD
  pathologic gambling disorder
PGR
  psychogalvanic reflex
  psychogalvanic response
PGSR
  psychogalvanic skin resistance
PGT
  play group therapy
PH
  past history
  personal history
Phaedra complex
phagomania
phagotherapy
phallic
  p. character
  p. level
  p. love
  p. mother
  p. overbearance
  p. partner
  p. phase
  p. pride
  p. primacy
  p. sadism
  p. stage
  p. stage psychosexual development
  p. symbol
  p. woman
phallicism, phallism
phallic-narcissistic character
phallic-oedipal phase
phalliform
phallism (*var. of* phallicism)
phallism
phallocentric culture
phalloid

phalloides
  Amanita p.
phallometry
phallus, pl. **phalli**
  p. envy
  p. girl
phaneromania
phanerothyme
phantasia
phantasm
phantasmagoria
phantasmatomoria
phantasmology
phantasmoscopia
phantasmoscopy
phantastica (*var. of* fantastica)
phantasy (*var. of* fantasy)
phantogeusia
phantom
  p. boarders
  p. extremity
  p. limb
  p. limb pain
  p. lover syndrome
  p. reaction
  p. sensation
  sensory p.
  p. speech
  p. vision
phantomize
pharmaceutical
  p. alternative
  p. equivalent
pharmacist
pharmacodynamic
  p. change
  p. tolerance
pharmacodynamics
  age-related p.
pharmacoeconomics
pharmacogenetics
pharmacogenic orgasm
pharmacogenomics
pharmacogeriatrics
pharmacokinetic
  p. change
  p. parameter
  p. reason
pharmacologic
  p. factor
  p. impact
  p. intervention

NOTES

P

pharmacologic *(continued)*
    p. prophylaxis
    p. sensitivity
    p. treatment
pharmacological
    p. agent
    p. approach
    p. armamentarium
    p. difference
    p. experimentation
    p. management
    p. mechanism
    p. predictor
    p. property
    p. provocation
    p. stimulus
pharmacologically induced penile erection (PIPE)
pharmacology
    p. of abuse
    p. of abuse and dependence
    nicotine p.
    serotonergic p.
pharmacomania
pharmacopedia
Pharmacopeia
    United States P. (USP)
pharmacophilia
Pharmacopoeia
pharmacopsychosis
pharmacotherapeutic
    p. intervention
pharmacotherapy
    antipsychotic p.
    conventional p.
    p. regimen
pharmacothymia
pharmacy
    online p.
pharyngeal
    p. psychophysiologic reaction
pharyngismus
pharyngoplegia
pharyngospasm
phase
    active p.
    acute p.
    p. advance
    anal p.
    appetitive p.
    ascension p.
    autistic p.
    circadian rhythm sleep disorder, delayed sleep p.
    p. cue
    p. delay
    delayed sleep p.
    dementia p.

depressive p.
developmental p.
    p. difference
    p. disparity
endogenous circadian rhythm p.
equatorial p.
excitement p.
follicular p.
genital p.
group p.
hypomanic p.
illness p.
insomnia p.
    p. lag on EEG
latency p.
libidinal p.
    p. of life
    p. locking
luteal p.
magic p.
manic p.
moon p.
normal autistic p.
oedipal p.
opposite p.
oral p.
oral-eroticism p.
oral-incorporative p.
orgasmic p.
phallic p.
phallic-oedipal p.
plateau p.
    p. position
post contraction recovery p.
preambivalent p.
pregenital p.
preoedipal p.
preoperational p.
presuperego p.
prodromal p.
recovery p.
reference p.
relaxation p.
residual p.
resolution p.
    p. reversal
rhythm p.
schizophrenia p.
second negative p.
    p. of seizure
sensorimotor p.
separation-individuation p.
    p. sequence
    p. shift
    p. shift of sleep-wake cycle
sleep p.
    p. spike on EEG
symbiotic p.

treatment p.
urethral p.
phase-of-life problem
phasic
    p. activation
    p. function
    p. reflex
phasophrenia
phencyclidine (PCP)
    analog of p.
    p. delusional disorder
    p. dependence
    p. intoxication
    p. intoxication delirium
    p. intoxication, with perceptual
      disturbance
    p. mixed organic brain
    p. mixed organic brain syndrome
    p. use disorder
phencyclidine-associated psychosis
phencyclidine-induced
    p.-i. disorder
    p.-i. psychosis
    p.-i. psychotic disorder with
      delusions
    p.-i. psychotic disorder with
      hallucinations
phencyclidine-related
    p.-r. disorder
    p.-r. disorder NOS
phenocopy
phenogenetic
phenology
phenomena (*pl. of* phenomenon)
phenomenal
    p. absolutism
    p. field
    p. motion
    p. pattern
    p. regression
    p. report
    p. self
phenomenalism
phenomenalistic
    p. introspection
    p. thought
phenomenistic
    p. causality
    p. thought
phenomenological
    p. analysis
    p. characteristic

p. feature
p. measure
p. reality
p. subgroup
phenomenology
    clinical p.
    existential p.
phenomenon, pl. **phenomena**
    abstinence p.
    arm p.
    autoscopic p.
    Bezold-Brucke p.
    breakaway p.
    breakoff p.
    breast-phantom p.
    Capgras p.
    choo-choo p.
    clasp-knife p.
    clinical p.
    cogwheel p.
    constancy p.
    crossed phrenic p.
    cultural p.
    dissociative p.
    disturbance associated with
      conversion p.
    Doppelganger p.
    echo p.
    escape p.
    facialis p.
    Fere p.
    finger p.
    freezing p.
    Fregoli p.
    gestalt p.
    Grasset-Gaussel p.
    hesitation p.
    hidden observer p.
    Hoffmann p.
    hypofrontality p.
    identification p.
    p. identification
    implausible p.
    interactive p.
    Isakower p.
    jamais p.
    jet lag p.
    knee p.
    Kohnstamm p.
    leg p.
    Leichtenstern p.
    mental p.

NOTES

P

phenomenon *(continued)*
    misdirection p.
    motor p.
    napping p.
    normal voluntary napping p.
    panic-spectrum p.
    panum p.
    paradoxical pupillary p.
    paranormal p.
    paroxysmal p.
    peroneal p.
    phi p.
    Pool p.
    psi p.
    psychic p.
    psychomotor p.
    psychotic-like p.
    radial p.
    rebound p.
    release p.
    riddance p.
    Ritter-Rollet p.
    Schüller p.
    sensory p.
    soft psychotic-like p.
    split screen p.
    Tarchanoff p.
    thought transfer p.
    tip-of-the-tongue p.
    toe p.
    tongue p.
    trailing p.
    transference p.
    transient p.
    transvestic p.
    voluntary napping p.
    Westphal p.
    Westphal-Piltz p.
    Wever-Bray p.
    Zeigarnik effect p.
phenomotive
phenoplegia
phenotype
    alcohol-related p.
    clinical p.
    membrane p.
phenotypic
    p. factor
    p. marker
    p. study
phenylpyruvic
    p. amentia
    p. oligophrenia
pheromone
PHI
    physiological hyaluronidase inhibitor
philandering
philanthropy

philobat
philology
philomimesia
philoneism
philopatridomania
philoprogenitive
philosophical
    p. analysis
    p. decision
    p. discussion
    p. inclination
    p. psychology
philosophize
philosophy
    analytical p.
    anthropological p.
    coercive p.
    humanistic p.
    p. of life
    moral p.
    treatment p.
philter, philtre
philtrum
phi phenomenon
phlegm
phlegmatic constitutional type
phobanthropy
phobia
phobia-induced migraine headache
phobic
    p. anxiety
    p. attitude
    p. avoidance
    p. avoidant behavior
    p. character
    p. companion
    p. desensitization
    p. neurotic disorder
    nongeneral p.
    p. obsessional neurosis
    p. psychogenic disorder
    p. psychoneurotic reaction
    p. situation
    p. state
    p. stimulus
    p. syndrome
    p. trend
phobic-anxiety-depersonalization neurosis
phoesthesia
pholcodine
phonasthenia
phonation
phonatory theory
phoneme
    anterior feature English p.
    diffuse p.
phoneme-grapheme association

phonemic
    p. analysis
    p. awareness
phonetic
    acoustic p.'s
    p. analysis
    p. babble
    p. clarity
    p. information
    p. input
    p. noise
phonetically balanced words
phoniatrics
phonic spasm
phonism
phonogram
phonological
    p. agraphia
    p. analysis
    p. disorder
    p. processing
phonologically
    p. irregular words
    p. regular words
phonologic assembly impairment
phonomania
phonomyoclonus
phonomyography
phonopathy
phonopsia
phosphatase
    alkaline p.
phosphorus
phosphorylation
photalgia
photesthesia
photic
    p. driving
    p. epilepsy
    p. stimulation
photism
photoaxis
photodynia
photodysphoria
photoesthetic
photogenic
    p. epilepsy
    p. seizure
photographic memory
photography
    pornographic p.
photokinetic

photolabile
photoma
photomania
photomyoclonus
photon
photopathy
photophilic
photophobic
photopic vision
photopilic
photoptarmosis
photoreceptor cell
photosensitive epilepsy
photosensitivity
phototherapy
phrase
    coin new p.'s
    p. construction (PC)
phren
phrenalgia
phrenectomy
phrenemphraxis
phrenetic
phrenic
phrenicectomy
phreniclasia
phrenicoexeresis
phreniconeurectomy
phrenicotomy
phrenicotripsy
phrenitica
    aphrodisia p.
phrenitis
phrenocardia
phrenoglottic
phrenologist
phrenology
phrenoplegia
phrenoplegy
phrenopraxic
phrenospasm
phrenotropic
phrictopathia
phrictopathic
phronemomania
phronesis
phthinoid
phthisica
    spes p.
phthisicus
    habitus p.
phyloanalysis

NOTES

P

phylobiology
phylogenesis
phylogenetic
    p. mneme
    p. predecessor
    p. principle
    p. symptoms
phylogenetically
phylogeny
physaliformis
    ecchordosis p.
physiatrics
physiatry
physic
physical
    p. abuse
    p. activity
    p. aggression
    p. agitation
    p. anergia
    p. anthropology
    p. appearance
    p. assault
    p. attack
    p. bondage
    p. capacity
    p. change
    p. comorbid disorder
    p. concern
    p. concomitant of anxiety
    p. condition organic psychosis
    p. danger
    p. defect
    p. dependence
    p. discipline
    p. discomfort
    p. disturbance
    p. education
    p. environment
    p. examination (PE)
    p. exercise
    p. experience
    p. fight
    p. fitness
    p. harm
    history and p. (H&P)
    p. impairment
    p. independence
    p. injury
    p. integrity
    p. intersex condition
    p. manifestation of pain
    p. medicine
    p. problem
    p. psychogenic disorder
    p. restraint
    p. sensation
    p. sign

    p. signs and symptoms
    p. skills
    p. strain
    p. stress
    p. support
    p. symptom distress
    p. symptoms adjustment reaction
    p. tension
    p. therapist
    p. therapy
    p. trauma
    p. withdrawal
physically aggressive behavior
physician
    American Society of
      Psychoanalytic P.'s (ASPP)
    p. assistant (PA)
    attending p.
    family p.
    general medical p.
    house p.
    National Association of
      Inpatient P.'s (NAIP)
    primary care p.
    resident p.
physician-assisted suicide
physician-expert
physician-patient
    p.-p. communication
    p.-p. encounter
    p.-p. relationship
    p.-p. scenario
Physicians'
    P. Desk Reference (PDR)
physiodrama
physiogenesis
physiogenetic depression
physiogenic
physiognomic
    p. perception
    p. thinking
physiognomy
physiognosis
physiologica
    alalia p.
physiological, physiologic
    p. age
    p. amenorrhea
    p. arousal
    p. aspect
    p. basis
    p. basis of personality
    p. component
    p. dependence
    p. drive
    p. effect
    p. feedback
    p. functional variation

p. hyaluronidase inhibitor (PHI)
p. hyperarousal
p. intoxication
p. limit
p. maintenance
p. manifestation
p. measure
p. mechanism
p. memory
p. motive
p. need
p. norm
p. paradigm
p. process
psychogenic p.
p. psychology
p. reactivity
p. reflex
p. response
p. response specificity
p. risk factor
p. sleepiness
p. sleepiness index
p. tremor

physiology
ejaculation p.
sexual p.
p. of women

physiomedical
physioneurosis
physiopathologic
physiopathology
physioplastic stage
physiopsychic
physiotherapy
physique type
physocephaly
phytochemicals
phytogenous
PI
paradoxical intention
present illness
proactive inhibition

Piaget cognitive development stage
piagetian theory of moral reasoning development
pianist's cramp
piano player's cramp
PIAPACS
psychological information, acquisition, processing, and control system

piblokto, pibloktog
p. syndrome
pica
p. disorder
paper p.
Picchu
Pick
P. atrophy
P. disease dementia
P. syndrome
picking
orifice p.
skin p.
pickwickian syndrome
picky eater
picrotoxin
PICSYMS
picture symbols
pictogram
pictograph
pictophilia
pictorial
p. aphasia
p. imagery
picture
p. arrangement
p. arrangement subtest
p. assembly
clinical p.
p. completion (PC)
p. completion subtest
concrete p.
p. frustration study (PFS)
p. inventory
inward p.
p. in picture technique
p. symbols (PICSYMS)
p. vocabulary test
picture-caption pair
PICU
psychiatric intensive care unit
piercing
body p.
piesesthesia
piety
filial p.
PIF
premorbid inferiority feeling
Pigem question
pigeon
stool p.

NOTES

P

PIL
  purpose in life
pilfer
pilgrimage
    spiritual p.
pill
    birth control p. (BCP)
    morning-after p.
    pop p.'s
    p. rolling
    sleeping p.
pillage
pillow
    psychological p.
pill-rolling tremor
piloerection
piloid
pilojection
pilomotor
    p. pathway
    p. reflex
    p. response
pilot
    p. interview
    p. program
    p. study
pimp
pimping
pineal
    p. body
    p. substance
    p. therapy
pinealopathy
Pinel-Haslam syndrome
Pinel system
ping-pong gaze
pinheaded
pining
pink
    p. collar worker
    p. noise
    p. spot
pinpoint pupils
pins-and-needles sensation
pins-sticking sensation
pious
PIPE
    pharmacologically induced penile
    erection
pipe
    p. dream
    peace p.
piperidyl derivative
Piportil Depot
pipotiazine
pique
Pisa syndrome

pistol
    snub-nose p.
pit
    snake p.
pitch
    absolute p.
    basal p.
    p. discrimination
pithecoid idiot
pithiatism
pithiatric
pitiable
pitiful
Pitres
    P. law
    P. rule
    P. sign
pitting edema
pituitary
    p. basophilia
    p. cachexia
    p. eunuchism
    p. prolactin release
    p. stalk section
pityrodes
    alopecia p.
piuturi
pivotal role
pixelated parietotemporal perfusion deficit
pixie
pixieish
pixilated
PK
    psychokinesis
    psychokinetic
PKC
    protein kinase C
PL
    psychosocial-labile
placate
place
    p. blame
    closed p.
    crowded p.
    deep p.
    p. deixis
    deserted p.
    p. identity
    open p.
    oriented to time and p.
    safe p.
    sense of p.
    p. theory
    unfamiliar p.
placebo
    active p.
    balanced p.

p. effect
p. medication trial
p. reactor
p. response rate
placebo-controlled
p.-c. drug study
p.-c. trial
placement
p. counseling
electrode p.
foster care p.
home p.
job p.
nursing home p.
personnel p.
residential p.
sheltered workshop p.
skilled nursing facility p.
therapeutic school p.
therapeutic vocational p.
unavoidable p.
place-specific event
placid disposition
plagiocephalic idiocy
plain-folks technique
plaintive
plaiser
maitre de p.
plan
absence of eating p.
acceptable treatment p.
complete treatment p.
cottage p.
electronic disaster recovery p.
family health insurance p. (FHIP)
game p.
homicidal p.
life p.
multidisciplinary treatment p.
  (MTP)
organizational p.
overcontrolled eating p.
realistic p.
rigid eating p.
subjective, objective, assessment, p.
  (SOAP)
suicidal p.
suicide p.
treatment p. (TRPL)
plane
coronal p.
median sagittal p.

sagittal p.
subjective p.
planigraphy
planned
p. after-school activity
p. course
p. learning environment
P. Parenthood
p. pregnancy
planner
planning
career p.
comprehensive treatment p.
conceptual p.
p. disturbance
family p.
lack of future p.
motor p.
operational p.
permanent p.
poor motor p.
social policy p.
strategic p.
treatment p.
uninhibited motor p.
planomania
planophrasia
planotopokinesia
plant
loco p.
plantalgia
plantar
p. response
planum
p. temporale
p. temporale morphology
plaque
argentophilic p.
neuritic p.
senile p.
plasma
p. cortisol
p. leptin level
plastic
p. arts therapy
p. compensatory mechanism
p. reorganization
p. surgery
p. tonus
plasticity
decerebrate p.
functional p.

NOTES

P

plasticity *(continued)*
    hippocampal synaptic p.
    p. of libido
    neural p.
    neuronal p.
    synaptic p.
plat
plateau
    p. in improvement
    p. masking technique
    p. method
    p. phase
    p. speech
platelet
    p. monoamine oxidase
platform
    orgasmic p.
platitude
platonic
    p. friendship
    p. love
    p. nymphomania
    p. relationship
platonism
platonization
platybasia
plausible
plausive
play
    p. acting
    associative p.
    p. both ends against the middle
    dramatic p.
    extended p.
    fantasy p.
    p. the field
    foul p.
    free p.
    p. the game
    games people p.
    group p.
    p. group psychotherapy
    p. group therapy (PGT)
    imaginative p.
    independent p.
    joint p.
    make-believe p.
    p. on words
    organized p.
    parallel p.
    peer p.
    repetitive p.
    rough-and-tumble p.
    p. session
    sex p.
    shadow p.
    symbolic p.
    p. technique

    p. therapy
    verbal p.
    p. with oneself
player
    game p.
    team p.
    war-game p.
playfulness
playing
    p. dead
    game p.
    multiple role p.
    role p.
playroom
PLC
    personal locus of control
plea
    p. bargain
    p. for help
    p. of insanity
plead
pleasant
    p. memory
    p. stimuli
pleasantness rating
pleasurable
    p. affect
    p. emotion
    p. stimuli
pleasure
    activity p.
    aesthetic p.
    p. center
    p. ego
    p. experience
    p. fear
    function p.
    loss of p.
    muscle p.
    organ p.
    organic p.
    p. principle
    sensual p.
    sexual p.
pleasure-oriented behavior
pleasure-pain principle
pleasuring
pledge
plenary indulgence
pleniloquence
plentitude
pleonasm
pleonexia
plethysmograph
    penile p.
    vaginal p.
plethysmography
pleurothotonos, pleurothotonus

pleusirs
    folie a p.
plexectomy
plexiform
plexitis
pliable
plight
PLISSIT Model
plod
plot
    funnel p.
ploy
plucking
    p. at clothes
    hair p.
plucky
plumbism
plunder
plunge
    postpartum psychological p.
pluralism
    p. marriage
    p. utilitarianism
pluralistic utilitarianism
plutocracy
plutomania
p.m.
    afternoon
PMA
    paramethoxyamphetamine
    positive mental attitude
PMDD
    premenstrual dysphoric disorder
PMI
    petition of mental illness
PMS
    premenstrual syndrome
PMTS
    premenstrual tension syndrome
PN
    pontine nucleus
    psychoneurotic
PNAvQ
    positive-negative ambivalent quotient
PND
    postnatal depression
pneumatocele
pneumocele
pneumocephalus
pneumophonia
pneumorhachis

PNI
    psychoneuroimmunology
PNP
    psychogenic nocturnal polydipsia
PNS
    parasympathetic nervous system
    peripheral nervous system
pococurante
podismus
Poggendorf illusion
poiesis
poignancy
poignant
poikilothymia
point
    apophysary p.
    beside the p.
    case in p.
    change p.
    choice p.
    critical p.
    end p.
    p. fear
    fixation p.
    flicker-fusion p.
    p. of honor
    indifference p.
    p. localization
    p. localization test
    moot p.
    motor p.
    p. of no return
    painful p.
    pressure p.
    p. prevalence
    racial saturation p.
    p. of regard
    p. resolved spectroscopy (PRESS)
    p. scale
    p. of subjective equality (PSE)
    tender p.
    time p.
    to the p.
    trigger p.
    Trousseau p.
    Valleix p.
    p. of view
point-and-shoot video game
pointed object
pointes
point-for-point correspondence

NOTES

P

pointing
 bone p.
 p. of the bone
 finger p.
pointless
7-point scale
poise
 tough p.
poison
 cultural p.
 p. hemlock
 social p.
poisoning
 acetaminophen p.
 acute amphetamine p.
 acute lead p.
 alcohol p.
 alcoholic p.
 amphetamine p.
 aspirin p.
 blood p.
 bromide p.
 carbon dioxide p.
 carbon monoxide p.
 chronic lead p.
 deadly nightshade p.
 food p.
 gas p.
 lead p.
 narcotic p.
 nicotine p.
 nightshade p.
 opiate p.
 opioid p.
 opium p.
 paregoric p.
 thallium p.
poisonous
Poisson distribution
poker
 p. face
 p. spine
polacrilex
polar
 p. opposite
 p. zone
polarity
 p. response
 sorting p.'s
polarization
 mass p.
 principle of dynamic p.
 sexual p.
polemic
polemicize
police power
policy
 p. analysis

 health p.
 p. implication
 Office of National Drug
  Control P.
 open-door p.
 social p.
polioclastic
politeness
politesse
politic
political
 p. affiliation
 p. genetics
 p. group
 p. mania
 p. psychiatry
 p. value
politically incorrect
politico-economic-conservatism (PEC)
 p.-e.-c. scale
politicomania
politikon
 zoon p.
poll
 opinion p.
pollodic
pollution
Pollyanna-like view
Pollyanna mechanism
poltergeist
polyandry
polyarteritis
 p. nodosa dementia
Polybus love
polyclonia
Polycrates complex
polycratism
polydipsia
 hysterical p.
 psychogenic p.
 psychogenic nocturnal p. (PNP)
 psychosis-induced p.
polydrug
 p. abuse
 p. addiction
polydystrophic oligophrenia
polyesthesia
polyethic criteria set
Polyfactorial Study of Personality
polygamist
polygamous
polygamy
polygenic
 p. inheritance
 p. trait
polyglot
 p. amnesia
 p. neophasia

polygraph
>Keeler p.

polygynous
polygyny
polygyria
polyideic somnambulism
polyleptic
polylogia
polymatric
polymorphism
>insertion-deletion p.
>restriction fragment length p.
>(RFLP)

polymorphous
>p. perverse disposition
>p. perverse sexuality
>p. perversion

polyneuritica
>psychosis p.

polyneuritic alcoholic psychosis
polyneuritiformis
>heredopathia atactica p.

polyneuritis
>acute idiopathic p.
>chronic familial p.

polyneuronitis
polyneuropathy
>buckthorn p.
>critical illness p. (CIP)
>nutritional p.

polyopia
polyparesis
polyphagia
polyphallic
polypharmacy
polyphasic
>p. activity
>p. potential
>p. sleep rhythm

polyphrasia
polyphyria
polyplegia
polypnea
polyposia
polypsychism
polysemous
polysemy
polysensory unit
polyserositis
polysomnogram (PSG, PSM)
polysomnograph, polysomnography (PSG)

polysteraxic
polysubstance
>p. abuse
>p. addiction
>p. dependence
>p. use disorder

polysubstance-related disorder
polysymptomatic syndrome
polytheism
polythetic
polytomography
polytomous regression
polytoxicomanic
polytrophic defect
polytropic defect
polyvalent
POM
>prescription-only medicine

Pompadour fantasy
pomposity
pompous
pompousness
ponder
ponderous
ponopathy
pons, pl. **pontes**
pontifical
pontificate
pontine
>p. nucleus (PN)
>p. sleep

pontocerebellar angle syndrome
pool
>autonomic motor p.
>dirty p.
>gene p.
>P. phenomenon

pooling
poor
>p. academic preparation
>p. attachment
>p. body image
>p. eating habit
>p. form response (F-)
>p. genital response
>p. historian
>p. hygiene
>p. impulse control
>p. insight
>p. judgment
>p. language skills
>p. law

NOTES

P

poor *(continued)*
- p. motor planning
- p. mouth
- p. peer relationship
- p. performance evaluation
- p. prognosis
- p. reasoning ability
- p. response to medication
- p. school performance
- p. sleep quality

poorly
- p. developed
- p. groomed
- p. systematized delusion

poorness of fit

pop
- p. culture
- p. off
- p. pills
- p. psychology

popper

poppy
- opium p.

popular
- p. culture
- p. response

population
- adolescent p.
- p. cage
- clinical p.
- clinic patient p.
- community p.
- criminal p.
- culturally diverse p.
- p. density
- general p.
- p. genetics
- geriatric p.
- high-risk p.
- outpatient patient p.
- partial hospital patient p.
- primary care patient p.
- prison p.
- p. research
- p. setting
- p. standard deviation
- p. stratification
- target p.

POR
- problem-oriented record

porencephalia *(var. of* porencephaly)

porencephalic, porencephalous

porencephalitis

porencephalopathy

porencephalous *(var. of* porencephalic)

porencephaly, porencephalia

poriomania

poriomanic fugue

porn
- kiddie p.

pornerastic

pornographic
- p. illustration
- p. mania
- p. photography
- p. writing

pornography
- child p.
- p. dependence
- dependence on p.
- Internet child p.
- online p.
- paraphiliac p.

pornolagnia

porosis, pl. poroses
- cerebral p.

porphobilinogen (PBG)

porphyria
- hepatic p.

porphyrismus

porropsia

portal systemic encephalopathy (PSE)

portend

portent

portentous

Posey restraint

posiomania

position
- p. agnosia
- p. of attack
- body p.
- coital p.
- cortical thumb p.
- depressive p.
- information optimization p.
- observer p.
- ordinal p.
- paranoid-schizoid p.
- phase p.
- p. response
- p. of responsibility
- rigid body p.
- schizoid p.
- p. sense
- sociopolitical p.
- subordinate p.
- sustained p.

positional tremor

positive
- p. acceleration
- p. adaptation
- p. afterimage
- p. attention behavior (PAB)
- p. attitude
- p. attitude change
- p. cathexis

p. communication skills
p. comparison
p. conditioned reflex
p. correlation
p. effect
p. emotion
p. emotionality
p. eugenics
p. event
false p.
p. feedback
p. feeling
p. frontal release sign
guaiac p.
p. image
p. incentive
p. induction
p. mental attitude (PMA)
p. motivation
p. parenting
p. picture-caption pair
p. predictive power
p. recency
p. regard
p. reinforcement
p. reinforcement therapy
p. reinforcer
p. relationship
p. response
p. result
p. schizophrenia
p. schizophrenic symptoms
p. score
p. speech content
p. spike pattern
p. symptom dimension
p. symptoms psychosis
p. thought disorder
p. transfer
p. transference
true p.
p. valence
positively
p. bathmotropic
p. correlated region
positive-negative ambivalent quotient (PNAvQ)
positivism
logical p.
positivity
positron emission tomography technique
possessed by spirit

possessing agent
possession
demonic p.
drug p.
handgun p.
spirit p.
spiritual p.
p. trance
p. trance disorder
p. trance state
p. trance symptom
possessor-possession
possibility
causal p.
noncausal p.
possible
as soon as p. (ASAP)
possumus
non p.
post
p. ambivalence
p. ambivalent phase stage
p. baseline visit
p. coitum triste
p. contraction recovery phase
p. contusion syndrome
p. contusion syndrome encephalopathy
p. hoc analysis
p. hoc comparison
p. hoc explanation
p. hoc stratification
p. rape syndrome
p. recovery
p. relevant history (PRH)
p. September 11 consciousness
p. stroke depression
p. TIA depression
postabortion syndrome
postadrenalectomy syndrome
postanalytic supervision
postanoxic
p. encephalopathy
p. epilepsy
postapoplectic
postbasic stare
post-binge anguish
postcentral sulcus
postcoital
p. euphoria
p. headache
postconcentration camp syndrome

NOTES

P

postconcussion
- p. amnesia
- p. disorder
- p. headache
- p. neurosis
- p. syndrome

postconvulsive stupor

postdisaster
- p. psychosocial intervention
- p. stress

postdischarge

postdivorce depression

postdormital
- p. chalastic fit
- p. depression
- p. sleep paralysis

postdormitum

post-ECT
- p.-E. amnesia
- p.-E. seizure

postelectroconvulsive
- p. amnesia
- p. therapy

postemotive schizophrenia

postencephalitic
- p. parkinsonism
- p. syndrome

postepileptic twilight state

posterior
- p. alexia
- p. cingulate
- p. cingulate region
- p. frontal hypoperfusion
- p. hypothalamus
- p. inferior cerebellar artery syndrome
- p. language zone

posteriori
- a p.

posterodorsal temporal lobe

postexertional malaise

postfebrile dementia

posthallucinogen
- p. perception
- p. perception disorder

posthemiplegic

posthion

posthypnotic
- p. amnesia
- p. psychosis
- p. suggestion

posthysterectomy depression

postictal
- p. confusion
- p. depression
- p. depression phase of seizure
- p. psychosis
- p. state

posticus
- p. palsy
- p. paralysis
- tetanus p.

postinfectious
- p. depression
- p. psychosis

postketamine

postleukotomy syndrome

postlobotomy syndrome

postmature

postmortem
- p. brain tissue
- p. data
- p. finding
- p. investigation
- p. study
- p. technique

postnatal
- p. depression (PND)
- p. development

postoperative
- p. confusional state
- p. pressure alopecia
- p. psychosis
- p. status
- p. tetany

postparalytic

postpartum
- p. alopecia
- p. blues
- p. depression (PPD)
- p. major depression
- p. mania
- p. psychiatric problem
- p. psychological plunge
- p. psychosis (PPP)
- p. syndrome

postpsychotic
- p. depression
- p. depressive disorder

postpubertal social decline

postpuberty

postpubescence

postpubescent

postreceptor
- heterotrimeric p.
- p. information transduction

postrema

postsaccadic neuronal response

postschizophrenic depression

postsurgical loss

postsynaptic
- p. compensatory mechanism
- p. 5-HT-2 receptor
- p. 5-HT-3 receptor
- p. potential (PSP)
- p. stimulation

posttermination
boundaries p.
p. boundary
posttest level
posttraumatic
p. amnesia (PTA)
p. amnestic syndrome
p. brain syndrome
p. chronic disability
p. cortical dysfunction
p. delirium
p. dementia
p. deterioration
p. disorientation
p. dissociative disorder
p. distress
p. disturbance
p. encephalopathy
p. hallucination
p. headache
immediate p.
p. neurosis
p. organic psychosis
p. osteoporosis
p. pain
p. patient
p. personality
p. personality disorder
p. psychopathic
p. psychopathic constitution
p. seizure
p. stress disorder (PTSD)
p. stress disorder complex
p. stress disorder by proxy
p. stress symptom
p. stress syndrome
p. symptom formation
posttreatment
postural
p. awareness
p. hypotension
p. instability
p. myoneuralgia
p. reflex
p. seizure
p. set
p. syncope
p. tremor
p. unsteadiness
p. vertigo
posture
bent p.

bizarre p.
body p.
curled-into-fetal-position p.
decerebrate p.
inappropriate p.
open p.
rigid p.
sagging p.
p. sense
sleep p.
slumped p.
unusual sleep p.
posturing
bizarre p.
catatonic p.
cerebrate p.
decorticate p.
dystonic p.
sexual p.
post-Vietnam psychiatric syndrome (PVNPS)
potassium chloride elixir
potatorum
potence
potency
orgastic p.
sexual p.
potent
potential
abuse p.
acoustic evoked p.
acting out p.
action p.
p. adverse effect
auditory evoked p. (AEP)
bioelectric p.
biotic p.
brain p.
brain evoked p. (BEP)
brainstem auditory evoked p.
cerebral p.
p. correlation
cortical p.
cortical evoked p.
demarcation p.
early latency p.
effective-reaction p.
electrical p.
p. energy
estimated learning p. (ELP)
event-related p. (ERP)
evoked p. (EP)

NOTES

P

potential *(continued)*
>excitatory postsynaptic p. (EPSP)
>p. external award
>p. external reward
>extrapyramidal symptom p.
>extreme somatosensory evoked p. (ESEP)
>far-field evoked p.
>glossokinetic p.
>graded p.
>high tolerance p.
>human p.
>p. impact
>inhibitory postsynaptic p. (IPSP)
>injury p.
>p. intellectual capacity
>lack of performing to p.
>leadership p.
>local p.
>low tolerance p.
>motor evoked p. (MEP)
>multimodality evoked p. (MEP)
>polyphasic p.
>p. positive event
>postsynaptic p. (PSP)
>p. predisposing factor
>pretreatment binding p.
>resource holding p.
>resting p.
>sensory evoked p. (SEP)
>somatosensory evoked p. (SEP)
>specific action p.
>suicidal p.
>suicide p.
>p. suicide victim
>p. target
>tolerance p.
>visual evoked p. (VEP)
>weight gain p.

potentially
>p. dangerous patient
>p. fatal complications of illicit drug use

potentiate

potentiation
>long-term p. (LTP)

potentiometer

potlatch

potomania

potu
>delirium e p.
>mania a p.
>manie a p.

potus
>fastidium p.

pounding
>p. heart
>p. pain

pourquoi
>folie du p.

poverty
>clinical p.
>p. of content
>p. of content of speech
>p. of content of thought
>p. delusion
>delusion of p.
>p. of idea
>Liddle psychomotor p.
>p. of movement
>psychomotor p.

POW
>prisoner of war
>POW syndrome

powdered opium

power
>combined predictive p.
>delusion of p.
>distribution of p.
>p. dynamic
>higher p.
>illusion of p.
>inflated p.
>instantaneous p.
>mind p.
>negative predictive p.
>perceived p.
>police p.
>positive predictive p.
>predictive p.
>special p.
>p. struggle
>p. struggle leadership pattern
>p. theme
>war p.
>will to p.

powerless

powerlessness
>overt signs of p.

PPAR
>peroxisomal proliferator receptor

PPD
>packs per day
>postpartum depression

PPP
>postpartum psychosis

PR
>psychotherapy responder

practical
>p. counseling
>p. reasoning
>p. social judgment score

practice
>clinical diagnostic p.
>contemporary p.
>contraceptive p.

p. effect
p. experience
group p.
p. guideline
massed negative p.
negative p.
parental feeding p.
programmed p.
reinforced p.
religious p.
P. Research Network
rigid sleep p.
spiritual p.
standard p.
practice-based learning and improvement
practiced task
practicing period
practitioner
p. data bank
general psychiatric p.
mental health p.
nurse p.
psychiatric p.
psychodynamic p.
praecocissima
dementia p.
praecox
dementia p.
ejaculatio p.
heboid p.
neurasthenia p.
predementia p.
pubertas p.
senium p.
pragmatagnosia
pragmatamnesia
pragmatic
p. aphasia
p. level
p. structure
p. text
pragmatics
pragmatism
prameha
sukra p.
Pranayama
praxiology
praxis
ideokinetic p.
prayer
healing p.

prayerful life
PRE
partial-reinforcement effect
preadaptive attitude
preadolescence
preambivalence
preambivalent phase
prearchaic thinking
preataxic
preattachment stage
precausal thinking
precaution
suicide p.
preceding association
precentral
p. seizure
p. sulcus
precipices
precipitant
precipitate
precipitating
p. crisis
p. of epilepsy
p. event
p. factor
p. stress
p. tremor
precipitous mood shift
precision
law of p.
p. therapy
preclinical
p. medicine
p. observation
p. stage
precocious
p. aging
p. puberty
p. sexual interest
precocity
islet of p.
precognition
preconcept
preconceptual stage
precondition
preconsciousness
preconscious thinking
precontemplation
preconvulsive
precuneus
precursor load strategy
predation

NOTES

P

predator
sexual p.
predatory
p. delinquent
p. violence
predecessor
phylogenetic p.
predelay reinforcement
predementia praecox
predestination
predeterminism
predicate thinking
predictability
establish p.
predictable
predictably
prediction
clinical p.
p. of dangerousness
p. of mortality
p. study
predictive
p. characteristic
p. factor
p. power
p. property
p. relationship
p. validity
p. value
predictor
early p.
independent p.
peritraumatic p.
pharmacological p.
psychometric p.
suicide p.
symptom-related p.
p. variable
predispose
predisposed
p. individual
situationally p.
predisposing
p. factor
p. socioculture factors for violence
predisposition
p. to attachment
biologic p.
fundamental p.
genetic p.
p. to suicidal acts
suicide p.
predominant
p. affect
p. current defense level
p. feature
p. mood disturbance
p. symptom presentation

predominate
predormital sleep paralysis
predormitum
preemployment drug screening
preepisode status
preexisting
p. condition
p. dementia
p. emotional problem
p. illness
p. mental disorder
p. mental disorder symptom
p. representation
p. tremor
p. underlying emotional issue
preference
color p.
conditioned place p. (CPP)
eye p.
food p.
hand p.
paraphiliac p.
risk p.
sexual p.
preferential occupancy
preferred
least p.
p. method
p. provider organization
p. representational system
prefrontal
p. cortex
p. cortex activation
p. cortex of the brain
p. cortical activity dysregulation
p. cortical area
p. cortical volume
p. flow
p. hyperactivity
p. hypermetabolism
p. hypofunction
p. lobe
p. lobotomy
p. metabolism
p. region
p. sonic treatment (PST)
pregenital
p. factor
p. love
p. organization
p. phase
p. stage
pregnancy
accidental p.
adolescent p.
anxiety during p.
p. and birth complication
depression during p.

false p.
p. fear
hysterical p.
p. loss
planned p.
psychosis in p.
psychosis during p.
termination of p.
unplanned p.
untimely p.
unwanted p.
voluntary interruption of p. (VIP)
preindustrial
prejudice
age p.
ethnic p.
expression of p.
lifestyle p.
radial p.
roots of p.
preliminary analysis
prelingual deafness
preliterate
prelogical
p. mind
p. thinking
Premack principle
premaniacal
premarital
p. counseling
p. sex
prematura
alopecia p.
premature
p. alopecia
p. birth
p. confrontation
p. death
p. discharge
p. ejaculation
p. ejaculation psychosexual
dysfunction
p. female orgasm
p. male orgasm
prematurity
premeditation
premenopausal amenorrhea
premenstrual
p. dysphoria
p. dysphoric disorder (PMDD)
p. syndrome (PMS)
p. tension

p. tension state
p. tension syndrome (PMTS)
premise
premium
incitement p.
premonition of seizure
premonitory
p. feeling
p. sigh
p. sign
p. symptom
p. urge
premorality
premorbid
p. adjustment
p. asociality
p. inferiority feeling (PIF)
p. intellectual function
p. level of functioning
p. personality
p. personality trait
p. psychiatric history
p. state
p. trauma
premotor
p. area
p. syndrome
prenatal
p. history
p. illicit drug use
p. period
prenubile
preoccupation
p. of bodily functions
control p.
death p.
defect p.
delusion-like p.
gambling p.
homicidal p.
hypochondriacal p.
lists p.
obsessive p.
orderliness p.
organization p.
pathologic p.
pathological p.
perfectionism p.
rule p.
schedules p.
sexual p.
stalker p.

NOTES

preoccupation (*continued*)
  suicidal p.
  p. of thought
  unshakable p.
  p. with death
  p. with defect
  p. with defect in appearance
  p. with detail
  p. with guilt
  p. with sameness
  p. with worthlessness
preoccupied
preoedipal, pre-oedipal
  p. factor
  p. level
  p. phase
  p. stage
preoperational
  p. development
  p. phase
  p. thinking
  p. thought
  p. thought period
  p. thought stage
preorgasmic
preparalytic
preparation
  academic p.
  antipsychotic p.
  atypical antipsychotic p.
  drug p.
  herbal p.
  marijuana p.
  poor academic p.
  split-brain p.
preparedness
  anxiety p.
  principle of p.
prephallic
preponderance of the evidence
prepotent
prepsychotic
  p. pain
  p. personality
  p. psychosis
  p. schizophrenia
prepubertal
  p. borderline psychosis
  p. child
  p. children
  p. mania
  p. psychopathology
prepuberty
prepubescent
preputial sensation
presbyophrenia
presbyophrenic psychosis
preschizophrenic ego

preschool child
preschooler
prescience
prescribed treatment
prescribing
  p. consultant
  p. privilege
prescription (Rx)
  p. drug
  p. drug abuse
  p. drug addiction
  p. drug dependence
  p. drug-related disorder
  p. forgery
  p. medication
prescription-only medicine (POM)
prescriptive authority
preselection
  sex p.
presence of frenzy
presenile
  confusional state p.
  p. dementia
  p. dementia confusional state
  p. mental disorder
  p. organic psychotic state
  p. paraphrenia
  p. psychosis
presenilis
  alopecia p.
  anxietas p.
  dementia p.
presenility
presenium
present
  p. distress
  p. illness (PI)
  p. oriented
present-absent dichotomy
presentation
  atypical p.
  catatonic p.
  clinical p.
  conversion disorder with mixed p.
  depressed p.
  distinct depressed p.
  distinct dysphoric p.
  distinct euphoric p.
  dysphoric p.
  equivalent symptomatic p.
  euphoric p.
  heterogeneous clinical p.
  historical p.
  histrionic p.
  mixed p.
  pain p.
  predominant symptom p.
  psychotic p.

substance-induced p.
subthreshold p.
symptom p.
symptomatic p.
typical p.
presentational ritual
presenting
p. characteristic
p. personality
p. psychopathology
p. symptom
present-oriented
preservation of affect
PRESS
point resolved spectroscopy
press
environmental p.
pressing thought
pressure
acoustic p.
ambient air p.
p. anesthesia
blood p.
cerebral perfusion p. (CPP)
cerebrospinal p.
cranial perfusion p. (CPP)
environmental p.
group p.
p. of ideas
intracranial p. (ICP)
job p.
minimal audible p.
p. palsy
p. paralysis
peer p.
p. point
p. sense
social p.
p. of speech
systolic p. (SP)
thought p.
time p.
pressured
p. behavior
p. speech
pressure-volume index
prestige suggestion
presumed
p. causality
p. etiology

presumption
p. of competence
tender years p.
presumptive basis
presuperego phase
presupposition
presynaptic
p. functional deficit
p. neuron
pretense
false p.
pretraumatic
p. risk factor
p. vulnerability
pretreatment
p. binding potential
p. measure
prevalence
cross-sectional p.
differential p.
gambling p.
lifetime p.
period p.
point p.
p. rate
suicide p.
treated p.
prevalent
prevention
accident p.
American Foundation for
Suicide P.
anxiety p.
Centers for Disease Control and P.
disease p.
dropout prediction and p. (DPP)
exposure and response p. (ERP)
new age suicide p.
Office of Juvenile Justice and
Delinquency P.
primary p.
relapse p.
response p.
ritual p.
secondary p.
stress p.
suicide p.
tertiary p.
p. and treatment of depression
(PTD)
violence p.

NOTES

P

preventive
  p. intervention
  p. medicine
  p. psychiatry
preverbal attentional processing
previous
  p. attempt
  p. history
  p. treatment
previously stabilizing social situations
prewiring
PRH
  post relevant history
priapism
pride
  brute p.
  domesticated p.
  excessive p.
  moral p.
  penis p.
  phallic p.
  p. in self
  p. system
priest
primacy
  complete genital p.
  early genital p.
  genital p.
  oral p.
  phallic p.
prima donna
primal
  p. anxiety
  p. fantasy
  p. father
  p. libido
  p. repression
  p. sadism
  p. scene
  p. scream
  p. scream therapy
  p. trauma
primary
  p. active compound
  p. affective disorder (PAD)
  p. affective witzelsucht
  p. amentia
  p. anesthesia
  p. anxiety
  p. anxiety disorder
  p. auditory cortex
  p. autism
  p. autonomous function
  p. behavior
  p. behavior disorder
  p. care
  p. care evaluation of mental
    disorders (PRIME-MD)

  p. caregiver
  p. care patient population
  p. care physician
  p. care setting
  p. caretaker
  p. circular reaction
  p. color
  p. complaint
  p. defense symptom
  p. degenerative dementia (PDD)
  p. degenerative dementia of
    Alzheimer type (PDDAT)
  p. diagnosis
  p. disorder of sleep
  p. disorder of wakefulness
  p. drives
  p. dysthymia
  p. effect
  p. efficacy outcome
  p. encopresis
  p. enduring negative symptom
  p. feeblemindedness
  p. gain
  p. generalized epilepsy
  p. hue
  p. hypersomnia
  p. hypersomnia, recurrent type
  p. ictal automatism
  p. identification
  p. identity
  p. impotence
  p. insomnia
  p. integration
  p. mechanism
  p. memory
  p. mental ability
  p. mental image
  p. mood disorder
  p. motivation
  p. motor deficit
  p. narcissism
  p. need
  p. neurasthenia
  p. nocturnal enuresis
  p. nonenduring negative symptom
  p. object-love
  p. oppositional attitude
  p. orgasmic dysfunction
  p. personality trait
  p. pharmacological approach
  p. prevention
  p. process thinking
  p. psychiatric disorder
  p. psychic process
  p. purpose
  p. quality
  p. reinforcement
  p. reinforcer

p. repression
p. responsibility
p. retarded ejaculation
p. reward conditioning
p. risk factor
p. schizophrenia
p. seizure
p. senile dementia
p. sensation
p. sensory cortex
p. sex character
p. sex characteristic
p. sexual deviation
p. sexual relationship
p. shock
p. somatic problem
p. stress
p. support group
p. task
p. thought disorder
p. tic
p. transitional object
p. victim
p. zone

primary-secondary distinction
prime of life
PRIME-MD
primary care evaluation of mental
disorders
priming
p. dose
p. memory
primitivation
primitive
p. aggressive self-organization
(PASO)
p. emotional level
p. idealization
p. narcissism
p. psychosomatic language
p. reflex
p. superego
primitivization
primordial
p. delusion
p. panic
primrose
evening p.
primum non nocere
principal
p. diagnosis
p. focus

p. investigation
p. objective
p. symptom
principal-components analysis (PCA)
principle
anticipatory-maturation p.
p. of anticipatory maturation
authority p.
binary p.
Bolam P.
p. of Buddhist meditation
closure p.
communion p.
consistency p.
disuse p.
dynamic p.
p. of dynamic polarization
echo p.
economic p.
epigenetic p.
ethical p.
homeopathic p.
homeostatic p.
p. of inertia
intimacy p.
isopathic p.
least-effort p.
moral p.
morality of self-accepted moral p.
nirvana p.
normalization p.
optimal-stimulation p.
organizing p.
pain p.
pain-pleasure p.
Peter P.
phylogenetic p.
pleasure p.
pleasure-pain p.
Premack p.
p. of preparedness
psychophysiologic p.
reality p.
rebus p.
repetition-compulsion p.
self-chosen ethical p.
talion p.
Tarasoff p.
transfer of p.
treble safeguard p.
p. of truth telling
utilitarian p.

NOTES

P

principle *(continued)*
>von Domarus p.
>weighted-harm p.
>wellness p.

principlism

prion
>p. analog
>p. disease

prior
>p. to admission (PTA)
>p. violence

priori
>a p.
>p. expectation of gratitude

prioritize

pris
>parti p.

prison
>p. confinement
>Federal Bureau of P.'s
>p. inmate
>maximum-security p.
>p. neurosis
>p. population
>p. psychiatry
>p. psychologist
>p. psychosis
>p. sentence

prisoner
>p. privileges
>p. of war (POW)
>p. of war syndrome

Pritikin diet

privacy
>p. clearinghouse
>p. compliance
>erosion of p.
>invasion of p.
>p. right

private
>p. belief system
>p. psychiatric hospital
>p. psychosis

privilege
>bathroom p.'s
>lost p.'s (LP)
>prescribing p.
>prisoner p.'s
>psychotherapist-patient p.
>testimonial p.

privileged
>p. communication
>p. information

prn, PRN
>as needed

PRO
>peer review organization

proactive inhibition (PI)

probabilistic fashion

probability
>conditional p.
>p. curve
>p. learning
>transitional p.

probable error (PE)

proband
>adult-onset p.
>autistic p.
>p. condition
>p. diagnosis
>p. method
>p. status

probation
>p. officer
>special needs p.
>standard p.
>supervised p.
>p. violation

probe
>indirect p.
>radiolabeled p.

problem
>academic p.
>acculturation p.
>addiction-related p.
>affect intensity p.
>aggregation p.
>alcohol p.
>alcohol-related physical p.
>alcohol-related psychiatric p.
>arithmetic p.
>attention p.
>attentional p.
>p. behavior
>behavior p.
>p. behavior clusters
>p. child
>p.'s of childhood
>conceptual p.
>concurrent psychiatric p.
>conduct p.
>core p.
>court-related p.
>daily record of severity of p.'s (DRSP)
>developmental learning p. (DLP)
>Diagnosis and Remediation of Handwriting P.'s
>disciplinary p.
>p. drinker (PD)
>p. drinking
>emotional p.
>employment p.

enduring p.
environmental p.
faith conversion p.
familial aggregation p.
feeding p.
fundamental conceptual p.
fundamental psychometric p.
gait p.
p. gambler
human p.
hyperactivity p.
identity p.
impulse control p.
International Statistical Classification
  of Diseases and Related
  Health P.'s
interpersonal cognitive p.
language p.
learning p.
life circumstance p.
marital p.
medical p.
mind-body p.
nuclear p.
occupational p.
orgasmic p.
other interpersonal p.
p. parent
parental control p.
parental marital p.
parent-child relational p.
partner relational p.
p. patient
personality p.
pervasive p.
phase-of-life p.
physical p.
postpartum psychiatric p.
preexisting emotional p.
primary somatic p.
psychiatric p.
psychological p.
psychometric p.
psychophysiological p.
psychosocial p.
questioning faith p.
real-life p.
p.'s related to abuse
p.'s related to neglect
relational p.
religious or spiritual p.
retrieval p.

school discipline p.
school entering p.
secondary emotional p.
sibling relational p.
sleep p.
social p.
p. solving
somatic p.
stress-related psychophysiological p.
substance-related legal p.
subtle memory p.
workplace p.
problematic sexual behavior
problem-based learning
problem-oriented record (POR)
problem-solving
  p.-s. communication
  group p.-s.
  p.-s. negotiation
  p.-s. skills
  p.-s. skills training
  p.-s. strategy
  p.-s. style
procedure
  age correction p.
  analysis p.
  assessment p.
  attention-focusing p.
  blocking p.
  carotid Amytal p. (CAP)
  clinical p.
  cloze p.
  commitment p.
  Committee on Standards and
    Survey P.'s
  decremental p.
  diagnostic p.
  functional pragmatic p.
  Mitofsky-Aaksberg random digit
    dialing p.
  prototype matching p.
  psychological p.
  Q-Sort p.
  rating p.
  recording p.
  standard rating p.
  surgical p.
  SWAP-200 assessment p.
  test orientation p. (TOP)
  time-out p.
proceeding
  care and protection p.

NOTES

proceeding *(continued)*
    incompetency p.
    protection p.
process
    action-group p.
    active pathophysiologic p.
    adaptive p.
    adjustment p.
    affective p.
    age-related developmental p.
    analytical p.
    automatic psychological p.
    biologic p.
    bizarre thought p.
    brain p.
    central timing p.
    children's language p.'s
    circumstantial thought p.
    closure p.
    cognitive p.
    collaborative treatment p.
    common central p.
    complex learning p.
    comprehensive identification p.
      (CIP)
    computational p.
    concrete thought p.
    conscious p.
    consciously accessible p.
    consciously inaccessible p.
    counseling p.
    cultural p.
    decision-making p.
    declarative memory p.
    defensive p.
    dementia p.
    dementing p.
    deterioration p.
    developmental p.
    diagnostic p.
    disease p.
    due p.
    egocentric thought p.
    elementary p.
    p. of elimination
    emotional memory p.
    emotive p.
    empirical p.
    environmental p.
    ergotropic p.
    evidence-based p.
    excitatory-inhibitory p.
    executive p.
    explicit p.
    family p.
    fantasy p.
    feature contrasts p.

    feeling of being detached from
      one's mental p.
    free access to p.
    fundamental cognitive p.
    fundamental response p.
    goal-oriented p.
    group p.
    harmony p.
    healing p.
    higher mental p.
    identification p.
    idiosyncratic p.
    imaginable p.
    imaginal p.
    implicit p.
    information input p.
    interpersonal p.
    intracellular metabolic p.
    p. issue
    judicial p.
    linear thought p.
    p. mania
    memory p.
    mental p.
    metabolic p.
    motivational p.
    motoric reproduction p.
    neurocognitive p.
    neurodegenerative p.
    neurodevelopmental telencephalic
      ontogenic p.
    neuronal p.
    neurotic p.
    normative aging p.
    ongoing cognitive p.
    ontogenic p.
    pathologic p.
    pathophysiologic p.
    pathophysiological p.
    perceptual p.
    personality p.
    physiological p.
    primary psychic p.
    psychobiological p.
    psychological p.
    p. psychosis
    psychosocial p.
    psychotic p.
    reactivation p.
    revision p.
    p. schizophrenia
    schizophrenic p.
    secondary psychic p.
    self-limited p.
    semantic p.
    sensory p.
    separation-individuation p.

social p.
stress-illness p.
switch p.
systematic p.
therapeutic p.
p. thinking
thought p.
transition p.
unconscious p.
withdrawal p.
processed cocaine
processing
affective p.
affect-related p.
altered tau p.
p. area
attentional p.
attention-information p.
auditory p.
declarative emotional memory p.
p. disorder
distributed p.
emotional information p.
emotional memory p.
higher integrative language p.
information p.
language p.
lexical p.
memory p.
normal affective p.
parallel p.
phonological p.
preverbal attentional p.
receptive language p.
semantic p.
speech p.
speed of p.
tau p.
p. time
unconscious p.
visual p.
visuospatial p.
word p.
p. word class
procrastination
proctoparalysis
proctoplegia
proctospasm
procursiva
aura p.

procursive
p. chorea
p. epilepsy
prodigy
child p.
idiot-p.
idiotic p.
prodromal
p. episode
p. period
p. phase
p. phase of schizophrenia
p. psychotic symptom
prodromata
prodrome
visual p.
product
end p.
nicotine replacement p.
nutriceutical p.
production
divergent p.
emotion p.
language comprehension and p.
word p.
productive
p. love
p. personality
p. symptoms
p. thinking
productivity of thought
product-moment correlation
profession
medical p.
professional
allied health p.
p. burnout
child mental health p.
p. code
p. counselor
p. criticism
p. dishonesty
p. distance
p. ethics
p. exploiter
p. gambler
p. gambling
health p.
p. help
medical p.
mental health p.
mental health care p.

NOTES

P

professional *(continued)*
    p. negligence
    p. neurasthenia
    p. neurosis
    p. patient syndrome
    p. spasm
    P. Standards Review Organization
      (PSRO)
professional-family relation
proficiency
profile
    adaptability p.
    anxiety p.
    clinical p.
    criminal p.
    development p.
    diagnostic p.
    employment p.
    high p.
    inhibition p.
    left-out sibling p.
    low p.
    metapsychological p.
    mood p.
    neurotic direction p.
    personality disorder p.
    psychodiagnostic p.
    psychotic direction p.
    Q-score p.
    risk p.
    risk-benefit p.
    sibling p.
    side effect drug p.
    spiked p.
    structural p.
    symptom p.
    therapeutic p.
    trait p.
profiling
    ethnic p.
    facial p.
    racial p.
profound
    p. amnesia
    p. anxiety
    p. dementia
    p. idiocy
    p. mental subnormality
    p. sadness
    p. shame
profoundly retarded
prognosis (Px, px)
    direction p.
    extent p.
    poor p.
prognostic
    p. status
    p. value

program
    behavior modification p.
    career planning p. (CPP)
    child and adolescent fear and
      anxiety treatment p.
    clinical intervention p.
    coercion p.
    College Outcome Measures P.
    community-based psychiatric p.
    community outreach p.
    community treatment and
      reintegration p.
    comparative guidance and
      placement p. (CGPP)
    cooperative institutional research p.
      (CIRP)
    day-care p.
    day treatment p.
    development p.
    Dole-Nyswauder p.
    drug abuse rehabilitation p.
    drug court p.
    dual diagnosis p.
    educational p.
    Employee Assistance P. (EAP)
    enhanced standard methadone
      maintenance treatment p.
    enrichment p.
    entitlement p.
    fast track p.
    Frostig-Horne training p.
    GROW The Marriage
      Enrichment P.
    Head Start p.
    individual p.
    individualized education p.
    infant stimulation p.
    intensive day treatment p.
    jail-based treatment p.
    jail diversion p.
    long-term detoxification p.
    long-term mental health p.
    maintenance treatment p.
    mentoring p.
    methadone maintenance treatment p.
    multicomponent p.
    National Institute of Mental Health
      - Epidemiologic Catchment
      Area P.
    National Institute of Mental
      Health-Epidemiologic Catchment
      Area P.
    outpatient p.
    outreach p.
    PAR Admissions Testing p.
    parent therapist p.
    pilot p.
    research p.

residential OCD p.
reward and punishment p.
standard methadone maintenance
   treatment p.
12-step p.
supported employment p.
tertiary intervention p.
therapeutic p.
Transformational Leadership
   Development P.
transitional p.
treatment p.
Treatment of Depression
   Collaborative Research P.
weight-control p.
weight-loss p.
work-study p.

programmed
p. practice
p. therapy

programming
genotypic p.
neurolinguistic p.

progredient neurosis

progress
p. chart
treatment p.

progression
clinical p.
dementia p.
obstinate p.
symptom p.

progressiva
dementia paratonia p.
dysbasia lordotica p.
dyssynergia cerebellaris p.
paratonia p.

progressive
p. assimilation
p. bulbar paralysis
p. cerebellar tremor
p. degenerative
p. degenerative subcortical
p. degenerative subcortical
   encephalopathy
p. dementia
p. dementing illness
p. deterioration
p. disability
p. disease
p. education
p. lingual hemiatrophy

p. muscular relaxation
p. paratonia
p. paratonia dementia
p. psychosis
p. teleologic regression
p. torsion spasm
p. traumatic encephalopathy

prohormone

project
adolescent diversion p.
Aptitude Research P. (ARP)
Harvard-Brown Anxiety Disorders
   Research P. (HARP)
Human Genome P.
live in the p.
Menninger Clinic Treatment
   Intervention P.
National Mental Illness
   Screening P.
Oregon Adolescent Depression P.
Stony Brook High Risk P.

projected jealousy

projection
applied extrasensory p. (AESP)
astral p.
p. defense mechanism
delusional p.
dopamine p.
eccentric p.
impersonal p.
maximum intensity p.
minimum intensity p.
p. neuron
optical p.
retrospective p.
ventral amygdaloid fugal p.

projectional paranoia

projective
p. identification
p. personality assessment
p. technique

prolactin
p. elevation
p. release

proliferation
T-cell p.

prolongata
alalia p.

prolongation

prolongatus
coitus p.

NOTES

P

525

prolonged
p. depressive reaction
p. exposure
p. grief
p. grief reaction
p. nocturnal sleep
p. nocturnal sleep episode
p. posttraumatic stress disorder
p. prodrome of schizophrenia
p. sadness
p. sedation
p. separation
p. situational depression
p. sleep latency
p. sleep therapy
p. sleep treatment
p. transition to fully awake state

prominent
p. anxiety
p. aspect
p. deterioration
p. grimacing
p. hallucination
p. irritable mood
p. mood symptom
p. narcissistic dynamics
p. phobic anxiety component

promiscuity
conjugal consequences of p.
ego-dystonic p.
protracted p.
sexual p.

promiscuous
p. act
p. sex
p. sexual behavior

promise
broken p.
false p.

promotion neurosis

prone
accident p.
p. to relapse

proneness
p. to addiction

pronoun
anaphoric p.

pronounced improvement

proof
forensic p.
incontrovertible p.
obvious p.
p. of paternity
scientific p.

propaganda

propensity for depression

proper
ego p.
p. repression

property
affective p.
anticholinergic p.
p. damage
destruction of p.
p. destruction
field p.
hebbian p.
pharmacological p.
predictive p.
psychometric p.
receptor-binding p.
reinforcing p.
sedative p.
social p.
thermoregulatory p.
thermosensory p.

propfschizophrenia

prophase

prophecy
self-fulfilling p.

prophetic dream

prophylactic treatment

prophylaxis
pharmacologic p.

propionic acidemia

propizepine

proportion
delusional p.
p. of survivors affected (PSA)

propositus

propriem

proprioception

proprioceptive
p. feedback
p. perception
p. sensation
p. sensibility

propulsion

proscription
religious p.

prosocial
p. behavior
p. motivation

prosodic feature

prosody

prosopagnosia

prosopalgia

prosopodiplegia

prosoponeuralgia

prosopoplegia

prosopospasm

prospective
p. experimental study design

p. memory
p. study
prospermia
prosternation
prosthesis, pl. **prostheses**
behavioral p.
penile p.
prostrate
prostration
protagonist
protaxic mode
protease
protected file
protection
p. factor
p. proceeding
protective
p. barrier
p. effect
p. survival strategy
protector
p. identity
p. role
protein
beta-amyloid p.
cAMP response element binding p.
growth-associated p. (GAP)
heterotrimeric G p.
p. kinase C (PKC)
N p.
signal-transducing guanine-nucleotide
binding p.
protensity
protest
body p.
masculine p.
p. psychosis
separation p.
Protestant
white Anglo-Saxon P.
prothipendyl
prothymia
protocol
Managed Care Appropriateness P.
surveillance p.
test p.
treatment p.
protomasochism
protopathic
p. sensibility
protophallic
protoplasmic

protospasm
prototaxic mode
prototype
borderline diagnosis p.
diagnostic p.
p. matching
p. matching procedure
schizoid diagnostic p.
prototypical
p. course pattern
p. schizophrenia
protracta
catatonia p.
protracted
p. detoxification
p. difficulty
p. difficulty
p. promiscuity
p. reactive paranoid psychosis
p. withdrawal syndrome
protracts
provacateur
agent p.
provider
general medical p.
medical p.
mental health p.
provisional diagnosis
proviso
parapathetic p.
provocation
aggression without p.
minimal p.
pharmacological p.
sexual p.
provocative
p. behavior
p. clowning
p. diagnosis
provoked
p. anxiety
easily p.
provoking
p. stimulus
thought p.
prowess
sexual p.
proxemic
proxibarbal
proximal
p. receptor

NOTES

P

proximity
    mother-infant p.
proximoataxia
proxy
    factitious disorder by p.
    factitious illness by p.
    healthcare p.
    Munchausen disease by p.
    Munchausen syndrome by p.
    posttraumatic stress disorder by p.
    p. symptom
proxy-for-deficit syndrome
PRT
    psychotic trigger reaction
prude
prudery
prudish
pruritic psychosomatic disorder
pruritus
    generalized p.
    psychogenic p.
PS
    psychiatric
PSA
    proportion of survivors affected
PSAN, PSAn, PsAn
    psychoanalysis
    psychoanalyst
PSE
    point of subjective equality
    portal systemic encephalopathy
psellism
pseudagraphia
pseudaphia
pseudesthesia
pseudo
    p. as-if
    p. psychosis
pseudoaddiction
pseudoaggression
pseudoagrammatism
pseudoagraphia
pseudoamnesia
pseudoapoplexy
pseudoapraxia
pseudoataxia
pseudoathetosis
pseudoauthenticity
pseudoautosomal locus for schizophrenia
pseudocatatonia
    traumatic p.
pseudochorea
pseudochromesthesia
pseudoclonus
pseudocollusion
pseudocoma
pseudocombat fatigue
pseudocommunity

pseudoconvulsion
pseudocyesis syndrome
pseudodebility
pseudodelirium
pseudodementia
    depressive p.
    hysterical p.
pseudodepression
pseudoesthesia
pseudofeeblemindedness
pseudoflexibilitas
pseudogeusesthesia
pseudogeusia
pseudogiftedness
pseudo-Graefe sign
pseudographia
pseudohallucination
    ego dystonic p.
    image p.
    manipulative p.
pseudohermaphrodite
pseudohermaphroditism
pseudohomosexual
pseudohypersexuality
pseudohypertrophic muscular paralysis
pseudohypnosis
pseudohypnotics
pseudoidentification
pseudoillusion
pseudoimbecility
pseudoinsomnia
pseudointoxication
pseudo-irreversible mechanism of action
pseudolalia
pseudolobulated
pseudologia fantastica
pseudologue
pseudomalignancy
pseudomania
pseudomasturbation
pseudomelancholia
pseudomelia paraesthetica
pseudomeningitis
pseudomnesia
pseudomotivation
pseudonarcotic
pseudonarcotism
pseudonecrophilia
pseudoneurogenic bladder
pseudoneuroma
pseudoneurotic schizophrenia
pseudonomania
pseudonym
pseudonymity
pseudonymous
pseudoparalysis
    congenital atonic p.
pseudoparameter

pseudoparanoia
pseudoparaplegia
pseudoparesis
    alcoholic p.
pseudoparkinsonism
pseudopellagra
pseudoperitonitis
pseudopersonality
pseudophotesthesia
pseudoplegia
pseudopsia
pseudopsychopathic schizophrenia
pseudopsychosis
pseudoquerulant
pseudoreminiscence
pseudorosette
pseudosauthenticity
pseudoschizophrenia
pseudoscience
pseudosclerosis
    Westphal p.
pseudoseizure
pseudosenility
pseudosexuality
pseudosmia
pseudosocial personality disorder
pseudosphresia
pseudotabes
    pupillotonic p.
pseudothrill
pseudotransference
pseudotumor
pseudoventricle
pseudovomiting
PSG
    polysomnogram
    polysomnograph
P&SH
    personal and social history
PSI
    psychosomatic inventory
psi
    p. phenomenon
    p. system
psilocin
psilocybin dependence
psittacism
PSM
    polysomnogram
PSMed
    psychosomatic medicine
psopholalia

PSP
    postsynaptic potential
PSRO
    Professional Standards Review
      Organization
PSS
    psychiatric services section
PST
    prefrontal sonic treatment
PSUD
    psychoactive substance use
PSV
    psychological, social, and vocational
Psy, psy
    psychiatry
    psychology
psych
    psychiatry
psychagogy
psychalgalia
psychalgia, psychalgalia
psychalgic
psychalia
psychanalysis
psychanopsia
psychasthene
psychasthenia
    compulsive p.
    mixed compulsive states p.
    obsession p.
    p. scale
psychasthenic
    p. delirium
    p. neurosis
psychataxia
psychauditory
psyche
    contrasexual component of p.
psycheclampsia
psychedelia
psychedelic
    p. agent
    p. agent dependence
    p. therapy
psychehormic
psycheism
psychelytic
psychentonia
psychephoric
psycheplastic
psycherhexic

NOTES

P

psychezymic
psychiatric (PS)
  p. admission
  p. anaphylaxis
  p. assessment
  p. assistant
  p. care
  p. case register
  p. chemistry
  p. clinician
  p. comorbid disorder
  p. comorbidity
  p. complication
  p. condition
  p. conflict
  p. consequence
  p. consultation
  p. CPT code
  p. criterion
  p. data
  p. deviance
  p. diagnosis
  p. disability
  p. disease
  p. disorder associated with
    alcoholism
  p. disorders in the elderly
  p. disturbance
  p. education
  p. effect
  p. emergency
  p. emergency department
  p. emergency service (PES)
  p. emergency team (PET)
  p. epidemiologist
  p. epidemiology
  p. evaluation
  p. evidence
  p. examination
  p. facility
  p. family history
  p. genetics
  p. ghetto
  p. help
  p. hospital
  p. hospitalization
  p. illness
  p. inpatient
  p. intensive care unit (PICU)
  p. intervention
  p. interview
  p. manifestation
  p. medication
  p. morbidity
  p. nomenclature
  p. nosology
  p. nurse
  p. parameter

  p. patient
  p. practitioner
  p. problem
  p. rating scale
  p. rationale
  p. reacting scale
  p. referral
  p. research
  p. researcher
  p. risk
  p. risk factor
  p. services section (PSS)
  p. setting
  p. severity
  p. severity rating
  p. social work
  p. social worker
  p. somatic therapy
  p. statistics
  p. symptom
  p. syndrome
  p. system interface disorder
  p. technician
  p. testimony
  p. treatment
  p. trend
  p. unit
  p. variable
  p. ward
psychiatrically
  p. demanding temperament
  p. disabled
psychiatrism
psychiatrist
  academic p.
  American Academy of Clinical P.'s
    (AACP)
  American Association of
    Community P.'s
  American Board of Forensic P.'s
    (ABFP)
  American College of P.'s (ACP)
  Association for Child P.
  biologic p.
  board certified p.
  board eligible p.
  child p.
  clinical p.
  Commission on Psychotherapy
    by P.'s
  consultation p.
  consulting p.
  court-appointed p.
  DO p.
  forensic p.
  geriatric p.
  liaison p.

National Guild of Catholic P.'s
(NGCP)
psychodynamic p.
Royal College of P.'s (RCP)
psychiatrize
psychiatry (Psy, psy, psych)
ABCs of geriatric p.
   affect, behavior, cognition
academic p.
addiction p.
administrative p.
adolescent p.
adulthood p.
American Academy of
  Addiction P. (AAAP)
American Academy of Child P.
American Academy of Child and
  Adolescent P. (AACAP)
American Association of
  Emergency P.
American Association for
  Geriatric P. (AAGP)
American Board of P. (ABP)
American Board of Forensic P.
American Society for
  Adolescent P. (ASAD)
analytic p.
Archives of General P.
Association of Directors of
  Medical Student Education in P.
  (ADMSEP)
behavioral p.
biologic p.
British Journal of P.
Canadian Academy of Child P.
child p. (CHP, CP)
child and adolescent p.
clinical p.
Clunis inquiry forensic p.
common sense p.
community p.
comparative p.
consultation p.
consultation-liaison p.
contractual p.
correctional p.
criminal p.
cross-cultural p.
cross-culture p.
cultural p.
descriptive p.
dynamic p.

ecological p.
p. emergency team
evidence-based p.
existential p.
experimental p.
folk p.
forensic p.
genetic-dynamic p.
geriatric p.
gerontologic p.
gerontological p.
gestalt p.
Group for the Advancement of P.
  (GAP)
hospital-based p.
hospital and community p.
industrial p.
infant p.
p. inpatient service
International Society for
  Adolescent P.
interpersonal p.
legal p.
liaison p.
military forensic p.
minority group p.
modern p.
molecular p.
multidisciplinary group p.
National Association of Veterans
  Affairs Chiefs of P. (NAVACP)
neuropsychiatric p.
occupational p.
old-age p.
organic p.
organized care p.
orthomolecular p.
outpatient-based p.
pastoral p.
pediatric p.
political p.
preventive p.
prison p.
psychoanalytic p.
psychopharmacologic p.
public p.
rehabilitation p.
rural p.
social p.
Society of Biological P.
spiritual dimension in p.
Standard System of P. (SSOP)

NOTES

P

psychiatry *(continued)*
    transcultural p.
    urban p.
    World Association for Social P.
      (WASP)
    World Congress of P.
    young adult p.
psychic
    p. ability
    p. aftershock
    p. anaphylaxis
    p. apparatus
    p. blindness
    p. censor
    p. contagion
    p. deafness
    p. dependence
    p. determinism
    p. disorder
    p. distress
    p. disturbance
    p. divorce
    p. dualism
    p. dysuria
    p. energizer
    p. energy
    p. epilepsy
    p. equivalent
    p. experience
    p. factor
    p. force
    p. helplessness
    p. impotence
    p. inertia
    p. masturbation
    p. numbing
    p. numbness
    p. ontogeny
    p. organization
    p. overtone
    p. pain
    p. phenomenon
    p. reality
    p. reflex
    p. reward
    p. scar
    p. seizure
    p. shock
    p. shock syndrome
    p. suicide
    p. tic
    p. trauma
    p. vaginismus
    p. wound
psychical reality
psychicism
psychinosis
psychism

psychnosia
psychoacoustics
psychoactive
    p. chemical
    p. drug
    p. drug abuse
    p. effect
    p. ingredient
    p. medication
    p. substance
    p. substance abuse
    p. substance abuse disorder
    p. substance delirium
    p. substance dementia
    p. substance dependence
    p. substance hallucinosis
    p. substance-induced organic
    p. substance-induced organic mental
      disorder
    p. substance intoxication
    p. substance use (PSUD)
    p. substance use disorder
    p. substance withdrawal
psychoaffective disorder (PAD)
psychoalgalia
psychoallergy
psychoanaleptic
psychoanaleptica
psychoanalysis (PA, PSAN, PSAn,
  PsAn)
    active p.
    adlerian p.
    American Academy of P. (AAP)
    applied p.
    Association for the Advancement
      of P. (AAP)
    boundaries in p.
    existential p.
    freudian p.
    fundamental rule of p.
    jungian p.
    National Psychological Association
      for P.
    The American Academy of P.
    wild p.
psychoanalyst (PA, PSAN, PSAn, PsAn)
    medical p.
psychoanalytic
    p. concept
    p. group
    p. group psychotherapy
    p. interpretation
    p. investigation
    p. neurosis
    p. pathography
    p. perspective
    p. psychiatry
    p. situation

p. technique
p. therapy
psychoanalytical
p. pathography
p. theory
**psychoanalytically oriented
psychotherapy**
psychoanalyze
psychoanopsia
psychoasthenics
psychoataxia
psychoauditory
psychobabble
psychobacillosis
psychobioanalysis
psychobiogram
psychobiological
p. process
p. process of dementia
psychobiology
clinical p.
development p.
objective p.
psychocardic reflex
psychocatharsis
psychocentric
psychochemistry
psychochrome
psychochromesthesia
psychocinesia
psychocoma
psychocortical center
psychocutaneous
psychodiagnosis
psychodiagnostic profile
psychodietetics
psychodometer
psychodometry
psychodrama
American Society of Group
Psychotherapy and P. (ASGPP)
forms of p.
p. group therapy
psychodramatic
p. catharsis
p. shock
psychodynamic
p. approach
p. cerebral system
p. clinician
p. concept
p. conflict

p. denial
p. effect
p. formulation
p. group psychotherapy
p. interpretation
p. interpretation and treatment
p. interview
p. origin
p. practitioner
p. psychiatrist
p. research orientation
p. theory
psychodynamic-experiential model
psychodynamics
adaptational p.
cognitive p.
psychodysleptica
psychodysleptic drug
psychoeducational
p. evaluation
p. group
p. test
psychoeducation group therapy
psychoendocrinology
psychoepilepsy
psychoexploration
psychogalvanic
p. reflex (PGR)
p. response (PGR)
p. skin reaction
p. skin resistance (PGSR)
psychogalvanometer
psychogender
psychogenesis
psychogenetic
psychogenia
psychogenic
p. air hunger
p. alopecia
p. amnesia
p. anxiety
p. aphagia
p. aphasia
p. aspermia (PA)
p. asthenia
p. ataxia
p. backache
p. cardiac nondisease
p. cardiospasm
p. chest pain
p. confusion
p. constipation

NOTES

P

psychogenic *(continued)*
- p. cough
- p. cyclical vomiting
- p. deafness
- p. depression
- p. depressive psychosis
- p. dermatitis
- p. diarrhea
- p. drug
- p. duodenal ulcer
- p. dysmenorrhea
- p. dyspareunia
- p. dyspepsia
- p. dystonia
- p. dysuria
- p. eczema
- p. effort syndrome
- p. enuresis
- p. excitation
- p. excoriation
- p. fatigue
- p. fugue
- p. gastric ulcer
- gastrointestinal functional p.
- p. headache
- p. hearing impairment
- p. hearing loss
- p. hiccup
- p. hyperventilation
- p. illness
- p. impotence
- p. learning disorder
- p. limb disorder
- p. megacolon
- p. motor disorder
- p. muscle disorder
- p. musculoskeletal disorder
- p. neurocirculatory disorder
- p. nocturnal polydipsia (PNP)
- p. nocturnal polydipsia syndrome
- p. obesity
- p. obsessional disorder
- p. oculogyric crisis
- p. origin
- p. overlay
- p. pain disorder
- p. painful coitus
- p. painful erection
- p. painful menstruation
- p. paralysis
- p. paranoid nonorganic
- p. paranoid nonorganic psychosis
- p. paroxysmal
- p. paroxysmal tachycardia
- p. pelvic pain
- p. penis pain
- p. peptic ulcer
- p. phobic disorder

- p. physical symptom
- p. physiological
- p. physiological manifestation
- p. polydipsia
- p. precordial pain
- p. pruritus
- p. purpura syndrome
- p. reaction
- p. respiratory disorder
- p. retention
- p. rheumatic disorder
- p. rumination
- p. seizure
- p. sexual disorder
- p. skin disorder
- p. sleep disorder
- p. stomach disorder
- p. stupor
- p. testicular pain
- p. testis pain
- p. tic
- p. torticollis
- p. twilight state
- p. urticaria
- p. uterus pain
- p. vertigo
- p. yawning

psychogenous
psychogeny
psychogeriatrics
psychogerontology
psychogeusic
psychognosia
psychognosis
psychognostic
psychogogic
psychogonical
psychogony
psychogram
psychograph
psychographic disturbance
psychography
psychohistory
psychoimmunology
psychoinfantile personality
psychoinfantilism
psychokinesia
psychokinesis (PK)
psychokinetic (PK)
psychokym
psychokyme
psycholagny
psycholepsis
psycholepsy
psycholeptica
psycholeptic episode
psycholinguistic
- p. ability

p. test
p. theory
psychologic
  p. adjustment
  p. defense system
  p. desensitization
  p. factor affecting physical
    condition
  p. medicine
  p. programming therapy
  p. rating scale
  p. test
  p. tremor
psychological
  p. abuse
  p. acculturation
  p. addiction
  p. autopsy
  p. autopsy study
  p. basis
  p. birth of the human infant
  p. burden
  p. capacity
  p. cause
  p. change
  p. characteristic
  p. concern
  p. consequence
  p. construct
  p. debriefing
  p. defense system
  p. defensiveness
  p. deprivation
  p. description
  p. determinant
  p. distortion
  p. distress
  p. disturbance
  p. dysfunction
  p. dysfunction symptom
  p. effect
  p. evaluation
  p. examination
  p. factor
  p. factors affecting medical
    condition (PFAMC)
  p. factors affecting a mental
    condition
  p. feature
  p. field
  p. foundation
  p. game

p. health
p. impact
p. information, acquisition,
  processing, and control system
  (PIAPACS)
p. intervention
p. interview
p. inventory
p. issue
p. loaner
p. loner
p. management
p. marker
p. maturation
p. maturity
p. meaning
p. mindedness
p. model
p. motivation
p. need
p. pain
p. pillow
p. problem
p. procedure
p. process
p. rapport
p. reaction
p. refractory period
p. related symptoms
p. research
p. resource
p. response
p. scars
p. signs and symptoms
p., social, and vocational (PSV)
p. state
p. strain
p. strength
p. stress
p. suicide
p. syndrome
p. technique
p. test
p. testing
p. theory
p. therapy
p. toll
p. toner
p. trait
p. trauma
p. trauma depressive
p. trauma depressive psychosis

NOTES

P

psychological *(continued)*
    p. warfare (PW)
    p. weakness
psychologically
    p. insightful
    p. mediated response
    p. overwhelming experience
    p. stressful
psychological-physiological arousal
psychologist
    adolescent p.
    Association of Correctional P.'s
    child p.
    clinical p.
    consulting p.
    counseling p.
    engineering p.
    environmental p.
    geriatric p.
    industrial organizational p.
    licensed p.
    pediatric p.
    personality p.
    prison p.
    social p.
psychology (Psy, psy)
    abnormal p.
    p. act
    adlerian p.
    adolescent p.
    advertising p.
    analytic p.
    analytical p.
    animal p.
    applied p.
    atomistic p.
    behavioral p.
    behaviorism school of p.
    behavioristic p.
    blame p.
    centralist p.
    child p. (CP)
    clinical p.
    cognitive p.
    community p.
    comparative p.
    constitutional p.
    consumer p.
    content p.
    correctional p.
    counseling p.
    courtroom p.
    criminal p.
    depth p.
    developmental p.
    dynamic p.
    educational p.
    ego p.

engineering p.
environmental p.
existential p.
experimental p.
faculty p.
folk p.
forensic p.
functional p.
general p.
genetic p.
geriatric p.
gestalt p.
health p.
health-related p.
holistic p.
human factor p.
humanistic p.
id p.
individual p.
industrial p.
Journal of Consulting and
    Clinical P.
jungian p.
legal p.
mass p.
medical p.
military p.
mob p.
objective p.
organismic p.
organizational p.
pediatric p.
perceptual p.
peripheralist p.
personality p.
personnel p.
philosophical p.
physiological p.
pop p.
rational p.
p. of scent
self p.
social p.
Society for Industrial and
    Organizational P.
subjective p.
topographical p.
topological p.
transpersonal p.
uprooted p.
victim p.
p. of women
psychomathematics
psychometer
psychometric
    p. advantage
    p. evaluation
    p. measure

p. performance
p. performance characteristic
p. predictor
p. problem
p. property
p. setting
p. standard
p. term
p. test
p. testing
p. validity
psychometrician
psychometry
psychomimetic
psychomimic syndrome
psychomotility
psychomotor
p. abnormality
p. activity
p. agitation
p. attack
p. behavior
p. change
p. convulsion
p. development
p. disorder
p. disturbance
p. disturbance stress reaction
p. epilepsy
p. excitement
p. fit
p. intelligence
p. measurement
p. overactivity
p. performance
p. phenomenon
p. poverty
p. restlessness
p. retardation
p. seizure
p. slowing
p. stimulant
p. stupor
p. symptom
p. test
psychoneural parallelism
psychoneuroimmunology (PNI)
psychoneurologist
psychoneurology
psychoneurosis, pl. **psychoneuroses**
anxiety p.
battle p.

climacteric p.
compensation p.
compulsion p.
conversion hysteria p.
defense p.
depersonalization p.
depressive-type p.
dissociative hysteria p.
hypochondriac p.
hypochondriacal p.
hysteria p.
p. maidica
mixed p.
neurasthenic p.
obsessional p.
obsessive-compulsive p.
occupational p.
paranoid p.
personality p.
senile p.
psychoneurotic (PN)
depersonalization p.
p. depression
p. depressive reaction
p. mental disorder
p. personality
psychonoetism
psychonomic
psychonomics
psychonomy
psychonosis
psychonosology
psychonoxious
psychooncology
psychooptical reflex control
psychoorganic
p. brain syndrome
nonpsychotic severity p.
psychoparesis
psychopath
criminal sexual p. (CSP)
industrial p.
sexual p.
workplace p.
psychopathia
p. partialis
p. sexualis
psychopathic
antisocial trends p.
p. constitution
p. deviance

NOTES

P

psychopathic *(continued)*
    p. deviance scale
    p. deviant (PD)
    p. diathesis
    p. inferiority
    mixed-type p.
    p. personality
    posttraumatic p.
    p. state
    p. trait
psychopathist
psychopathologic
    p. accompaniment
    p. deterioration
psychopathological thought
psychopathologist
psychopathology
    acute p.
    adult p.
    child p.
    coexisting p.
    comorbid p.
    disinhibitory p.
    p. of epilepsy
    general p.
    general adult p.
    global p.
    impulsive-compulsive p.
    p. level
    p. measure
    overall p.
    prepubertal p.
    presenting p.
    p. rating scale
    related p.
    p. of retardation
    retardation p.
    scientific p.
    stress-related p.
psychopathosis
psychopathy
    autistic p.
    benign p.
    passive parasitic p.
    workplace p.
psychopedagogy
psychopenetration test
psychopetal
psychopharmaceutical intervention
psychopharmaceuticals
psychopharmacologic
    p. agent
    p. intervention
    p. psychiatry
psychopharmacological
    p. therapy
    p. treatment
psychopharmacologist

psychopharmacology
    adolescent p.
    P. Bulletin
    child p.
    clinical p.
    p. consultation
    essential p.
    gender-sensitive p.
    geriatric p.
    pediatric p.
psychophonasthenia
psychophylaxis
psychophysical
    p. function
    p. parallelism
psychophysics
psychophysiologic
    p. correlate
    p. disorder
    p. manifestation
    p. principle
    p. reaction
psychophysiological
    p. change
    p. insomnia
    p. problem
    p. test
psychophysiology
psychoplegia
psychoplegic
psychopneumatology
psychoprophylactic treatment
psychoprophylaxis
psychoreaction
psychorelaxation
psychorhythm
psychormic
psychorrhythmia, psychorhythmia
psychosedation
psychosedative
psychosensorial
psychosensory
    p. aphasia
    p. epilepsy
    p. stimulus
    p. symptom
psychose passionelle
psychoses (*pl. of* psychosis)
psychosexual
    p. development
    p. dysfunction
    p. factor
    p. gender identity disorder
    p. history
    p. identity
    p. identity crisis
    p. moratorium
    p. sphere

p. stage
p. symptom
psychosexuality
psychosis, pl. **psychoses**
accidental p.
active p.
acute delusional p.
acute hysterical p.
acute infective p.
acute paranoid reaction
  nonorganic p.
acute posttraumatic organic p.
acute psychogenic paranoid p.
acute shock p.
addiction organic p.
addiction-type organic p.
affective alcoholic p.
affective paranoid organic p.
affective schizophreniform p.
akinetic p.
alcoholic Korsakoff p.
alcoholic liver disease-type
  organic p.
alcoholic paranoid p.
alcoholic polyneuritic p.
alcoholism organic p.
alternating p.
alternative p.
Alzheimer p.
amnestic confabulatory alcoholic p.
amphetamine p.
anergastic organic p.
anxiety-blissfulness p.
arteriosclerotic brain disease-type
  organic p.
p. of association
atropine p.
atypical childhood p.
autistic p.
autoscopic p.
barbed-wire p.
biogenic p.
bipolar affective p.
birth brain trauma organic p.
black patch p.
borderline p.
brain disease organic p.
brain infection organic p.
brain trauma organic p.
brief reactive p.
buffoonery p.
cannabis p.

cardiac p.
cerebral glucose metabolic-type
  organic p.
cerebrovascular disease organic p.
Cheyne-Stokes p.
child p.
p. in childbirth
childbirth organic p.
childhood p.
p. of childhood
childhood-onset p.
chronic p.
chronic paranoid p.
circular p.
circulatory p.
climacteric paranoid p.
cocaine p.
collective p.
confusional schizophreniform p.
confusion reactive p.
conjugal p.
constitutional p.
cycloid p.
degeneration p.
degenerative p.
delirious transient organic p.
delirium state drug p.
delirium transient organic p.
delirium tremens alcoholic p.
delusional syndrome drug p.
delusional transient organic p.
dementia state drug p.
dependence organic p.
dependence-type organic p.
depressed bipolar affective p.
depressive transient organic p.
depressive-type nonorganic p.
disintegrative childhood p.
drug p.
drug-induced p.
p. due to physical condition
p. during pregnancy
dysmnesic p.
p. in the elderly
electrical current brain trauma
  organic p.
electroshock-induced p.
embarrassment p.
emotional stress depressive p.
endocrine disease organic p.
endocrine type organic p.
epilepsy organic p.

NOTES

P

539

psychosis *(continued)*

epileptic transient organic p.
excitation p.
excitative p.
excitative-type nonorganic p.
exhaustion p.
exhaustive p.
exogenous p.
exotic p.
p. factor
familial p.
febrile p.
first-episode p.
florid p.
full-blown p.
functional p.
furlough p.
gender ambiguity p.
gestational p.
governess p.
group p.
hallucinatory state drug p.
hallucinatory transient organic p.
hallucinosis alcoholic p.
heredofamilial p.
housewife p.
Huntington chorea organic p.
hypochondriacal p.
hypomanic p.
hyposomnia associated with p.
hysteria p.
hysterical p.
iatrogenic p.
ICU p.
idiopathic p.
idiophrenic p.
incipient schizophrenia p.
incipient schizophrenic p.
induced p.
infantile p.
infection-exhaustion p.
infection organic p.
infectious-exhaustive p.
infective p.
influenced p.
insomnia associated with p.
interactional childhood p.
interictal p.
intermittent p.
interval p.
intoxication organic p.
intoxication-type organic p.
intracranial infection organic p.
invocational p.
involutional paranoid p.
ischemia organic p.
Jakob-Creutzfeldt disease organic p.
juvenile p.

koro p.
Korsakoff alcoholic p.
Korsakoff nonalcoholic p.
kraepelinian view of p.
latent p.
liver disease organic p.
major depressive affective p.
malignant p.
manic p.
manic-depressive affective p.
marijuana p.
melancholia affective p.
meningismus p.
menopausal paranoid p.
metabolic disease organic p.
migration p.
mixed bipolar affective p.
mixed manic-depressive p.
mixed schizophrenic-affective p.
model p.
monosymptomatic
  hypochondriacal p.
mood swing affective p.
motility p.
motor p.
multi-infarct p.
multiple sclerosis-type organic p.
nonaffective p.
nonorganic p.
organic p.
paranoiac p.
paranoid schizophrenic p.
paranoid transient organic p.
paranoid-type alcoholic p.
paranoid-type arteriosclerotic p.
paranoid-type senile p.
paretic p.
paroxysmal p.
pathologic drug intoxication
  drug p.
pathologic intoxication alcoholic p.
perplexed manic-depressive p.
perplexed-type manic-depressive p.
perplexity p.
phencyclidine-associated p.
phencyclidine-induced p.
physical condition organic p.
p. polyneuritica
polyneuritic alcoholic p.
positive symptoms p.
posthypnotic p.
postictal p.
postinfectious p.
postoperative p.
postpartum p. (PPP)
posttraumatic organic p.
p. in pregnancy
prepsychotic p.

prepubertal borderline p.
presbyophrenic p.
presenile p.
prison p.
private p.
process p.
progressive p.
protest p.
protracted reactive paranoid p.
pseudo p.
psychogenic depressive p.
psychogenic paranoid nonorganic p.
psychological trauma depressive p.
puerperal p.
p. in puerperium
purpose p.
reactive confusion nonorganic p.
reactive depressive p.
reactive paranoid p.
recurrent episode depressive p.
refractory p.
scale of p. (SP)
schizoaffective p.
schizophrenia p.
schizophrenic-affective p.
schizophrenic paranoid p.
schizophreniform p.
semantic p.
senile paranoid p.
senile paroxysmal p.
senility organic p.
sensory p.
septicemia p.
shock p.
simple deterioration senile p.
simple-type arteriosclerotic p.
single-episode depressive p.
situational p.
sleeplessness associated with p.
somatic p.
status epilepticus organic p.
stigma p.
stigma of p.
stress p.
stuporous manic-depressive p.
stuporous-type manic-depressive p.
subacute posttraumatic organic p.
substance-induced chronic p.
surgical brain trauma organic p.
symbiotic infantile p.
symptomatic p.
p. of syphilis

tabetic p.
toxic p.
toxic-infectious p.
transient organic p.
transitory p.
trauma organic p.
traumatic p.
uncomplicated arteriosclerotic p.
unipolar manic-depressive p.
untreated p.
Windigo p.
withdrawal syndrome alcoholic p.
withdrawal syndrome drug p.
p. with mental retardation
Wittigo p.
zoophile p.
psychosis-induced polydipsia
psychosocial
p. assessment (PA)
p. complication
p. deprivation
p. development
p. dwarfism
p. event
p. factor
p. factor evaluation
p. functioning
p. history
p. intervention
p. issue
p. management
p. moratorium
p. morbidity
p. pain
p. pathology
p. perspective
p. problem
p. process
p. rehabilitation
p. residential care
p. retardation
p. service
p. setting
p. skill acquisition
p. stigma
p. stress
p. stressor
p. symptom outcome
p. treatment
p. turbulence
psychosocial-environmental
psychosocial-labile (PL)

NOTES

P

psychosocially determined short stature
psychosolytic
psychosoma
psychosomatic
  p. illness
  p. inventory (PSI)
  p. medicine (PSMed)
  p. paralytic disorder
  p. pruritic disorder
  p. reaction
  p. skin disorder
  p. symptom
psychosomaticist
psychosomimetic
psychostimulant
  p. dependence
  p. drug
  p. effect
psychostimulation
  subjective p.
psychosuggestive
psychosuggestivity
psychosurgeon
psychosurgery
  seed p.
psychosyndrome
  algogenic p.
  focal organic p.
  organic p.
  partial organic p.
psychosynthesis
psychotaxis
psychotechnics
psychotherapeusis
psychotherapeutic
  p. approach
  p. background
  p. drug
  p. intervention
  p. measure
  p. neuroscience
  p. spectrum
  p. therapy
  p. treatment
psychotherapist
  American Academy of P.'s (AAP)
  American Association of P.'s
psychotherapist-patient privilege
psychotherapy
  active analytic p.
  activity group p.
  activity-interview group p. (A-IGP)
  adlerian p.
  adolescent p.
  p. alternative
  anaclitic p.
  analytic group p.

Association for the Advancement of P. (AAP)
autonomous p.
behavioral p.
bioenergetic p.
brief dynamic p.
client-centered p.
cognitive p.
cognitive-behavioral p.
cognitive behavioral analysis system of p. (CBASP)
contractual p.
cooperative p.
crisis-intervention group p.
didactic group p.
directive p.
dyadic p.
dynamic p.
educational p.
ego p.
emergency p.
existential p.
experiential p.
exploratory insight-oriented p. (EIO)
family p.
family and systemic p.
focal p.
freudian p.
gestalt p.
group p.
group analytic p.
heteronomous p.
hypnotic p.
individual p.
insight-oriented p.
intensive p.
interactional group p.
International Association of Group P.
Internet p.
interpersonal p. (IPT)
interview group p.
long-term p.
manual-based interpersonal p.
marathon group p.
medical p.
Morita p.
multiple p.
nondirective p.
objective p.
outpatient p.
patterning p.
play group p.
psychoanalytically oriented p.
psychoanalytic group p.
psychodynamic group p.
rational p.
rational-emotive p.

reciprocal inhibition p.
reconstructive p.
regressive-inspirational group p.
relationship p.
remedial p.
repressive-inspirational group p.
p. responder (PR)
p. session
short-contact p.
short-term anxiety-provoking p.
  (STAPP)
short-term dynamic p.
specific p.
structured interactional group p.
suggestive p.
superficial p.
supportive p.
supportive-expressive p.
terminal reinforcement p.
time-limited p. (TLP)
traditional p.
transactional p.

psychothymia
psychotic
p. aggressive behavior
p. Alzheimer patient
p. attack
p. break
p. catatonia
p. decompensation
p. delusions scale
p. denial
p. depression (PD)
p. depression scale
p. depressive reaction
p. depressive subtype
p. dimension of schizophrenia
p. direction
p. direction profile
p. disease
p. disorder due to a general
  medical condition
p. disorder not otherwise specified
p. disorder with delusions
p. disorder with hallucinations
p. disorganization
p. disorganization in schizophrenia
p. disruptive behavior
p. distortion
p. disturbance
p. episode
p. exacerbation

p. factor
p. feature
p. fugue
p. illness
p. inpatient
p. manifestation
p. mental disorder
p. posttraumatic brain syndrome
p. presenile mental disorder
p. presentation
p. process
recurrent episode p.
p. relapse
p. schizophrenic episode
p. signs and symptom
p. speech
p. state
p. symptomatology
p. thinking
p. thinking scale
p. trigger reaction (PRT, PTR)

psychotica
psychotic-like
p.-l. idea
p.-l. phenomenon
psychotogen
psychotogenic
psychotoid
psychotomimetic
p. agent dependence
p. drug
psychotonic
psychotoxicomania
psychotropic
p. agent
p. drug (PTD)
p. medication
p. metabolism
psychroalgia
psychroesthesia
pt
patient
PTA
posttraumatic amnesia
prior to admission
PTCA
parent-to-child aggression
PTD
prevention and treatment of depression
psychotropic drug
ptosis sympathetica

NOTES

P

543

PTR
    psychotic trigger reaction
PTSD
    posttraumatic stress disorder
      complex PTSD
puberal
puberism
    persistent p.
pubertal
    p. sexual recapitulation
    p. stage
pubertas praecox
puberty
    atypical p.
    p. melancholia
    periodic psychosis of p.
    precocious p.
    p. rite
pubescence
pubescency
pubescent
public
    p. display of emotion
    p. drunkenness
    p. health
    p. health issue
    p. health model
    p. health mood
    p. image
    p. masturbation
    p. opprobrium
    p. psychiatry
    p. residential treatment center
    p. sentiment
pudding opium
pudendum, pl. pudenda
puer
    p. aeternus
    p. eternus
Pueraria lobata
puericulture
puerile
puerilism
    hysterical p.
puerperal
    p. convulsion
    p. delirium
    p. dementia
    p. mania
    p. melancholia
    p. psychosis
    p. seizure
puerperium
    psychosis in p.
puesto
    mal p.
puffy eye

pugilistica
    dementia p.
pulling
    p. of clothes
    ear p.
    hair p.
pulsating
    p. headache
    p. neurasthenia
    p. pain
pulsation
pulse
    alternating p.
    chest p.
    p. rate
    p. waveform
pulveratum
    opium p.
pulvinar
    p. nucleus
    p. nucleus of thalamus
pump
punch-drunk
    p.-d. encephalopathy
    p.-d. syndrome
punch-drunkenness
puncture
    cisternal p.
    Quincke p.
    suboccipital p.
punishment
    contingent p.
    corporal p.
    cruel p.
    deserved p.
    p. dream
    expiatory p.
    Midas p.
    need for p.
    petty p.
    reciprocal p.
    unconscious need for p.
    unusual p.
punitive psychologic attitude
punk music
punning
pupil
    constricted p.
    dilated p.'s
    fixed p.
    Hutchinson p.
    paradoxical p.
    pinpoint p.'s
    rigid p.
    Robertson p.
    tonic p.
pupillary
    p. constriction

p. reaction
p. skin reflex
pupillomotor
pupilloplegia
pupillotonia
pupillotonic pseudotabes
pupil-teacher fit
puppy love
purchase
pure
p. absence
p. agraphia
p. alexia
p. aphasia
p. aphemia
p. depressive disease
p. line
p. mania
p. mood
p. obsession
purgation
purge
binge and p.
bulimic p.
purging
p. behavior
eating and p.
p. method
purging-type bulimia
purified pleasure ego
purine metabolism
purist
language p.
puritanical aversion to intercourse
Purkinje afterimage
Purmann method
purple
p. heart
p. people syndrome
purpose
clinical p.
dual p.
p. in life (PIL)
primary p.
p. psychosis
purposeful
p. behavior
p. movement
purposeless
p. activity
p. agitation
p. movement

purposive movement
purpura simplex
purse snatcher
pursing
lip p.
pursuit
p. abnormality
family p.
purveyor of mysticism
pusher
putamen
putative
p. adoptee
p. adoptee vulnerability
p. effect
p. index
p. influence
p. insult
p. neurotransmitter
**putatively poor-prognosis deficit
syndrome**
putting
p. affairs in order
off p.
putty
p value
PVNPS
post-Vietnam psychiatric syndrome
PVS
persistent vegetative state
PW
psychological warfare
PWA
person with AIDS
PWP
Parents Without Partners
Px, px
prognosis
pyencephalus
Pygmalion effect
pygmalionism
pyknic
p. constitutional type
pyknophrasia
pylorospasm
pyocephalus
circumscribed p.
pyogenic
p. pachymeningitis
pyogenica
pyramidal
p. decussation

NOTES

P

pyramidotomy
    spinal p.
pyrimidine metabolism
pyritinol
pyrolagnia
pyromania
    p. disorder
    erotic p.

pyromaniac
pyroptothymia
pyrosis
pyruvate

Q
clerical perception
quantitative test
   Q data
   Q factor
   Q method
   Q methodology
   Q score
   Q technique
QALY
quality-adjusted life year
QEEG
quantitative electroencephalogram
quantitative electroencephalography
Qi Gong movement-based meditation
qi-gong psychotic reaction
Q-score profile
Q-Set
California Child Q-S
Q-Sort
California Q.-S.
Q.-S. description
Q.-S. method
Q.-S. procedure
Q.-S. technique
qt
quiet
QTL
quantitative trait loci
quack
quadrangular therapy
quadrantanopia
quadrantanopsia
quadrigemina
corpora q.
quadriparesis
quadriplegia
quale
qualitative
q. approach
q. difference
q. impairment in communication
q. judgment
quality
Agency for Healthcare Research and Q.
q. of caring
compulsive q.
determining q.
exaggerated negative q.
exaggerated positive q.
histrionic q.
hypomanic q.
q. of life
q. of life measure

q. of life rehabilitation assessment
q. of mood
narcissistic q.
negative q.
q. of obsession
q. of performance
poor sleep q.
primary q.
semiautomatic q.
q. of sexual functioning
q. of sleep
sleep q.
q. of speech
q. time
uncontrollable q.
quality-adjusted life year (QALY)
quanta (*pl. of* quantum)
quantal hypothesis
quantification
quantified
q. clinical observation
q. cognitive assessment
quantitative
q. approach
q. data
q. electroencephalogram (QEEG)
q. electroencephalography (QEEG)
q. electrophysiological battery
q. judgment
q. measure
q. morphometric technique
q. score
q. semantics
q. test (Q)
q. trait loci (QTL)
q. variable
quantity
absolute q.
q. of speech
sufficient q.
quantum, pl. **quanta**
libido q.
q. theory
quarrel
domestic q.
quarrelsomeness
quarter-way house
quartile deviation (q)
quasi-action
quasi-experimental
q.-e. design
q.-e. research
quasi-expert
Quasimodo complex
quasi-need

quasi-purposive movement
quasi-representative
quasi-rhythmic
quaternity
quatre
    delire a q.
    folie á q.
quavering voice
querulans
    paranoia q.
querulent
querulous paranoia
query
    close-ended q.
quest
    q. for attention
question
    actively phrased q.
    closed-ended q.
    direct q.
    empirical q.
    end-of-life q.
    exception q.
    generic q.
    key q.
    open-ended q.
    passively phrased q.
    Pigem q.
    screening q.
    self-help q.
    q. stage
    unanswered q.
    yes-no q.
questioning
    q. faith problem
    socratic q.
    q. under hypnosis
questionnaire
    assessment q.
    depression q.
    description q.
    development q.
    memory q.
    opinion q.
    pain q.
    personal history q.
    personality q.
    self-report q.
    status q.
quick and dirty
quickening
quick-tempered
quick-witted
quick-wittedness
quid pro quo harassment

quiescent
quiet (qt)
    q. biting attack
    q. niche
    q. room
    q. sleep
    wakefulness q.
    q. wakefulness mode
quieting
quietism
quietude
Quincke
    Q. puncture
quintessential
Quixote
    Don Q.
quixotic
quixotism
quo
    status q. (SQ)
quoque
quota system
quotient
    accomplishment q. (AQ)
    achievement q. (AQ)
    activity q.
    adolescent language q.
    ambivalent q.
    aphasia q. (AQ)
    brain age q. (BAQ)
    circadian q. (CQ)
    cognitive laterality q. (CLQ)
    conceptual q. (CQ)
    custody q.
    deterioration q.
    deviation q.
    education q. (EQ)
    educational q. (EQ)
    expressive language q.
    full-scale intelligence q. (FIQ, FSIQ)
    language q.
    listening language q.
    memory q. (MQ)
    open q.
    positive-negative ambivalent q. (PNAvQ)
    reading language q.
    receptive language-processing q.
    social q. (SQ)
    speed q.
    spoken language q.
    verbal language q.
    vocabulary language q.
    written language q.

R

    relapse
    relation
    remission

90-R
rabbi
rabble-rouser
rabid
rabies
raccoon eye
race
    rat r.
race-ethnicity
racemic amphetamine
rachicentesis
rachigraph
rachitome
racial
    r. bias
    r. discrimination
    r. memory
    r. minority
    r. profiling
    r. saturation point
    r. slur
racing thought
racism
    aversive r.
racist
racket
racketeer
raconte
    déjà r.
racy
radar
    interpersonal r.
radial
    r. phenomenon
    r. prejudice
radiant
radiation
    acoustic r.
    auditory r.
    visual r.
radiation-induced mental deterioration
radical
    r. behaviorism
    r. fringe
    r. therapy
radiculalgia
radiculopathy
radioactive count
radioimmunoassay
radioisotope brain scanning
radiolabeled probe

radioligand
radiological
    chemical, bacteriological, r. (CBR)
radionuclide
radioreceptor
Rado view of depressive disorder
raffish
rage
    r. attack
    defiant r.
    driver's r.
    explosive r.
    feeling of r.
    hidden r.
    jealous r.
    narcissistic r.
    overt r.
    retributive r.
    retroflexed r.
    road r.
    sham r.
    unconscious r.
rageful feeling
raging parent
railroad neurosis
raise
    r. Cain
    r. hell
raising
    consciousness r.
raison d'etre
raisonnante
    folie r.
RAM
    rapid alternating movement
ramble
rambling
    r. flow of thought
    r. speech
rambunctious
ramification
ramisection
ramitis
rampage
    murder r.
    shooting r.
rampant
ramrod
ramshackle
rancorous
random
    r. activity
    r. act of violence
    r. assignment
    r. digital dialing (RDD)

random (*continued*)
    r. mating
    r. model
    r. movement
    r. noise
    r. observation
    r. sample
    r. urine testing
    r. variable
    r. wave
randomization
randomized
    r. clinical trial (RCT)
    r. controlled trial (RCT)
    r. group design
range
    r. of affect
    affect within normal r.
    borderline r.
    bright normal r.
    dose r.
    dull normal r.
    dynamic r.
    emotional r.
    extreme r.
    r. of feeling
    r. of interests
    normal r.
    significant r.
    some degree of r.
    subclinical r.
    therapeutic r.
    tolerance r.
    wide r.
rank
    r. correlation
    r. and file
    r. order
    percentile r.
rank-difference correlation
rankian
    r. theory
ranking
    merit r.
rankle
ransom
rant
rap
    r. group
    r. music
    r. session
    r. song
rape
    r. act
    anal r.
    r. crisis center
    date r.
    r. fantasy

    gang r.
    heterosexual r.
    male r.
    sadistic act of r.
    spouse r.
    statutory r.
    r. trauma syndrome
    r. victim
rapid
    r. alternating movement (RAM)
    r. change in activity
    r. cycler
    r. cycling
    r. eye movement (REM)
    r. eye movement latency
    r. eye movement sleep
    r. eye movement state
    r. fine movement
    r. metabolizer patients
    r. motor movement
    r. neuroleptization
    r. repetitive movement
    r. shift in affective expression
    r. speech
    r. time-zone change syndrome
    r. tranquilization
    r. tremor
    r. vocalization
rapid-change theory
rapid-cycling
    r.-c. bipolar disorder
    r.-c. course
    r.-c. pattern
rapidity
    r. of analyzing information
    r. of assimilating information
    r. of reinforcement
rapid-smoking theory
rapist
    adolescent r.
rapper
rapport
    en r.
    inadequate r.
    interpersonal r.
    parent-child r.
    psychological r.
rapprochement
    r. crisis
    r. subphase
rapture
rapture-of-the-deep syndrome
raptus
    r. action
    r. of attention
    impulsive r.
    r. melancholicus
    status r.

R

rare detail response
rarefaction
RAS
    reality-adaptive supportive
    reticular activating system
rasa
    tabula r.
rash
    r. decision-making
    glue sniffer's r.
rat
    r. race
    smell a r.
ratchet rigidity
rate
    accelerated heart r.
    age-specific cumulative incidence r.
    alternate motion r. (AMR)
    attrition r.
    basal metabolic r. (BMR)
    base r.
    birth r.
    case fatality r.
    compliance r.
    concordance r.
    r. control
    cumulative incidence r.
    cure r.
    death r.
    decline r.
    divorce r.
    dropout r.
    drug response r.
    exacerbation r.
    r. of fluency disturbance
    homicide-suicide r.
    hospital mortality r.
    incidence r.
    long-term mortality r.
    maturation r.
    mentation r.
    metabolic r.
    mortality r.
    mutation r.
    nonspecific response r.
    placebo response r.
    prevalence r.
    r. of production of speech
    pulse r.
    r. of recovery
    r. of recovery at discharge
    relapse r.

    response r.
    suicide attempt r.
    treatment completion r.
    treatment response r.
ratification theory
rating
    baseline r.
    behavior r.
    Bunney-Hamburg global
      psychosis r.
    Bunney-Hamburg nurse r.
    clinician r.
    daily symptom r.
    desire-for-death r.
    dimensional r.
    employment problem r.
    evaluative r.
    global clinician r.
    grade r.
    hyperintensity r.
    r. instrument
    intent r.
    internalized-state r.
    lethality r.
    maturity r.
    maximum intent r.
    maximum lethality r.
    merit r.
    r. method
    nonrandom r.
    peer r.
    pleasantness r.
    r. procedure
    psychiatric severity r.
    risk rescue r. (RRR)
    r. scale
    sexual maturity r.
    social impairment r.
    subjective unit of distress r.
    symptom r.
    three-factor model of global r.
    trait r.
ratio
    achievement r. (AR)
    affective r.
    affectivity r.
    age r.
    association sensation r.
    brain-to-plasma r.
    correlation r.
    critical r.
    dopamine r.

NOTES

ratio *(continued)*
 extinction r.
 fixed r. (FR)
 high affectivity r.
 odds r. (OR)
 oral-nasal acoustic r.
 risk r. (RR)
 risk-benefit r.
 r. scale
 sex r.
 stimulation r.
 T r.
 variable r. (VR)
 ventricle-to-brain r. (VBR)
rational
 r. cognitive coping
 r. emotive therapy (RET)
 r. medicine
 r. problem solving
 r. psychology
 r. psychotherapy
 r. suicide
 r. therapy (RT)
rationale
 psychiatric r.
rational-emotive
 r.-e. behavior
 r.-e. psychotherapy
rationality
rationalization defense mechanism
rationalize
rattle
 death r.
raucous
raunchy
rauwolfia
Rauwolfia serpentina
ravage
rave
 r. drug
 r. gathering
 r. party
ravenous
raver
raving madness
ravish
raw
 r. personality disorder score
 r. volume
Ray
 R. syndrome
razor
RBD
 REM behavior disorder
rCBF
 regional cerebral blood flow
RCP
 Royal College of Psychiatrists

RCT
 randomized clinical trial
 randomized controlled trial
RD
 reaction of degeneration
 reward dependence
RDA
 recommended daily allowance
RDD
 random digital dialing
rea
 mens r.
reach
 grasp and r.
reacquaint
reactance
 inductive r.
reaction
 Abderhalden-Fauser r.
 abnormal r.
 accelerated r.
 acute anxiety r.
 acute maladjustment situational r.
 acute organic r.
 acute paranoid r.
 acute paranoid schizophrenic r.
  (APSR)
 acute stress situational r.
 acute undifferentiated
  schizophrenic r. (AUSR)
 adaptation r.
 adjustment situational r.
 r. of adolescence
 adolescent turmoil r.
 adult situational stress r. (ASSR)
 adverse drug r. (ADR)
 affective depressive r.
 aggressive undersocialized r.
 agitated r.
 alarm r. (AR)
 alcohol-Antabuse r.
 allergic r.
 all-or-none r.
 anergastic r.
 anesthetic conversion r.
 anger r.
 angry r.
 anniversary r.
 antigen-antibody r.
 antisocial r.
 anxiety panic r.
 anxiety psychoneurotic r.
 anxious mood adjustment r.
 arousal r.
 arrest r.
 Asian alcohol flush r.
 associative r.
 asthenic r.

R

autonomic conversion r.
aversion r.
behavior r.
brief depressive r.
brief psychotic r.
cancer r.
cardiac r.
catastrophic r.
r. of childhood
choice r.
chronic paranoid r.
chronic paranoid schizophrenic r.
  (CPSR)
chronic stress r.
chronic undifferentiated
  schizophrenic r.
circular r.
civilian-catastrophe r.
climacteric paranoid r.
combat r.
compulsive psychoneurotic r.
conduct disturbance adjustment r.
confusional psychotic r.
consciousness disturbance stress r.
consensual r.
conversion psychoneurotic r.
cutaneous r.
dangerous behavior r.
r. to death
defense r.
defensive r.
deferred r.
r. of degeneration (RD)
dehydration r.
delayed r.
delirious r.
dental patient r.
depersonalization psychoneurotic r.
depressed mood adjustment r.
depressive psychoneurotic r.
depressive psychotic r.
depressive situational r.
dissociate-dysmnesic substitution r.
dissociative psychoneurotic r.
doll's eye r.
duplicative r.
dysergastic r.
dyssocial r.
dysthymic adjustment r.
dystonic r.
echo r.
elective mutism adjustment r.

emotional disturbance adjustment r.
emotional disturbance stress r.
emotionally unstable immaturity r.
emotional stress r.
emotions-conduct adjustment r.
escape r.
excitation psychotic r.
fear r.
fight or flight r.
fixation r.
r. formation
r. formation defense mechanism
galvanic skin r.
gemistocytic r.
general adaptation r.
grief r.
gross stress r.
group delinquent r.
group stress r.
hand-to-mouth r.
heel-tap r.
hyperkinetic conversion r.
hypochondriacal psychoneurotic r.
hypochondriac psychoneurotic r.
hypomanic-depressive r.
hypomanic manic-depressive r.
hysterical conversion r. (HCR)
hysterical psychoneurotic r.
idiosyncratic r.
immaturity r.
initial stress r.
intensity of r.
intermittent emotional conflicts
  or r.
involutional paranoid r.
involutional psychotic r.
Jolly r.
justifiable r.
laryngeal psychophysiologic r.
late r.
latent schizophrenic r.
lengthening r.
r. to life stress
LSD r.
magnet r.
maladaptive r.
maniacal grief r.
manic r.
manic-depressive r.
melancholic involutional r.
menopausal paranoid r.
r. to minor stimuli

NOTES

reaction *(continued)*
    mixed disturbance stress r.
    mixed paralytic conversion r.
    mobilization r.
    myasthenic r.
    negative therapeutic r.
    neurasthenic psychoneurosis r.
    neurasthenic psychoneurotic r.
    neurogenic r.
    neurotic r.
    neurotic-depressive r.
    nonpathological r.
    obsessional psychoneurotic r.
    obsessive-compulsive r.
    obsessive psychoneurotic r.
    organic r.
    overanxious r.
    pain r.
    paradoxical r.
    paranoid involutional r.
    paresthetic conversion r.
    passive r.
    passive-aggressive r.
    passive-dependent r.
    pathological grief r.
    pathologic grief r.
    personality r.
    phantom r.
    pharyngeal psychophysiologic r.
    phobic psychoneurotic r.
    physical symptoms adjustment r.
    primary circular r.
    prolonged depressive r.
    prolonged grief r.
    psychogalvanic skin r.
    psychogenic r.
    psychological r.
    psychomotor disturbance stress r.
    psychoneurotic depressive r.
    psychophysiologic r.
    psychosomatic r.
    psychotic depressive r.
    psychotic trigger r. (PRT, PTR)
    pupillary r.
    qi-gong psychotic r.
    recurrent episode psychotic r.
    repetition r.
    runaway r.
    r. scale
    schizophrenic r. (SR, S/R)
    schizophrenic reaction circular r.
    senile paranoid r.
    shock r.
    shortening r.
    simple paranoid r.
    single-episode psychotic r.
    situational stress r.

    sleeplessness associated with acute emotional conflicts or r.
    sleeplessness associated with intermittent emotional conflicts or r.
    socialized runaway r.
    somatization r.
    spite r.
    spoiled child r.
    startle r.
    stress situational r.
    subacute organic r.
    suspected adverse drug r. (SADR)
    sympathetic stress r.
    symptomatic r.
    task-oriented r.
    tension state psychoneurotic r.
    tertiary circular r.
    r. test
    therapeutic r. (TR)
    thymonoic r.
    r. time (RT)
    toxic r.
    transference r.
    transient depressive r.
    transplantation r.
    trigger r.
    r. type
    unaggressive undersocialized r.
    undersocialized, aggressive r.
    undersocialized nonaggressive r.
    undersocialized runaway r.
    unsocialized aggressive r.
    visual disorientation r.
    Wernicke r.
    withdrawal adjustment r.

reactional biography
reactions biography
reaction-type deterioration
reactivation process
reactive
    acute schizophrenic r.
    r. alcoholism
    r. attachment disorder
    r. attachment disorder of infancy
    r. attachment disorder of infancy or early childhood
    r. attachment disorder of infancy or early childhood, disinhibited type
    r. attachment disorder of infancy or early childhood, inhibited type
    r. bowel
    r. cell
    r. clinical depression
    r. confusion
    r. confusional state
    r. confusion nonorganic psychosis

R

r. depression and anxiety
r. depressive psychosis
r. ego alteration
r. epilepsy
r. exaltation
r. excitation
r. inhibition
r. mania
r. measure
r. melancholia
r. mental excitement
r. paranoid psychosis
r. psychotic depression
r. reinforcement
r. response
r. schizophrenia
symptomatically r.
r. thought

reactivity
affective r.
automatic r.
autonomic r.
emotional r.
lack of r.
mood r.
physiological r.

reactor
placebo r.

readaptation
neurobehavioral r.

reader
mind r.

readiness
complex r.
explosion r.
r. inventory
reading r.
r. test

reading
r. achievement
r. activities in life
r. backwards
r. comprehension impairment
delusions of mind r.
r. developmental delay disorder
r. disability
r. epilepsy
r. grade equivalent
r. language quotient
lip r.
mind r.
r. readiness

r. skills acquisition
r. skills learning retardation
thought r.

readjust
readmission
readout, read out
reaffirm
real
r. abandonment
r. anxiety
r. external stimulus
feeling that self is not r.
feeling that things are not r.
r. image
r. life
r. loss
r. self

realignment
circadian r.

realism
experimental r.
moral r.
mundane r.

realistic
r. expectation
r. fear
r. guilt
r. plan
r. thinking

reality
r. ability testing
r. adaptation
r. anxiety
r. assumption
r. awareness
break with r.
r. confrontation
contact with r.
deficient sense of r.
r. denial
denial of external r.
disconnection with r.
distorted perception of r.
r. distortion
escape from r.
external r.
flight from r.
independent physical r.
r. issue
r. life of ego
objective r.
r. orientation (RO)

NOTES

reality *(continued)*
    r. oriented (RO)
    r. oriented therapy
    out of touch with r.
    perceived r.
    perception of r.
    phenomenological r.
    r. principle
    psychic r.
    psychical r.
    relativity of r.
    retreat from r.
    sense of r.
    sociopolitical r.
    r. system
    r. test
    r. testing ability
    r. ties
    ties with r.
    transcendent r.
    unseen r.
reality-adaptive supportive (RAS)
reality-oriented supportive strategy
realization
    symbolic r.
real-life
    r.-l. behavior
    r.-l. circumstance
    r.-l. decision making
    r.-l. emotional episode
    r.-l. problem
    r.-l. stimuli
realm
    interpersonal r.
real-word cocaine cue
real-world
    r.-w. setting
    r.-w. situation
reanalysis strategy
reanalyzed data
reaper
    grim r.
reappear
rearing
    child r.
reason
    r.'s for living
    medical r.
    pharmacokinetic r.
    r. for visit
reasonable
    r. ego
    r. fear
    r. willingness
    r. zest
reasoning
    r. ability
    abstract r.

    age of r.
    arithmetical r.
    clinical r.
    conceptual r.
    deductive r.
    r. disturbance
    dynamic r.
    ethical r.
    evaluative r.
    exonerative moral r.
    hypothetical r.
    hypothetical-deductive r.
    idiosyncratic r.
    illogical r.
    inductive r.
    r. mania
    r. and memory skills
    nonverbal r.
    practical r.
    syllogistic r.
    verbal r.
    verbal, numerical, and r. (VNR)
reassessment
    attitude r.
    sexual attitude r. (SAR)
reassignment
    gender r.
    hormonal sex r.
    hormonal sexual r.
    sex r.
    sexual r.
    surgical sex r.
reassociation
reassurance sensitivity
reassure
reassuring explanation
reattribution technique
rebel against authority
rebellion
    adolescent r.
rebellious
    r. teen
    r. youngster
rebelliousness
rebirth fantasy
reborn
rebound
    r. effect
    r. hyperthermia
    r. insomnia
    r. mood swing
    r. phenomenon
    REM sleep r.
    r. suppression
rebreathe
rebreathing
rebuild
rebuke

rebus principle
rebuttal
recalcitrant pain
recall
 body-image r.
 delayed r.
 digit r.
 diminished r.
 dream r.
 event r.
 r. failure
 free r.
 inconsistent r.
 r. of information test
 r. 5 items after 5 minutes test
 r. memory
 memory r.
 r. method
 r. performance
 recognition vs r.
 recollection and r.
 remote r.
 retention and r.
 rote r.
 total r.
 verbatim r.
 vivid dream r.
recall-accuracy
 code substitution-immediate r.-a.
 (CDS-ACC)
recall-generated
 r.-g. emotion
 r.-g. sadness
recalling new information disturbance
recant
recap
recapitulation
 pubertal sexual r.
recapture
recathexis
recede
receiver operating characteristic (ROC)
receiving type
recency
 positive r.
recent
 r. life event (RLE)
 r. loss
 r. past memory
recent-onset schizophrenia
receptive
 r. aphasia

 r. character
 r. dysphasia
 r. function
 r. language development
 r. language disorder
 r. language processing
 r. language-processing quotient
 r. orientation
 r. personality
receptive-expressive observation (REO)
receptor
 acetylcholine cholinergic r.
 adenosine r.
 r. affinity
 alpha adrenergic r.
 alpha-2 adrenergic r.
 r. alteration
 beta adrenergic r.
 catecholamine r.
 cholinergic r.
 9-cis retinoic acid r. (RXR)
 delta opiate r.
 distance r.
 dopamine D_2 r.
 r. functioning
 5-HT-1 r.
 5-HT$_{2C}$ r.
 kappa opiate r.
 limbic dopamine r.
 mu opiate r.
 muscarinic cholinergic r.
 neurotransmitter r.
 nicotinic cholinergic r.
 noradrenergic r.
 r. occupancy
 opiate r.
 opioid r.
 pain r.
 peripheral catecholamine r.
 peroxisomal proliferator r. (PPAR)
 postsynaptic 5-HT-2 r.
 postsynaptic 5-HT-3 r.
 proximal r.
 sensory r.
 serotonergic r.
 serotonin 5-HT$_2$ r.
 sigma r.
 unencapsulated joint r.
 r. up-regulation
 vitamin D r. (VDR)
receptor-binding property

NOTES

recessive
- autosomal r.
- r. gene
- r. trait

recessiveness

recidivation

recidivism
- r. in schizophrenia
- victim r.

recidivist

recidivity

recipient
- action r.

recipiomotor

reciprocal
- r. agreement
- r. assimilation
- r. circuitry
- r. communication
- r. connection
- r. determinism
- r. inhibition
- r. inhibition and desensitization
- r. inhibition psychotherapy
- r. parenting
- r. punishment
- r. regulation
- r. social interaction

reciprocate

reciprocity
- behavioral r.
- emotional r.
- overadequate-inadequate r.

recitation

recitative

recite
- survey, question, read, review, r. (SQ3R)

reckless
- r. behavior
- r. driving

recline

recluse

recognition
- facial r.
- r. memory
- pattern r.
- r. of people
- r. site
- r. time
- visual pattern r.
- r. vs recall
- r. in wit

recognizable

recognizance

recognize
- r., empathize, think, hear, integrate, notice, keep (RETHINK)

recoil

recollection
- intrusive r.
- r. and recall
- r. of trauma

recommencement mania

recommendation

recommended
- r. daily allowance (RDA)
- r. dose

recommission

recommit

recompensation

reconcile

reconciliation attempt

reconditioning
- orgasmic r.
- r. therapy

reconnaissance
- fausse r.

reconnoiter

reconsider

reconstituted family

reconstruct

reconstruction
- cosmetic r.
- r. dream
- r. method
- pathology-induced memory r.

reconstructive
- r. psychotherapy
- r. therapy

record
- activity r.
- automated clinical r.
- Bayley behavior r.
- behavior r.
- chronological drinking r.
- confidential r.
- criminal r.
- cumulative r.
- hospital r.
- infant behavior r.
- medical r.
- mental status examination r.
- problem-oriented r. (POR)
- r. review

recording
- behavior specimen r.
- depth r.
- r. procedure

recount

recoup

recourse

recover

recovered memory

recovery
- adolescent r.

r. from delinquency
full r.
r. of function
r. issue
language r.
partial r.
personal r.
r. phase
post r.
rate of r.
r. and reorganization
social r.
spontaneous r.
r. stage
uncomplicated r.
r. wish
recreate
recreation
active r.
passive r.
therapeutic r.
recreational
r. drinking
r. drug
r. drug use
r. gambler
r. service
r. therapy (RT)
recriminate
recruit
recruiting response
rectal psychogenic disorder
rectify
rectitude
rectum, pl. **recta, rectums**
per r.
recur
recurred
recurrence
likelihood of r.
r. risk
recurrent
r. abuse
r. brief depressive disorder
r. catatonia
r. course
r. depersonalization
r. dream
r. encephalopathy
r. episode
r. episode chronic mania
r. episode depressive psychosis

r. episode psychotic
r. episode psychotic depression
r. episode psychotic reaction
r. illusion
major depressive disorder, r.
r. melancholia
r. migraine headache
r. mood disorder
r. motor movement
r. nightmare
r. panic attack
r. seizure
r. suicidal ideation
r. thought
r. vocalization
recurring
r. dream
r. idea
r. symptom
r. theme
recursion
recursive autoassociative memory
recutita
Matricaria r.
recycled air
redescribe
red-handed
redintegration
redirect
redirecting anger
redirection
red-light district
redneck
reduce
reduced
r. aggression level
r. agitation
r. anxiety
r. attention ability
r. awareness of surroundings
r. gratification
r. intellectual function
r. level of consciousness
r. motivation
r. rapid eye movement latency
r. responsiveness
r. sodium diet
r. verbal output
reduction
accident r.
anxiety r.
r. of anxiety

R

NOTES

reduction *(continued)*
    cluster r.
    cue r.
    cumulative medication r.
    dose r.
    drive r.
    gambling r.
    medication r.
    meditation-based stress r.
    mindfulness-based stress r.
    risk r.
    ritual r.
    smoking-related r.
    stress r.
    symptom r.
    tension r.
    tobacco use r.
reductionism
    biologic r.
reductive
redundancy
    correlation r.
    genetic r.
    r. rule
redundant
reduplicated babbling
reduplicative paramnesia
reeducation
    emotional r.
reeducative therapy
reefer
reemergence
reemploy
reenact
reenactment
    emotional r.
    trauma-specific r.
reenforce
reenforced thought
reentry
reestablish
reevaluation counseling
reexperienced
    r. trauma
    r. traumatic event
reexperiencing
    r. category
    r. perceptual symptom
referee
reference
    cultural frame of r.
    delusion of r.
    r. delusion
    distorted ideas of r.
    frame of r.
    r. group
    ideas of r.
    memory r.

    r. phase
    Physicians' Desk R. (PDR)
    r. picture-caption pair
    standard r.
    transient ideas of r.
    r. zero level
referential
    r. attitude
    r. delusion
    r. function
    r. idea
    r. index
    r. semantics
referral
    psychiatric r.
referred
    r. pain
    r. sensation
refined
reflect
reflection
    factor r.
    r. of feeling
reflective
reflex, pl. **reflexes**
    acquired r.
    acromial r.
    r. act
    acute affective r.
    allied r.
    antagonistic r.
    r. arc
    r. asymmetry
    attention r.
    attitudinal r.
    bar r.
    behavior r.
    brisk r.
    r. center
    chain r.
    r. change
    conditioned r. (CR)
    consensual r.
    contralateral r.
    r. control
    r. convulsion
    convulsive r.
    coordinated r.
    cry r.
    darwinian r.
    r. decay
    deep tendon r. (DTR)
    defecation r.
    defense r.
    delayed r.
    depressed r.
    diffused r.
    diminished r.

diving r.
doll's eye r.
dorsal r.
ejaculatory r.
emptying r.
eye-closure r.
gag r.
galvanic skin r.
grasp r.
grasping and groping r.
gustatory-sudorific r.
r. hallucination
r. headache
inborn r.
r. incontinence
r. inhibition of epilepsy
innate r.
intrinsic r.
inverted radial r.
ipsilateral r.
jaw r.
jaw-working r.
labyrinthine righting r.
r. latency
latent r.
laughter r.
lip r.
magnet r.
mass r.
Mendel instep r.
milk-ejection r.
r. movement
muscular r.
neck r.
r. neurogenic bladder
orienting r.
palmar r.
parachute r.
pathologic r.
r. pattern
phasic r.
physiological r.
pilomotor r.
positive conditioned r.
postural r.
primitive r.
psychic r.
psychocardic r.
psychogalvanic r. (PGR)
pupillary skin r.
r. seizure
r. sensation

startle r.
stress-altered startle r.
r. therapy
r. threshold
r. time
unconditional r.
unconditioned r. (UCR)
upper abdominal periosteal r.
utricular r.
vomiting r.
withdrawal r.
reflexive movement
reflexogenic zone
reflexogenous
reflexograph
reflexology
reflexometer
reflexotherapy
reflux
    ejaculation r.
    r. management
reform
    mental health r.
    thought r.
reformation
reformatory
    r. paranoia
    r. paranoiac
reformist delusion
reformulation
    sequential diagrammatic r. (SDR)
refractoriness
    medication r.
refractory
    r. depression
    r. erectile dysfunction
    r. mental illness
    r. period
    r. psychosis
    r. schizophrenia
    r. state
    treatment r.
refraining
reframing
    context r.
    meaning r.
refreshed
refreshing sleep attack
refrigerator
    r. parent
    r. parenting
refuge

NOTES

refugee
refusal
    r. to eat
    medication r.
    school r.
    treatment r.
    r. of treatment
regard
    field of r.
    mutual r.
    point of r.
    positive r.
    unconditional positive r.
regardant
regardless
regenerate
regeneration
    aberrant r.
regime
regimen
    birth control r.
    drug r.
    holistic r.
    medication r.
    multiple-dose r.
    pharmacotherapy r.
    steady-state r.
    treatment r.
region
    anterior insula r.
    auditory r.
    bilateral r.'s
    brain r.
    central gray matter r.
    cerebellar r.
    cerebral r.
    circumscribed r.
    comparison r.
    cortical r.
    critical r.
    deep white matter r.
    dorsal anterior cingulate r.
    dorsal limbic r.
    dorsal neocortical r.
    frontal brain r.
    gray matter r.
    inferior parietal r.
    interconnected cerebral r.
    limbic brain r.
    limbic-related r.
    motor r.
    negatively correlated r.
    neocortical r.
    orbitofrontal r.
    paralimbic r.
    perceptual-motor r.
    periventricular gray r.
    positively correlated r.

    posterior cingulate r.
    prefrontal r.
    septal r.
    speech perception r.
    subcortical gray r.
    subgenual cingulate r.
    temporal speech r.
    terminal r.
    thalamic r.
    ventral paralimbic r.
    visual r.
    white matter r.
regional
    r. background
    r. blood flow
    r. brain glucose metabolism
    r. brain lactate
    r. cerebral blood flow (rCBF)
    r. differentiation
    r. distribution
    r. epilepsy
    r. glucose metabolism at rest
register
    case r.
    psychiatric case r.
registered
    Music Therapist, R. (MTR)
    r. nurse (RN)
    r. recreation therapist (RRT)
    r. sex offender
registration
    image r.
    imperfect image r.
registry
    Clozaril National R.
regnancy
regress
regressed
regression
    age r.
    r. analysis
    atavistic r.
    r. defense mechanism
    Galton law of r.
    logistic r.
    multiple r.
    r. neurosis
    partial r.
    past-life hypnotic r.
    phenomenal r.
    polytomous r.
    progressive teleologic r.
    teleologic r.
regressive
    r. alcoholism
    r. assimilation
    r. behavior
    r. electroshock treatment (REST)

r. infantilism
r. substitute
r. symptoms of schizophrenia
r. transference neurosis
regressive-inspirational
r.-i. group
r.-i. group psychotherapy
regressive-reconstructive approach
regret
regrettable
regrettably
regroup
regular
r. caffeine consumption
r. caffeine user
r. diet
r. drug user
r. eating schedule
r. gambler
r. sleeping schedule
r. waking schedule
regularity
regularly
regulation
emotional r.
immune system r.
impulse r.
reciprocal r.
self-esteem r.
sexual r.
top-down r.
weight r.
regulator
mood r.
regulatory
r. center
r. input
r. role
regurgitation
rehab
rehabilitate
rehabilitation
acoupedic r.
alcoholic r.
r. assessment
r. behavior
Boston University Model of
Psychiatric R.
cognitive r.
r. counselor
r. evaluation
r. facility

geriatric r.
neuromuscular r.
occupational r.
r. psychiatry
psychosocial r.
sexual r.
social r.
r. stage
testing, orientation, and work
evaluation for r. (TOWER)
r. treatment
vocational r. (VR)
rehabilitative issue
rehashing
rehearsal
behavior r.
behavioral r.
cognitive r.
obsessional r.
thought r.
reign of terror
reimbursement
ICD-9 diagnostic codes for
Medicare r.
r. issue
rein
free r.
reincarnation
reindoctrination
reinforce
reinforced
r. practice
r. thought
reinforcement
adventitious r.
aperiodic r.
chained r.
concurrent r.
conjunctive r.
contingency r.
continuous r.
r. counseling
covert r.
delayed r.
differential r.
drug r.
fixed r.
homogeneous r.
homogenous r.
intermittent r.
interval r.
mixed r.

NOTES

reinforcement *(continued)*
 multiple r.
 negative r.
 partial r.
 periodic r.
 positive r.
 predelay r.
 primary r.
 rapidity of r.
 reactive r.
 schedule of r.
 r. schedule
 secondary r.
 self-managed r.
 social r.
 systematic r.
 tandem r.
 terminal r.
 time out from r.
 variable r.
 verbal r.
reinforcer
 conditioned r.
 negative r.
 positive r.
 primary r.
 secondary r.
reinforcing
 r. agent
 r. drug response
 r. effect
 r. property
 r. stimulus
reinsert
reinstatement
 job r.
reinstinctualization
reintegrate
reintegration
reinterpret
reinterpretation
reintroduction
reintrojection
Reitan
 R. rules to assess learning disorder
reiterate
reject
rejecting-neglecting parent
rejecting parent
rejection
 r. fear
 feeling of r.
 interpersonal r.
 r. of intimacy
 maternal r.
 parental r.
 paternal r.
 r. by peers

 perceived interpersonal r.
 r. sensitivity
rejoice
rejuvenate
rejuvenation fantasy
relabeling
relapse (R)
 full r.
 impending r.
 r. mechanism
 r. prevention
 prone to r.
 psychotic r.
 r. rate
relapse-prevention
 r.-p. counseling
 r.-p. technique
relapsing
related
 alcohol r. (AR)
 drug r.
 r. psychopathology
 r. sleep disorder
 transformational r.
 transformationally r.
relatedness
 developmentally inappropriate
  social r.
 disturbed social r.
 failure to develop r.
 functional r.
 inappropriate social r.
 semantic r.
 social r.
 symbiotic r.
relating
 disordered r.
 forms of satisfactory r.
 r. to others
 time periods of satisfactory r.
relation (R)
 afferent r.
 r. to age
 community-institutional r.'s
 court of domestic r.'s
 dose-response r.
 efferent r.
 extramarital r.'s
 family r.
 human r.
 intergenerational r.
 interpersonal r.
 intimate human r.
 negative r.
 object r.
 perception of spatial r.'s
 professional-family r.
 sexual r.

R

sibling r.
step r.
r.'s test
relational
   r. alliance
   r. behavior
   r. efficacy
   r. opposite
   r. problem
   r. threshold
   r. unit
relationship
   r. addiction
   addiction r.
   adversarial r.
   anaclitic r.
   appropriate r.
   attachment r.
   r. behavior
   bisexual r.
   brain-behavior r.
   causal r.
   cause-effect r.
   chewing-speech r.
   chronological r.
   clearly demarcated r.
   collaborative r.
   competent r.
   complainant-listener r.
   complex r.
   complicated r.
   conflictual r.
   consistent r.
   consultative r.
   counseling r.
   dating r.
   demarcated r.
   dependent r.
   dependent-protective r.
   destructive r.
   detachment from social r.
   disrupted r.
   disturbed attachment r.
   disturbed interpersonal r. (DIR)
   doctor-patient r.
   dose-response r.
   dramatic interpersonal r.
   dual r.
   dysfunctional r.
   early r.
   email r.
   etiological r.

failure to sustain a monogamous r.
family r.
fantasy-based elements of the
   doctor-patient r.
forced r.
former r.
genetic r.
harmful sexual r.
helping r.
heterosexual r.
r. history
homosexual r.
human r.
hypnotic r.
I-it r.
imaginary r.
impaired r.
impersonal r.
inappropriate r.
incestuous r.
independent r.
initiate r.
instability in interpersonal r.
intense interpersonal r.
Internet r.
interpersonal r.
intimate r.
intrafamilial r.
intrinsic r.
r. inventory
inverse r.
inversion r.
I-thou r.
live-in r.
loss of r.
love r.
love-hate r.
maternal r.
meaningful interpersonal r.
monogamous r.
mother-child r. (MCR)
mother-infant r.
multiple r.
negative r.
no-win r.
nurturing r.
object r.
online r.
optimal r.
parent-child r.
paternal r.
peer r.

NOTES

relationship *(continued)*
    perfect negative r.
    perfect positive r.
    periodic reinforcement r.
    personal r.
    physician-patient r.
    platonic r.
    poor peer r.
    positive r.
    predictive r.
    primary sexual r.
    r. problems of childhood
    r. psychotherapy
    replacement r.
    required r.
    romantic r.
    sadomasochistic r.
    r. satisfaction
    semantic r.
    sexual r.
    shared r.
    spectral r.
    stress-strain r.
    supervisory r.
    supportive r.
    teacher-student r.
    temporal r.
    terminate r.
    therapeutic r.
    therapist-patient r.
    r. therapy
    r. tool
    transference r.
    troubled r.
    trusting physician-patient r.
    unsatisfactory r.
    unstable interpersonal r.
    r. with God
    working r.
relative
    death of r.
    r. dementia
    r. elective mutism
    first-degree biological r.
    r. frequency
    r. hypoxia
    r. impotence
    r. risk
    r. scotoma
    r. slow-wave sleep stability
relativism
    cultural r.
    moral r.
relativistic
relativity
    law of r.
    r. of reality
    special theory of r.

relaxant
    depolarizing muscle r.
relaxation
    applied r. (AR)
    r. constant
    differential r.
    r. phase
    progressive muscular r.
    r. response
    state of mindful r.
    r. technique
    r. technique training
    therapeutic r.
    r. therapy
    r. time
    r. training
    r. training in adolescence
    r. training in children
relaxation-induced anxiety (RIA)
relaxed
    squarely (face person), open
        posture, lean (toward person), eye
        (contact), r. (SOLER)
relay station
relearning method
release
    dopamine r.
    emotional r.
    r. of information
    orgastic r.
    r. phenomenon
    pituitary prolactin r.
    prolactin r.
    r. therapy
releaser
relegate
relent
relentless
relevance
    clinical r.
    personal r.
    r. of spirituality
relevant diagnostic criteria
reliability
    r. coefficient
    equivalent form r.
    index of r.
    interjudge r.
    interobserver r.
    interrater r.
    split-half r.
    test-retest r.
reliable
    r. diagnosis
    r. history
reliance
    hemispheric r.
reliant

relief
    comic r.
    pain r.
    symptom r.
relieve
reliever
religion
    Eastern r.
    influence of r.
    organized r.
    salience of r.
religiosa
    melancholia r.
religiosity
religio-terror
religious
    r. activity
    r. affiliation
    r. approach
    r. attitude
    r. background
    r. behavior
    r. belief
    r. commitment
    r. community
    r. conflict
    r. conviction
    r. cult
    r. delusion
    r. denomination
    r. difference
    r. dynamics
    r. ecstasy
    r. experience
    explicitly r.
    r. faith
    r. fasting
    r. healer
    r. influence
    r. insanity
    r. institution
    r. interest
    r. intervention
    r. language
    r. life
    r. mania
    r. metaphor
    r. nonbelief
    r. object
    r. obsession
    r. organization
    r. orientation
    r. orthodoxy factor
    r. person
    r. perspective
    r. practice
    r. proscription
    r. or spiritual problem
    r. teachings
    r. tenet
    r. theme
    r. tradition
    r. upbringing
    r. values
    r. value system
religiously devout
relinquish
relinquishment
    custody r.
relive
relocate
relocation
    frequent r.
reluctance
reluctant
REM
    rapid eye movement
        REM behavior disorder (RBD)
        REM period
        REM sleep
        REM sleep activity
        REM sleep behavior
        REM sleep behavior disorder
        REM sleep efficiency
        REM sleep rebound
        REM sleep-related disorder
        REM state
remand
remark
    caustic r.
    derogatory r.
    disparaging r.
    self-deprecatory r.
remarkable
remarriage
remarried
remarry
rematch
remedial
    r. intervention
    r. psychotherapy
    r. teaching
remediation
    cognitive r.

NOTES

remedy
    herbal r.
remilitarize
reminder
reminisce
reminiscence therapy
reminiscent
    r. aura
    r. neuralgia
remission (R)
    early full r.
    full r.
    partial r.
    periods of r.
    spontaneous r.
    sustained full r.
    sustained partial r.
    transference r.
remitted substance abuser
remittent
remitting
    r. dementia
    r. schizophrenia
REM-onset sleep
remonstrate
remorse
    feeling of r.
    lack of r.
remorseful
remorseless
remote
    r. attempter
    r. memory
    r. recall
    r. suicide attempt
remotivation
removed affect
remover
remuneration
rename
render
rendezvous
renegade
renege
renegotiable
renew
renewal
renifleur
renitent
Renpenning syndrome
renunciation
    instinctual r.
REO
    receptive-expressive observation
    REO Scale
reorganization
    plastic r.
    recovery and r.

reorient
reorientation
reparation
reparative response
reparenting
repartee
repay
repeat
    r. abuser
    r. sex offender
    r. tendency
repeated
    r. abuse
    r. bullying
    r. handwashing
    r. heavy drinker
    r. infarct dementia
    r. painful experience
    r. REM sleep interruptions
    r. shift in affective expression
    r. substance self-administration
repeatedly
repeater
    accident r.
repeating
    r. pattern
    r. ritual
repent
repentance
repentant
repercussion
repersonalization
repertoire
    r. of aggressive behavior
    behavioral r.
repertory
repetition
    r. compulsion
    compulsive r.
    r. by imitation
    needless r.
    r. reaction
    senseless imitative word r.
    sentence r. (SR, S/R)
    r. of sound
    stereotyped r.
    r. test
    trauma-related r.
repetition-compulsion
    r.-c. principle
repetitious
    r. activity
    r. behavior
    r. request
repetitive
    r. checking behavior
    r. convulsion
    r. idea

r. imitative movement
r. impulse disorder
r. lying
r. motor activity
r. partial seizure
r. pattern
r. pattern of behavior
r. play
r. rumination
r. task
r. transcranial magnetic stimulation (rTMS)
r. violence
r. watching
replaceable
replacement
electrolyte r.
r. formation
hormone r.
r. memory
r. relationship
r. technique
r. therapy
repletion
replication
reply
latency of r.
report
case r.
r. criminal
informant r.
mental status examination r. (MSER)
paucity of r.'s
phenomenal r.
retrospective r.
reportedly
repose
reprehend
reprehension
representation
coitus r.
collective r.
concrete r.
internal r.
preexisting r.
representational
abstract-versus-r.
r. system
representative
instinct r.

r. intelligence
r. sample
repress
repressed
r. feeling
r. impulse
r. instinctual drive
r. need
return of the r.
repression
cognitive approaches to dreaming and r.
emotional r.
organic r.
primal r.
primary r.
proper r.
r. resistance
r. scale
secondary r.
repression-sensitization scale
repressive
r. behavior
r. personality
repressive-inspirational group psychotherapy
repressor
reprieve
reprimand
reprisal
reproach
reprobate
reprocessing
eye movement r.
eye movement desensitization and r. (EMDR)
reproduce
reproduction
chain r.
visual r.
reproductive
r. assimilation
r. facilitation
r. failure
r. mortality
reprove
reptilian stare
repudiate
repugnance
repugnant
repulse
repulsion

NOTES

repulsive
reputable
reputation
    evil r.
repute
request
    repetitious r.
required
    r. guardianship
    r. relationship
    r. task
requirement
    performance r.
requisite
rescind
rescission
rescue fantasy
rescuer
research
    action r.
    advocacy r.
    Agency for Health Care Policy
     and R.
    applied r.
    r. assistant
    behavioral r.
    biologic r.
    brain r.
    r. clinic
    comparative r.
    consumer r.
    cross-sectional r.
    empirical r.
    epidemiological r.
    ethics of psychiatric r.
    evaluation r.
    ex post facto r.
    field r.
    genetic r.
    infancy r.
    r. initiative
    Institute of Educational R. (IER)
    Institute of Personality and R.
     (IPAR)
    International Society for Sexually
     Transmitted Disease R.
    intervention r.
    r. interview
    Journal of Psychiatric R.
    motivation r.
    neurochemical r.
    nonspecific r.
    normatological r.
    r. observation
    operational r.
    operations r. (OR)
    personality r.
    population r.

    r. program
    psychiatric r.
    psychological r.
    quasi-experimental r.
    specificity of r.
    taxonomic r.
    twin r.
researcher
    personality r.
    psychiatric r.
resemblance
    clinical r.
resemble
resent
resentful
resentment
    covert r.
reservatus
    coitus r.
reserve
    cognitive r.
    operant r.
reserved
reservist
reside
residence
    intensive care community r.
residential
    r. center
    r. OCD program
    r. placement
    r. setting
    r. treatment
    r. treatment center (RTC)
    r. treatment facility
resident physician
residual
    r. amnesia
    r. disability
    r. impairment
    r. negative symptom
    r. pain
    r. phase
    r. phase of schizophrenia
    r. positive symptom
    r. psychotic symptom
    r. state
residual-type
    r.-t. schizophrenia
    r.-t. schizophrenic disorder
residue
    archaic r.
    day r.
    night r.
resignation
    neurotic r.
resilience
resilient

resistance
analysis of the r.
character r.
compliance masking covert r.
conscious r.
covert r.
ego r.
environmental r. (ER)
r. to extinction
galvanic skin r.
id r.
least r.
r. level
level of r.
manifestations of r.
overt compliance masking covert r.
passive r.
patient r.
psychogalvanic skin r. (PGSR)
repression r.
social r.
state of r.
superego r.
r. to thyroid hormone (RTH)
transference r.
unconscious r.
violent r.
resistant
r. attachment
r. depression
r. mood disorder
r. schizophrenia
seizure r. (SR, S/R)
treatment r.
resistentiae
locus minoris r.
resistiveness
resocialization
resolute
resolution
anxiety r.
conflict r.
crisis r.
r. of crisis
peer-to-peer conflict r.
r. phase
r. phase of sexual response cycle
temporal r.
resolve conflict
resolving conflict skills

resonance
acoustic r.
r. disorder
resource
community r.'s
r.'s for coping
deep inner r.
r. holding potential
human r.'s
intellectual r.
mental health r.
neuropsychologic r.
psychological r.
r. state
resourceful
respect
mutual r.
respectable
respectful
respiration
Biot r.
bronchial r.
Cheyne-Stokes r.
diffusion r.
electrophrenic r.
internal r.
opposition r.
temperature, pulse, r. (TPR)
tissue r.
respiratory
r. anosmia
r. impairment sleep disorder
r. pause
r. psychogenic disorder
respite
resplendent
respondeat superior
respondent
r. behavior
r. condition
r. conditioning
respond to environment
responder
psychotherapy r. (PR)
response
abnormal r.
abnormal muscle r. (AMR)
achromatic color r.
r. acquiescence
acute stress r.
adaptive r.
adverse autonomic r.

NOTES

response *(continued)*

adverse psychological r.
affect r.
aggressive r.
agitation r.
amygdala r.
anamnestic r.
anticipatory r.
antidepressant r.
antipsychotic r.
anxiety relief r.
anxiolytic r.
appropriate r.
appropriateness of emotional r.
auditory brainstem r. (ABR)
auditory evoked r.
autonomic r.
aversion r.
avoidance r.
barrier r.
blink r.
blunted r.
brain metabolic r.
brainstem auditory evoked r.
caffeine r.
catastrophic r.
cellular immunologic r.
center-surround r.
chaining r.
chromatic r.
chronic r.
cingulate r.
circular-pattern r.
clasp-knife r.
clerical r.
clinical r.
cocaine-related r.
color r.
conditioned avoidance r.
conditioned drug r.
conditioned emotional r. (CER)
conditioned escape r.
confabulated detail r. (dD)
confabulated whole r. (DW)
consistent r.
coping r.
cortical-evoked r.
covert r.
criminal r.
culturally sanctioned r.
culturally unsanctioned r.
cumulative r.
r. curve
Cushing r.
delayed r.
r. deviation
differential r.
discrete emotional r.

r. dispersion
dissociative r.
dysphoric r.
dyspnea r.
dysregulated stress r.
electrodermal r. (EDR)
emotional r.
r. to environment
evoked r. (ER)
evoked potential r. (EPR)
evoked somatosensory r.
exaggerated startle r.
extensor plantar r.
eye-blink r.
false-negative r.
false-positive r.
fastigial pressor r. (FPR)
fear r.
flight or fight r.
form r. (F)
free r.
frequency r.
frustration r.
galvanic skin r. (GSR)
generalization r.
genital r.
good form r. (F+)
heat-defense r.
hedonic r.
r. hierarchy
hostile r.
human r. (h)
human figure parts r.
human movement r.
hyperactive sympathetic r.
hypnotic r.
immune r.
implicit r.
inadequate r.
inappropriate r.
incompatible r.
inconsistent r.
r. index
individual r.
inhibited sexual r.
instrumental r.
intropunitive r.
involuntary r.
latency of r.
latent r.
level of r.
local r.
long latency r.
loss of r.
low-key r.
maladaptive r.
marriage r.
mediated r.

metabolic r.
morbid r.
motor r.
negative r.
negativistic r.
no r.
oculomotor r.
orienting r.
original r.
overt r.
r. to pain
paradigmatic r.
paradoxical r.
pathological r.
r. pattern
penetration r.
perseverative r.
personal r.
physiological r.
pilomotor r.
plantar r.
polarity r.
poor form r. (F-)
poor genital r.
popular r.
position r.
positive r.
postsaccadic neuronal r.
r. prevention
r. processing time
psychogalvanic r. (PGR)
psychological r.
psychologically mediated r.
rare detail r.
r. rate
reactive r.
recruiting r.
reinforcing drug r.
relaxation r.
reparative r.
reward-irrelevant r.
satiety r.
r. set
sexual r.
shading r. (ShR)
skin conductance orienting r.
  (SCOR)
small detail r.
somatosensory evoked r. (SER)
sonomotor r.
space r.
r. specificity

startle r.
stimulus r.
stress effect and immune r.
stress-related physiological r.
sympathetic r.
r. system
target r.
texture r.
thalamic r.
r. theory
therapeutic r.
thermoeffector r.
thermoregulatory r.
tissue-type metabolic r.
total r. (lz R)
treatment r.
unconditioned r. (UCR)
unexpected r.
unsanctioned r.
unusual detail r. (Dd)
unusual rare detail r. (dr)
vibrotactile r.
vista r.
visual evoked r. (VER)
whole r. (W, WR)
response-produced cue
response-specificity
individual r.-s.
responsibility
ascriptive r.
assigned r.
clinical r.
community r.
criminal r.
denial of r.
diminished r.
disavows r.
distribution of r.
excessive r.
feeling of r.
generational r.
homemaking r.
household r.
increased r.
individual r.
interpersonal r.
legal r.
limited r.
minimizes r.
new r.
obsessive feelings of r.
patient r.

NOTES

responsibility *(continued)*
    personal r.
    position of r.
    primary r.
    sense of r.
    serotonergic r.
    sexual r.
    social r.
    test of criminal r.
responsible
    r. eating habit
    r. sexual behavior
responsive
    treatment r.
responsiveness
    abnormal r.
    absence of emotional r.
    affective r.
    diminished r.
    emotional r.
    facial r.
    mutual affective r.
    OCD r.
    reduced r.
    threshold of r.
responsivity
    emotional r.
    mood r.
    neuroleptic r.
    treatment r.
REST
    regressive electroshock treatment
    restricted environment stimulation
     therapy
rest
    r. home
    metabolism at r.
    r. pain
    regional glucose metabolism at r.
    r. tremor
restatement
rest-cure technique
restful
resting
    r. anterior cingulate flow
    r. energy expenditure
    r. PET study
    r. potential
    r. state
    r. tremor
    wakefulness r.
restitution
    cognitive r.
    neurologic r.
restitutional symptoms of schizophrenia
restitutive therapy
restless
    r. behavior

    r. legs syndrome
    r. pacing
restlessness
    motor r.
    nocturnal r.
    psychomotor r.
restrain
restraining
    r. order
    r. order violation
    r. therapy
restraint
    chemical r.
    chest r.
    compulsive r.
    ethical r.
    four-point r.
    1-hour r. rule
    lack of r.
    r. law
    leather r.
    physical r.
    Posey r.
    seclusion and r. (S&R)
    situational r.
    soft r.
    wrist r.
restrict
restricted
    r. access to food
    r. activity
    r. behavior
    r. diet
    r. environment stimulation therapy
     (REST)
    r. focus
    r. interest
    r. range of affect
    r. range of emotional expression
restricters
restricting
    r. behavior
    cognitive r.
    r. type
restriction
    activity r.
    building r.
    close watch r.
    dietary r.
    ego r.
    r. endonuclease
    r. fragment length polymorphism
     (RFLP)
    open seclusion r.
    shoe r.
    unit r.

restrictive
    r. behavior
    r. criterion
restructuring
    attitude r.
    cognitive r.
    perceptual r.
    sexual attitude r. (SAR)
    systematic rational r. (SRR)
restzustand schizophrenia
result
    anomalous r.
    biometric r.
    concordant r.
    positive r.
resumption
resurgence
resuscitate
    do not r. (DNR)
resuscitation
    cardiopulmonary r.
resuscitative snores
resymbolization
RET
    rational emotive therapy
Ret, ret
    retarded
retaliate
retaliation
retardata
    ejaculatio r.
retardate
    ejaculatio r.
retardation
    American Association of Mental R. (AAMR)
    arithmetical skills learning r.
    borderline mental r.
    cultural-familial mental r.
    developmental r.
    r. developmental delay disorder
    idiopathic language r.
    incidental learning language r.
    language skills learning r.
    learning r.
    mental r. (MR)
    moderate mental r.
    motor r.
    perceptual r.
    psychomotor r.
    psychopathology of r.
    r. psychopathology

    psychosis with mental r.
    psychosocial r.
    reading skills learning r.
    severe mental r.
    simple r.
    trichorrhexis nodosa with mental r.
    unspecified mental r.
retarded (Ret, ret)
    r. depression
    r. development
    educationally mentally r. (EMR)
    r. ejaculation
    r. maturation
    mentally r.
    profoundly r.
    r. schizophrenia
    trainable mentally r. (TMR)
retch
retell
retention
    r. control training
    r. defect
    fluid r.
    informal r.
    involuntary r.
    memory r.
    psychogenic r.
    r. and recall
    selective r.
    r. in treatment
    voluntary r.
retentive
    anal r.
retest
RETHINK
    recognize, empathize, think, hear, integrate, notice, keep
reticence
reticent
reticula (*pl. of* reticulum)
reticular
    r. activating system (RAS)
    r. thalamic nucleus
reticuloendothelial system
reticulum, pl. **reticula**
retifism
retinopathy
retirement
    job r.
    r. neurosis
    r. syndrome
retiring

NOTES

R

retort

retour
> age de r.

retrace

retract

retraction nystagmus

retrain

retraining
> breathing r.
> r. emotion

retreat
> r. from reality
> vegetative r.
> York r.

retrenchment
> ego r.

retribution

retributive rage

retrieval
> information r.
> limited-capacity r.
> r. problem
> r. task
> word r.

retroactive
> r. amnesia
> r. displacement
> r. inhibition (RI)

retroanterograde amnesia

retrocollic spasm

retrocollis

retrocursive absence

retroflexed rage

retroflexion

retrogasserian

retrogenesis
> law of r.

retrograde
> r. amnesia
> r. degeneration
> r. ejaculation
> r. loss of memory
> r. memory interference

retrography

retrogression

retropulsion of gait

retropulsive epilepsy

retrospect

retrospection

retrospective
> r. experimental study design
> r. falsification
> r. gaps in memory
> r. projection
> r. report
> r. ruminative jealousy
> r. study

retrosplenial cingulate

Rett
> R. disorder
> R. syndrome

return
> law of diminishing r.
> point of no r.
> r. of the repressed

returning to home

reuniens
> nucleus r.

reunion

reunite

reuptake
> r. blockade
> dopamine r.
> r. inhibitor

reus
> actus r.

revamp

revelation

revenant

revenge
> desire for r.
> r. obsession

revengeful

reverberating circuit

revere

reverence

reverent

reverie
> hypnagogic r.

reversal
> r. of affect
> behavior r.
> deficit r.
> r. formation
> habit r.
> r. learning
> phase r.
> role r.
> sex r.
> sudden financial r.
> r. test

reverse
> r. causality
> r. digit span recall test
> r. discrimination
> r. diurnal variation
> r. orientation
> r. vegetative symptoms

reversed orientation

reversibility

reversible
> r. affective disorder syndrome
> r. amnesia
> r. cholinesterase inhibitor
> r. cognitive impairment of depression

R

r. decortication
r. intoxication
r. memory impairment
r. schizophrenia
r. shock
reversion
revert
review
claims r.
clinical record r.
comprehensive r.
computer-assisted r.
concurrent r.
continued stay r. (CSR)
contract r.
critical r.
drug use r. (DUR)
empirical r.
extended-care r.
extended-stay r.
literature r.
medical r.
r. method
peer r.
record r.
systematic r.
r. of systems (ROS)
treatment services r.
utilization r. (UR)
revile
revindication
revision
r. process
secondary r.
revisionism
revitalize
revive
revocable
revocation of driver's license
revoke
revolution
sexual r.
revolutionary
revolutionist
revolutionize
revolver
.22-caliber r.
revolving
r. door
r. door syndrome
revulsion
sexual stimuli r.

rewake
reward
r. circuitry
consummatory r.
delayed r.
r. dependence (RD)
external r.
extrinsic r.
feeling frightened; expecting bad
things to happen; attitudes and
actions that help; results and r.
(FEAR)
intrinsic r.
potential external r.
psychic r.
r. and punishment program
r. by the superego
r. system
token economy r.
reward-associated behavior
rewarding effect
reward-irrelevant response
RFLP
restriction fragment length polymorphism
rhathymia
rhembasmus
rheobase
rheoencephalogram
rheoencephalography
rheumatica
tetania r.
rheumatic psychogenic disorder
rheumatism
rheumatoid
rhigosis
rhigotic
rhinencephalon
rhinolalia clausa
RHMI
family history of mental illness
rho
Spearman r.
rhombencephalic sleep
rhomboidalis
rhomboidal sinus
rhotacism
rhyme
rhyming
r. delirium
r. slang
word r.
rhypophagy

NOTES

rhythm
    alpha r.
    beta r.
    bicircadian r.
    biologic r.
    cardiac r.
    circadian r.
    circannual r.
    circaseptan r.
    delta r.
    endogenous r.
    erratic speech r.
    infradian r.
    r.'s of lags and spurts in
      development
    r. method
    r. method of contraception
    r. phase
    polyphasic sleep r.
    sleep-wake r.
    theta r.
    ultradian r.
rhythmic
    r. chorea
    r. contraction
    r. mood
    r. sensory bombardment therapy
      (RSBT)
    r. slow eye movement
    r. tremor
rhythmical twitch
RI
    retroactive inhibition
RIA
    relaxation-induced anxiety
ribald
ribonucleic acid (RNA)
Ribot law
Richardson-Steele-Olszewski syndrome
Richards-Rundel syndrome
riche
    nouveau r.
riddance
    r. phenomenon
ridden
    instinct r.
riddling
rider
    night r.
ridicule
ridiculous
Riese hearing
rifle
    assault r.
rift
right (rt)
    bill of r.'s
    birth r.
    civil r.'s
    fight for r.'s
    gay r.'s
    r. hemisphere
    r. hemisphere cognitive skills
    r. hemisphere dominance
    human r.
    r. to life
    mentally retarded persons' r.'s
    moral r.
    parental r.'s
    patient r.'s
    Patient's Bill of R.'s
    privacy r.
    r. to refuse treatment
    visitation r.'s
    r. wing authoritarianism (RWA)
righteous
right-footed
right-hand dominant
right-handed
right-handedness
right-left
    r.-l. confusion
    r.-l. discrimination
    r.-l. disorientation
right-minded
right-to-lifer
right-to-work
right-wrong test
rigid
    r. akinetic syndrome
    r. attitude
    r. body position
    r. control
    r. eating plan
    r. family
    r. posture
    r. pupil
    r. sleep practice
rigidity
    affective r.
    catatonic r.
    cerebellar r.
    clasp-knife r.
    cogwheel r.
    decerebrate r.
    excessive r.
    extensor r.
    extrapyramidal r.
    intellectual r.
    lead-pipe r.
    muscle r.
    mydriatic r.
    nuchal r.
    ratchet r.
rigor
Riley-Day syndrome

ring
    international child pornography r.
    Kayser-Fleischer r.
    multistate drug distribution r.
ringleader
riot
    r. gun
riotous
rip
    r. off
rip-off
ripped
rip-roaring
rip-snorting
risible
risk
    accident r.
    r. activity
    addictive r.
    adolescent at r.
    at r.
    attributable r.
    averse to r.
    r. aversion
    children at r.
    depression r.
    elevated r.
    empiric r.
    r. factor
    r. factor for mortality
    r. factors for violence
    falling r.
    health r.
    high r.
    r. indicator
    infant at r.
    r. inventory
    level of r.
    r. level
    lifetime r.
    long-term r.
    minimal r.
    morbid r.
    mortality r.
    r. paradigm
    parents at r.
    r. preference
    r. profile
    psychiatric r.
    r. ratio (RR)
    recurrence r.
    r. reduction

    relative r.
    r. rescue rating (RRR)
    schizophrenia r.
    significant r.
    suicide r.
    r. of suicide
    r. of suicide attempt
    r. taker
    underestimating r.
    violence r.
    women at r.
risk-benefit
    r.-b. assessment
    r.-b. profile
    r.-b. ratio
risk-reduction counseling
risk-taking
    r.-t. behavior
    sex-related r.-t.
    sexual r.-t.
risky
    r. sexual activity
    r. sexual behavior
risque
risus
    r. caninus
    r. sardonicus
rite
    r. of passage
    puberty r.
Ritter
    R. law
    R. opening tetanus
Ritter-Rollet phenomenon
ritual
    r. abuse
    accepted r.
    ADHD r.'s
    r. behavior
    centro r.
    checking and touching r.'s
    cognitive r.
    compulsive r.
    degrading r.
    handwashing r.
    healing r.
    r. injury in OCD
    marriage r.
    masochistic r.
    painful r.
    presentational r.
    r. prevention

NOTES

ritual *(continued)*
  r. reduction
  repeating r.
  self-damage r.
  touching r.'s
ritualism
ritualistic
  r. behavior
  r. fashion
  r. thinking
ritualized makeup application
ritualizer
ritual-making
rival normative theory
rivalry
  perceptual r.
  sibling r.
rive
riverboat gambling
RLE
  recent life event
RN
  registered nurse
RNA
  ribonucleic acid
   heterogeneous nuclear RNA
   messenger RNA
RO
  reality orientation
  reality oriented
R/O
  rule out
roached out
road
  r. rage
  yellow brick r. (YBR)
robbery
Robertson pupil
robin complex
robotic
robotism
robotize
robust
robustious
ROC
  receiver operating characteristic
Rochester method
rock
  acid r.
  hard r.
  r. and roll
  soft r.
rocker
rocking
  body r.
rodomontade
rodonalgia

rogerian
  r. group therapy
  r. theory
rogue's gallery
roister
rolandic
  r. epilepsy
  r. fissure
Rolando
  fissure of R.
  R. zone
role
  alternating r.
  altruistic r.
  r. ambiguity
  anticipation of r.
  attacker r.
  behavior r.
  r. boundary
  caretaking r.
  central r.
  community r.
  complementary r.
  r. conflict
  r. confusion
  contributing r.
  cross-sex r.
  cultural r.
  r. demand
  dependent patient r.
  r. deprivation
  r. deviance
  r. diffusion
  discomfort with gender r.
  etiologic r.
  r. experimentation
  explicit r.
  feminine social r.
  r. fixation
  follower r.
  r. function
  gender r.
  helper r.
  implicit r.
  r. insufficiency
  integral r.
  interpersonal r.
  interpreter r.
  leader r.
  leadership r.
  masculine social r.
  maternal r.
  r. model
  noncomplementary r.
  r. obligation
  r. obsolescence
  pathophysiological r.
  r. pattern

peacemaker r.
pivotal r.
r. playing
protector r.
regulatory r.
r. reversal
sex r.
r. shift
sick r.
social r.
r. specialization
spectator r.
stereotypical gender r.'s
r. strain
thematic r.
r. theory of personality
therapeutic r.
r. therapy
r. transition
victim r.
women's r.
role-enactment theory
role-play
role-playing
rolfing
roll
rock and r.
Spiegel eye r.
roller
high r.
roller-coaster emotion
rollick
rolling
head r.
pill r.
romance
family r.
r. fantasy
memory r.
Roman holiday
romantic
r. disappointment
r. fantasy
r. intrigue
r. relationship
romanticism
romanticize
Romberg
R. sign
R. symptom
R. test
Romberg-Howship symptom

rombergism
roof
rookie
room
behavior control r. (BCR)
r. and board
chill-out r.
consulting r.
dead r.
emergency r. (ER)
free field r.
Internet suicide chat r.
locked r.
padded r.
quiet r.
semiprivate r.
roomer
roommate conflict
root
addiction r.
conjoined nerve r.
cultural r.'s
developmental r.'s
r. doctor
nerve r.
r.'s of prejudice
r. sign
rootedness
rooted obsession
Rorschach
R. card
R. projective technique
ROS
review of systems
rosa
mal de la r.
rose-colored glasses
Rosenbach law
Rosenthal syndrome
Rosenzweig Picture-Frustration Study (RPFS)
rosso
mal r.
Rossolimo
rostral
r. medial prefrontal cortex
r. supplementary motor area
rostrum, pl. **rostra, rostrums**
rotary
r. nystagmus
r. vertigo
rotated factor

NOTES

rotation
    factor r.
    r. test
    varimax r.
rotatoria
    chorea r.
rotatory
    r. spasm
    r. tic
rote
    r. memory
    r. recall
    r. verbal learning
rotoscoliosis
rotted obsession
rotunda
    fenestra r.
rough-and-tumble play
roughness
roughshod
roulette
    Russian r.
rounds
    grand r.
Rouse vs Cameron
route
    cognitive r.
    oral r.
routine
    agreed-on r.
    r. clinical care
    complex finger r.
    complex hand r.
    constant r.
    family r.
    grimly adhered-to r.
    negligible r.
    r. skill
    r. use
roving
    r. eye movement
    r. ocular movement
row
    death r.
    skid r.
Royal College of Psychiatrists (RCP)
RPFS
    Rosenzweig Picture-Frustration Study
RR
    risk ratio
RRR
    risk rescue rating
RRT
    registered recreation therapist
RSBT
    rhythmic sensory bombardment therapy
RT
    rational therapy

    reaction time
    recreational therapy
rt
    right
RTC
    residential treatment center
RTH
    resistance to thyroid hormone
rTMS
    repetitive transcranial magnetic
      stimulation
rub
    r. out
    r. up
rubber
    burning r.
rubbing
    coin r.
rubella
Rubinstein-Taybi syndrome
Rubin vase
rubout
rubric
ruckus
rudeness
rudimentary paranoia
rue
rueful
rugged
ruination
ruinous
rule
    r. of abstinence
    American Law Institute R.
    analytic r.
    Anstie r.
    assimilation r.
    base r.
    basic r.
    r. bending
    r. breaker
    disregard for r.'s
    dissimilation r.
    Durham r.
    r. of evidence
    grandma r.
    ground r.
    group r.
    Hebb r.
    1-hour restraint r.
    house r.
    Jackson r.
    mature minor r.
    M'Naghten r.
    morphological r.
    neutralization r.
    New Hampshire r.
    OHIO r.

only handle it once r.
r. out (R/O)
Pitres r.
r. preoccupation
redundancy r.
seclusion and restraint r.
sequencing r.
serious violations of r.'s
r. skills
syntactic r.
Tarasoff r.
r. of thumb
transformational r.
r. utilitarianism
violation of r.'s

ruler

ruling
r. of the court
r. in tics

rumble

rumbling

rum fit

ruminate

rumination
anxious r.
behavioral theory of r.
r. disorder
r. disorder of infancy
guilty r.
homicidal r.
manie de r.
morbid r.
neurotic r.
obsessional r.
obsessive r.
persistent r.
psychogenic r.
repetitive r.
suicidal r.
r. syndrome

ruminative
r. coping style

r. depression
r. idea
r. tension state
r. thought

rumormonger

rumor spreading

run
r.'s in family
r. in
trial r.

runabout

runaround

runaway
habitual r.
r. hotline
r. reaction

running
r. commentary
r. commentary hallucination
r. fit

rural
r. psychiatry
r. society

ruralist

rush

Russell
R. sign
R. syndrome

Russia

Russian
R. roulette

russomania

ruthful

ruthless

RWA
right wing authoritarianism

Rx
prescription
therapy

RXR
9-cis retinoic acid receptor

NOTES

SA
Schizophrenics Anonymous
self-analysis
sensory awareness
Sexaholics Anonymous
social acquiescence
social age
suicide attempt
SAA
Sex Addicts Anonymous
sabotage
masochistic s.
s. of therapy
saboteur
sabulous
saccade
saccadic
s. eye movement
s. tracking
saccharate
sacerdotal
sacerdotalism
sacrament
sacramental
sacramentalist
sacrifice
sacrificial
sacrilege
sacrolisthesis
sacrosanct
SAD
seasonal affective disorder
separation anxiety disorder
social avoidance and distress
sadism
anal s.
id s.
infantile s.
larval s.
manual s.
omnipotent infantile s.
oral s.
phallic s.
primal s.
sexual s.
superego s.
sadist
sexual s.
sadistic
s. act of rape
s. behavior
s. mutilation
s. patient
s. personality
s. personality disorder

s. rape act
s. sexual abuse
SADL, SADLs
simulated activities of daily living
sad mood
sadness
frequent s.
induced s.
normal s.
s. period
profound s.
prolonged s.
recall-generated s.
sadomasochism (SM, S/M)
sexual s.
sadomasochistic
s. personality disorder
s. relationship
s. sex
SADR
suspected adverse drug reaction
Saenger sign
SAFE
support, autonomy, fusioning, empathy
safe
s. place
s. sex
safeguard
safekeeping
safety
community s.
contract for s.
s. device
s. of ego
factor of s. (FS)
s. motive
sense of s.
therapeutic s.
s. valve
workplace s.
sagging posture
sagittal
s. orientation
s. plane
SAID
sexually acquired immunodeficiency
Saint
S. Dymphna disease
S. John's dance
S. Louis Criteria for Schizophrenia
S. Martin disease
S. Mathurin disease
saintly
salaam
s. convulsion

S

salaam *(continued)*
    s. seizure
    s. spasm
salacious
salad
    word s.
salax
    paroneiria s.
    paroniria s.
sales
    illegal drug s.
Saleto
salicylate
    ammonium s.
    amyl s.
salience
    emotional s.
    s. of religion
    s. of spirituality
salient loading
saliva
    s. screen for alcohol
    s. smearing
sallow
saltation
saltatoria
saltatory
    s. chorea
    s. evolution
    s. spasm
salt-free diet
salubrious
salute
salvation
salvo
SAM
    sex arousal mechanism
SAMe
    S-adenosylmethionine
sameness
    preoccupation with s.
same-sex
    s.-s. group composition
    s.-s. harassment
    s.-s. marriage
    s.-s. orientation
    s.-s. peer
    s.-s. sexual experience
    s.-s. twins
sample
    cocaine-free urine s.
    random s.
    representative s.
    s. standard deviation
sampling
    area s.
    behavior s.

    block s.
    controlled s.
samsara
SAN
    slept all night
sanatorium, sanitarium
sanctification
sanctimonious
sanctimony
sanction
    legal s.
    social s.
sanctioned
    culturally s.
sanctity
sanctuary
sanctum
sandbox marriage
Sander disease
Sandhoff disease
Sandler
    S. triad
    S. view of depressive disorder
sandwich generation
sane
Sanfilippo
    S. disease
    S. syndrome
sangue dormido
sanguine constitutional type
sanguineous
sanitarium *(var. of* sanatorium)
sanity
SANS
    Scale for the Assessment of Negative
      Symptoms
      SANS total score
SAPD
    self-administration of psychoactive drug
sapience
sapphism
SAR
    sexual attitude reassessment
    sexual attitude restructuring
sarcasm
sarcastic
sardonic
    s. grin
    s. laugh
sardonicus
    risus s.
sarmassation
SAT
    systematized assertive therapy
satanic
    s. cult
    s. worship
satanism

satanist
Satan worship
satellite
    s. clinic
    s. housing
satellitosis
satiable
satiate
satiation
    eating without s.
    food s.
satiety
    s. center
    s. response
satisfaction
    decreased job s.
    impaired orgasm s.
    s. inventory
    job s.
    marital s.
    orgasm s.
    patient s.
    personal s.
    relationship s.
sativa
    Cannabis s.
Saturday night palsy
saturnine
    s. encephalopathy
satyriasis
satyrism
satyromania
sauced
Saunders-Sutton syndrome
savage attack
savagely
savagery
savant
    idiot s.
    linguistic s.
save face
savoir faire
savvy
Saxonius
    coitus S.
SBB
    stimulation-bound behavior
SBD
    supervisory behavior description
SBS
    social breakdown syndrome
scabiomania

scaffolding
scale
    absolute rating s.
    achromatic-chromatic s.
    AD S.
    adaptive behavior s.
    ADL s.
    age s.
    aggression s.
    aggressive s.
    alcohol abuse s.
    antisocial s.
    anxiety rating s.
    AO s.
    A-S s.
    assessment s.
    S. for the Assessment of Negative
      Symptoms (SANS)
    attitude s.
    autonomy s.
    avoidant s.
    balance s.
    Barratt s.
    behavioral rating s.
    behavior rating s.
    borderline s.
    brief psychiatric rating s. (BPRS)
    brief psychiatric reacting s. (BPRS)
    Bunney-Hamburg global
      psychosis s.
    Buss-Durkee s.
    childhood autism rating s.
    chromatic s.
    clinical s.
    clinician-rated s.
    clinician rating s.
    coma s.
    communication s.
    compulsive s.
    content s.
    cumulative s.
    Cumulative Illness Rating S.
    dependent s.
    depression s.
    deterioration s.
    development s.
    developmental s.
    development language s.
    dichotomous s.
    disability status s. (DSS)
    discrepancy s.
    drug abuse s.

S

NOTES

scale *(continued)*
dysthymia s.
E s.
E-F s.
efficacy s.
ego strength s.
Environment S.
equal interval s.
ethnocentrism s.
family evaluation s.
global clinician-rated s.
grade s.
graphic rating s.
histrionic s.
hypochondriasis s.
hypomania s.
hypomanic s.
hysteria s.
I-E s.
impulsivity s.
inferred self-concept s.
infrequency s.
intelligence s.
interest s.
internal versus external s.
interval s.
introversion-extroversion s. (IES)
s. item
language s.
lethality s.
lie s.
masculinity-femininity s.
maturity s.
memory s.
mental s.
movement s.
narcissistic s.
paranoid s.
parent anxiety rating s.
passive-aggressive s.
PEC s.
personality disorders s.
point s.
7-point s.
politico-economic-conservatism s.
psychasthenia s.
psychiatric rating s.
psychiatric reacting s.
psychologic rating s.
psychopathic deviance s.
psychopathology rating s.
s. of psychosis (SP)
psychotic delusions s.
psychotic depression s.
psychotic thinking s.
rating s.
ratio s.
reaction s.

REO S.
repression s.
repression-sensitization s.
schizoid s.
schizophrenia s.
schizotypal s.
school readiness s.
s. scores subtest
self-esteem s.
sensory s.
sexual differentiation s. (SDS)
social introversion s.
social readjustment rating s.
sociotropy s.
somatoform s.
special s.
state-dependent psychopathology
  rating s.
status s.
suicide prediction s.
suppressor s.
test point s.
total s.
trait-dependent psychopathology
  rating s.
tridimensional evaluational s.
validity s.
verbal s. (VS)
vocabulary s.
well-being s.

Scale–Adolescents
scaling
age-grade s.
item s.
scalp
s. contusion
s. lock
scam
SCAN
suspected child abuse/neglect
scan
baseline s.
brain s.
brain SPECT s.
CAT s.
computerized tomography s.
emission tomography s.
eye s.
longitudinal s.
single photon emission CT s.
scandal
sex s.
scandale
succes de s.
scandalize
scandalmonger
scandalous

scanning
    s. communication board
    comparative s.
    eye s.
    radioisotope brain s.
    s. speech
    s. visage
scapegoat
scapegoating communication pattern
scaphocephalic idiocy
scar
    emotional s.'s
    psychic s.
    psychological s.'s
scare
scared
scaremonger
scarify
scarlet letter
Scarpa method
scary
scathe
scathing
scatologia
    telephone s.
scatologic
scatological language
scatology
scatophagy
scatter
    s. child
    s. diagram
scatteration
scatterbrained
scattering
scavenger
    free radical s.
SCD
    service-connected disability
scelalgia
scelotyrbe
scenario
    physician-patient s.
scene
    high-emotion s.
    primal s.
    traumatic s.
scent
    psychology of s.
schadenfreude
schedule
    S. I–IV

abnormal sleep-wake s.
altered sleep s.
continuous reinforcement s.
developmental s.
s. drug
fixed-interval reinforcement s.
fixed-ratio reinforcement s.
interest s.
intermittent reinforcement s.
medication taper s.
mental status s. (MSS)
National Institute of Mental
    Health-Diagnostic Interval S.
    (NIMH-DIS)
s.'s preoccupation
regular eating s.
regular sleeping s.
regular waking s.
reinforcement s.
s. of reinforcement
shifting sleep-work s.
sleep-wake s.
status s.
s. II substance
variable-interval reinforcement s.
vocational interest s. (VIS)
work s.
Scheid
    cyanotic syndrome of S.
    S. cyanotic syndrome
schema, pl. **schemata**
    body s.
    cognitive s.
    Kraepelin s.
    perceptual s.
schematic mental model
scheme
Schicksal analysis
Schirmer
    S. syndrome
    S. test
schism
    marital s.
schismatic
schismatize
schizencephalic microcephaly
schizencephaly
schizoaffective
    s. disorder
    s. disorder, bipolar type
    s. disorder, depressed
    s. disorder, manic

NOTES

schizoaffective *(continued)*
    s. episode
    s. psychosis
    s. schizophrenia
    s. syndrome
schizobipolar
schizocaria
schizogen
schizogyria
schizoid
    s. composite description
    s. diagnostic prototype
    s. disorder of childhood
    s. fantasy
    s. feature
    s. neurotic personality disorder
    s. personality
    s. position
    s. Q factor
    s. scale
schizoidia
schizoidism
schizoid-schizotypal personality disorder (SSPD)
schizomania
schizomanic
schizomimetic
schizophasia
schizophrasia
schizophrene
schizophrenese
schizophrenia (SZ)
    active phase of s.
    active-phase symptoms of s.
    acute simple-type s.
    acute undifferentiated s.
    adult s.
    agitation catatonic s.
    alternative dimensional descriptors for s.
    ambulatory s.
    Andreasen positive and negative symptoms of s.
    arrest of s.
    atypical s.
    behavioral disorganization in s.
    borderline s. (BS)
    burned-out anergic s.
    catalepsy s.
    catastrophic s.
    catatonic s.
    cenesthopathic s.
    childhood s.
    childhood-onset s.
    chronic undifferentiated s.
    clear-cut s.
    coenesthetic s.
    compensation s.

cyclic s.
deficit s.
s. deliriosa
depressed schizoaffective s.
diathesis-stress theory of s.
disorganized factor in s.
disorganized speech in s.
disorganized-type s.
distorted communication in s.
distorted language in s.
double bind theory of s.
early-onset s.
engrafted s.
exaggerated communication in s.
exaggerated inferential thinking in s.
excited schizoaffective s.
3-factor dimensional model of s.
familial transmission of s.
Finnish Adoptive Family Study of S.
first-episode s.
flexibilitas cerea s.
fragmentary hallucinations in s.
grandiose-type s.
hebephrenic s.
hyofrontality hypothesis in s.
iatrogenic s.
incipient s.
s. index
individual with s.
induced s.
jealous-type s.
larval s.
late-life s.
latent s.
late-onset s.
medication-resistant s.
mixed s.
mixed-type s.
negative-symptom s.
nondeficit s.
non-kraepelinian chronic s.
nonregressive s.
nonsystematic s.
nuclear s.
oneiroid s.
paranoid s.
paranoid-type s.
paraphrenic s.
Pavlov theory of s.
persecutory-type s.
s. phase
positive s.
postemotive s.
prepsychotic s.
primary s.
process s.

prodromal phase of s.
prolonged prodrome of s.
prototypical s.
pseudoautosomal locus for s.
pseudoneurotic s.
pseudopsychopathic s.
s. psychosis
psychotic dimension of s.
psychotic disorganization in s.
reactive s.
recent-onset s.
recidivism in s.
refractory s.
regressive symptoms of s.
remitting s.
residual phase of s.
residual-type s.
resistant s.
restitutional symptoms of s.
restzustand s.
retarded s.
reversible s.
s. risk
Saint Louis Criteria for S.
s. scale
schizoaffective s.
schizophreniform s.
schizophreniform-type s.
Schneider diagnostic system for s.
Selvini-Palazzoli model of s.
simple s.
simple-type s.
s. simplex
somatic s.
s. spectrum
s. spectrum disorder
stupor catatonic s.
subchronic s.
s. symptom
systematic s.
three-day s.
total push treatment of s.
toxic s.
treatment-refractory s.
treatment-resistant s.
undifferentiated s.
undifferentiated-type s.
unspecified s.
water balance in s.
withdrawn catatonic s.
s. with premorbid asociality (SPA)

s. with premorbid association
  (SPA)
schizophrenia-prone individual
schizophrenic
s. affect
anergic s.
S.'s Anonymous (SA)
s. attack
burned-out s.
s. catalepsy
s. catatonia
s. defect state
s. dementia
s. diagnosis
s. disorder
s. episode
s. exacerbation
s. excitement
s. factor
s. genotype
s. illness
s. inpatient
International Society for the
  Psychological Treatments of S.'s
neuroleptic-resistant s.
s. paranoid psychosis
s. patient
s. personality
s. process
s. reaction (SR, S/R)
s. reaction, acute, paranoid
  (SR/AP)
s. reaction, acute, undifferentiated
  (SR/AU)
s. reaction, chronic, paranoid
  (SR/CP)
s. reaction, chronic, undifferentiated
  (SR/CU)
s. reaction circular reaction
s. residual state (SRS)
s. spectrum (SS)
subchronic s.
s. surrender
s. symptom
s. syndrome
s. syndrome of childhood
  treatment-resistant s.
schizophrenic-affective psychosis
schizophreniform
s. attack
confusional s.
s. diagnosis

NOTES

schizophreniform *(continued)*
 s. disorder
 s. patient
 s. psychosis
 s. schizophrenia
schizophreniform-type schizophrenia
schizophrenoides
 delirium s.
schizophrenosis
schizotaxia
schizothemia
schizothyme
schizothymia
 introverted s.
 schizotypal s.
schizothymic personality
schizotonia
schizotypal
 s. category
 s. patient
 s. personality disorder
 s. scale
 s. schizoid personality
 s. schizothymia
schlock
schmaltz
schmoozer
schmuck
schnauzkrampf
Schneider
 S. definition of personality
 S. diagnostic system for
  schizophrenia
 S. first rank symptom
schneiderian
 s. criteria for depressive personality
 s. delusion
 s. first-rank symptom
 s. type I
schnook
scholarly
school
 s. achievement
 s. adjustment
 s. advisor
 s. age
 alternative s.
 s. aversion
 s. counselor
 s. culture
 day s.
 s. difficulty
 s. discipline problem
 s. dropout
 s. dysfunction
 s. entering problem
 existential s.
 s. functioning

 s. functioning impairment
 s. handicap condition
 s. history
 humanistic s.
 s. language
 middle s.
 missed s.
 s. nurse
 s. performance
 s. readiness scale
 s. refusal
 s. refusal syndrome
 senior high s.
 s. sickness
 s. support system
 s. of thought
 s. truancy
school-age
 s.-a. child
 s.-a. testing
school-based
 s.-b. child-and-parent focused
  psychosocial treatment
 s.-b. intervention
Schooler-Kane criteria
schooling
 home s.
Schreber case
Schuele sign
Schüller phenomenon
Schutz measure
schwannoma
sciatica
science
 applied s.
 Bachelor of Medical S.
 behavioral s.
 cognitive s.
 exact s.
 s. research associates (SRA)
 social s.
scientific
 s. empiricism
 s. method
 s. proof
 s. psychopathology
scientism
scientist
scierneuropsia
scieropia
sciolism
sciosophy
scissor gait
SCL-90 subscale
scleresis
 pavor s.
sclerneuropsia

scleropia
sclerosis, pl. **scleroses**
    Canavan s.
    combined s.
    diffuse s.
    focal s.
    hippocampal s.
    insular s.
    lobar s.
    mantle s.
    s. of white matter
sclerotica
    eutonia s.
scleroticans
sclerotic area
sclerotome area
scoliosis
scoop
SCOPE
    systematic, complete, objective, practical,
      empirical
scope of treatment
scopolagnia
scopolamine
    transdermal s.
scopomorphinism
scopophilia
scoptophilia
SCOR
    skin conductance orienting response
scoracratia
scorch
score
    age s.
    avoidance s.
    Barnes global s.
    borderline personality style s.
    BPRS anxiety-depression s.
    BPRS total s.
    BPRS withdrawal/retardation s.
    chronic disease s.
    clinical performance s. (CPS)
    cognitive s.
    composite s.
    compulsion s.
    conservative cutoff s.
    critical s.
    cutoff s.
    depression s.
    descriptor s.
    dichotomization of s.
    s. discrimination

    elevated s.
    emotional memory s.
    endpoint CGI s.
    event recall s.
    factor s.
    finger-tapping s.
    general knowledge s.
    global clinical impression s.
    histrionic personality disorder s.
    intelligence s.
    intrusion s.
    liberal cutoff s.
    logarithm of the odds s.
    logical memory subtest s.
    mania rating s.
    mean total weighted sum s.
    memory s.
    mood cluster s.
    narcissistic Q s.
    negative s.
    numerical s.
    overprotection s.
    pain and distress s.
    peak s.
    percentile s.
    performance s.
    personality disorder s.
    personal memory s.
    positive s.
    practical social judgment s.
    Q s.
    quantitative s.
    raw personality disorder s.
    SANS total s.
    Simpson-Angus total s.
    social judgment s.
    speech discrimination s. (SDS)
    standard s.
    subclinical s.
    subtest scale s.
    sum s.
    summary s.
    T s.
    total AIMS s.
    total emotional memory s.
    total symptom s.
    total weighted sum s.
    verbal weighted sum s.
    weighted sum s.
    word discrimination s.
    z s.
scorecard

S

NOTES

scoring
    s. coefficient
    objective s.
scorn
scornful
Scorpio
scotoma, pl. **scotomata**
    absolute s.
    cecocentral s.
    central s.
    dense s.
    flittering s.
    fortification s.
    homogenous scintillating s.
    mental s.
    negative s.
    paracentral s.
    relative s.
scotomata (*pl. of* scotoma)
scotomization
scotophilia
scourge
scowl
scrappy
scratch fear
scratching
    excessive skin s.
scrawny
scream
    primal s.
screamer
screaming meemies
screech
screen
    blank s.
    blood drug s.
    cocaine-free urine s.
    s. defense
    dream s.
    drug s.
    s. fantasy
    gambling s.
    heavy metal s.
    memory s.
    s. memory
    opiate-free urine s.
    s. out irrelevant stimulus
    simple drug s.
    smoke s.
    toxicology s.
    urine drug s.
    urine toxicology s.
screener
screening
    developmental s.
    s. examination
    fetal s.
    genetic s.

    illiteracy s.
    language s.
    organicity s.
    periodic s.
    preemployment drug s.
    s. question
    s. test
screw around
screwball
screwy
scribble
scribblemania
scribomania
script
    s. analysis
    life s.
    sexual s.
scriptorius
    tic s.
    tric s.
scrotal pain
scrounge
scrub
scruffy
scruple
    decoration s.
    defloration s.
    virginity s.
scrupulosity
scrupulous
scrutinize
scrutiny
SCS
    subacute confusional state
sculpting
    family s.
scum
scurrile
scurrility
scurrilous
scurry
Scutellaria lateriflora
S-D
    suicide-depression
Sd
    stimulus drive
SDAT
    senile dementia of Alzheimer type
SDB
    sleep disordered breathing
SDD
    specific developmental disorder
    sporadic depressive disease
SDL
    self-directed learning
SDR
    sequential diagrammatic reformulation

SDS
    sensory deprivation syndrome
    sexual differentiation scale
    speech discrimination score
seaman mania
seamstress cramp
seamy
sear
search
    s. for parent
    strip s.
    transderivational s.
    s. warrant
    word s.
searching
    symptom s.
searchingly
searing pain
seasonal
    s. affective disorder (SAD)
    s. affective disorder syndrome
    s. energy syndrome
    s. migraine
    s. migraine headache
    s. mood disorder
    s. mood swing
    s. pattern
seasonal-related psychosocial stressor
season of birth
seasoned
seat
    driver's s.
Seattle Longitudinal Study
secandi
    mania s.
secern
secession
Seckel syndrome
seclude
seclusion
    s. law
    locked door s.
    s. need
    office s.
    s. and restraint (S&R)
    s. and restraint rule
    unlocked s.
seclusive personality
second
    s. childhood
    s. fiddle
    s. generation
    s. guess

    s. messenger
    s. messenger system
    s. negative phase
    s. opinion
    s. signaling system
    s. thought
secondary
    s. amenorrhea
    s. anorgasmia
    s. autism
    s. autoerotism
    s. care
    s. defense symptom
    s. degeneration
    s. delirium
    s. dementia
    s. depression
    s. deviance
    s. diagnosis
    s. disorder
    s. drives
    s. effect
    s. elaboration
    s. elaboration of dream
    s. emotional problem
    s. environment
    s. erectile dysfunction
    s. fantasy
    s. gain
    s. generalized epilepsy
    s. identification
    s. impotence
    s. integration
    s. mania
    s. mental deficiency
    s. mood disorder
    s. motivation
    s. narcissism
    s. orgasmic dysfunction
    s. pain
    s. personality
    s. personality trait
    s. prevention
    s. process
    s. process thinking
    s. psychic process
    s. reinforcement
    s. reinforcer
    s. repression
    s. retarded ejaculation
    s. revision
    s. reward conditioning

S

NOTES

595

secondary (*continued*)
    s. self
    s. sensation
    s. sex character
    s. sex characteristic
    s. sleep disorder
    s. stress
    s. syphilis
    s. transitional object
    s. verbal memory
second-class
second-generation
    s.-g. antipsychotic
    s.-g. antipsychotic drug
second-line
    s.-l. agent
    s.-l. therapy
second-order conditioning
second-rate
secrecy
secret
    s. ceremony
    s. control
    s. society
secretary
    unit s.
secretin
secretion
    cortisol s.
    leptin s.
secretive manner
sect
sectarian
section
    axial s.
    coronal s.
    S. Eight
    pituitary stalk s.
    psychiatric services s. (PSS)
sectionalism
sector
secularism
secularist
secular trend
secure
    s. attachment
    s. base effect
    s. communication
    s. correspondence
    s. environment
    s. file transfer
security
    s. blanket
    s. breach
    breach of s.
    computer s.
    emotional s.
    false sense of s.

    maximum s.
    s. operation
sedate
sedation
    acute s.
    daytime s.
    prolonged s.
    s. threshold
    unnecessary s.
sedative
    s. abuse
    s. activity
    s. addiction
    s. antihistamine
    Battley s.
    s. delirium
    s. dependence
    s. drug
    s. effect
    s. hallucinogen
    s. hypnotic
    s., hypnotic, or anxiolytic-induced anxiety disorder
    s., hypnotic, or anxiolytic-induced persisting dementia
    s., hypnotic, or anxiolytic-induced sexual dysfunction
    s. intoxication
    s. occupation
    s. overdose
    s. property
    s. use disorder
    s. withdrawal
sedative-hypnotic
    s.-h. agent
    s.-h. drug
    s.-h. withdrawal symptom
sedative-induced
    s.-i. anxiety
    s.-i. disorder
    s.-i. persisting dementia
    s.-i. psychotic disorder with delusions
    s.-i. psychotic disorder with hallucinations
sedativism
sedentary lifestyle
sedimentation
sedition
seditious
seduce
seducement
seducer
seduction
    infantile s.
seductive
    s. behavior
    s. personality

s. personality disorder
s. tendency
seductress
sedulous
seed psychosurgery
seedy
seeker
care s.
fact s.
spiritual s.
seeking
help s.
novelty s.
outpatient psychiatric help s.
sympathy s.
seeming
seemingly
seer
seeress
seethe
seething
Seglas-type paranoia
segment
adrenal s.
segmental
s. analysis
s. anesthesia
s. neuritis
s. neuropathy
segmentation
segregate
segregated community
segregation
administrative s.
s. analysis study
disciplinary s.
s. hypothesis
perceptual s.
segregationist
SEH
severe emotional handicap
Seitelberger disease
seizure
absence s.
s. activity
acute s.
akinetic s.
alcohol as cause of s.
alcohol-related s.
alcohol withdrawal s.
aphasic s.
apneic s.

apoplectiform s.
asteric s.
asymptomatic s.
atonic absence s.
atypical absence s.
audiogenic s. (AGS)
auditory s.
automatic s.
autonomic s.
bilateral myoclonic s.
brain s.
cardiovascular s.
central s.
centrencephalic s.
cephalic s.
cerebellar s.
cerebral s.
cerebrospinal s.
clonic s.
clonic-tonic-clonic s.
complex partial s. (CPS)
continuing petit mal s.
conversion s.
convulsive s.
coordinate s.
cryptogenic s.
diencephalic s.
drug-induced s.
drug withdrawal s.
s. dyscontrol
elementary partial s.
emotional cause of s.
epilepsia partialis continua s.
s. epilepsy
epileptic s.
epileptiform s.
erotic s.
essential s.
febrile s.
fluent aphasic s.
focal s.
fragmentary s.
s. frequency (SF)
generalized tonic-clonic s.
grand mal s.
gustatory s.
s. history
hysterical s.
iatrogenic s.
ictal confusional s.
ictal depression phase of s.
infantile s.

NOTES

seizure *(continued)*
    jackknife s.
    jacksonian s.
    major motor s.
    s. management
    massive s.
    maximal electroshock s. (MES)
    mimetic s.
    mimic s.
    s. monitoring
    myoclonic s.
    new-onset s.
    nocturnal s.
    nonfluent aphasic s.
    olfactory psychomotor s.
    paroxysmal s.
    partial complex s.
    partial sensory s.
    partial tonic s.
    petit mal variant s.
    phase of s.
    photogenic s.
    post-ECT s.
    postictal depression phase of s.
    posttraumatic s.
    postural s.
    precentral s.
    premonition of s.
    primary s.
    psychic s.
    psychogenic s.
    psychomotor s.
    puerperal s.
    recurrent s.
    reflex s.
    repetitive partial s.
    s. resistant (SR, S/R)
    salaam s.
    s. sensitive (SS)
    sensory-evoked s.
    simple partial s. (SPS)
    situation-related s.
    sleep-related epileptic s.
    somatosensory s.
    spasmodic s.
    spontaneous s.
    subclinical s.
    subjective s.
    symptomatic s.
    temporal lobe s.
    tetanic s.
    s. threshold
    tonic s.
    tonic-clonic s.
    traumatic s.
    typical absence s.
    uncinate s.
    unilateral s.
    uremic s.
    vertiginous s.
    visual s.
    withdrawal s.

sejunction

sejunctiva
    dementia s.

selection
    adverse s.
    s. bias
    internal s.
    item s.
    ligand s.
    natural s.
    personnel s.

selective
    s. amnesia
    s. attachment
    s. attention
    s. auditory agnosia
    s. deafness
    s. inattention
    s. memory
    s. mutism
    s. norepinephrine reuptake inhibitor
    s. preventive intervention
    s. retention
    s. serotonin reuptake inhibitor (SSRI)
    s. service
    s. silence
    s. speech perception alteration

selectivity
    s. of attention
    mesolimbic s.
    motivational s.

self, pl. **selves**
    acceptance of s.
    actual s.
    bad s.
    bipolar s.
    s. centered
    creative s.
    danger to s.
    dangerous to one's s.
    death of s.
    deformation of s.
    disturbed sense of s.
    empirical s.
    ethical s.
    faith in s.
    fragile sense of s.
    fragmented sense of s.
    glorified s.
    grandiose s.
    harming s.
    hidden s.
    idealized s.

looking-glass s.
multiple domains of s.
nonturning against self (NTS)
not turning against the s.
personified s.
phenomenal s.
pride in s.
s. psychology
real s.
secondary s.
sense of s.
subconscious s.
subliminal s.
true s.
turning against s. (TAS)
turning aggression against s.
self-abandoned
self-abasement
self-abnegation
self-absorbed tendency
self-absorption
    intimacy versus s.-a.
self-abuse
self-acceptance
self-accusation
    delusion of s.-a.
self-actualization
self-administer
self-administration
    s.-a. of psychoactive drug (SAPD)
    repeated substance s.-a.
self-aggrandizement
self-aggrandizing
self-alienation
self-analysis (SA)
self-anger
self-annoyance
self-appointed
self-appraisal
self-assertion
self-assessment
self-assurance
self-assured
self-attribution of guilt
self-aware
self-awareness
    objective s.-a.
self-blaming depression
self-burning
self-care
    s.-c. activity
    s.-c. deficit

    s.-c. dysfunction
    impaired s.-c.
    s.-c. skill
self-censure
self-centered attitude
self-centeredness
self-chosen ethical principle
self-commitment
self-comparison
    negative s.-c.
self-concept
    narcissistic s.-c.
    negative s.-c.
self-condemnation
self-condemning
self-confidence
    lack of s.-c.
    low s.-c.
self-conflict
    undisciplined s.-c.
self-contained
self-content
self-control
    s.-c. technique
    s.-c. therapy
self-correlation
self-critical attitude
self-criticism
    pervasive s.-c.
self-cutting
self-damage ritual
self-damaging
    s.-d. behavior
    s.-d. impulsivity
self-debasement
self-deceiving
self-deception
self-defeat
self-defeating
    s.-d. behavior
    s.-d. personality
    s.-d. personality disorder
    s.-d. thinking
    s.-d. trait
self-defense
    fighting, injuries, sex, threats, s.-d. (FISTS)
self-deluding
self-denial
self-deprecating thought
self-deprecation
self-deprecatory remark

NOTES

S

self-deprivation
self-derogation
self-derogatory
    s.-d. concept
    s.-d. content
    s.-d. theme
self-described agnostic
self-desensitization
self-destruction
self-destructive
    s.-d. adolescent
    s.-d. behavior
    s.-d. hallucination
    s.-d. impulse
    s.-d. patient
self-destructiveness
self-determination
self-development
self-devoted
self-differentiation
self-directed
    s.-d. aggression
    s.-d. exposure
    s.-d. learning (SDL)
    s.-d. writing
self-direction
self-disapproval
self-discipline
    lack of s.-d.
self-disciplined
self-disclosure anxiety
self-discovery
self-distrust
self-doubt
self-dramatization
self-dramatizing behavior
self-dynamism
self-effacement
self-efficacy
self-emancipation
self-employed
self-energizing
self-enrichment
self-esteem
    denigrated s.-e.
    inflated s.-e.
    s.-e. regulation
    s.-e. scale
self-evident
self-examination
self-excoriation
self-exiled
self-experience
self-exposure therapy
self-expression
self-extension
self-extinction
self-feeding

self-fellator
self-fulfilling prophecy
self-fulfillment
self-given
self-guided
self-handicapping strategy
self-harm
    s.-h. behavior
    contract against s.-h.
    deliberate s.-h. (DSH)
self-harming act
self-hate
self-hatred
self-healing
self-help
    belief system of s.-h.
    s.-h. clearinghouse
    s.-h. group
    s.-h. manual
    s.-h. participant
    s.-h. question
    s.-h. skill
self-helper
    inner s.-h.
self-hypnorelaxation
self-hypnosis
self-identification
self-identity
self-image
    impaired s.-i.
    negative s.-i.
    unstable s.-i.
self-importance
self-imposed fasting
self-impression
self-incriminating
self-incrimination
self-induced
    s.-i. alopecia
    s.-i. dermatitis artefacta
    s.-i. disease
    s.-i. factitial dermatitis
    s.-i. hair loss
    s.-i. injury
    s.-i. vomiting
self-indulgence
self-inflicted (SI)
    s.-i. bodily injury
    s.-i. chemical injury
    s.-i. dermatitis neglecta
    s.-i. gunshot wound
    s.-i. hair cutting
    s.-i. head shaving
    s.-i. lesion
    s.-i. physical injury
    s.-i. stab wound
    s.-i. thermal injury

s.-i. trauma
s.-i. wound (SIW)
self-injurious behavior (SIB)
self-injury
adult s.-i.
method of s.-i.
motivation for s.-i.
pattern of s.-i.
self-interest
self-inventory
selfish
self-knowledge
selfless
self-limited process
self-limiting
self-loathing
self-love
self-made
self-managed reinforcement
self-management
self-manipulation
self-maximation
self-medicate
self-medication
self-mutilation
history of s.-m.
self-mutilative behavior
self-mutilator
self-neglect
selfobject
self-object transference
self-observation
self-opinionated
self-organization
primitive aggressive s.-o. (PASO)
self-painting
self-peeping
narcissistic s.-p.
self-perceived cognitive disorder
self-perception
self-perpetuated disease
self-pity
self-pitying constellation
self-portrait
self-possessed
self-preservation
self-pressuring
self-pride
self-produced
self-protective
self-psychology
self-punish

self-punishing behavior
self-punishment
expiatory s.-p.
illness as s.-p.
self-rated
s.-r. impact of disease
s.-r. improvement
self-rating
s.-r. test
self-realization
self-recognition
self-reference value
self-referential
self-reflection
self-regard
self-regulation
self-regulatory capacity
self-reinforcement
cognitive s.-r.
self-related thought
self-reliance training
self-reliant
self-renewal
self-report
s.-r. data
s.-r. format
s.-r. measure
s.-r. personalities inventory
s.-r. psychological inventory
s.-r. questionnaire
s.-r. study
Young Adult s.-r.
Youth s.-r.
self-reported
s.-r. anxiety
s.-r. case
s.-r. guilt
s.-r. helplessness
s.-r. pessimism
s.-r. sinfulness
s.-r. symptom
s.-r. worthlessness
self-reporting
self-reproach
self-restraint
self-revealing
self-ridicule
self-righteous
self-role concept
self-sacrifice
self-satisfaction
self-searching

S

NOTES

self-seeking
self-sentience
self-serving
self-soothing
    s.-s. capacity
    s.-s. coping skill
    impaired s.-s.
    s.-s. technique
self-starter
self-starvation
self-stimulating
self-stimulation
self-stimulatory behavior
self-study
self-styled
self-sufficient
self-supportive
self-suspicion
self-sustaining
self-system
self-talk
self-taught
self-titrate
self-tolerance
self-torture
self-treatment
self-trust
self-understanding
self-will
self-worship
self-worth
Seligman view of depressive disorder
sella, pl. sellae
sell short
Selter disease
Selvini-Palazzoli model of schizophrenia
Selye
    adaptation syndrome of S.
SEM
    standard error of the mean
semantic
    s. aberration
    s. activation
    s. aphasia
    s. argument
    s. argument communication pattern
    s.'s of autism
    behavioral s.'s
    s. category
    s. clustering
    s. cue
    s. dementia
    s. differential
    s. dissociation
    extension s.'s
    general s.'s
    generative s.'s
    s. jargon

    s. memory
    s. memory function
    s. pragmatic disorder
    s. process
    s. processing
    s. psychosis
    quantitative s.'s
    referential s.'s
    s. relatedness
    s. relationship
    s. therapy
semantogenic disorder
semblance
semeiopathic, semiopathic
semeiosis, semiosis
semeiotic (*var. of* semiotic)
semen
    s. fear
    loss of s.
    s. loss
semiautomated spatial normalization
    technique
semiautomatic
    s. quality
semi-autonomous systems concept of
    brain function
semicomatose
semiconscious
semicretinism
semidarkness
semideify
semidominant
semierect
semi-independent
semilethal
semiliterate
semimystical
seminarcosis
seminomad
seminude
semiobsession a deux
semiopathic (*var. of* semeiopathic)
semiosis (*var. of* semeiosis)
semiotic, semeiotic
    s. function
semipermeable
semiprivate room
semiquantitative
semireligious
semiretirement
semisacred
semisecret
semiskilled employee
semisleep
    state of s.
semistructured diagnostic interview
semitendinous
Semon-Hering theory

Semon law
Semon-Rosenbach law
send up
senectitude
senescence
senescent pedophilia
senile
    s. brain syndrome
    s. chorea
    s. degeneration
    s. delirium
    s. dementia
    s. dementia of Alzheimer type
      (SDAT)
    s. dementia confusional state
    s. depression
    s. deterioration
    s. epilepsy
    s. imbecility
    s. insanity
    s. involution
    s. mania
    s. melancholia
    s. memory
    s. neurosis
    s. organic psychotic state
    s. osteoporosis
    s. paranoia
    s. paranoid psychosis
    s. paranoid reaction
    s. paranoid state
    s. paraplegia
    s. paroxysmal psychosis
    s. plaque
    s. psychoneurosis
    s. psychotic mental disorder
    s. tremor
senilis
    alopecia s.
    paranoia s.
    sexualitas s.
senility organic psychosis
senior
    s. citizen
    s. citizen community
    s. high school
seniority
senium praecox
sensate
    s. focus
    s. focus approach
    s. focus learning

sensate-focus-oriented therapy
sensation
    abnormal tactile s.
    altered s.
    anxiety-related s.
    buzzing s.
    creeping-crawling s.
    delayed s.
    diminished s.
    drug-induced floating s.
    s. of ejaculatory inevitability
    epicritic s.
    facial s.
    feeling s.
    fine tactile s.
    girdle s.
    s. increment
    kinesthetic s.
    light touch s.
    loss of s.
    numbing s.
    objective s.
    out-of-body s.
    out-of-mind s.
    peripheral s.
    phantom s.
    physical s.
    pins-and-needles s.
    pins-sticking s.
    preputial s.
    primary s.
    proprioceptive s.
    referred s.
    reflex s.
    secondary s.
    sexual s.
    smothering s.
    special s.
    sticking s.
    subjective s.
    superficial s.
    tactile s.
    taste s.
    temperature s.
    tingling s.
    touch s.
    transferred s.
    visual s.
sensational
sensationalism
sensationalize
sensation-focused apprehension

S

NOTES

sensation-seeking trait
sense
- s. of alienation
- s. of apprehension
- s. of arousal
- s. of attachment
- s. of belonging
- s. of betrayal
- s. of bodily change
- chemical s.
- s. of commitment
- common s.
- s. of community
- s. of concern
- s. of continuity
- s. of control
- s. of detachment
- s. of empowerment
- s. of entitlement
- equilibratory s.
- s. of equilibrium
- s. of estrangement
- external s.
- s. of failure
- s. of fatigue
- s. of a foreshortened future
- s. of humor
- s. of identity
- s. of impending doom
- internalized s.
- s. of intimacy
- joint s.
- kinesthetic s.
- labyrinthine s.
- make s.
- muscular s.
- no s.
- s. of numbing
- obstacle s.
- s. of ownership
- s. of place
- position s.
- posture s.
- pressure s.
- s. of reality
- s. of responsibility
- s. of righteous indignation
- s. of safety
- s. of self
- seventh s.
- s. of shame
- sixth s.
- space s.
- special s.
- static s.
- stimulation of s. (SOS)
- street s.
- s. of superiority

- tactile s.
- temperature s.
- thermal s.
- thermic s.
- time s.
- touch s.
- s. of trust
- visceral s.
- s. of well-being
- s. of wellness
- s. of wholeness

senseless imitative word repetition
sensibilia
sensibility
- articular s.
- bone s.
- cortical s.
- deep s.
- dissociation s.
- epicritic s.
- mesoblastic s.
- proprioceptive s.
- protopathic s.
- splanchnesthetic s.
- vibratory s.

sensible
sensiferous
sensigenous
sensimeter
sensitiva
sensitive
- s. Beziehungswahn paranoid
- s. measure
- seizure s. (SS)

sensitiver Beziehungswahn paranoid state
sensitivity
- absolute s.
- alcohol s.
- anxiety s. (AS)
- cold s.
- contrast s.
- cosmic s.
- cultural s.
- deep-pressure s.
- s. to diversity
- dopamine receptor s.
- enhanced s.
- feedback s.
- general stress s.
- s. group
- high s.
- interpersonal s.
- loss of s.
- pharmacologic s.
- s. reaction of adolescence
- s. reaction of childhood
- reassurance s.

rejection s.
separation s.
substance s.
s. training
warm s.
sensitivity-training group
sensitization
behavioral s.
covert s.
overt s.
perceptual s.
sensomobility
sensomotor
sensoria (*pl. of* sensorium)
sensorial
s. epilepsy
s. idiocy
sensorimotor
s. act
s. arc
s. development
s. intelligence period
s. phase
s. skill
s. stage
s. system
s. theory
sensorium, pl. **sensoria, sensoriums**
clear s.
clouded s.
cloudy s.
sensorivasomotor
sensor operation
sensory
s. acuity
s. alexia
s. amusia
s. anesthesia
s. aphasia
s. apraxia
s. association area
s. ataxia
s. aura
s. awareness (SA)
s. bondage
s. charge
s. conversion symptom
s. cortex
s. cue
s. defect
s. deficit
s. deprivation

s. deprivation syndrome (SDS)
s. difficulty
s. dimension
s. discrimination
s. dissociation
s. dissociation syndrome
s. disturbance
s. environment
s. evoked potential (SEP)
s. experience
s. extinction
s. function
s. functioning
s. image
s. impairment
s. impression
s. inattention
s. information
s. integration
s. integration dysfunction (SID)
s. interface
s. level
s. load
s. modality
s. neglect
s. nerve
s. neuron
s. neuronopathy
s. overload
s. paralysis
s. perception
s. phantom
s. phenomenon
s. precipitated epilepsy
s. process
s. processing area
s. psychosis
s. receptor
s. scale
s. shock
s. stimulation
s. stimulus
s. threshold
transcortical s.
sensory-evoked seizure
sensory-induced epilepsy
sensory-motor behavior
sensory-perceptual test
sensualism
sensuality
sensualize
sensual pleasure

NOTES

S

sensum
sensuosity
sensuous
sentence
    s. completion
    complex s.
    death s.
    jail s.
    life s.
    prison s.
    s. repetition (SR, S/R)
sentence-closure task
sentence-repetition task
sentencing
senticosus
    Eleutherococcus s.
sentience
sentient
sentiment
    public s.
sentimentality
sentimental value
sentinel activity
SEP
    sensory evoked potential
    somatosensory evoked potential
separable
separate
separated
    s. from spouse
    legally s. (LS)
    s. status
separation
    affective s.
    s. agreement
    s. anxiety
    s. anxiety disorder (SAD)
    s. anxiety disorder of childhood
    s. distress
    early s.
    family s.
    s. from parent
    legal s.
    parental s.
    prolonged s.
    s. protest
    s. sensitivity
    sibling s.
    traumatic s.
    trial s.
    twin s.
separation-individuation
    s.-i. phase
    s.-i. process
separative
separator state

septal
    s. area
    s. region
September
    S. 11
    S. 11, 2001
septicemia psychosis
septooptic dysplasia
septuagenarian
septum pellucidum
sepulture
sequela, pl. sequelae
    caffeine s.
    caffeine-related s.
    clinical s.
    clinically adverse s.
    underdiagnosed s.
    untreated s.
sequence
    elaborate dream s.
    s. of events
    genetic s.
    s. memory
    phase s.
    storylike dream s.
sequencing
    s. ability
    auditory s.
    s. disability
    letter-number s.
    s. rule
    s. task
sequential
    s. diagrammatic reformulation (SDR)
    s. dose
    s. memory
    s. multiple analysis (SMA)
sequester
sequestrate
sequestration
sequitur
    non s.
SER
    somatosensory evoked response
serendipity
serene
serenity
serge
sergeant
    gunnery s.
serial
    s. assaulter
    s. child molester
    s. epilepsy
    s. killer
    s. linguistic expectation
    s. list learning

s. murderer
s. observation
s. problem-solving approach
s. 7's (sevens)
seriatim function
series
 experimental s.
 s. of numbers
serious
 s. assaultive act
 s. consequence
 s. desire for death
 s. impairment
 s. traumatic stress
 s. violations of rules
seriously wounded in action (SWA)
serious-minded
sermon fear
sermonize
serology
serostatus
serotonergic
 s. activity
 s. agent
 s. antidepressant
 s. anxiolytic
 s. deficiency hypothesis
 s. deficit
 s. neuron
 s. neurotransmission
 s. pathway
 s. pharmacology
 s. raphe nuclei
 s. receptor
 s. responsibility
 s. side effect
 s. synapse
 s. system
 s. tract
serotonin
 s. 5-HT$_2$ receptor
 s. level
 s. reuptake inhibitor (SRI)
 s. stimulation
 s. system
serotonin-dopamine
serotonin-norepinephrine reuptake inhibitor
serpent
serpentina
 Rauwolfia s.
serum, pl. **sera**

s. diagnosis
s. level
s. sickness
s. testosterone
truth s.
s. vitamin A
server
 file s.
service
 access to health care s.'s
 adjunctive mental health s.
 Adult Protective S.'s (APS)
 ambulatory mental health s.
 American Psychiatry Association-Center for Mental Health S.'s
 basic methadone s.
 Center for Mental Health S.'s (CMHS)
 child inpatient s.
 child outpatient s.'s
 Children's Protective S. (CPS)
 Civilian Health and Medical Program of the Uniformed S. (CHAMPUS)
 community s.
 comprehensive s.
 consultation-liaison s.
 Council on Psychiatric S.'s
 counseling s.
 Department of Health and Human S.'s (DHHS)
 disability determination s. (DDS)
 emergency s. (ES)
 enhanced standard methadone s.
 environment-centered s.
 geriatric psychiatry inpatient s.
 Health and Human S.'s (HHS)
 Indian Health S. (IHS)
 inpatient s.
 Memphis Educational Model Providing Handicapped Infant S.'s (MEMPHIS)
 mental health s.
 mutual-help s.'s
 outreach s.'s
 patient-centered s.'s
 patient and family s.'s (PFS)
 peer-helping s.
 psychiatric emergency s. (PES)
 psychiatry inpatient s.
 psychosocial s.
 recreational s.

S

NOTES

service (continued)
    selective s.
    sleep disorder s.
    social s. (SS)
    social and rehabilitation s. (SRS)
    special educational s.
    system to plan early childhood s.'s (SPECS)
    The Center for Mental Health S.'s
    United States Public Health S. (USPHS)
    vocational s.
service-connected disability (SCD)
servile
servitude
SES
    socioeconomic status
session
    adjunctive individual s.
    buzz s.
    dyadic s.
    education-focused s.
    fixed-ended s.
    four-way s.
    group psychotherapy s.
    individual psychotherapy s.
    learning s.
    marathon s.
    open-ended s.
    orientation s.
    play s.
    psychotherapy s.
    rap s.
    skull s.
    therapy s.
SET
    support, empathy and truth
set
    s. about
    acquiescent-response s.
    s. aside
    s. back
    data s.
    difficulty in changing response s.
    empty s.
    s. eyes on
    s. foot on
    Health Plan Employer Data and Information S.
    jet s.
    learning s.
    mental s.
    mind s.
    s. in motion
    s. one straight
    s. in one's ways
    perceptual s.
    perseveration s.

    polyethic criteria s.
    postural s.
    response s.
    single criteria s.
    s. the stage
    substance-specific intoxication criteria s.'s
    substance-specific withdrawal criteria s.'s
    SWAP-200 item s.
set-by-age dosing
setter
    fire s. (FS)
setting
    behavior s.
    clinical practice s.
    community s.
    Consortium on Special Psychiatric Delivery S.
    dimensional s.
    educational s.
    emergency psychiatric s.
    experimental psychometric s.
    fire s.
    forensic s.
    geriatric health care s.
    goal s.
    group s.
    home s.
    hospitalized s.
    inpatient psychiatric s.
    institutional s.
    intentional fire s.
    limit s.
    outpatient mental health clinic s.
    partial hospital s.
    population s.
    primary care s.
    psychiatric s.
    psychometric s.
    psychosocial s.
    real-world s.
    residential s.
    social s.
    vocational goal s.
settle
sevens
    serial 7's (s.)
seventh sense
sever
severable
severalty
severance
severe
    s. anxiety
    s. ataxia
    s. dementia
    s. depression

s. diffuse brain dysfunction
s. disability
s. dissociative symptom
s. emotional handicap (SEH)
s. environmental deprivation
s. impairment
s. intoxication
s. life stress
s. mental retardation
s. mental subnormality

severely

s. compromised
s. mentally impaired (SMI)

severity

addiction s.
baseline s.
compulsive s.
dementia s.
depression s.
disease s.
hyperintensity s.
s. of intent
s. of lethality
objective s.
psychiatric s.
s. specifier
s. of worry

sewing spasm

sex

s. addict
S. Addicts Anonymous (SAA)
adult-child s.
anal s.
s. appeal
s. arousal mechanism (SAM)
assigned s.
s. assignment
biologic s.
casual s.
s. change
s. characteristic
s. chromatin
s. chromosome
s. clinic
compulsive s.
s. counseling
s. determination
s. deviant
s. differentiation
s. drive
s. education
extramarital s.

fair s.
s. fear
forced s.
s. hormone
indeterminate s.
s. infantilism
S. Information and Education
  Council of the US (SIECUS)
s. interest
intermediate s.
Internet s.
s. inventory (SI)
s. kitten
s. limitation
s. linkage
900 number s.
s. object
s. offender (SO)
s. offense
opposite biological s.
oral s.
orogenital s.
parental attitudes toward s.
s. perversion
s. play
s. play with peers
s. play with siblings
premarital s.
s. preselection
promiscuous s.
s. ratio
s. reassignment
s. reassignment surgery (SRS)
s. reversal
s. role
s. role inversion
sadomasochistic s.
safe s.
s. scandal
s. specific
s. steroid
s. symbol
telephone s.
s. therapy
third s.
s. toy
trading s.
s. typing
unprotected s.
Sexaholics Anonymous (SA)
sex-conditioned character
sexism

NOTES

sexist
sexless
sex-limited character
sex-linked character
sexological examination
sexology
sexopathy
sexploitation
sexpot
sex-related
    s.-r. HIV risk behavior
    s.-r. risk-taking
sex-role
    s.-r. behavior
sexual
    s. aberration
    s. abstinence
    s. abuse
    s. abuse of adult
    s. abuse of child
    s. abuse history
    s. abuse status
    s. acting out
    s. activity
    s. adaptation
    s. addiction
    s. adjustment
    s. advances
    s. aid
    s. anesthesia
    s. anomaly
    s. anxiety
    s. arousal
    s. arousal disorder
    s. assault
    s. attitude
    s. attitude reassessment (SAR)
    s. attitude restructuring (SAR)
    s. attraction
    s. aversion
    s. aversion disorder
    s. boundary violation
    s. climax
    s. coercion
    s. commentary
    s. compulsion
    s. concern
    s. contact
    s. curiosity
    s. delusion
    s. demand
    s. desire
    s. desire disorder
    s. desire disturbance
    s. development
    s. deviance
    s. deviance disorder
    s. deviant

s. deviation
s. deviation neurotic disorder
s. differentiation
s. differentiation scale (SDS)
s. dimorphism
s. discrimination
s. domination
s. dysfunction
s. dysfunction due to a general
  medical condition
s. encounter
s. energy
s. erethism
s. escapade
s. excitement
s. exhibition
s. experience
s. experimentation
s. expression
s. fantasy
s. favor
s. fear
s. feeling
s. frequency
s. frigidity
s. function
s. functioning
s. and gender identity disorder
s. gratification
s. harassment (SH)
s. high-risk behavior
s. identity
s. impotence
s. inappropriateness
s. incident
s. indifference
s. indiscretion
s. infantilism
s. inhibition
s. instinct
s. interaction
s. intercourse
s. interest
s. intimacy
s. intrigue
s. inversion
s. learning
s. libido
s. life
s. love
s. maladjustment
s. masochism
s. maturity rating
s. melancholia
s. misbehavior
s. misconduct
s. mores
s. motivation

s. motive state
s. myth
s. nature
s. negativism
s. neurasthenia
s. neurosis
s. obsession
s. opportunity
s. orientation
s. orientation distress
s. orientation disturbance
s. pain
s. pain disorder
s. partner
s. performance
s. perversion
s. pervert
s. physiology
s. pleasure
s. polarization
s. posturing
s. potency
s. predation behavior
s. predator
s. preference
s. preoccupation
s. promiscuity
s. provocation
s. prowess
s. psychogenic disorder
s. psychopath
s. reassignment
s. regulation
s. rehabilitation
s. relation
s. relationship
s. response
s. response cycle
s. responsibility
s. revolution
s. risk-taking
s. sadism
s. sadist
s. sadomasochism
s. script
s. sensation
s. side effect
s. soliloquy
s. stimulation
s. stimuli revulsion
s. stimulus
s. surrogate

s. symptom
s. symptom grouping
s. synergism
s. tension
s. thought
s. touching
s. trauma
s. urge
s. vandalism

sexualis
psychopathia s.

sexualism

sexualitas senilis

sexuality
s. conversion therapy
extramarital s.
human s.
inappropriate s.
index of s. (IS)
s. index
infantile s.
pathologic s.
pathological s.
perverted s.
polymorphous perverse s.
three essays on the theory of s.

sexualization

sexualize

sexually
s. abused child
s. acquired immunodeficiency (SAID)
s. arousing behavior
s. arousing fantasy
s. charged magazines
s. charged movies
s. charged television
s. dangerous
s. dimorphic
s. gratified
s. inappropriate behavior
s. intimate
s. involved
s. maladjusted
s. seductive behavior
s. stimulated
s. suggestive
s. transmitted condition (STC)
s. transmitted disease (STD)
s. violated
s. violent nature

S

NOTES

SF
seizure frequency
S factor
SFLE
stress from life experience
SH
sexual harassment
social history
state hospital
S&H
speech and hearing
sha
gwa s.
shabby
shabu
shackle
shack up
shading
emotional s.
s. response (ShR)
s. response to black areas (Fc)
s. response to gray areas (Fc)
shadow
s. dance
object s.
s. play
shadowing masking technique
shake
fair s.
shakes
shakily
shakiness
shaking
hand s.
s. palsy
s. tremor
s. voice
shaky
shallow
s. affect
s. expression
sham
s. disorder
s. feeding
s. rage
shaman
shamanism
shamanistic thought disorder
shambles
shame
feeling of s.
overt signs of s.
profound s.
sense of s.
shame-aversion therapy
shamefaced
shameful
sham-movement vertigo

shamus
shanghai
shape
body s.
good s.
shaping
behavior s.
shared
s. delusional belief
s. grammar
s. mechanism
s. paranoid disorder
s. phenomenological feature
s. psychotic disorder
s. relationship
s. thought pattern
s. understanding
sharing
expression of s.
needle s.
s. of values
sharp
intellectually s.
s. object
sharpen
sharp-eyed
sharp-sighted
sharp-tongued
sharp-witted
shatter
shaving
s. cramp
self-inflicted head s.
SHCU
state hospital children's unit
sheepish
sheet
personal data s.
s. sign
timed behavioral rating s. (TBRS)
shellacking
shell-shock
shell-shocked
shelter
battered women's s.
s. facility
homeless s.
sheltered
s. home
s. life
s. workshop
s. workshop placement
shelve
shenjing shuairuo
shen-k'uei, shenkui
shield
ideational s.

shift
    s. ability
    abrupt topic s.
    binaural s.
    biobehavioral s.
    Doppler s.
    functional s.
    gradual topic s.
    s. masking technique
    s. in mood
    mood s.
    paradigm s.
    paradigmatic s.
    phase s.
    precipitous mood s.
    s. referential index
    role s.
    temporary threshold s. (TTS)
    s. work-related sleep disorder
    s. work-type dyssomnia

shifting
    associative s.
    idiosyncratic topic s.
    s. sleep-work schedule
    topic s.

shiftless

shin-byung

shinkeishitsu

shivering thermogenesis

shock
    break s.
    cultural s.
    culture s.
    deferred s.
    delayed s.
    delirious s.
    electrical s.
    electric skin s.
    electroconvulsive s. (ECS)
    erethismic s.
    s. exhibitionism
    s. fear
    future s.
    insulin s.
    irreversible s.
    mental s.
    neurogenic s.
    primary s.
    psychic s.
    psychodramatic s.
    s. psychosis
    s. reaction

    reversible s.
    sensory s.
    spinal s.
    s. stage
    s. syndrome
    s. therapy (ST)
    transplantation s.
    s. treatment
    s. troops
    vasogenic s.

shocky

shoddy

shoe
    s. fetish
    s. restriction

shook-up

shook yong

shoot
    s. down
    s. from the hip
    s. up

shooting
    accidental s.
    Columbine High School s.
    drive-by s.
    s. gallery
    s. pain
    s. rampage
    s. spree

shoot-up

shopaholic

shoplift

shoplifting

shopping
    doctor s.
    s. spree

shore up

short
    s. cycle
    fall s.
    s. fuse
    s. orientation-memory-concentration test (OMC)
    s. REM latency
    sell s.
    s. shrift
    s. sleep duration
    s. sleeper
    s. sleep latency
    s. stare epilepsy
    s. stature

S

NOTES

short *(continued)*
    stop s.
    s. temper
short-acting
    s.-a. benzodiazepine
    s.-a. hypnotic agent
shortcoming
short-contact psychotherapy
shortening reaction
shortfall
short-lasting drug effect
short-lived schizophrenic affect
shortness of breath
short-sighted
short-spoken
short-tempered
short-term
    s.-t. anxiety-provoking
      psychotherapy (STAPP)
    s.-t. care facility
    s.-t. commitment
    s.-t. consequence
    s.-t. declarative memory
    s.-t. dynamic psychotherapy
    s.-t. goal (STG)
    s.-t. hospitalization
    s.-t. hypoxia
    s.-t. insomnia
    s.-t. insurance
    s.-t. maintenance
    s.-t. memory (STM)
    s.-t. psychotherapy technique
    s.-t. therapy
    s.-t. treatment
short-timer
shot in the arm
shotgun
    .410-caliber s.
    .410-gauge s.
    s. marriage
    s. wedding
shoulder
    cold s.
    stooped s.'s
shouldered
showdown
shower
showman
show one's hand
showy
ShR
    shading response
shrapnel
shrewd
shrewish
shriek
shrift
    short s.

shrill
shrink
shrinking retrograde amnesia
shroud
shrug off
shuairuo
    shenjing s.
shuffling
    s. gait
    s. steps
shuk yang
shun
shunt
shut
    s. in
    s. out
    s. up
shut-eye
shut-in personality
shyness
    s. disorder
    s. disorder of childhood
shyster
SI
    self-inflicted
    sex inventory
    social introversion
    stimulation index
    structure of intellect
    systematic inquiry
sialidosis
sialoaerophagy
sialorrhea
Siamese twins
SIB
    self-injurious behavior
Siberian ginseng
sibling
    biologic s.
    s. bond
    childhood loss of a s.
    s. jealousy
    s. profile
    s. relation
    s. relational problem
    s. rivalry
    s. separation
    sex play with s.'s
    s. subsystem
sibship method
sicchasia
sick
    s. headache
    s. leave
    s. role
    s. thought
sicken
sickening

sickle flap
sickness
    altitude s.
    chronic African sleeping s.
    decompression s.
    falling s.
    ghost s.
    laughing s.
    motion s.
    school s.
    serum s.
    sleeping s.
sick-out
SID
    sensory integration dysfunction
side
    deep s.
    s. effect
    s. effect drug profile
sideburns
side-glance
sideline
sideration
siderodromomania
sidetrack
SIDS
    sudden infant death syndrome
SIECUS
    Sex Information and Education Council
    of the US
sigh
    premonitory s.
sighing
sighted
sightedness
    close s.
sightless
sigil
sigma receptor
sigmatism
sign
    accessory s.
    s. of alcohol intoxication
    arithmetic s.
    autonomic hyperactivity s.
    Battle s.
    s. blindness
    brainstem s.
    Cantelli s.
    cardinal s.
    cerebellar s.
    cerebral s.

    characteristic s.
    Claude hyperkinesis s.
    clinical s.
    contralateral s.
    conventional s.
    s. depression
    doll's eye s.
    early warning s.
    echo s.
    Escherich s.
    extrapyramidal s.
    eyelash s.
    eye-roll s.
    fan s.
    frontal release s.
    Gordon s.
    Gorlin s.
    Hoffmann s.
    iconic s.
    s. of impending violence
    indexical s.
    Jackson s.
    Joffroy s.
    Kernig s.
    s. language
    Legendre s.
    Leichtenstern s.
    Leri s.
    Lichtheim s.
    local s.
    Macewen s.
    Magnan s.
    Mannkopf s.
    matchbox s.
    mirror s.
    motor s.
    neurovegetative s.
    nonextrapyramidal neurologic s.
    objective s.
    Omega s.
    operational s.
    s. of the orbicularis
    s. out
    pathognomonic s.
    physical s.
    Pitres s.
    positive frontal release s.
    premonitory s.
    pseudo-Graefe s.
    Romberg s.
    root s.
    Russell s.

S

NOTES

sign *(continued)*
Saenger s.
Schuele s.
sheet s.
Signorelli s.
Simon s.
spine s.
telltale s.
Uhthoff s.
vital s. (VS)
von Graefe s.
Westphal s.
withdrawal s.
Woltman s.

signal
acoustic s.
s. anxiety
bilateral contralateral routing of s.'s
(BICROS)
s. detection
focal contralateral routing of s.'s
(FOCALCROS)
s. hyperintensity
ideomotor s.
increased s.
ipsilateral frontal routing of s.'s
(IFROS)
leptin s.
s. theory of anxiety

signaling
chemical s.
intraceptive s.

signalize

signalment

signal-noise characteristic

signal-transducing
s.-t. guanine-nucleotide binding
protein

signed
s. communication
s. consent form
s. out against medical advice
(SOAMA)

significance
affective s.
clinical s.
emotional s.
s. level
nonparametric tests of s.
parametric test of s.
statistical s.
test of s.

significant
clinically s.
s. conflict
s. deterioration
s. difference
s. impairment

s. loss
not s. (NS)
s. other
s. range
s. risk
s. risk factor
statistically s.
s. supporting person
s. trend

signify

Signorelli sign

siknis
grisi s.

silence
code of s.
s. communication pattern
electrocerebral s. (ECS)
selective s.
teen s.
tyranny of s.

silencer

silent
s. area
s. blocking in speech
s. cerebral infarction
s. generation
s. period
s. speech blockade
s. treatment

silicone implant

silliness
childlike s.

silly affect

silver
s. bullet
s. cord syndrome
s. lining

silver-tongued

similarity
assumed s.
s. disorder of aphasia
s.'s mental status test
s.'s subtest
vocabulary, information, block
design, s. (VIBS, vibs)

simmer down

Simon sign

simple
s. absence
s. affective depression
s. alcoholic drunkenness
s. aphasia
s. aspect of fear conditioning
s. confrontation
s. depressive dementia
s. deterioration
s. deterioration senile psychosis
s. deteriorative disorder

s. drug screen
s. figure
s. hallucination
s. motor tic
s. obesity
s. paranoid reaction
s. paranoid state
s. partial seizure (SPS)
s. retardation
s. schizophrenia
s. senile dementia
s. task
s. vocal tic
simpleminded
simpleness
simple-type
s.-t. arteriosclerotic psychosis
s.-t. schizophrenia
simplex
melancholia s.
paranoia s.
purpura s.
schizophrenia s.
Simpson-Angus total score
simulant
simulate
simulated
s. activities of daily living (SADL, SADLs)
s. presence therapy
simulation
conscious s.
simulee
folie s.
simulis
simultanagnosia, simultagnosia
simultanee
folie s.
simultaneous insanity
sin
capital s.
cardinal s.
deadly s.
mortal s.
perceived s.
venial s.
sine
s. delirio
s. delirium
s. qua non
s. wave
s. wave unilateral ECT

sinful feeling
sinfulness
delusion of s.
self-reported s.
single
s. combat
s.'s community
s. criteria set
s. custody
s. diagnosis
s. episode
s. photon emission CT scan
s. word stage
single-agent oral strategy
single-episode
s.-e. chronic mania
s.-e. depressive psychosis
s.-e. psychotic depression
s.-e. psychotic reaction
single-handed
single-major-locus (SML)
s.-m.-l. model
single-minded
singleness
single-parent
s.-p. family
s.-p. home
single-track
single-valued
singly
singsong fashion
singularity
singultus
sinica
Ephedra s.
sinister
sinistrad
sinistral
sinistrality
sinistromanual
sinistropedal
sinkable
sinkage
sinking feeling
sinner
sinning
sinography
sinus, pl. sinus, sinuses
rhomboidal s.
siren song
sissified
sissy behavior

S

NOTES

sister
    weak s.
sisterhood
sister-in-law
sisterly
sister-sister dyads
Sisyphus dream
SIT
    stress inoculation training
sit
    s. in
    s. out
site
    binding s.
    dopamine uptake s.
    recognition s.
    uptake s.
sitieirgia
sitomania, sitiomania
sitting
    s. balance
    s. fear
situation
    acute maladjustment s.
    s. anxiety
    anxiety-provoking s.
    Asch s.
    clinical s.
    s. cluster
    cluster of s.'s
    conflictual s.
    crisis s.
    danger s.
    dangerous s.
    direful s.
    dreaded s.
    educational s.
    either-or s.
    emergency s.
    emotion-laden s.
    s. ethics
    family s.
    feared single performance s.
    high-risk gambling s.
    histrionic s.
    living s.
    low-activity s.
    low-stimulation s.
    s. neurosis
    oedipal s.
    one-to-one s.
    open-cue s.
    peer interactional s.
    performance s.
    phobic s.
    previously stabilizing social s.'s
    psychoanalytic s.
    real-world s.

    social s.
    stabilizing social s.'s
    sticky s.
    triage s.
    triggering s.
    volatile s.
situational
    s. anger disorder with aggression
    s. anger disorder without
      aggression
    s. attribution
    s. crisis
    s. depression
    s. disturbance
    s. ethics
    s. homosexuality
    s. hypoactive sexual desire
    s. insomnia
    s. orgasmic dysfunction
    s. panic
    s. perception
    s. posttraumatic neurosis
    s. psychosis
    s. restraint
    s. sexual dysfunction
    s. stressor
    s. stress reaction
    s. test
    s. therapy
    s. tic variation
    s. trigger
    s. variable
situationally
    s. appropriate atmosphere
    s. bound
    s. bound panic attack
    s. optimistic atmosphere
    s. predisposed
    s. predisposed panic attack
situational-type
    s.-t. dyspareunia
    s.-t. female orgasmic disorder
    s.-t. female sexual arousal disorder
situation-related
    s.-r. epilepsy
    s.-r. seizure
situs analysis
sitzkrieg
SIW
    self-inflicted wound
six-gun
six-pack
sixth sense
size
    class s.
    effect s.
    internal architecture neuronal s.
    neuronal s.

optimal group s.
s. perception
ventricle s.

skeptic
skeptical
skepticism
adolescent s.
sketchy
skew
s. deviation
s. distribution
marital s.
SKI
skill indicators
skid-row
s.-r. bum
s.-r. derelict
skid row
skill
abstraction s.'s
activities of daily living s.'s
adaptation s.
adaptive s.
s. area
assertiveness s.
attentional s.'s
auditory s.
basic s.'s
calculation s.
communication s.'s
conceptual s.
conflict resolution s.'s
coping s.
core mindfulness s.'s
decision-making s.
decoding s.
developmental s.'s
distress tolerance s.'s
ego-coping s.
encoding s.
expressive language s.
fine motor s.
functional s.
generic s.
gross motor s.
health literacy s.'s
higher level s.
improved communication s.'s
s. indicators (SKI)
intellectual s.
interpersonal effectiveness s.
s. inventory

leisure s.
mathematical s.
memory s.
mental s.'s
mindfulness s.'s
motor s.
negotiating goals s.'s
negotiating routines s.'s
negotiating rules s.'s
nonconfrontational
communication s.'s
numerical reasoning s.'s
oral language s.
organizational s.'s
parenting s.
people s.'s
perceptual s.
perceptual-motor s.
perspective-taking s.'s
physical s.'s
poor language s.'s
positive communication s.'s
problem-solving s.'s
reasoning and memory s.'s
resolving conflict s.'s
right hemisphere cognitive s.'s
routine s.
rule s.'s
self-care s.
self-help s.
self-soothing coping s.
sensorimotor s.
social s.
socialization s.'s
stress adaptability s.'s
s. training
uncoordinated motor s.'s
unrefined motor s.
visual perceptual s.
visuomotor problem-solving s.
vocabulary s.'s
word-attack s.
word-finding s.
word-recognition s.
skilled
s. nursing care (SNC)
s. nursing facility placement
s. worker
skillful
skill-less
skimming
skimpy

NOTES

skin
    clammy s.
    s. conductance orienting response (SCOR)
    s. disease fear
    s. erotism
    glossy s.
    s. injury fear
    on the s.
    s. picking
    s. psychogenic disorder
    taut facial s.
    under the s.
skinhead gang member
Skinner box
skinnerian conditioning
skinny
skip
    s. bail
    s. class
    s. meals
    s. out
    s. town
skipping
    grade s.
skirmish
skirt the issue
skittish
skulk
skull
    s. asymmetry
    cloverleaf s.
    s. and crossbones
    maplike s.
    s. session
    steeple s.
skullcap
sky-high
sky marshal
skyscraper fear
slacken
slain
slammer
slander
slanderous
slang
    rhyming s.
slap down
slaphappy
slasher
slashing
    throat s.
slattern
slatternly
slaughter
slaughterous

slave
    s. driver
    s. system component
slavery
slavish
slay
slayer
SLC
    sociopolitical locus of control
sleaze
sleazy
sledgehammer
sleep
    abnormal behavior during s.
    s. abnormality
    abnormal physiological event during s.
    activated s.
    active s.
    s. activity
    alcohol-induced nighttime s.
    s. arousal
    arousal from s.
    s. attack
    s. behavior disorder
    circadian phase of s.
    s. complaint
    confusional arousals from s.
    consolidated s.
    s. continuity
    s. continuity disturbance
    continuous s.
    crescendo s.
    curtailed s.
    s. cycle
    decreased need for s.
    deep s.
    s. deficit
    delta-wave s.
    s. deprivation
    s. deprived EEG
    depth of s.
    s. diary
    s. disorder due to a general medical condition
    s. disordered breathing (SDB)
    disorder of initiating and maintaining s. (DIMS)
    s. disorder insomnia
    s. disorder service
    s. disruption
    s. dissociation
    disturbed s.
    dreamless s.
    s. drunkenness
    s. dysfunction
    easily disturbed s.
    s. efficiency

electric s.
electrotherapeutic s.
environmental disturbance of s.
s. epilepsy
s. erection
erratic s.
s. fear
fitful s.
forced s.
fragmented nighttime s.
s. hygiene
hypnotic s.
indeterminate s.
insufficient nocturnal s.
s. interference
s. inversion
irresistible s.
s. latency
light s. (LS)
s. loss
s. mechanism
s. movement
need for s.
negative conditioning for s.
nonrestorative s.
NREM s.
s. numbness
onset of s.
s. onset REM period
s. organization
paradoxical s.
s. paralysis
paroxysmal s.
s. pattern
s. phase
s. phase dyssomnia
s. phase syndrome
pontine s.
s. posture
primary disorder of s.
s. problem
prolonged nocturnal s.
s. psychogenic disorder
quality of s.
s. quality
quiet s.
rapid eye movement s.
REM s.
REM-onset s.
S. Research Society
rhombencephalic s.
slow-wave s. (SWS)

s. spindle on EEG
s. stage
s. starts disorder
s. state
s. state misperception
telencephalic s.
s. tendency
s. terror
s. terror disorder
s. terror episode
s. therapy
transitional s. (TS)
s. treatment
twilight s.
undisturbed nocturnal s.
unintended s.
yen s.
sleep-electroshock therapy
sleeper
short s.
sleep-induced respiratory impairment
sleep-inducing peptide
sleepiness
disorder of excessive s.
excessive daytime s. (EDS)
pathologic s.
pathological s.
physiological s.
sleeping
s. drunkenness
s. partner
s. pill
s. sickness
sleepless
sleeplessness
s. associated with acute emotional
    conflicts or reaction
s. associated with anxiety
s. associated with conditional
    arousal
s. associated with depression
s. associated with intermittent
    emotional conflicts or reaction
s. associated with psychosis
sleep-onset
s.-o. episode
s.-o. insomnia
sleep-related
s.-r. abnormal swallowing syndrome
s.-r. asthma
s.-r. bruxism
s.-r. cluster headache

NOTES

S

sleep-related *(continued)*
    s.-r. epilepsy
    s.-r. epileptic seizure
    s.-r. hallucination
    s.-r. head banging
    s.-r. myoclonus syndrome
sleeptalking disorder
sleep-terror event
sleep-wake
    s.-w. abnormality
    s.-w. cycle
    s.-w. rhythm
    s.-w. schedule
    s.-w. schedule disorder
    s.-w. system
    s.-w. transition
    s.-w. transition disorder
sleepwalker
sleepwalking
    s. behavior
    s. disorder
sleeve graft
sleight
slept all night (SAN)
SLI
    speech and language impaired
slice-of-life
slicker
sliding of meanings
slight
    s. defect
    inner s.
slink
slip
    freudian s.
slippage
    cognitive s.
slipshod
slope
    gradient s.
sloppy appearance
slothful
slot machine gambling
slough
    s. off
    s. over
slovenly
slow
    s. double taper
    s. learner
    s. metabolizer patients
    s. rate of language development
    s. speech
    start low and go s.
    s. virus
slowed gait
slow-frequency EEG activity

slowing
    motor s.
    psychomotor s.
slowness
    obsessional s.
    s. of thought
slow-tempered
slow-wave
    s.-w. sleep (SWS)
    s.-w. sleep stability
slow-witted
sluggard
sluggish
sluggishness
slum
slumber
    affective s.
slumlord
slumming
slump
slumped posture
slur
    racial s.
    verbal s.
slurred speech
slut
sly
SM, S/M
    sadomasochism
SMA
    sequential multiple analysis
    supplementary motor area
smacking
    lip s.
small
    s. detail response
    s. minded
    s. mindedness
    s. penis complex
    s. talk
small-amplitude rapid tremor
small-time
smashing
SMD
    stereotypic movement disorder
smear
    blood s.
smearing
    saliva s.
smell
    s. a rat
    s. blindness
    s. imagery
SMH
    state mental hospital
SMI
    severely mentally impaired

smile
- endogenous s.
- exogenous s.
- forced s.
- social s.

smirk

smite

Smith-Lemli-Opitz syndrome

SML
- single-major-locus
- SML model

smoke
- s. screen

smoker
- abstinent tobacco s.
- acutely abstinent tobacco s.
- chain s.
- heavy s.
- s. syndrome
- tobacco s.

smoking
- s. cessation
- health risks from s.
- s. history

smoking-related reduction

smooth pursuit eye movement (SPEM)

smooth-tongued

smothering sensation

smother love

smug

smuggle

smuggler

smut

smutty

snake
- s. pit
- s. symbol

snap
- s. back
- s. finger

snappish

snappy

snapshot
- cross-sectional s.

snare

snarl

snatcher
- child s.
- purse s.

snatching
- body s.

SNC
- skilled nursing care

sneaky

snicker

snide

sniff

sniffing
- s. death
- glue sniffing
- inhalant sniffing

sniffy

snipe

snippy

snit

snitch

snivel

snob appeal

snobbery

snobbish

snobby

snooping
- data s.

snoopy

snore
- resuscitative s.

snorting

snow
- s. fear
- s. job
- s. under

snowbird

SNR
- specific neurotic syndrome

SNS
- sympathetic nervous system

snub-nose pistol

snuff
- cohoba s.

SO
- sex offender

SOAMA
- signed out against medical advice

SOAP
- subjective, objective, assessment, plan

soapbox

soaring

sobbing

sober

soberness

sobersided

sobriety
- s. test

NOTES

sobriety *(continued)*
    white knuckling s.
    Youth Enjoying S. (YES)
sob story
SOC
    state of consciousness
so-called
sociability
sociable
social
    s. abulia
    s. acquiescence (SA)
    s. acting out
    s. activity
    s. adaptation
    s. adjustment
    s. adjustment measure
    s. age (SA)
    s. alienation
    s. anhedonia
    s. anorexia
    s. anthropology
    s. anxiety
    s. anxiety disorder
    s. apprehensiveness
    s. atom
    s. attachment
    s. attribution
    s. avoidance and distortion
    s. avoidance and distress (SAD)
    s. awkwardness
    s. babbling
    s. barrier
    s. beverage
    s. breakdown syndrome (SBS)
    s. casework
    s. causation theory
    s. class
    s. class and mental illness
    s. climber
    s. club
    s. cognition
    s. communication
    s. competence
    s. compliance
    s. concern
    s. conformity
    s. connectedness
    s. connection
    s. consciousness
    s. consequence
    s. contact
    s. context
    s. control
    s. cripple
    s. cue
    s. darwinism
    s. dependence

s. deprivation
s. deprivation syndrome
s. desirability
s. detachment
s. development
s. deviance
s. diagnosis
s. disability syndrome
s. disconnection
s. disease
s. distance
s. dominance
s. dominance theory
s. drinker
s. drinking
s. dyad
s. dysfunction
s. dysmaturation
s. engineering
s. environment
s. evaluation
s. facilitation
s. function
s. functioning
s. functioning impairment
s. functioning level
s. gambling
s. gesture speech
s. goal
s. harmony
s. hierarchy
s. history (SH)
s. hunger
s. identification
s. identity
s. immaturity
s. impairment rating
s. inappropriateness
s. ineptness
s. inhibition
s. insecurity
s. instinct
s. integration
s. integration-disintegration model
s. intelligence
s. interaction
s. interaction therapy
s. interest
s. introversion (SI)
s. introversion scale
s. island
s. isolate
s. isolation
s. judgment
s. judgment score
s. justice
s. learning experience
s. learning group therapy

s. learning theory
s. maladjustment
s. masochism
s. medicine
s. minded
s. mores
s. network therapy
s. niche
s. norm
s. objective
s. opportunity
s. outcast
s. overdependence
s. perception
s. performance
s. persecution
s. phobic-like behavior
s. poison
s. policy
s. policy planning
s. pressure
s. problem
s. process
s. property
s. psychiatry
s. psychologist
s. psychology
s. quotient (SQ)
s. readjustment rating scale
s. recovery
s. reference group
s. rehabilitation
s. and rehabilitation service (SRS)
s. reinforcement
s. relatedness
s. relatedness disturbance
s. relations deficit
s. resistance
s. responsibility
s. risk factor
s. role
s. role disability
s. sanction
s. science
s. selection theory
s. service (SS)
s. service agency
s. service consultation
s. setting
s. situation
s. situation avoidance
s. skill

s. skills deficit
s. skills deterioration
s. skills training (SST)
s. smile
s. standard
s. status
s. stereotypical behavior
s. stimulation
s. strata
s. stress
s. stress and functionability inventory (SSFI)
s. stress and functionality inventory
s. stressor
s. structure
s. support
s. support after treatment
s. support during treatment
s. taboo
s. tension
s. tolerance
s. toxicity
s. trap
s. type
s. undesirable
s. value
s. viscosity
s. welfare
s. welfare organization
s. withdrawal
s. withdrawal of childhood
s. work
s. worker
s. Zeitgebers
s. zone

social-emotional functioning
social-isolation syndrome
socialist
socialistic
socialite
sociality
socialization
   adult s.
   s. skills
socialize
socialized
   s. childhood truancy
   s. conduct disorder
   s. delinquency
   s. dementia
   s. disturbance

S

NOTES

socialized *(continued)*
    s. medicine
    s. runaway reaction
socially
    s. acceptable behavior
    s. adhesive
    s. alienated
    s. beneficial
    s. disabling
    s. disruptive environment
    s. dysfunctional
    s. dysfunctional adolescent
    s. effective
    s. functional
    s. harmful
    s. intimate model
    s. neutral
    s. unacceptable behavior
    s. undesirable behavior
social-minded
societal
    s. bias
    s. force
    s. implication
    s. norm
    s. reaction theory
    s. structure
society
    American Pain S. (APS)
    American Psychological S. (APS)
    American Psychosomatic S.
    Behavior Therapy and Research S.
     (BTRS)
    S. of Biological Psychiatry
    demand of s.
    S. for Developmental and
     Behavioral Pediatrics
    Hemlock S.
    S. for Industrial and Organizational
     Psychology
    s. level
    majority s.
    Orphan Train Heritage S.
    rural s.
    secret s.
    Sleep Research S.
    traditional s.
    Vienna Psychoanalytic S.
    Wednesday Evening S.
sociobiology
sociocenter
sociocentric
sociocentrism
sociocosm
sociocultural
    s. ambiance
    s. background
    s. foundation

    s. milieu
    s. trend
sociodemographic
    s. composition
    s. feature
    s. measure
    s. variable
socioeconomic
    s. background
    s. class
    s. group
    s. life change
    s. status (SES)
socioenvironmental therapy
sociofugal space
sociogenesis
sociogenic
sociogram
    objective s.
    perceptual s.
sociolinguistics
sociologese
sociologic
sociological
sociology
    clinical s.
    industrial s.
    medical s.
sociomedical
sociometric distance
sociometrist
sociometry
sociopath
sociopathic
    s. behavior
    s. personality
    s. personality disorder (SPD)
    s. personality disturbance (SPD)
sociopathology
sociopathy
sociopolitical
    s. agenda
    s. locus of control (SLC)
    s. position
    s. reality
sociopsychological
socioreligious
sociosexual
sociotaxis
sociotherapy
sociotropy scale
socratic questioning
sodium
    s. barbital
    s. valproate
sodium-responsive periodic paralysis
sodomist
sodomize

sodomy
soft
- s. chancre
- s. diet
- s. line
- s. psychotic-like phenomenon
- s. psychotic symptom
- s. restraint
- s. rock
- s. speech
- s. spot
- s. touch

Softab
softheaded
softhearted
softliner
soft-pedal
soft-spoken
soiled
soiling
solace
soldier
- s. of fortune
- s. heart

soldiering
solely
solemn
- s. affect
- s. vow

solemnity
solemnize
SOLER
  squarely (face person), open posture, lean (toward person), eye (contact), relaxed

solicit
solicitation
solicitous
solicitude
solidarity
solidify
soliloquize
soliloquy
  sexual s.

solipsism
solitariness
solitary
- s. activity
- s. aggressive type conduct
- s. aggressive-type conduct disorder
- s. confinement
- s. hunter syndrome
- s. stealing

solitude
solitudinarian
solution
- s. analysis
- auxiliary s.
- comprehensive s.
- expansive s.
- major s.
- The Centre for Mental Health S.'s

solution-focused therapy
solvable
solve
solvent
- s. dependence
- volatile s.

solving
- failure of problem s.
- inductive problem s.
- interpersonal cognitive problem s. (ICPS)
- problem s.
- rational problem s.
- visuospatial problem s.

soma
somata
- neuronal s.

somatagnosia
somatalgia
somatesthesia
somatesthetic
- s. area

somatic
- s. antidepressant
- s. antidepressant treatment
- s. category
- s. cell
- s. complaint
- s. delusion
- s. focus
- s. hallucination
- s. memory
- s. obsession
- s. paranoid disorder
- s. problem
- s. psychosis
- s. schizophrenia
- s. subtype
- s. symptom
- s. therapy
- s. treatment for depression
- s. type

somatist

NOTES

S

somatization
    s. neurotic disorder
    s. pain symptoms
    s. pseudoneurological symptoms
    s. reaction
    s. sexual symptoms
    s. tendency
somatized plea for treatment
somatizing
    s. clinical depression
    s. disorder
somatoform
    s. interface disorder
    s. pain
    s. pain disorder (SPD)
    s. scale
somatognosia
somatology
somatometry
somatomotor epilepsy
somatopathic drinking
somatophrenia
somatopsychiatric comorbidity
somatopsychic disorder
somatopsychosis
somatosensory
    s. cortices of the right hemisphere of the brain
    s. epilepsy
    s. evoked potential (SEP)
    s. evoked response (SER)
    s. seizure
    s. system
somatosexual
somatosexuality
somatotherapy
somatotonia
somatotopagnosia
somatotopagnosis
somatotopic
somatotype
somatotypology
somatron table
somber mood
some degree of range
somesthesia
somesthetic
    s. area
    s. system
sommeil
    tic de s.
somnambulance
somnambulant
somnambulate
somnambulic epilepsy
somnambulism
    cataleptic s.

    monoideic s.
    polyideic s.
somnambulist
somnambulistic trance
somnial
somnifacient
somniferous
somniferum
    Papaver s.
somnific
somnifugous
somniloquence, somniloquism
somniloquist
somniloquy
somnipathist
somnipathy
somnocinematograph
somnolence, somnolency
    daytime s.
    disorders of excessive s. (DOES)
    excessive daytime s.
    treatment-emergent s.
somnolent detachment
somnolentia
somnolescent
somnolism
somopsychosis
son
    favorite s.
song
    s. and dance
    rap s.
    siren s.
son-in-law
sonogram
sonomotor response
sonorous
soothe
soothing
soothsayer
sophism
sophist
sophistic
sophisticate
sophistication
sophistry
sophomania
sophomoric
sopiet
sopor
soporiferous
soporifical
soporific drug dependence
soporose, soporous
sorbitol
sorcerer
sorceress
sorcerous

sorcery
sordid
sore
    venereal s.
sorehead
sororate
sorority
sorrow
    overt signs of s.
sorrowful
sorrow-provoking stimuli
sortie
sortilege
sorting
    s. polarities
    s. test
SOS
    stimulation of sense
sosies
    illusion des s.
SOT
    stream of thought
sot
soteira
Sotos syndrome
soul
    s. blindness
    folk s.
    s. loss
    s. mate
    negative ruler of the s.
    s. pain
    world s.
soulful
soulless
soul-searching
sound
    abnormal stoppage of s.
    air-blade s.
    s. analysis
    attention to s.
    s. blending
    clucking s.
    coconut s.
    s. fear
    s. inside the head
    opening s.
    s. outside the head
    perception of s.
    repetition of s.
    s. symbolism
    s. therapy

sounding board
soundless voice
soundly
soundness
sound-symbol association
soup kitchen
source
    anxiety s.
    collateral s.'s
    external s.
    nonself s.
    s.'s of sexual knowledge
sour grapes
sour-grapes mechanism
sourness fear
soused
SP
    scale of psychosis
    systolic pressure
SPA
    schizophrenia with premorbid asociality
    schizophrenia with premorbid association
space
    brain s.
    s. context
    defensible s.
    detail response to small white s.
    (Dds)
    enclosed s.
    ethological models of personal s.
    inner s.
    life s.
    s. perception
    personal s.
    s. response
    s. sense
    sociofugal s.
spaced-out
spacer
spacing
span
    apprehension s.
    attention s.
    s. of attention
    auditory s.
    auditory memory s. (AMS)
    comprehension s.
    digit s. (DS)
    eye-voice s.
    life s.
    liver s.
    memory s.

NOTES

S

span (*continued*)
    narrowed attention s.
    s. recall test
spank
spanking
spar
Spartan diet
spasm
    affect s.
    anorectal s.
    canine s.
    carpopedal s.
    clonic s.
    cynic s.
    dancing s.
    functional s.
    habit s.
    hemifacial s.
    histrionic s.
    infantile s.
    intention s.
    masticatory s.
    mimic s.
    mobile s.
    muscle s.
    nictitating s.
    nodding s.
    occupational s.
    phonic s.
    professional s.
    progressive torsion s.
    retrocollic s.
    rotatory s.
    salaam s.
    saltatory s.
    sewing s.
    synclonic s.
    tailor's s.
    s. tic
    s. and tic
    tonic s.
    tonoclonic s.
    tooth s.
    vasomotor s.
    winking s.
spasmodic
    s. convulsion
    s. diathesis
    s. laughter
    s. laughter syndrome
    s. mydriasis
    s. seizure
    s. tic
    s. winking syndrome
spasmodica
    tabes s.
spasmodicus
spasmology

spasmolygmus
spasmolysis
spasmolytic
spasmophemia
spasmophenia
spasmophilia
spasmus
    s. caninus
    s. coordinatus
    s. nictitans
    s. nutans
spastic
    s. abasia
    s. amaurotic axonal idiocy
    s. aphonia
    s. diplegia
    s. dysphonia
    s. gait
    s. hemiplegia
    s. micosis
    s. miosis
    s. mydriasis
    s. state
spastica
    dysphonia s.
spasticity
    clasp-knife s.
    s. of conjugate gaze
    flexor s.
spat
spate
spatial
    s. ability
    s. agnosia
    s. agraphia
    s. aptitude
    s. balance
    s. behavior
    s. contiguity
    s. disorganization
    s. disorientation
    s. distortion
    s. music
    s. neglect
    s. nonrecognition
    s. organization
    s. orientation
    s. summation
    s. task
spatially
spatial-temporal context
SPD
    sociopathic personality disorder
    sociopathic personality disturbance
    somatoform pain disorder
speak
    s. out
    s. up

speaker
speaking
　　avoidance s.
　　s. capacity
　　novelty s. (NS)
spearhead
Spearman
　　S. rho
　　S. two-factor theory
special
　　s. education
　　s. educational service
　　s. jury
　　s. needs probation
　　s. power
　　s. relationship to deity theme
　　s. relationship to famous person theme
　　s. scale
　　s. sensation
　　s. sense
　　s. talent
　　s. theory of relativity
specialist
　　addiction s.
　　learning disabilities s.
　　mental health s.
specialization
　　role s.
specialized
　　s. foster care
　　s. language assessment
specially
specialty
　　American Board of Medical S.'s
　　s. mental health treatment
species
　　allopatric s.
specific
　　s. academic or work inhibition
　　s. action potential
　　s. culture, age, and gender feature
　　s. delay
　　s. developmental disorder (SDD)
　　s. dynamic pattern
　　s. effect
　　s. gender feature
　　s. learning disability
　　s. neurotic syndrome (SNR)
　　s. neurotransmitter
　　s. pathophysiological mechanism
　　s. psychotherapy

s. reading difficulty (SRD)
s. reading disability
s. sensory cue
sex s.
s. situational stressor
s. symptom
s. system
specification
　　job s.
specificity
　　criterion of s.
　　s. hypothesis
　　I-R s.
　　physiological response s.
　　s. of research
　　response s.
　　stimulus s.
　　symptom s.
　　treatment s.
specified
　　depressive disorder not otherwise s.
　　disorders of extreme stress not otherwise s. (DESNOS)
　　eating disorders not otherwise s. (EDNOS)
　　not otherwise s. (NOS)
　　psychotic disorder not otherwise s.
specifier
　　course s.
　　longitudinal course s.
　　severity s.
　　subtype and/or s.
　　type s.
specify
speciosity
specious
SPECS
　　system to plan early childhood services
spectacle
spectacular
spectator
　　s. role
　　s. therapy
spectin
　　brain s.
spectra (*pl. of* spectrum)
spectral
　　s. relationship
　　s. relationship to deity
　　s. relationship to famous person
spectrometry

NOTES

spectroscopy
  magnetic resonance s. (MRS)
  point resolved s. (PRESS)
spectrum, pl. **spectra, spectrums**
  acoustic s.
  band s.
  bulimic-anorexic s.
  s. disorder
  fortification s.
  impulsive s.
  panic-agoraphobic s.
  psychotherapeutic s.
  schizophrenia s.
  schizophrenic s. (SS)
speculate
speculation
speculative
speech
  absent s.
  accelerated s.
  s. act
  agrammatic s.
  alaryngeal s.
  alteration in rate of s.
  antiexpectancy s.
  s. apraxia
  s. aprosody
  s. arrest
  arrest of s.
  articulation of s.
  s. aspect
  ataxic s.
  audible blocking in s.
  automatic s.
  s. behavior
  bilateral s.
  bizarre s.
  blocked s.
  buccal s.
  cerebellar s.
  circumstantial s.
  cleft-palate s.
  clipped s.
  condescending s.
  confused s.
  s. content
  cued s.
  delayed s.
  s. derailment
  s. developmental delay disorder
  s. difficulty
  digressed s.
  s. disability
  disconnect s.
  s. discrimination score (SDS)
  s. discrimination test
  s. disfluency
  disorganized s.

s. disorientation
distractible s.
s. disturbance
disturbance in s.
dramatic s.
s. in dream
droning s.
dysarthric s.
s. dysfunction
s. dyspraxia
dysrhythmic s.
echo s.
egocentric s.
emotional s.
emotive s.
emphatic s.
euphoric s.
excessively impressionistic s.
excessively loud s.
excessively soft s.
executive s.
explosive s.
external s.
fast s.
figure of s.
flaccid s.
s. fluency
fluent aphasic s.
fluent paraphasic s.
s. hallucination
halting s.
s. and hearing (S&H)
hesitant s.
hyperkinetic s.
hypokinetic s.
imitative s.
s. impairment
impoverished s.
incessant s.
incoherent s.
incomprehensible s.
increased s.
infantile s.
s. inflection
s. intention center
internalized s.
involuntary pauses in s.
labyrinthine s.
lack of s.
laconic s.
s. and language behavior
s. and language disorder
s. and language impaired (SLI)
loud s.
manic s.
s. mannerism
mimic s.
mirror s.

s. monitoring center
monosyllabic s.
monotone s.
monotonous s.
s. and motor mapping
narrative s.
nonfluent aphasic s.
nonsensical s.
odd s.
organ s.
organic s.
overconcrete s.
over-elaborate s.
parasocial s.
s. pattern
paucity of s.
pause in s.
s. perception
s. perception region
s. perception system
performative s.
perseverative s.
phantom s.
plateau s.
poverty of content of s.
pressure of s.
pressured s.
s. processing
s. processing alteration
s. processing impairment
psychotic s.
quality of s.
quantity of s.
rambling s.
rapid s.
rate of production of s.
s. reading aphasia
s. reception threshold (SRT)
scanning s.
silent blocking in s.
slow s.
slurred s.
social gesture s.
soft s.
spoken s.
spontaneous s.
staccato s.
stilted s.
s. structure
subvocal s.
syllabic s.
tangential s.

s. therapy
s. tracking
s. tracking alteration
s. tracking task
tremulous s.
underproductive s.
unintelligible s.
unstoppable flow of s.
vague s.
well-articulated s.
whispered s.
speechless
speech-motor deficit
speed
    s. freak
    s. of information processing
      disturbance
    mental s.
    motor s.
    perceptual s.
    s. of processing
    s. quotient
    s. of thought
    verbal perceptual s.
    visual perceptual s.
speedball
spell
    crying s.
    dizzy s.
    doubting s.
    s.'s of doubting and brooding
    s. out
    staring s.
    vacant s.
spellbind
spellbound
spelling
    s. dyspraxia
    finger s.
    s. grade equivalent
SPEM
    smooth pursuit eye movement
spender
    binge s.
spending
    excessive s.
    s. spree
spent
spes phthisica
sphere
    conflict-free s.
    oriented in all s.'s

NOTES

sphere *(continued)*
    personality s.
    psychosexual s.
spheresthesia
sphincter
    s. control
    s. morality
spider fantasy
Spiegel eye roll
Spielmeyer acute swelling
spike
    peak absorption s.
spike-and-wave complex
spiked
    s. hair
    s. profile
spina
spinal
    s. anesthesia
    s. ataxia
    s. paralysis
    s. pyramidotomy
    s. shock
    s. stroke
    s. tap
    s. trigeminal nucleus
spinale
spinalis
    commotio s.
    tabes s.
spinant
spindle
spine
    poker s.
    s. sign
spineless
spinifugal
spinipetal
spinogalvanization
spinoreticulothalamic pathway
spinothalamic
spinster
spiperone
spiral
spirit
    acquisitive s.
    ancestral s.
    community s.
    controlling external s.
    evil s.
    external s.
    neutral s.
    possessed by s.
    s. possession
    s. writing
spirited
spiritism
spiritless

spiritual
    s. advice
    s. advisor
    s. approach
    s. assessment
    s. attitude
    s. awareness
    s. behavior
    s. concern
    s. counselor
    devoutly s.
    s. dimension
    s. dimension in psychiatry
    s. direction
    s. distress
    s. domain
    s. emergence syndrome
    s. emergency
    s. emptiness
    s. exercise
    s. factor
    s. focus group
    s. function
    s. guidance
    s. guide
    s. healing
    s. impairment
    s. intervention
    s. issue
    s. leadership
    s. medium
    s. orientation
    s. pain
    s. person
    s. pilgrimage
    s. possession
    s. possession experience
    s. practice
    s. seeker
    s. strength
    s. value
spiritualism
spirituality
    awareness of s.
    personal s.
    relevance of s.
    salience of s.
spiritually homeless
spiteful
spite reaction
spitting
splanchnesthesia
splanchnesthetic sensibility
splanchnic anesthesia
splenetic
splenium, pl. **splenia**
    s. tissue

splinter
    s. function
    s. group
split
    s. brain
    s. custody
    s. in the ego
    s. half reliability coefficient
    s. personality
    s. screen phenomenon
split-brain preparation
split-half reliability
split-off and denied experience
splitting
    s. behavior
    ego s.
    time s.
splurge
    stealing s.
spoiled child reaction
spoken
    fair s.
    s. language
    s. language disorder
    s. language impairment
    s. language quotient
    s. speech
spontaneity
    parental s.
    s. state
    s. test
    Theater of S.
    s. training
spontaneous
    s. abortion
    s. convulsion
    s. dyskinesia
    s. imitation
    s. improvement
    s. laughter
    s. movement
    s. narrative discourse
    s. panic attack
    s. recovery
    s. remission
    s. seizure
    s. speech
spoon
spoonerism
sporadic
    s. depression
    s. depressive disease (SDD)

sporotrichositic chancre
sports
    s. betting gambling
    wheelchair s.
spot
    blind s.
    cold s.
    figurative blind s.
    hypnogenic s.
    mental blind s.
    pink s.
    soft s.
    temperature s.
    touch s.
    Trousseau s.
spousal
    s. abuse
    s. loss
    s. loss through death
spouse
    s. abuse
    s. abuse index
    s. abuser
    battered s.
    distraught s.
    dominant s.
    s. rape
    separated from s.
    s. subsystem
spread
spreading
    s. depression
    rumor s.
spree
    buying s.
    shooting s.
    shopping s.
    spending s.
spring finger
springing mydriasis
sprouting
    hippocampal s.
spurious
    s. finding
spurt
    end s.
    initial s.
SQ
    social quotient
    status quo
SQ3R
    survey, question, read, review, recite

S

NOTES

squander mania
squarely (face person), open posture, lean (toward person), eye (contact), relaxed (SOLER)
SR, S/R
　schizophrenic reaction
　seizure resistant
　sentence repetition
S&R
　seclusion and restraint
SRA
　science research associates
SR/AP
　schizophrenic reaction, acute, paranoid
SR/AU
　schizophrenic reaction, acute, undifferentiated
SR/CP
　schizophrenic reaction, chronic, paranoid
SR/CU
　schizophrenic reaction, chronic, undifferentiated
SRD
　specific reading difficulty
SRI
　serotonin reuptake inhibitor
SRR
　systematic rational restructuring
SRS
　schizophrenic residual state
　sex reassignment surgery
　social and rehabilitation service
SRT
　speech reception threshold
SS
　schizophrenic spectrum
　seizure sensitive
　social service
SSFI
　social stress and functionability inventory
SSN
　superior salivary nucleus
SSOP
　Standard System of Psychiatry
SSPD
　schizoid-schizotypal personality disorder
SSRI
　selective serotonin reuptake inhibitor
　　SSRI discontinuation
SSRI-induced
　　S.-i. anorgasmia
　　S.-i. bruxism
　　S.-i. erectile dysfunction
　　S.-i. sexual disturbance
　　S.-i. sexual side effect
SST
　social skills training

ST
　shock therapy
　standardized test
St.
　　St. Louis hysteria
　　St. Vitus dance
stabbing pain
stability
　　behavioral s.
　　clinical s.
　　s. of ego
　　emotional s.
　　family s.
　　job s.
　　marital s.
　　s. of marriage
　　mental s.
　　occupational s.
　　personality trait s.
　　relative slow-wave sleep s.
　　slow-wave sleep s.
stabilization
　　acute s.
　　crisis s.
　　in-home crisis s.
　　mood s.
stabilize
stabilizer
　　mood s.
stabilizing social situations
stable
　　s. ego structure
　　emotionally s.
　　s. personality
　　s. sleep difficulty
　　s. sleep-wake pattern
staccato speech
stacking anchor
staff
　　consulting s.
　　medical s.
　　s. member
stage
　　adolescence developmental s.
　　adulthood developmental s.
　　alarm reaction s.
　　anal s.
　　anal-expulsive s.
　　attending to language s.
　　autonomous s.
　　biting s.
　　childhood developmental s.
　　cognitive development s.'s (Period I–IV)
　　concrete operation s.
　　concrete operational s.
　　confrontation s.
　　dementia s.

developmental s.
equality s.
equity s.
exhaustion s.
s. of exhaustion
formal operations s.
s. fright
functional assessment s.
genital s.
grammar development s.
grammar formation s.
group s.
heteronomous s.
HIV illness s.
individuation s.
infancy developmental s.
initial s.
intuitive s.
late life developmental s.
latency s.
life s.
locomotor-genital s.
s. 3 mania
manipulation s.
muscular-anal s.
oedipal s.
oral s.
oral-sensory s.
phallic s.
physioplastic s.
Piaget cognitive development s.
post ambivalent phase s.
preattachment s.
preclinical s.
preconceptual s.
pregenital s.
preoedipal s.
preoperational thought s.
psychosexual s.
pubertal s.
question s.
recovery s.
rehabilitation s.
sensorimotor s.
set the s.
shock s.
single word s.
sleep s.
symbiotic s.
symptom experience s.
toddler s.
true communication s.

two-word messages s.
urethral s.

stagger
staggering gait
stagnation
generativity versus s.
stake
stalemate
analytic s.
stalk
stalker
nonviolent s.
violent s.
stalker preoccupation
stalking
s. behavior
s. laws
s. victim
violence in s.
stammer
stammering
s. of the bladder
stamp
date s.
digit s.
stance
approach-avoidance s.
defensive adultomorphic s.
norm-assertive s.
stand
one-night s.
s. out
standard
s. antipsychotic therapy
s. behavior
s. of care
competency s.
s.'s development
s. deviation
s. dose
s. dose administration
double s.
s. error
s. error of difference
s. error of the mean (SEM)
foreign s.
s.'s implementation
s. kinetic model
s. laboratory test
legal s.
s. of living
living s.

NOTES

S

standard (*continued*)
    s. methadone maintenance treatment program
    s. neuropsychological battery
    s. of performance
    s. practice
    s. probation
    s. psychiatric nomenclature
    psychometric s.
    s. rating procedure
    s. reference
    s. score
    social s.
    S. System of Psychiatry (SSOP)
standardization of a test
standardize
standardized
    s. assessment
    s. cognitive assessment technique
    s. test (ST)
standing balance
standoff
stapes
STAPP
    short-term anxiety-provoking psychotherapy
starch eater
starch-eating
stare
    blank s.
    s. down
    empty s.
    manic s.
    postbasic s.
    reptilian s.
    vacant s.
star fear
staring
    s. face
    s. facial expression
    s. spell
starter marriage
startle
    s. abnormality
    acoustic s.
    s. epilepsy
    s. reaction
    s. reaction/response
    s. reflex
    s. response
    s. syndrome
    s. technique
startling stimulus
start low and go slow
starvation fasting
starve
stash

stasis
    libido s.
stat
state
    absent s.
    across identity s.
    activated s.
    active s.
    acute s.
    acute confusional s. (ACS)
    adrenergic-response s.
    adult ego s.
    affect s.
    affective and paranoid s.
    agitated s.
    alcoholic confusional s.
    alcoholic paranoid s.
    alcoholic twilight s.
    alcohol-induced paranoid s.
    alcohol paranoid s.
    alert awake s.
    s. of alertness
    alpha s.
    altered s.
    amnesic s.
    amnestic s.
    anxiety s. (AS)
    anxiety tension s. (ATS)
    apallic s.
    appetitive s.
    apprehension s.
    arousal s.
    arteriosclerotic dementia confusional s.
    arteriosclerotic paranoid s.
    arteriosclerotic psychosis confusional s.
    atypical neurotic anxiety s.
    awake s.
    borderline s.
    break s.
    calm wakefulness s.
    catatonic s.
    central excitatory s.
    central motive s.
    chronic deficit s.
    chronic delusional s.
    clear twilight s.
    climacteric paranoid s.
    clouded s.
    cognitive s.
    S. Comprehensive Mental Health Plan Act of 1986
    confusional twilight s.
    conscious s.
    s. of consciousness (SOC)
    consciousness s.
    constitutional psychopathic s. (CPS)

convulsive s.
delirium-like s.
s. dependence
depressed manic s.
depressive s.
depressive mixed s.
desire s.
dietary s.'s
diffusional s.
disorganized s.
dissociated s.
dissociative s.
dream s.
dreamlike s.
dreamy s.
drug-induced confusional s.
drug-induced hallucinatory s.
drug-induced paranoid s.
drug-induced semihypnotic s.
drug-like desire s.
drug psychosis hallucinatory s.
dysequilibrium s.
dysphoric manic s.
ego s.
elusive illness s.
emotional s.
end s.
epileptic clouded s.
epileptic confusional s. (ECS)
epileptic twilight s.
erotomanic delusional s.
euthymic s.
excited s.
exhaustion s.
explosive psychotic s.
s. factor
fatigue s.
fluctuating ego s.
fugue s.
fusion s.
generalized neurotic anxiety s.
general mood s.
global attractor s.
hallucinatory s.
s. of heightened attention
heightened attention s.
heightened awareness s.
s. of heightened awareness
homicidal s.
s. hospital (SH)
s. hospital children's unit (SHCU)
hyperadrenergic s.

hypereridic s.
hypnagogic s.
hypnoid s.
hypnopompic s.
hypnotic s.
hypodopaminergic s.
hysterical fugue s.
hysteric coma-like s.
identity s.
immobile s.
internal s.
involutional paranoid s.
lacunar s.
litigious delusional s.
local excitatory s.
locked in s.
manic s.
marasmic s.
s. markers of heavy drinking
menopausal paranoid s.
mental s.
s. mental hospital (SMH)
merger s.
s. of mind
s. of mindful relaxation
mixed bipolar s.
mixed mood s.
mood s.
moribund s.
multiple ego s.
mute s.
negative mood s.
neurotic anxiety s.
neurotic depressive s.
nonresponsive s.
obsessional s.
obsessive-ruminative tension s.
oneiroid s.
opposite affect s.
oral s.
organic psychotic s.
pain s.
panic attack neurotic anxiety s.
panic-free s.
paranoia paranoid s.
paranoia querulans paranoid s.
paranoid litigious s.
paraphonic s.
paraphrenia paranoid s.
parasomniac conscious s.
parent ego s.
pathological mood s.

NOTES

S

state *(continued)*
  perfection s.
  perplexity s.
  persistent vegetative s. (PVS)
  phobic s.
  possession trance s.
  postepileptic twilight s.
  postictal s.
  postoperative confusional s.
  premenstrual tension s.
  premorbid s.
  presenile dementia confusional s.
  presenile organic psychotic s.
  prolonged transition to fully
    awake s.
  s. psychiatric institution
  psychogenic twilight s.
  psychological s.
  psychopathic s.
  psychotic s.
  rapid eye movement s.
  reactive confusional s.
  refractory s.
  REM s.
  residual s.
  s. of resistance
  resource s.
  resting s.
  ruminative tension s.
  schizophrenic defect s.
  schizophrenic residual s. (SRS)
  s. of semisleep
  senile dementia confusional s.
  senile organic psychotic s.
  senile paranoid s.
  sensitiver Beziehungswahn
    paranoid s.
  separator s.
  sexual motive s.
  simple paranoid s.
  sleep s.
  spastic s.
  spontaneity s.
  s. statute
  steady s.
  subacute confusional s. (SCS)
  subacute delirious s.
  subacute irritable depressive s.
  subdelirious s.
  subdued s.
  substance-induced s.
  subsyndromal s.
  tension s.
  toxic confusional s.
  trance s.
  trancelike s.
  transcendental s.
  transient postictal confusional s.

  traumatic defect s.
  twilight confusional s.
  unresponsive s.
  vegetative s.
  visceral emotional s.
  wakeful s.
  withdrawal s.
stated
  s. age
  s. desire
state-dependent
  s.-d. learning
  s.-d. measure
  s.-d. memory
  s.-d. psychopathology rating scale
statement
  fashion s.
  nonsensical s.
  opening s.
  personality-descriptive s.
  suicidal s.
  SWAP-200 s.
state-of-the-art
  s.-o.-t.-a. analysis
  s.-o.-t.-a. analysis technique
state-trait interaction
static
  s. ataxia
  s. convulsion
  s. dementia
  s. demography
  s. encephalopathy
  s. infantilism
  s. sense
  s. tremor
station
  nurse's s.
  obligatory relay s.
  relay s.
  s. test
statistic
statistical
  s. artifact
  s. deviation
  s. inference
  s. mean
  s. median
  s. significance
  s. trend
statistically
  s. significant
  s. significant improvement
statistics
  s. collection
  descriptive s.
  inferential s.
  National Center for Health S.

psychiatric s.
vital s.

stature

psychosocially determined short s.
short s.

status

absence s.
acute change in mental s.
altered mental s.
ambulatory s.
s. aura
biologic s.
s. choreicus
clinical s.
cognitive s.
confident s.
s. cribrosus
s. criticus
current cognitive s.
Current, Global, Psychiatric-
Social S.
degenerative s.
s. degenerativus
s. deterioration
disordered mental s.
divorced s.
s. dysgraphicus
s. dysraphicus
elopement s. (ES)
s. epilepsy
s. epilepticus
s. epilepticus organic psychosis
s. examination
female biological s.
functional s.
general cognitive s.
grand mal s.
health s.
higher s.
s. hypoplasticus
immigrant s.
s. index
s. indicators
s. lacunaris
male biological s.
marital s.
menopausal s.
mental s.
s. nervosus
nutritional s.
s. offender
open-ward s.

petit mal s.
postoperative s.
preepisode s.
proband s.
prognostic s.
s. questionnaire
s. quo (SQ)
s. raptus
s. scale
s. schedule
separated s.
sexual abuse s.
social s.
socioeconomic s. (SES)
suicide s.
symptomatic s.
temporal lobe s.
uncertain biological s.
s. value
s. vertiginosus
widowed s.

statute

federal s.
state s.

statutory

s. offense
s. rape

statuvolence
statuvolent
Stauder lethal catatonia
staunch
stauroplegia
stay

estimated length of s.
inpatient s.
length of s. (LOS)
length of patient s. (LOPS)
s. on task

STC

sexually transmitted condition

STD

sexually transmitted disease

steady

s. gait
s. state

steady-state

s.-s. dose
s.-s. method
s.-s. regimen

stealing

s. an anchor
compulsive s.

S

NOTES

stealing *(continued)*
    s. impulse
    solitary s.
    s. splurge
stealth
steamy
Stearns alcoholic amentia
steatosis
    hepatic s.
Steele-Richardson-Olszewski disease
steeple skull
stem
    brain s.
stem-completion test
stenosis, pl. stenoses
    artery s.
stenostenosis
12-step
    -s. meetings
    -s. program
    -s. program for substance abuse
stepbrother
stepchild
stepdaughter
stepfather
stepmother
steppage gait
stepparent
steppingstone theory
step relation
steprelations
steps
    shuffling s.
stepsister
stepson
stepwise deterioration
stereoagnosis
stereoanesthesia
stereoelectroencephalography
stereoencephalometry
stereognosis
stereognostic perception
stereopathy
stereopsyche
stereoscopic vision
stereotaxic coordinate system
stereotaxis
stereotaxy
stereotype
    cultural s.
stereotyped
    s. activity
    s. attitude
    s. body movement
    s. interest
    s. motor movement
    s. movement disorder
    s. pattern of behavior

    s. repetition
    s. stress
    s. vocalization
stereotypic
    s. motor movement
    s. movement disorder (SMD)
stereotypical
    s. behavior
    s. gender roles
stereotypies
stereotypy
    s. and habit disorder
    oral s.
sterile
sterility
    elective s.
sterilization
    mental patient s.
sterilize
stern
sternutatory absence
steroid
    anabolic s.
    sex s.
    s. withdrawal syndrome
stethoparalysis
stethospasm
Stewart-Morel syndrome
STG
    short-term goal
stick
    needle s.
sticking sensation
sticky situation
stiff neck
stifle
stigma, pl. stigmas, stigmata
    external s.
    medication s.
    s. psychosis
    s. of psychosis
    psychosocial s.
stigmatic
stigmatization
stigmatized
stiletto
stillbirth
stilted
    s. attitude
    s. speech
    s. view
stimulant
    s. abuse
    beta s.
    s. challenge test
    chimeric s.
    CNS s.
    dopaminergic s.

s. effect
s. overdose
psychomotor s.
s. therapy
s. treatment
stimulant-dependent sleep disorder
stimulant-induced
s.-i. insomnia
s.-i. postural tremor
stimulate
stimulated
sexually s.
stimulating
s. environment
s. experience
s. occupation
stimulation
s. adjustment
amygdaloid s.
audiobrain s.
audiovisual s.
autogenital s.
brain s.
chemical s.
chimeric s.
clitoral s.
cocaine-induced dopamine s.
cognitive s.
s. condition
conditioned s.
dopamine s.
dorsal column s.
double simultaneous s. (DSS)
electrical intracranial s.
electrical transcranial s. (ETS)
emotional s.
endogenous s.
environmental s. (ES)
epileptogenic s.
exogenous s.
external s.
s. fatigue
fixed dose s.
functional electrical s. (FES)
genital s.
s. index (SI)
insufficient s.
intracranial s. (ICS)
manual s.
minimizing s.
noncoital s.
olfactory s.

oral s.
pathway s.
percutaneous s.
s. PET study
photic s.
postsynaptic s.
s. ratio
repetitive transcranial magnetic s.
  (rTMS)
s. of sense (SOS)
sensory s.
serotonin s.
sexual s.
social s.
subliminal s.
supranormal s.
sympathetic s.
synesthetic s.
tactile genital s.
tetanic s.
therapeutic electric s.
thyrotropin-releasing hormone s.
transcranial magnetic s. (TMS)
vagus nerve s. (VAS, VNS)
visual s.
stimulation-bound behavior (SBB)
stimulation-related adverse effect
Stimulator
Caldwell High Speed Magnetic S.
stimulus, pl. **stimuli**
accidental stimuli
adequate s.
alerting s.
ambiguous external stimuli
angry reaction to minor stimuli
anxiolytic stimuli
auditory s.
aversive s.
stimuli avoidance
chemical s.
conditioned s. (CS)
s. control
discriminant s.
discriminative s.
distracting stimuli
dream s.
s. drive (Sd)
effective s.
emotional s.
emotionally provoking s.
emotion-related feedback s.
emotive s.

NOTES

S

stimulus (*continued*)

environmental s.
epileptogenic s.
erotic s.
excitatory s.
external speech s.
s. fading
fatness s.
frightening s.
s. generalization
heterologous s.
homologous s.
inadequate s.
incidental s.
ineffective s.
internal s.
irrelevant external stimuli
liminal s.
masking s.
maximal s.
method of constant stimuli
minor s.
musical s.
neutral s.
novel s.
noxious s.
outside s.
s. overload
painful s.
paraphiliac s.
pedophilic s.
perceptual emotive s.
pharmacological s.
phobic s.
pleasant stimuli
pleasurable stimuli
provoking s.
psychosensory s.
reaction to minor stimuli
real external s.
real-life stimuli
reinforcing s.
s. response
screen out irrelevant s.
s. sensitive myoclonus
sensory s.
sexual s.
sorrow-provoking stimuli
s. specificity
startling s.
subliminal s.
s. substitution
subthreshold s.
summation of stimuli
supramaximal s.
tactile s.
target s.
s. tension

terrifying s.
s. therapy
thermal s.
threshold s.
s. threshold
train-of-four s.
triggering s.
unconditioned s. (UCS)
visual s.
visuospatial s.
s. word

stimulus-bound
stimulus-independent thought
stimulus-response theory
stinginess
stinging pain
stingy
stir fever
Stirling County study
stirred-up emotion
stitch
STM

short-term memory

Stockholm syndrome
stocking-and-glove

s.-a.-g. anesthesia
s.-a.-g. sensory loss

stocking anesthesia
stocking-glove
stoic
stoichiometric change
stoker's cramp
stolen
stomach

nervous s.

stoned
stonewall
Stony Brook High Risk Project
stooge
stool pigeon
stooped shoulders
stop

s., look and listen intervention
s. short

stop-and-think technique
stopping

thought s.

stop-start technique
storage

iconic s.
long-term s.
memory s.

store

cellular s.
high-energy cellular s.

storm

emotional s.
Operation Desert S. (ODS)

storm-and-stress period
stormed defense
storminess
stormy personality
story
    s. fear
    horror s.
    sob s.
storylike dream sequence
storyteller
strabismus
straight
    s. and narrow
    set one s.
strain
    interpersonal s.
    physical s.
    psychological s.
    role s.
    vocational s.
straitjacket
    chemical s.
straits
    dire s.
strangalesthesia
strangeness fear
stranger
    s. anxiety
    s. fear
strangle
stranglehold
strangulated affect
strangulation
strategic
    s. compliance
    s. family therapy
    s. intervention
    s. planning
strategically
strategist
strategy
    acceptance s.
    adjunctive s.
    age-appropriate s.
    alternative s.
    augmentation s.
    bibliotherapeutic s.
    candidate-gene s.
    challenge s.
    coactive s.
    cognitive s.
    combination s.

    conflict resolution s.
    coping s.
    crisis management s.
    data reanalysis s.
    defense s.
    dose reduction s.
    empirical-rational s.
    gambling s.
    genetic s.
    hockey-stick s.
    inference s.
    learning s.
    loading s.
    low-dose s.
    maladaptive problem-solving s.
    maternal problem-solving s.
    memory retrieval s.
    mnemonic s.
    optimal treatment s.
    precursor load s.
    problem-solving s.
    protective survival s.
    reality-oriented supportive s.
    reanalysis s.
    self-handicapping s.
    single-agent oral s.
    survival s.
    therapeutic s.
    treatment evaluation s.
    treatment package s.
    validation s.
    visual representation s.
stratification
    population s.
    post hoc s.
stratum, pl. **strata**
    social strata
straw
    last s.
stream
    breath s.
    s. of consciousness
    s. of mental activity
    s. of thought (SOT)
street
    s. addict
    s. drug
    s. fear
    s. gang
    s. people
    s. person

S

NOTES

street *(continued)*
    s. sense
    s. talk
streetperson
streetwalker
strength
    antagonistic muscle s.
    associative s.
    effective-habit s.
    ego s. (ES)
    fatigue s.
    habit s.
    human s.
    psychological s.
    spiritual s.
    s.'s and weaknesses
strenuous
streptodornase
stress
    acute foot-shock s.
    adaptability to s.
    s. adaptability skills
    s. audit
    biologic s.
    catastrophic s.
    causative s.
    chronic s.
    combat s.
    contrastive s.
    day-to-day s.
    disabling s.
    s. disorder
    s. effect and immune response
    s. effect in old age
    s. effect on adult
    s. effect on adult thinking
    s. effect on learning
    s. effect on memory
    effects of s.
    ego s.
    emotional s.
    environmental s.
    exceptional s.
    excessive s.
    executive s.
    exogenous s.
    family s.
    fatigue s.
    fight-or-flight s.
    s. from life experience (SFLE)
    s. and functionability inventory
    iambic s.
    identifiable s.
    s. immunity
    s. inoculation
    s. inoculation training (SIT)
    s. interview
    job s.

    job-related s.
    level of pychosocial s.
    life s.
    major life s.
    s. management
    s. management style
    marital s.
    maternal s.
    medical s.
    mental s.
    nonspecific s.
    occupational s.
    overwhelming s.
    physical s.
    postdisaster s.
    precipitating s.
    s. precipitating tremor
    s. prevention
    primary s.
    psychological s.
    s. psychosis
    psychosocial s.
    reaction to life s.
    s. reduction
    s. response syndrome
    secondary s.
    serious traumatic s.
    severe life s.
    s. situational reaction
    social s.
    stereotyped s.
    temporary s.
    tertiary s.
    transient emotional s.
    trauma-related s.
    traumatic s.
    trochaic s.
    war-related s.
    weak s.
stress-altered startle reflex
stress-diathesis model
stress-driven diathesis
stressful
    s. encounter
    s. environment
    s. event
    s. life experience
    psychologically s.
stress-illness process
stress-induced
    s.-i. alopecia
    s.-i. personality disorder
    s.-i. reactive bowel
stressor
    brief reactive psychosis with
      marked s.
    childhood s.
    cumulative s.

disaster s.
early life s.
educational s.
external s.
extreme s.
identifiable s.
internal s.
life s.
maladaptive reaction to a s.
psychosocial s.
seasonal-related psychosocial s.
situational s.
social s.
specific situational s.
traumatic s.
s. uncontrollability
stress-related
s.-r. amenorrhea
s.-r. disorder
s.-r. disturbance
s.-r. illness
s.-r. paranoid ideation
s.-r. physiological response
s.-r. psychopathology
s.-r. psychophysiological problem
stress-strain relationship
stria, pl. **striae**
acoustic s.
s. terminalis
striatal
s. hypometabolism
s. metabolism
striatocerebral tremor
striatofrontal
s. circuitry
s. dysfunction
striatum
corpus s.
striatus-orbitofrontal metabolism
stricken
pain s.
strict parent
strident
stridor
strife
family s.
strike
hunger s.
stringent
stripper
strip search
striptease

striving
conative appetitive s.
emancipatory s.
maintenance s.
superiority s.
s. for superiority
stroke
lacunar s.
National Institute of Neurological and Communicative Disorders and S.
spinal s.
stroking
strongly held idea
strong-minded
strong-willed
Stroop effect
structural
s. ambiguity
s. analysis of social behavior
s. atrophy
s. balance
s. brain abnormality
s. brain imaging
s. change
s. diagnosis
s. family therapy
s. gene
s. integration
s. magnetic resonance imaging
s. MRI
s. neuroimaging
s. pathology
s. profile
structuralism
structural-strategic therapy
structure
abnormal brain s.
alteration of memory s.
base s.
brain s.
character s.
cognitive s.
cooperative reward s.
cortical s.
deep s.
depressive character s.
dysphoric character s.
ego s.
external s.
field s.
functional superego s.

S

NOTES

structure *(continued)*
    group s.
    hierarchical s.
    hypoactive limbic s.
    individualistic reward s.
    initiating s.
    s. of intellect (SI)
    intermediate s.
    knowledge s.
    lack of s.
    limbic s.
    medial temporal s.
    mental s.
    narcissistic character s.
    neural s.
    organizational s.
    perceptual s.
    personality s.
    pragmatic s.
    social s.
    societal s.
    speech s.
    stable ego s.
    superego s.
    surface s.
    underlying s.
    white matter s.
structured
    s. clinical interview
    s. clinical interview method
    s. hallucination
    s. interactional group
    s. interactional group psychotherapy
    s. milieu
    s. task
    s. verbal information
structured-based ethics
struggle
    s. behavior
    leadership power s.
    power s.
strychnine
    aloin, belladonna, s. (ABS)
strychninism
strychnomania
stubborn
stubbornly defiant
student
    above-average s.
    at-risk high school s.
    at-risk middle school s.
    average s.
    below-average s.
    college s.
    s. disease
studies on hysteria
study
    adoption s.

Allport A-S Reaction S.
analog s.
autopsy s.
bidirectional selection s.
biochemical s.
biophysical s.
blind s.
brain imaging s.
brain potential s.
brain structure s.
case control s.
case history s.
Children's Health S. (CHS)
clinical comparison s.
cohort s.
community s.
correlation s.
crossover s.
cross-sectional s.
s. design
diachronic s.
double-blind drug s.
Dunedin Multidisciplinary Health
  and Development S.
ECA s.
ecological s.
electrodiagnostic s.
emotional fatigue s.
empirical s.
epidemiological s.
ethological s.
event-related brain potential s.
experimental s. (ES)
family risk s.
followup s.
functional brain imaging s.
functional imaging s.
genetic linkage s.
s. group
high-risk s.
hysteria s.
imaging s.
International Society for Traumatic
  Stress S.'s
Isle of Wight S.
laboratory s.
longitudinal s.
long-term naturalistic s.
Marcé s.
Masters and Johnson s.'s
Medical Outcomes S. (MOS)
Midtown Manhattan S.
moon-phase s.
multivariate s.
National Comorbidity S. (NCS)
National Vietnam Veterans
  Readjustment S.
naturalistic followup s.

nerve conduction s.
neurophysiological s.
New Haven s.
New York Longitudinal S. (NYLS)
nocturnal penile tumescence s.
noninvasive brain imaging s.
outcome s.
parametric s.
pathological s.
pedigree s.
phenotypic s.
picture frustration s. (PFS)
pilot s.
placebo-controlled drug s.
postmortem s.
prediction s.
prospective s.
psychological autopsy s.
resting PET s.
retrospective s.
Rosenzweig Picture-Frustration S. (RPFS)
Seattle Longitudinal S.
segregation analysis s.
self-report s.
stimulation PET s.
Stirling County s.
synchronic s.
systematic s.
time-motion s.
time and motion s.
twin s.'s
ultrastructural s.
United States-United Kingdom S.
S. of Values (SV)

stumbling
syllable s.

stump
s. hallucination
s. neuralgia

stun gun

stunt
dangerous s.

stupefacient, stupefactive

stupefaction

stupefy

stupemania

stupidity

stupor
affective s.
akinetic s.
alcoholic s.

anergic s.
benign s.
Cairns s.
catatonic s.
s. catatonic schizophrenia
delusion s.
depressive s.
diencephalic s.
emotional s.
epileptic s.
examination s.
exhaustive s.
frank catatonic s.
lethargic s.
malignant s.
s. mania
manic s.
postconvulsive s.
psychogenic s.
psychomotor s.

stuporosa
melancholia s.

stuporous
s. catatonia
s. depression
s. manic-depressive psychosis
s. melancholia
s. patient

stuporous-type manic-depressive psychosis

stutterer

stuttering
s. block theory
s. gait
hysterical s.
labiochoreic s.

style
adaptive s.
analysis of coping s.
arrogant s.
attachment s.
avoidance s.
borderline personality s.
cognitive s.
coping s.
deceitful s.
deception s.
dramatic interpersonal s.
dysfunctional family s.
dysfunctional personality s.
interpersonal s.
intrapsychic s.

NOTES

S

style (*continued*)
    introtensive personality s.
    introtensive problem-solving s.
    introversive problem-solving s.
    s. of leadership and management
    linguistic s.
    neurotic s.
    obsessive neurotic s.
    parenting s.
    perceptual s.
    problem-solving s.
    ruminative coping s.
    stress management s.
stymie
subacute
    s. confusional insanity
    s. confusional state (SCS)
    s. delirious state
    s. delirium
    s. irritable depressive state
    s. organic reaction
    s. posttraumatic organic psychosis
    s. psychoorganic syndrome
    s. spongiform encephalopathy
subaffective
    s. disorder
    s. dysthymia
subantigen
subaverage
    s. academic function
    s. academic functioning
    s. intellectual functioning
    s. motor coordination
subcategory
subception
subchronic
    s. schizophrenia
    s. schizophrenic
subclass
subclassification
subclavian steal syndrome
subclinical
    s. absence
    s. depressive symptom
    s. range
    s. score
    s. seizure
    s. syndrome
subcoma therapy
subconscious
    s. awareness
    s. memory
    s. mind
    s. perception
    s. self
subconsciousness
subcortical
    s. alexia

    s. arteriosclerotic encephalopathy
    s. brain involvement
    s. condition
    s. dementia
    s. dysfunction model
    s. gray matter
    s. gray matter area
    s. gray matter hyperintensity
    s. gray region
    s. motor aphasia
    s. pathology
    progressive degenerative s.
    s. white matter
subcortical-frontal lobe abnormality
subcultural language
subculture norm
subcutaneous
    s. injection
subdelirious state
subdelirium
subdivision
    hippocampal formation s.
subdue
    difficult to s.
subdued state
subdural
subfactor
    borderline s.
    dysphoric s.
subgenual cingulate region
subgroup
    cultural s.
    diagnostic s.
    phenomenological s.
subgrundation
subiculum, pl. **subicula**
subject
    s.'s as their own control
    caffeine-abstinent s.
    ego s.
    normal s.
subjective
    s. criticism
    s. depression
    s. distortion
    s. distress
    s. doubles
    s. drive
    s. effect
    s. emotional feeling
    s. equality
    s. error
    s. experience
    s. fear
    s. insomnia complaint
    s. manifestation
    s. mentation
    s. mood change

s., objective, assessment, plan (SOAP)
s. orientation
s. pain
s. plane
s. psychology
s. psychostimulation
s. seizure
s. sensation
s. symptom
s. unit of distress rating
s. vertigo
s. vision
s. well-being
subjectivism factor
subjectivity
overwhelmed s.
subject-verb agreement
subjugate
subjunctive mood
sublimate
sublimation
s. defense mechanism
s. difficulty
sublime
subliminal
s. behavior
s. consciousness
s. excitation
s. fringe
s. learning
s. message
s. perception
s. self
s. stimulation
s. stimulus
s. suggestion
s. thirst
sublimity
sublingual medication
submachine gun
submania
submerge
submerged individual need
submission
authoritarian s.
submissive behavior
submissiveness
submodalities
critical s.
subnormal
educationally s. (ESN)

subnormality
mental s.
moderate mental s.
profound mental s.
severe mental s.
subnucleus
amygdala s.
suboccipital
s. decompression
s. headache
s. neuralgia
s. neuritis
s. puncture
suboccipitale
suboptimal
s. treatment
s. treatment modality
subordinate
s. association
s. position
subordination
subphase
rapprochement s.
subplate zone
subpoena duces tecum
subpoenaed
subpotent
subpsyche
subscale
BPRS anxiety-depression s.
cognitive s.
depression s.
low-magnitude stressor s.
noncognitive s.
nonturbulence s.
SCL-90 s.
vegetative s.
subscribe
subsequent
s. amnesia
s. development
s. trauma
subservient
subshock therapy
subsidiation
subsidize
subsidy
subsist
subsistence diet
subsocial
subsonic
subspecialty

S

NOTES

substance
  s. abuse
  s. abuse counselor
  s. abuse and dependence
  s. abuse and dependence disorder
  s. abuser
  s. abuse treatment
  s. abuse treatment facility
  s. addiction
  amphetamine-like s.
  anxiety due to a s.
  anxiolytic s.
  behavior-altering s.
  caffeinated s.
  controlled s.
  ego s.
  endogenously produced s.
  s. group
  illicit psychoactive s.
  s. intoxication
  s. K
  long-half-life anxiolytic s.
  mind-altering s.
  mood-altering s.
  nontoxic s.
  pineal s.
  psychoactive s.
  schedule II s.
  s. sensitivity
  s. tolerance
  toxic s.
  s. use
  s. use disorder
  s. withdrawal tremor
substance-abuse persisting dementia
substance-abusing parent
substance-induced
  s.-i. anxiety
  s.-i. chronic psychosis
  s.-i. delirium
  s.-i. dystonia
  s.-i. etiology
  s.-i. intoxication
  s.-i. manic episode
  s.-i. organic mental disorder
  s.-i. perception
  s.-i. persisting dementia
  s.-i. presentation
  s.-i. psychotic disorder
  s.-i. sexual dysfunction
  s.-i. state
  s.-i. symptomatology
  s.-i. syndrome
substance-related
  s.-r. cause
  s.-r. disorder
  s.-r. legal problem
  s.-r. syndrome

substance-seeking behavior
substance-specific
  s.-s. intoxication criteria sets
  s.-s. withdrawal
  s.-s. withdrawal criteria sets
substandard
substantia
  s. innominata
  s. nigra
substantial comorbidity
substantive universals
substitute
  displacement s.
  father s.
  s. formation
  mother s.
  s. object
  opioid s.
  regressive s.
substituted amphetamine
substituting
  s. behavior
  s. feeling
  s. thought
substitution
  s. analysis
  s. defense mechanism
  digit symbol s.
  s. disorder
  dissociate-dysmnesic s.
  stimulus s.
  symptom s.
substitution-accuracy
  code s.-a. (CDS-ACC)
substitution-efficiency
  code s.-e. (CDS-EFF)
substitutive
  s. agent therapy
  s. medication
  s. reaction type
substrate
  biologic s.
  brain s.
  neural s.
subsultus
  s. clonus
  s. tendinum
subsume
subsyndromal
  s. bipolar mood fluctuation
  s. depression
  s. depressive symptom
  s. mood symptom
  s. state
  s. thought disorder
subsystem
  s. boundary
  cognitive s.

depreciated s.
individual s.
interacting cognitive s.
parallel s.
parent s.
sibling s.
spouse s.

subteen
subtemporal decompression
subtest

arithmetic s.
block design s.
comprehension s.
digit span s.
information s.
PC s.
picture arrangement s.
picture completion s.
s. scale score
scale scores s.
similarities s.
verbal s.
visual s.

subtetanic
subthalamic nucleus
subtherapeutic dose
subthreshold

s. presentation
s. stimulus

subtle

s. gesture
s. meaning
s. memory problem

subtype

s. and/or specifier
Central European s.
clinical s.
delusional s.
depression s.
diagnostic s.
disorganized s.
Eastern s.
erotomanic s.
grandiose s.
jealous s.
kraepelinian s.
male alcoholism s.
persecutory s.
psychotic depressive s.
somatic s.
Western s.

subunit

beta s.

suburban community
subversion
subversive
subvocal speech
subwaking
succedaneum

caput s.

succeed
succes de scandale
success

cumulative probability of s. (CPS)
s. experience
failure through s.
lack of academic s.
lack of vocational s.
s. neurosis
outlet for s.
therapeutic s.

successful suicide
successive approximation
succinct
succinimides
succorance need
succubus
succumb
sucking

s. behavior
finger s.
s. technique
thumb s.

suckling

eternal s.

sudden

s. cheerfulness
s. death
s. fear
s. financial reversal
s. infant death syndrome (SIDS)
s. insight
s. motor movement
s. onset
s. vocalization

sudden-onset headache
Sudeck syndrome
sudomotor component
suffer
suffering

anticipated emotional s.
s. death
ego s.

S

NOTES

suffering *(continued)*
    emotional s.
    mental s.
suffering-hero daydream
sufficient quantity
suffocate
suffocating attachment
suffocation
    s. fear
    s. hysterica
    s. hysterics
    s. panicker
    traumatic s.
suffrage
    female s.
sugar
    blood s.
suggestibility
    disturbance in s.
    s. effect
suggestible
suggestion
    affective s.
    hypnotic s.
    posthypnotic s.
    prestige s.
    subliminal s.
    s. therapy
    s. under hypnosis
    verbal s.
suggestive
    s. medicine
    s. psychotherapy
    sexually s.
suicidal
    s. act
    actively s.
    s. behavior
    s. crisis
    s. depressed patient
    s. emergency
    s. feature
    s. gesture
    s. ideation
    s. intent
    s. melancholia
    s. obsession
    s. plan
    s. potential
    s. preoccupation
    s. rumination
    s. statement
    s. thinking
    s. thought
suicidality
suicide
    accidental s.
    accomplished s.

s. act
adolescent s.
alcohol-related risk for s.
altruistic s.
anomic s.
assisted s.
s. attempt (SA)
s. attempter
s. attempt history
s. attempt rate
cluster s.
s. cluster
collective s.
completed s.
s. completion
contract against s.
copy-cat s.
deterrent to s.
Durkheim theory of s.
egotistic s.
elderly s.
focal s.
s. gesture
half-hearted attempt at s.
s. by hanging
s. hotline
impulsive s.
s. incidence
s. intent
s. inventory
s. lethality
s. method
s. motivation
s. pact
physician-assisted s.
s. plan
s. potential
s. precaution
s. prediction scale
s. predictor
s. predisposition
s. prevalence
s. prevention
s. prevention center
psychic s.
psychological s.
rational s.
risk of s.
s. risk
s. risk factor
s. status
successful s.
s. survivor syndrome
s. talk
teenage s.
s. tendency
thought of s.
s. threat

threat of imminent s.
s. victim
s. vulnerability
suicide-depression (S-D)
suicidology
American Association of S. (AAS)
suigenderism
suit
paternity s.
sukra prameha
sulcal prefrontal cortex
sulcus, pl. **sulci**
calcarine s.
callosal s.
central s.
cingulate s.
frontal s.
inferior frontal s.
inferior temporal s.
middle frontal s.
occipital s.
postcentral s.
precentral s.
superior frontal s.
superior temporal s.
temporal s.
terminal s.
sultry
summary score
summation
spatial s.
s. of stimuli
sum score
Sunday neurosis
sundowner
s. effect
s. syndrome
sundowning behavior
sundown syndrome
sunlight fear
sunrise fear
suo yang
superachiever
superambitious
supercautious
supercilious
superconfident
supercriminal
superego
s. anxiety
autonomous s.
s. control

s. disturbance
double s.
group s.
heteronomous s.
s. lacuna
parasites of the s.
parasitic s.
primitive s.
s. resistance
reward by the s.
s. sadism
s. structure
superexcitation
superficial
s. affect
s. charm
s. idiot
s. pain
s. psychotherapy
s. sensation
superfluous
superhit
superhuman
superimposed
s. delirium
s. dementia
superintelligent
superior
s. frontal sulcus
s. functioning
s. intelligence
s. manner
s. paraplegia
respondeat s.
s. salivary nucleus (SSN)
s. temporal auditory cortical area
s. temporal sulcus
superiority
s. complex
s. feeling
intellectual s.
sense of s.
striving for s.
s. striving
superlative
superman
supermoron
supermotility
supernatural
supernaturalism
supernormal
supernumerary

S

NOTES

superordinate
superpersonal **unconscious**
superpower
supersensible
supersensory
supersexuality
superstar
superstition
superstitious
  s. behavior
  s. control
supervalent **thought**
supervise
supervised
  s. after-school activity
  s. probation
supervision
  boundaries in postanalytic s.
  one-on-one s.
  person in need of s.
  postanalytic s.
supervisor
supervisory
  s. behavior description (SBD)
  s. relationship
superwoman
supinator **jerk**
supplement
  dietary s.
supplementary **motor area (SMA)**
supplementation
  oral s.
supplicate
supplicatory
supply
  drug s.
  emotional s.
support
  s., autonomy, fusioning, empathy
   (SAFE)
  behavioral s.
  child s.
  community s.
  considerable external s.
  constructive s.
  decision s.
  emotional s.
  s., empathy and truth (SET)
  empirical s.
  environmental s.
  external s.
  family s.
  financial s.
  s. group
  informational s.
  instrumental s.
  lack of family s.
  limited s.

  peer s.
  physical s.
  social s.
  s. system
  s. team
  youth self s. (YSR)
supported **employment program**
supporter
supporting
  s. data
  s. evidence
supportive
  s. confrontation
  s. ego
  s. group therapy
  s. medication
  s. medication clinic
  not s.
  s. psychotherapy
  reality-adaptive s. (RAS)
  s. relationship
  s. talk-down
supportive-expressive **psychotherapy**
suppressant
  appetite s.
suppressed **anger**
suppression
  conditioned s.
  s. neurosis
  rebound s.
  thought s.
suppressive **therapy**
suppressor **scale**
Supprettes
suppurative
suprachiasmatic **nuclei**
supraclinoid
supraindividual
supraliminal
supramarginal/angular **cortex**
supramaximal **stimulus**
supranormal **stimulation**
supranuclear
  s. gaze palsy
  s. paralysis
supraoptic **nucleus**
supraorbital **neuralgia**
suprarational
suprasegmental **analysis**
suprasellar
supratentorial **overlay**
suprathreshold **ECT**
supremacist
  white s.
supremacy
supreme
  s. being
  s. court

supremo
surcease
surdimutism
surdity
surety
surface
    s. affability
    s. ego
    s. structure
surfeit
surge
surgency
surgent growth
surgery
    gastric bypass s.
    plastic s.
    sex reassignment s. (SRS)
surgical
    s. addiction
    s. brain trauma organic psychosis
    s. procedure
    s. sex reassignment
surly
surmise
surmount
surpass
surreal
surrealism
surrealistic
surrender
    schizophrenic s.
    will to s.
surreptitious
surrogate
    father s.
    s. father
    mother s.
    s. mother
    s. parent
    sexual s.
    s. sexual partner
surroundings
    familiar s.
    indifferent to s.
    oblivious to s.
    reduced awareness of s.
surveillance protocol
survey
    s. data
    s., question, read, review, recite (SQ3R)
surveyor

survival
    s. of the fittest
    nerve cell s.
    s. skills workshop
    s. strategy
    s. time
survivalist
surviving
    s. family member
    s. parent
survivor
    s. of abuse
    s. of death
    s. guilt
    holocaust s.
    s. of neglect
    s. syndrome
    trauma s.
susceptibility
    environmental s.
    s. factor
    genetic s.
susceptible individual
suspect
    murder s.
suspected
    s. adverse drug reaction (SADR)
    s. awareness
    s. child abuse/neglect (SCAN)
    s. disease
suspended animation
suspension
suspicion
suspicious
    s. behavior
    s. ideation
suspiciousness
sustain
sustained
    s. attention
    s. belief
    s. compliance
    s. emotion
    s. fatigue
    s. full remission
    s. manner
    s. partial remission
    s. position
sustenance of life
sustentation
suturectomy

S

NOTES

SV
    Study of Values
SWA
    seriously wounded in action
swagger
swallow-belch method
swallowing
    air s.
    s. automatism
SWAP-200
    SWAP-200 assessment procedure
    SWAP-200 description
    SWAP-200 item
    SWAP-200 item set
    SWAP-200 statement
swastika
swat
swaying
    body s.
    s. gait
swear
swearing
    compulsive s.
sweatbox
sweep-cheek test
sweetheart contract
sweet-lemon mechanism
swelled head
swelling
    brain s.
    Spielmeyer acute s.
swill
swimming in the head
swindle
swindler
    epileptic s.
    pathologic s.
    pathological s.
swing
    compensatory mood s.
    cyclic mood s.
    decreased arm s.
    dramatic behavioral s.
    energy s.
    mood s.
    s. phase control
    rebound mood s.
    seasonal mood s.
swinging
switch
    s. process
    s. referential index
swollen eye
SWS
    slow-wave sleep
Sx
    symptom
sycophant

syllabic speech
syllable stumbling
syllogism
syllogistic reasoning
sylvian fissure
symbion
symbiosis
    dyadic s.
    triadic s.
symbiotic
    s. attachment
    s. infantile psychosis
    s. marriage
    s. phase
    s. psychosis of childhood
    s. relatedness
    s. stage
symbol
    association of sounds and s.'s
    digit s. (DS)
    mathematical s.
    memory s.
    phallic s.
    picture s.'s (PICSYMS)
    sex s.
    snake s.
    universal s.
    Wing s.
symbolia
symbolic
    s. anxiety
    s. categorization
    s. computation
    s. displacement
    s. elaboration
    s. function
    s. loss
    s. masturbation
    s. meaning
    s. persona
    s. play
    s. realization
    s. thinking
    s. thought
    s. value
    s. wounding
symbolically
    performing s.
symbolism
    anagogic s.
    cryptogenic s.
    dream s.
    functional s.
    material s.
    metaphoric s.
    sound s.
    threshold s.
    true s.

symbolization defense mechanism
symmetric distal neuropathy
symmetromania
symmetry obsession
sympathectomy
    chemical s.
    periarterial s.
sympathetic
    s. discharge
    s. dysfunction
    s. epilepsy
    s. hypertonia
    s. imbalance
    s. nerve ending
    s. nervous system (SNS)
    s. output
    s. response
    s. stimulation
    s. stress reaction
sympathetica
    ptosis s.
sympathetic-nervous-system-medicated
  vasoconstriction
sympathic
sympathiconeuritis
sympathicopathy
sympathicotonia
sympathicotonic
sympathicotripsy
sympathism
sympathist
sympathize
sympathizer
sympathoadrenal hyperactivity
sympathomimetic
    s. abuse
    s. addiction
    s. agent
    s. delirium
    s. delusional disorder
    s. drug
    s. effect
    s. intoxication
    s. withdrawal
sympathomimetic-induced thermogenesis
sympathy seeking
symptom (Sx)
    abstinence s.
    accessory s.
    active-phase s.
    active psychotic s.
    acute s.

adjustment reaction physical s.
adolescent depression s.
affective s.
alcoholic s.
s. amplification
anchor s.
anxiety s.
arousal s.
array of s.'s
s. assessment
attention deficit s.
atypical factitious disorder with
  physical s.'s
auditory s.
autoplastic s.
avoidance s.
avoidant s.
baseline s.
behavioral dysfunction s.
s. of bereavement
biologic dysfunction s.
biphasic s.
bodily s.
body-related obsessive-like s.
cardiac s.
catatonic s.
s. categorization
chronology of s.
clinical s.
clinician-rated cognitive s.
cluster of s.
cluster C, D s.
cocaine withdrawal s.
cognitive s.
s. complex
compulsive s.
constellation of signs and s.'s
conversion s.
s. criteria
s. crystallization
culturally sanctioned s.
cyclical pattern of s.'s
debilitating dysphoric s.
deficit s.
delusion s.
depression s.
depressive s.
s. diary
s. dimension
disaster-related avoidant s.
disaster-related intrusive s.
discrete s.

S

NOTES

symptom *(continued)*
dishonest simulation of s.
disorganization dimension of
  positive schizophrenic s.'s
dissociative s.
drug-induced negative s.
eclamptic s.
emotional s.
equivalent s.
s. evaluation
exacerbated s.'s
s. exacerbation
s. experience stage
extrapyramidal s. (EPS)
extrapyramidal syndrome s.
fatigue s.
feigned s.
first-rank s. (FRS)
first-rank psychotic s.
florid s.'s
food-related obsessive-like s.
s. formation
frank psychotic s.'s
s. free
Frenkel s.
fundamental s.
general s.
generic negative s.
Gordon s.
gramophone s.
s. group
s. grouping
Grund s.
hyperarousal s.
hypnotic withdrawal s.
hypochondriacal s.
impairment s.
individual depressive s.
induced factitious s.
insomnia s.
intentionally produced s.
intrusive s.
key s.
s. level
localization of s.'s
Macewen s.
manic s.
manifest s.
manifestly observable s.
s. measure
medical s.
mental s.
minimal residual s.
mood s.
motor conversion s.
movement s.
multiple medically unexplained s.
  (MMUS)

negative s.
neurobehavioral s.
s. neurosis
neurovegetative s.
nicotine withdrawal s.
nonbizarre s.
nonpsychotic onset of s.'s
nonpsychotic signs and s.
numbing s.
objective s.
obsessive-compulsive s.
onset of s.'s
overall depressive s.
s. overlap
pain s.
painful s.
panic s.
perceptual s.'s
phylogenetic s.'s
physical signs and s.'s
positive schizophrenic s.'s
possession trance s.
posttraumatic stress s.
preexisting mental disorder s.
premonitory s.
s. presentation
presenting s.
primary defense s.
primary enduring negative s.
primary nonenduring negative s.
principal s.
prodromal psychotic s.
productive s.'s
s. profile
s. progression
prominent mood s.
proxy s.
psychiatric s.
psychogenic physical s.
psychological dysfunction s.
psychological related s.'s
psychological signs and s.'s
psychomotor s.
psychosensory s.
psychosexual s.
psychosomatic s.
psychotic signs and s.
s. rating
recurring s.
s. reduction
reexperiencing perceptual s.
s. relief
s. relief through hypnosis
residual negative s.
residual positive s.
residual psychotic s.
s. response pattern
reverse vegetative s.'s

Romberg s.
Romberg-Howship s.
Scale for the Assessment of Negative S.'s (SANS)
schizophrenia s.
schizophrenic s.
Schneider first rank s.
schneiderian first-rank s.
s. searching
secondary defense s.
sedative-hypnotic withdrawal s.
self-reported s.
sensory conversion s.
severe dissociative s.
sexual s.
soft psychotic s.
somatic s.
somatization pain s.'s
somatization pseudoneurological s.'s
somatization sexual s.'s
specific s.
s. specificity
subclinical depressive s.
subjective s.
s. substitution
subsyndromal depressive s.
subsyndromal mood s.
target s.
tic s.
total s.
trauma-type s.
troublesome s.
unintentionally produced s.
vegetative s.
visual s.
withdrawal s.
worrying s.
s. worsening
symptomatic
s. act
acutely s.
s. depression
s. disadvantage
s. epilepsy
s. headache
s. impotence
s. indication
s. neuralgia
s. paramyotonia
s. patient
s. perspective
s. presentation

s. psychosis
s. reaction
s. seizure
s. status
s. therapy
s. treatment
symptomatica
alopecia s.
indicatio s.
symptomatically reactive
symptomatize
symptomatology
acute psychiatric s.
depressive s.
mood s.
negative s.
panic s.
psychotic s.
substance-induced s.
symptom-based drug choice
symptom-free
symptom-related predictor
symptom-sparing
extrapyramidal s.-s.
synagogue
synaphoceptor
synapse, pl. **synapses**
chemical s.
cholinergic s.
conjoint s.
dopaminergic s.
electrical s.
excitatory s.
noradrenergic s.
serotonergic s.
viable s.
synaptic
s. activity
s. compartment
s. compensation
s. plasticity
s. transmission
synaptobrevin
synaptogenesis
synaptotagmin
synchronic study
synchronous
synchrony
bilateral s.
synclonic spasm
synclonus
syncopal

S

NOTES

syncope
    hysterical s.
    laryngeal s.
    local s.
    micturition s.
    postural s.
    vasomotor s.
    vasopressor s.
    vasovagal s.
syncopic
syncretic
    s. thinking
    s. thought
syncretism
syndrome
    aberrant motivational s.
    absence s.
    abstinence s.
    abused-child s.
    Acosta s.
    acquired immunodeficiency s. (AIDS)
    acroparesthesia s.
    acute brain s. (ABS)
    acute organic brain s.
    acute posttraumatic stress s.
    acute psychoorganic s.
    Adams-Stokes s.
    adaptation s.
    addiction s.
    adiposogenital s.
    adjustment reaction physical s.
    adrenogenital s. (AGS)
    advanced sleep-phase s.
    affective disorder s.
    Aicardi s.
    air pollution s. (APS)
    akinetic-abulic s.
    alcohol abstinence s.
    alcohol amnestic s.
    alcohol dependence s.
    alcoholic brain s.
    alcoholic malabsorption s.
    alcohol-induced organic mental s.
    alcohol withdrawal s.
    Alice in Wonderland s.
    alveolar hypoventilation s.
    Alzheimer s.
    amnesic s.
    amnestic s.
    amnestic-confabulatory s.
    amotivational s.
    androgen insensitivity s.
    Angelucci s.
    anger and violence psychiatric s.
    angry woman s.
    anticholinergic s.
    antimotivational s.

    Anton s.
    anxiety s.
    anxiety-related psychiatric s.
    apallic s.
    apathy s.
    s. aphasia
    approximate answers s.
    s. of approximate relevant answers
    asphyctic s.
    atypical or mixed organic brain s.
    autoscopic s.
    aviator's effort s.
    avoidance s.
    Balint s.
    Bardet-Biedl s.
    battered child s. (BCS)
    battered spouse s.
    battered woman s. (BWS)
    behavioral reaction brain s.
    behavior, speech, and other s.'s (BSO)
    Behr s.
    benzodiazepine discontinuation s.
    Bianchi s.
    black patch s.
    blue velvet s.
    Bonnevie-Ullrich s.
    Bonnier s.
    Borjeson-Forssman-Lehmann s.
    bradykinetic s.
    brain psychoorganic s.
    Briquet s.
    Brissaud-Marie s.
    Bristowe s.
    Brown-Sequard s.
    buffoonery s.
    burnout s.
    callosal disconnection s.
    Capgras s.
    capsulothalamic s.
    cardiopulmonary-obesity s.
    carinatum s.
    catastrophic ancataplexy s.
    catatonic s.
    cat-cry s.
    cat's-eye s.
    characteristic withdrawal s.
    child abuse s.
    childhood-onset Tourette s.
    childhood Tourette s.
    China s.
    choreiform s.
    chromosome 21-trisomy s.
    chronic alcoholic brain s. (CABS)
    chronic brain s. (CBS)
    chronic fatigue s. (CFS)
    chronic hyperventilation s.
    Cinderella s.

Citelli s.
Claude s.
Clerambault erotomania s.
clinical poverty s.
cloverleaf skull s.
clumsiness s.
Cohen s.
Collet-Sicard s.
compulsive swearing s.
concentration camp s. (CCS)
concussion s.
confused language s. (CLS)
contralateral neglect s.
Cornelia de Lange s.
corpus callosum s.
Cotard s.
Creutzfeldt-Jakob s.
cri du chat s.
Crigler-Najjar s.
Crouzon s.
crush s.
crying-cat s.
culture-bound s.
culture-specific s.
DaCosta s.
de Clerambault s.
de Lange s.
delayed sleep phase s.
Delilah s.
delusional misidentification s.
dementia s.
dementia-aphonia s.
dementia-related psychiatric s.
denial visual hallucination s.
dependence s.
depersonalization s.
depression-related psychiatric s.
depressive s.
depressive-type psychoorganic s.
deprivation s.
De Sanctis-Cacchione s.
s. of deviously relevant answers
dialysis encephalopathy s.
dietary chaos s.
disconnection s.
disinhibition psychiatric s.
disorganization s.
displaced child s.
dissociation s.
Don Juan s.
drug abstinence s.
drug-induced s.

drug withdrawal s.
Dubowitz s.
dysmnesic s.
dyspraxia s.
ectopic ACTH s.
Edwards s.
effort s.
Ehret s.
Eisenlohr s.
Ekbom s.
electroshock-induced psychotic s.
Elpenor s.
elusive s.
empty nest s.
epileptic s. (ES)
episodic dyscontrol s.
Epstein-Barr s.
exhaustion s. (EPS)
extrapyramidal s. (EPS)
failure-to-grow s.
failure-to-thrive s.
false memory s.
fatigue s.
feminizing-testes s.
fetal alcohol s. (FAS)
fetal hydantoin s.
Figueira s.
flashing pain s.
fluid retention s. (FRS)
Flynn-Aird s.
fragile X s. (FMR1)
fragmented s.
Fregoli s.
Freud s.
Frohlich s.
frontal lobe s.
full s.
full-blown s.
functional psychiatric s.
Ganser s.
G-D s.
Gelineau s.
gender difference psychiatric s.
gender dysphoria s.
general adaptation s. (GAS)
Gilles de la Tourette s.
Gjessing s.
Goliath s.
Gowers s.
gray-out s.
Guillain-Barré s.
Gulf War s.

S

NOTES

663

syndrome *(continued)*

hallucinatory transient organic s.
hallucinatory-type psychoorganic s.
happy puppet s.
headache s.
head-bobbing doll s.
Heller s.
hepatorenal s.
Herrmann s.
holiday s.
hospital addiction s.
housewife s.
hyperactive child s. (HACS)
hyperkinetic s.
hyperkinetic behavior s. (HBS)
hypersensitivity s.
hyperventilation s. (HVS)
hypokinetic s.
immune deficiency s.
impostor s.
indifference to pain s.
infectious-exhaustive s.
intensive care s.
interictal behavior s.
intermediate brain s.
intoxication s.
irritable s.
irritable bowel s. (IBS)
isolation s.
Joubert s.
jumping Frenchmen of Maine s.
Kallmann s.
Kanner s.
Kleine-Levin s.
Klinefelter s.
Klippel-Feil s.
Klüver-Bucy s.
koro s.
Korsakoff s.
Krabbe s.
lacunar s.
Landau-Kleffner s.
Landry-Guillain-Barré s.
latah s.
Laurence-Biedl s.
Laurence-Moon s.
Laurence-Moon-Bardet-Biedl s.
Laurence-Moon-Biedl s.
laxative abuse s. (LAS)
Lesch-Nyhan s.
lobotomy s.
Louis-Bar s.
Madame Butterfly s.
Mad Hatter s.
Magenblase s.
Main s.
major psychiatric s.
male climacteric s.

manic s.
manic-depressive s.
Marie-Robinson s.
marker X s.
Martin-Bell s.
Mast s.
maternal deprivation s.
medial frontal lobe s.
medical s.
medullary s.
Millard-Gubler s.
Milles s.
mood swing s.
Moore s.
Morgagni s.
Moynahan s.
Muenzer-Rosenthal s.
multi-impulsivity s.
Munchausen by proxy s.
myasthenic s.
narcolepsy cataplexy s.
neglect s.
nest s.
Neumann s.
neurobehavioral s.
neurogenic shock s.
neuroleptic malignant s. (NMS)
neurotic reaction brain s.
Nielsen s.
night-eating s.
nocturnal drinking s.
nocturnal eating s.
non-24-hour sleep-wake s.
nonpsychotic posttraumatic brain s.
nonpsychotic severity
  psychoorganic s.
nonsense s.
nonspecific s.
nonspecific neurotic s. (NSN)
Nothnagel s.
obsession s.
obsessional s.
old-sergeant s.
olfactory reference s.
opiate abstinence s.
Oppenheim s.
orbitomedial s.
organic affective s.
organic-affective s.
organic amnestic s.
organic brain s. (OBS)
organic hallucinosis s.
organic mental s. (OMS)
organic mood s.
oriental nightmare-death s.
orofaciodigital s.
Othello s.
pain dysfunction s. (PDS)

pain, touch and stroke psychiatric s.
pallidal s.
paranoia and delusions psychiatric s.
paranoid-type psycho-organic s.
s. pattern
Pepper s.
persecution s.
Persian Gulf War s.
personality s.
phantom lover s.
phencyclidine mixed organic brain s.
phobic s.
piblokto s.
Pick s.
pickwickian s.
Pinel-Haslam s.
Pisa s.
polysymptomatic s.
pontocerebellar angle s.
postabortion s.
postadrenalectomy s.
postconcentration camp s.
postconcussion s.
post contusion s.
postencephalitic s.
posterior inferior cerebellar artery s.
postleukotomy s.
postlobotomy s.
postpartum s.
post rape s.
posttraumatic amnestic s.
posttraumatic brain s.
posttraumatic stress s.
post-Vietnam psychiatric s. (PVNPS)
POW s.
premenstrual s. (PMS)
premenstrual tension s. (PMTS)
premotor s.
prisoner of war s.
professional patient s.
protracted withdrawal s.
proxy-for-deficit s.
pseudocyesis s.
psychiatric s.
psychic shock s.
psychogenic effort s.
psychogenic nocturnal polydipsia s.

psychogenic purpura s.
psychological s.
psychomimic s.
psychoorganic brain s.
psychotic posttraumatic brain s.
punch-drunk s.
purple people s.
putatively poor-prognosis deficit s.
rape trauma s.
rapid time-zone change s.
rapture-of-the-deep s.
Ray s.
Renpenning s.
restless legs s.
retirement s.
Rett s.
reversible affective disorder s.
revolving door s.
Richardson-Steele-Olszewski s.
Richards-Rundel s.
rigid akinetic s.
Riley-Day s.
Rosenthal s.
Rubinstein-Taybi s.
rumination s.
Russell s.
Sanfilippo s.
Saunders-Sutton s.
Scheid cyanotic s.
Schirmer s.
schizoaffective s.
schizophrenic s.
school refusal s.
seasonal affective disorder s.
seasonal energy s.
Seckel s.
senile brain s.
sensory deprivation s. (SDS)
sensory dissociation s.
shock s.
silver cord s.
sleep phase s.
sleep-related abnormal swallowing s.
sleep-related myoclonus s.
Smith-Lemli-Opitz s.
smoker's s.
social breakdown s. (SBS)
social deprivation s.
social disability s.
social-isolation s.
solitary hunter s.

NOTES

S

syndrome (*continued*)
Sotos s.
spasmodic laughter s.
spasmodic winking s.
specific neurotic s. (SNR)
spiritual emergence s.
startle s.
steroid withdrawal s.
Stewart-Morel s.
Stockholm s.
stress response s.
subacute psychoorganic s.
subclavian steal s.
subclinical s.
substance-induced s.
substance-related s.
sudden infant death s. (SIDS)
Sudeck s.
suicide survivor s.
sundown s.
sundowner s.
survivor s.
tabagism s.
Taijin-Kyofusho s.
Tapia s.
tardive Tourette s.
tea and toast s.
temporal lobe s.
teratogenic s.
testicular feminization s. (TFS)
time zone-change s.
Todeserwartung s.
Tolosa-Hunt s.
Tourette s. (TS)
trait-like s.
trisomy s.
vasovagal s.
vibration s.
victim s.
Vietnam s.
VIP s.
visual hallucination denial s.
vulnerable child s.
Wernicke s.
Wernicke-Korsakoff s.
Werther s.
Westphal-Leyden s.
wet brain s.
Wilson s.
Windigo culture-specific s.
winking spasmodic s.
withdrawal s.
Wittmaak-Ekbom s.
wounded victim s.
Wyburn-Mason s.
Zange-Kindler s.
Zanoli-Vecchi s.
Zappert s.

syndromic
s. depression
s. pattern
synergetic
synergic
s. control
s. marriage
synergism
sexual s.
synergistic
synergy
synesthesia
s. algica
auditory s.
synesthesialgia
synesthetic stimulation
synkinesia
synkinesis
synkinetic motor movement
synonymous
synostosis
syntactic
s. aphasia
s. category
s. complexity
s. rule
syntality
syntaxic
s. language
s. mode
s. mode of experience
s. thought
synthesis, pl. **syntheses**
analysis by s.
analysis and s.
distributive analysis and s.
dopamine s.
illegal drug s.
illicit drug s.
perceptual s.
synthesizing ability
synthetic
s. drug dependence
s. function
s. heroin dependence
s. method
syntone
syntonic
ego s.
s. personality
syntropic
syntropy
syphilis
cerebral s.
CNS s.
meningovascular s.
psychosis of s.

secondary s.
tertiary s.
syphilitic
s. alopecia
s. cirrhosis
s. meningitis
s. meningoencephalitis
s. paralytic dementia
s. progressive dementia
syphilitica
alopecia s.
syphilology
syphilomania
syphilopsychosis
syringe
syringeal
syringobulbia
syringoid
syringomyelia
syringomyelic
syringomyelus
syringopontia
system
action s.
activity s.
adaptive control of thought s.
adolescent support s.
Aesculap ABC cervical plating s.
alcohol-metabolizing s.
antireward s.
ascending neurotransmitter s.
ascending reticular activating s.
auditory s.
autonomic nervous s. (ANS)
behavior s.
behavioral activation s. (BAS)
behavioral inhibition s. (BIS)
biomedical monitoring s. (BMS)
biophysical s.
Bleuler diagnostic s.
boarding-out s.
brain dopaminergic s.
Brown Schools Behavioral
Health S.
categorical s.
central nervous s. (CNS)
cerebrospinal s.
circadian s.
classification s.
closed-loop feedback s.
Committee on Information S.'s
community support s.

conceptual nervous s.
criminal justice s.
decision support s.
delusional s.
dimensional s.
direct motor s.
disposition s.
dopamine s.
dopaminergic s.
drug risk analysis message s.
(DRAMS)
Dyadic Parent-Child Interaction
Coding S.
dysfunctional dopamine s.
epicritic s.
ergotropic s.
ertotropid s.
esthesiodic s.
expert s.
external support s.
extrapyramidal s. (EPS)
extrapyramidal motor s.
Facial Action Coding S. (FACS)
family support s.
feedback s.
feeding s.
first-signal s.
five-axis s.
fixed delusional s.
focus of delusional s.
foster care s.
haptic s.
hemodynamic s.
honor s.
hypothalamic-pituitary-
adrenocortical s.
immune s.
incentive s.
indirect motor s.
innate response s.
integrated ECT s.
interactive voice response s.
internal second messenger s.
intracellular second messenger s.
justice s.
juvenile justice s.
kinship s.
knowledge information processing s.
(KIPS)
Kraepelin diagnostic s.
life support s.
limbic s.

NOTES

system *(continued)*
 malevolent thought s.
 man-machine s.
 medial temporal memory s.
 medical value s.
 memory s.
 mental health s.
 miniature s.
 mnemonic s.
 motor s.
 multiaxial classification s.
 multistate information s. (MSIS)
 National Association of Psychiatric
  Health S.'s (NAPHS)
 nervous s.
 neural s.
 neurotransmitter s.
 nicotine transdermal s.
 nonspecific s.
 noradrenergic s.
 norepinephrine neurotransmitter s.'s
 paranoid belief s.
 parasympathetic nervous s. (PNS)
 peripheral nervous s. (PNS)
 persecutory delusional s.
 personality assessment s. (PAS)
 Pinel s.
 s. to plan early childhood services
  (SPECS)
 preferred representational s.
 pride s.
 private belief s.
 psi s.
 psychodynamic cerebral s.
 psychological defense s.
 psychological information,
  acquisition, processing, and
  control s. (PIAPACS)
 psychologic defense s.
 quota s.
 reality s.
 religious value s.
 representational s.
 response s.
 reticular activating s. (RAS)
 reticuloendothelial s.
 review of s.'s (ROS)
 reward s.
 school support s.
 second messenger s.
 second signaling s.
 sensorimotor s.
 serotonergic s.
 serotonin s.
 sleep-wake s.
 somatosensory s.
 somesthetic s.
 specific s.
 speech perception s.
 stereotaxic coordinate s.
 support s.
 sympathetic nervous s. (SNS)
 thalamic reticular activating s.
 theoretical s.
 thermoregulatory s.
 third nervous s.
 thought s.
 transmitter s.
 value s.
 vegetative nervous s.
 ventricular s.
 villa s.
 visceral nervous s.
 welfare s.
 well-systematized delusional s.

systematic
 s. comparison
 s. desensitization
 s. drug administration
 s. family therapy
 s. followup
 s. inquiry (SI)
 s. method
 s. process
 s. quantitative observation
 s. rational restructuring (SRR)
 s. reinforcement
 s. review
 s. schizophrenia
 s. study
 s. vertigo

systematica
 paraphrenia s.

systematic, complete, objective, practical, empirical (SCOPE)

systematique
 delire chronique a evolution s.

systematization

systematized
 s. amnesia
 s. assertive therapy (SAT)
 s. delusion

systemic
 s. assertive therapy
 s. delusion
 s. desensitization
 s. family
 s. impact

systems-based learning

systolic pressure (SP)

SZ
 schizophrenia

T

T group
T ratio
T score
T score elevation

TA

test age
transactional analysis

TAB

therapeutic abortion

tabagism syndrome

tabes

juvenile t.
peripheral t.
t. spasmodica
t. spinalis

tabetic

t. crisis
t. cuirass
t. form paralytic dementia
t. psychosis

tabetiform
tabic
tabid
table

life t.
somatron t.

tablet
taboo, tabu

t. emotion
incest t.
social t.
virginity t.

taboparesis
tabula rasa
tabular index
tabulation
tache
tachistoscope
tachycardia

psychogenic paroxysmal t.

tachylalia
tachylogia
tachyphagia
tachyphasia
tachyphemia
tachyphrasia
tachyphrenia
tachyphylaxis
tachypnea
tachypneic
tachypragia
tachypsychia
tachytrophism
tactical maneuver
tactics

guerrilla t.

tactile

t. agnosia
t. alexia
t. amnesia
t. anesthesia
t. anomia
t. aphasia
t. aphonia
t. extinction
t. feedback
t. genital stimulation
t. hallucination
t. hyperactivity
t. hyperesthesia
t. illusion
t. image
t. imagery
t. kinesthetic perception
t. sensation
t. sense
t. sensory difficulty
t. sensory modality
t. stimulus

tactile-perceptual disorder
tactility
tactometer
tactual hallucination
Tadoma method
tae kwon do
tag

medical identification t.

tagger

graffiti t.

TAI

Test Anxiety Inventory

tai chi
Taijin-Kyofusho syndrome
tailor's

t. cramp
t. spasm

taint
take

t. advantage
t. charge
double t.
t. down
t. for granted
t. heart
t. issue
t. out

take-home pay
taken out of context
taker

risk t.

taking control

T

talbutal
tale
    tall t.'s
    tell a t. (TAT)
talent
    creative t.
    grandiose delusion of exceptional t.
    special t.
talion
    t. dread
    t. law
    t. principle
talionis
    lex t.
talipes spasmodicus
talisman
talk
    baby t.
    back t.
    t. down
    facial t.
    t. out
    t. over
    pep t.
    small t.
    street t.
    suicide t.
    t. therapy
    t. up
talkative
talkativeness
talk-down
    t.-d. from overdose
    supportive t.-d.
talking
    t. back behavior
    t. cure
    excessive t.
    t. fear
    t. it out
tall tales
tandem reinforcement
tangent
tangential
    t. association
    t. layer
    t. speech
    t. thinking
tangentiality
tangere
    noli me t.
tangle
tank
    think t.
tannate
tantalize
tantamount
tantra

tantric yoga
tantrum
    temper t.
taoism
taoist
tap
    glabellar t.
    heel t.
    spinal t.
taper
    double t.
    slow double t.
tapering
    drug t.
    medication t.
tapeworm fear
taphophilia
Tapia syndrome
tapping compulsion
TaqIA
Taractan
tarantism
tarantulism
Tarasoff
    T. case
    T. decision
    T. principle
    T. rule
    T. warning
Tarchanoff phenomenon
tarda
tardive
    t. dementia
    t. dyskinesia
    t. dystonia
    forme t.
    t. tic
    t. Tourette syndrome
tardy epilepsy
target
    t. of aggression
    t. behavior
    bullying t.
    t. language
    t. multiplicity
    t. organ
    t. patient
    t. population
    potential t.
    t. response
    t. stimulus
    t. symptom
    therapeutic t.
    t. weight
targeted
    t. approach
    t. intervention
    t. medication

tarot card
tartrate
TAS
    turning against self
task
    auditory continuous performance t.
    cognitive t.
    t. completion
    complex multistep t.
    developmental t.
    dichotic listening t.
    dot-probe t.
    t. of emotional development (TED)
    forced-choice span of
      apprehension t.
    t. force on electroconvulsive
      therapy
    t. force on local arrangements
    T. Force on Sexually Dangerous
      Offenders
    t. of independent living
    instrumental t.
    t. inventory
    lateralized rapid activating t.
    learning t.
    linguistic content of t.
    manipulatory t.
    memory t.
    mental status cognitive t.
    modal adaptive t.
    motor t.
    multistep t.
    necessary t.
    neuropsychologically relevant t.
    nine-digit t.
    nonverbal t.
    novel memory t.
    novel recall t.
    particular t.
    performance t.
    t. performance
    t. performance and analysis
    practiced t.
    primary t.
    repetitive t.
    required t.
    retrieval t.
    sentence-closure t.
    sentence-repetition t.
    sequencing t.
    simple t.
    spatial t.

    speech tracking t.
    stay on t.
    structured t.
    theory of mind t.
    three-step t.
    unemotional learning t.
    visual memory span t.
    visual-motor t.
    work-related t.
task-accuracy
    continuous performance t.-a. (CPT-
      ACC)
task-efficiency
    continuous performance t.-e. (CPT-
      EFF)
task-oriented
    t.-o. approach
    t.-o. assessment
    t.-o. group
    t.-o. reaction
taste
    t. blindness
    color t.
    t. fear
    t. imagery
    t. sensation
    t. threshold
TAT
    tell a tale
tattered clothing
tattle
tattletale
tattoo
tau
    t. processing
    t. protein peptide
taunt
taurine
taut facial skin
tautological
tautologous
tautology
tautophone
taxometric analysis
taxonic
taxonomic research
taxonomy
    t. of anger disorder
    biologic t.
    personality disorder t.
Taylor
    T. series linearization method

NOTES

taylorism
TBI
    traumatic brain injury
TBRS
    timed behavioral rating sheet
TC
    therapeutic community
TCA
    tricyclic antidepressant
    tricyclic antipsychotic
TCAD
    tricyclic antidepressant drug
T-cell proliferation
TCET
    transcerebral electrotherapy
TCP
    teacher-child-parent
TCSW
    thinking creatively with sounds and
      words
TD
    threshold of discomfort
TDE
    thiamine deficiency encephalopathy
TDF
    thinking disturbance factor
T&E
    testing and evaluation
Te
    tetanic contraction
tea and toast syndrome
teacher
    t. attitude inventory
    t. inventory
teacher-child-parent (TCP)
teacher-student
    t.-s. model
    t.-s. relationship
teaching
    clinical t.
    diagnostic t.
    t. hospital
    religious t.'s
    remedial t.
team
    t. building
    crisis t.
    interdisciplinary t. (IDT)
    t. leader (TL)
    t. member (TM)
    mobile crisis outreach t.
    t. player
    psychiatric emergency t. (PET)
    psychiatry emergency t.
    support t.
    treatment t.
    two-person interview t.
teammate
teamwork

tear
    t. at
    t. away
    crocodile t.'s
    t. down
    t. gas
    t. up
teardrop
tearfulness
    breakthrough t.
    momentary t.
    unexplained t.
tearful outburst
tea and toast syndrome
technicality
technical limitation
technician
    emergency medical t. (EMT)
    psychiatric t.
technique
    activation t.
    active daydream t.
    adaptive t.
    anxiety control t.
    arousal reduction t.
    ascending t.
    assets-liabilities t.
    average evoked response t.
    backward making t.
    ballet t.
    Bayesian t.
    behavioral t.
    bell and pad t.
    blind matching t.
    breathing t.
    brief stimuli t.
    capping t.
    clinical monitoring t.
    cognitive t.
    cognitive-behavioral t.
    compensatory t.
    corrective t.
    critical-incident t.
    descending t.
    differential diagnostic t.
    effective t.
    effort-shape t.
    empty-chair t.
    fast gradient recalled spectroscopic
      imaging t.
    feeding t.
    functional imaging t.
    glissando t.
    graphomotor t.
    Hartel t.
    head turn t.
    homogenate t.
    hot-seat t.

interview t.
interviewing t.
kinesthetic t.
Luria t.
manipulative t.
microelectrode t.
mirror t.
monitoring t.
morphometric t.
multiple regression t.
multivariate t.
observation t.
paradoxical t.
picture in picture t.
plain-folks t.
plateau masking t.
play t.
positron emission tomography t.
postmortem t.
projective t.
psychoanalytic t.
psychological t.
Q t.
Q-Sort t.
quantitative morphometric t.
reattribution t.
relapse-prevention t.
relaxation t.
replacement t.
rest-cure t.
Rorschach projective t.
self-control t.
self-soothing t.
semiautomated spatial
  normalization t.
shadowing masking t.
shift masking t.
short-term psychotherapy t.
standardized cognitive assessment t.
startle t.
state-of-the-art analysis t.
stop-and-think t.
stop-start t.
sucking t.
threshold shift-masking t.
time-out t.
uncovering t.
utilization t.
verbal t.
word association t.
technological
t. detection of deceit

t. illiteracy
t. limitation
technology
genetic t.
information t.
tecum
subpoena duces t.
TED
task of emotional development
tedious
tedium
teen
t.'s in crisis
frightened t.
t. killer
rebellious t.
t. silence
troubled t.
victimized t.
t. violence
teenage
t. father
t. smoking behavior
t. suicide
t. violence
teenager
antisocial t.
teetotaler
teetotalism
teetotalist
tegmental
teichopsia
telalgia
telangiectasia
teleceptor
telegnosis
telegrammatism
telehealth
telekinesis
telemnemonike
telencephalic
t. fusion
t. sleep
telencephalization
teleoanalysis
teleologic
t. hallucination
t. regression
teleological
teleology
teleonomic
teleonomy

T

NOTES

telepathic dream
telepathy
telephone
    t. scatologia
    t. sex
teleplasm
telepsychiatry
telergy
telescopia
telesis
telesthesia
teletactor
television
    closed-circuit t. (CCTV)
    sexually charged t.
    t. violence
    violent acts on t.
telling
    principle of truth t.
tell a tale (TAT)
telltale sign
temerarious
temerity
temper
    t. dyscontrol
    evil t.
    explosive t.
    hot t.
    t. outburst
    short t.
    t. tantrum
    violent t.
    volatile t.
temperament
    hyperaesthetic variant of schizoid t.
    hyperthymic t.
    manic t.
    psychiatrically demanding t.
    t. trait
temperamental
temperance
temperate
temperature
    ambient t.
    basal t.
    t. biofeedback
    core t.
    core body t.
    t. effect
    t. erotism
    t. fluctuation
    t., pulse, respiration (TPR)
    t. sensation
    t. sense
    t. spot
tempestuous course
template
    diagnostic t.

temple
tempo
    conceptual t.
temporal
    t. association
    t. characteristic
    t. contiguity
    t. cortex
    t. cortices
    t. course
    t. dynamics
    t. hallucination
    t. headache
    t. integration deficit
    t. lobe
    t. lobectomy
    t. lobe epilepsy (TLE)
    t. lobe illusion
    t. lobe seizure
    t. lobe status
    t. lobe syndrome
    t. neocortical association area
    t. organization
    t. orientation
    t. pattern
    t. perspective
    t. relationship
    t. resolution
    t. speech region
    t. sulcus
    t. tissue
temporale
    planum t.
temporal, occipital, parietal (TOP)
temporal-perceptual disorder
temporarily disabled
temporary
    t. admission
    t. commitment
    t. deafness
    t. disability
    t. epilation
    t. habit
    t. personality disorder
    t. stress
    t. threshold shift (TTS)
temporizer
temptation
    fits of horrific t.
    horrific t.
tempting
tenable
tenacious
tenacity
tenancy
tendency, pl. tendencies
    acting out t.
    t. of action

anagogic t.
antisocial t.
central t.
cognitive t.
dependence t.
destructive t.
dissociative t.
evasive t.
excitement-seeking t.
familial t.
final t.
hypomanic t.
impulsive t.
introversive t.
katagogic t.
measure of central t.
narcissistic t.
paranoid t.
repeat t.
seductive t.
self-absorbed t.
sleep t.
somatization t.
suicide t.
tender-minded t.
tough-minded t.
t. toward amelioration
t. wit
tendentious apperception
tender
t. loving care (TLC)
t. minded
t. point
t. years presumption
t. zone
tenderhearted
tender-minded tendency
tenderness
tendinum
subsultus t.
tremor t.
tendon
tenement
tenens
locum t.
tenesmus penis
tenet
t.'s of faith
religious t.
tense gaze
tenseness
tensile

tensiometer
tension
combat t.
conjugal t.
emotional t.
inner t.
instinctual t.
marked t.
mental t.
t. migraine
t. migraine headache
muscular t.
need t.
nervous t.
physical t.
premenstrual t.
t. reduction
t. reduction therapy
sexual t.
social t.
t. state
t. state psychoneurotic reaction
stimulus t.
tension-reduction theory
tension-vascular headache
tensity
tentative
t. diagnosis
t. finding
tenuous
tenure
job t.
teonanactl
tephromalacia
tephrylometer
teratogen
teratogenic
t. syndrome
teratogenicity
behavioral t.
morphologic t.
teratologic defect
teratology
mammalian t.
terephthalate
tergiversate
tergiversation
tergo
coitus a t.
term
abstract t.
coin new slang t.'s

T

NOTES

term *(continued)*
    intellectualized t.'s
    interaction t.
    psychometric t.
terminal
    t. achievement behavior
    axon t.
    delire t.
    t. dementia
    t. insomnia
    t. lag
    t. neuronal field
    t. region
    t. reinforcement
    t. reinforcement psychotherapy
    t. sulcus
    t. tremor
    video lottery t. (VLT)
terminalis
    stria t.
terminally ill
terminate relationship
termination
    t. issue
    t. of pregnancy
    t. of therapy
terminological obfuscation
terpin
terrestial
terrifying
    t. experience
    t. stimulus
territorial
    t. aggression
    t. dominance
territoriality
territorialize
territory
    interaction t.
    vascular t.
terror
    t. dream
    night t.
    reign of t.
    sleep t.
terrorism
    t. behavior
    fear of t.
    mass t.
terrorist
    t. attack
    t. violence
terrorize
terse
tertiary
    t. amine tricyclic antidepressant
      drug
    t. care

    t. circular reaction
    t. gain
    t. intervention program
    t. prevention
    t. stress
    t. syphilis
tertiary-process thinking
test
    ability t.
    absurdities t.
    accuracy t.
    achievement t. (AT)
    acid t.
    acoustic immittance measurement t.
    adrenaline-Mecholyl t.
    t. age (TA)
    aiming t.
    alpha verbal t.
    alternate response t.
    alternate uses t.
    amphetamine challenge t.
    analyst anchor t.
    anchor t.
    Anstie t.
    t. anxiety
    T. Anxiety Inventory (TAI)
    aphasia screening t.
    apperception t.
    apprehension t.
    aptitude t.
    art t.
    articulation t.
    association t.
    attention alertness t.
    ball-and-field t.
    baseline t.
    t. of basic experience
    t. battery
    battery of online t.
    beta t.
    binomial t.
    blind t.
    block design t.
    blood screen for drugs t.
    Bolgar-Fischer Word T.
    brain t.
    calculation t.
    cancellation t.
    carotid ultrasound t.
    Carrow Receptive Language T.
    t. case
    cause-and-effect t.
    ceruloplasmin t.
    challenge t.
    chi-square t.
    city and state t.
    classification t.
    clock face t.

code t.
cognitive t.
color sorting t.
combining power t. (CPT)
completion, arithmetic, vocabulary, and directions t.
complex thematic pictures t.
comprehensive t.
t. condition
confrontation naming t.
copy geometric designs t.
copy intersecting pentagons t.
could not t. (CNT)
count backwards from 100 t.
creativity t.
t. of criminal responsibility
criterion-referenced t.
cumulative t.
day of month t.
delayed-alteration t.
delayed-matching t.
development t.
developmental hand-function t. (DHFT)
digit repetition t.
digit reversal t.
dominance t.
drawing t.
Durham t.
educational t.
empirical t.
Expressive One Word Picture Vocabulary T.
eye blink conditioning t.
fables t.
face-hand t.
FES figure-drawing t.
finger-to-finger t.
fund of information t.
grip-strength t.
group t.
hand t. (HT)
head-dropping t.
heel-tap t.
heel-to-knee t.
hyperventilation t.
identification t.
immediate memory t.
individual t.
infant and preschool t.
intelligence t.
t. interpretation

interpretation t.
inventory t.
IQ t.
job-specific t.
knowledge t.
Knox Cube T.
literacy t.
liver function t.
logical memory t.
making change t.
matching t.
memory t.
mental status t.
methylphenidate challenge t.
misplaced objects t.
M'Naghten t.
motor performance t.
multi-item t.
multiplication table t.
Myers-Briggs psychological t.
neuropsychiatric t.
neuropsychologic t.
neuropsychometric t.
nocturnal penile tumescence t.
number 3 traced on patient's palm t.
t. object
object t. (OT)
objective t. (OT)
object reversal t.
occupational t.
oral t.
orientation-memory-concentration t.
t. orientation procedure (TOP)
paragraph-meaning t.
paragraph recall t.
paternity t.
perceptual-identification t.
performance t.
peripheral cue t.
personality t.
personnel t.
picture vocabulary t.
point localization t.
t. point scale
t. protocol
psychoeducational t.
psycholinguistic t.
psychologic t.
psychological t.
psychometric t.
psychomotor t.

T

NOTES

test *(continued)*
    psychopenetration t.
    psychophysiological t.
    quantitative t. (Q)
    reaction t.
    readiness t.
    reality t.
    recall of information t.
    recall 5 items after 5 minutes t.
    relations t.
    repetition t.
    reversal t.
    reverse digit span recall t.
    right-wrong t.
    Romberg t.
    rotation t.
    Schirmer t.
    screening t.
    self-rating t.
    sensory-perceptual t.
    Shortened Edinburgh Reading T.'s
    short orientation-memory-concentration t. (OMC)
    t. of significance
    similarities mental status t.
    situational t.
    sobriety t.
    sorting t.
    span recall t.
    speech discrimination t.
    spontaneity t.
    standardization of a t.
    standardized t. (ST)
    standard laboratory t.
    station t.
    stem-completion t.
    stimulant challenge t.
    sweep-cheek t.
    t. of syntactic ability (TSA)
    thematic picture t.
    tolerance t.
    visual choice reaction time t.
    visual distortion t. (VDT)
    visual threat t.
    vocabulary t.
    WAIS-R Block Design T.
    Weber t.
    Western blot t.
    word-building t.
    work-limit t.
testamentary capacity
testicular
    t. feminization mutation (TFM)
    t. feminization syndrome (TFS)
    t. hypofunction
testimonial privilege

testimony
    expert t.
    psychiatric t.
testing
    adaptive t.
    air conduction t.
    American College of T. (ACT)
    attention t.
    cognitive t.
    continuous cognitive t.
    cortical t.
    cross-cultural t.
    cultural t.
    demarcation in sensory t.
    diminished reality t.
    t. and evaluation (T&E)
    formal t.
    functional gain t.
    gross impairment of reality t.
    hypothesis t.
    mental t.
    motivation analysis t.
    multiple-choice t.
    neurophysiological t.
    neuropsychologic t.
    t., orientation, and work
    t., orientation, and work evaluation for rehabilitation (TOWER)
    psychological t.
    psychometric t.
    random urine t.
    reality ability t.
    school-age t.
    urine t.
testis
    irritable t.
testosterone
    serum t.
test-retest
    t.-r. reliability
    t.-r. reliability coefficient
testy
tetania
    t. parathyreopriva
    t. rheumatica
tetanic
    t. contraction (Te)
    t. convulsion
    t. seizure
    t. stimulation
tetaniform
tetanigenous
tetanilla
tetanism
tetanization
tetanode
tetanoid
    t. chorea

t. epilepsy
t. paraplegia
tetanometer
tetanomotor
tetanus
benign t.
cephalic t.
cerebral t.
drug t.
extensor t.
flexor t.
head t.
imitative t.
t. neonatorum
t. posticus
Ritter opening t.
toxic t.
tetany
t. of alkalosis
duration t. (DT)
hyperventilation t.
infantile t.
latent t.
manifest t.
postoperative t.
tetchy
tete-a-tete
tetrachloride
carbon t.
tetrad
narcoleptic t.
tetrahydrobiopterin
tetrahydrocannabinol (THC)
t. dependence
tetraparesis
tetrapeptide
tetraplegia
tetrasomy
teutonomania
text
t. blindness
pragmatic t.
textbook case
textual description
texture
causal t.
t. response
TF
transvestic fetishism
TFM
testicular feminization mutation

TFS
testicular feminization syndrome
TGA
transient global amnesia
thalamic
t. dementia
t. epilepsy
t. region
t. response
t. reticular activating system
thalamocortical activity
thalamus
anterior nucleus of t.
t. overactivity in OCD
pulvinar nucleus of t.
t. tissue
thalassomania
thalassoposia
thallium poisoning
thanatobiologic
thanatognomonic
thanatography
thanatology
thanatopsia
thanatopsis
thanatopsy
thanatos
thankless
thank-you theory
thaumaturgic
thaumaturgy
THC
tetrahydrocannabinol
THC dependence
Theater of Spontaneity
theatricalism
theatrics
theatromania
theft
drug t.
opportunity for t.
theism
thematic
t. paralogia
t. paraphasia
t. paraphrasia
t. picture test
t. role
thematically related groups
theme
central t.
common t.

T

NOTES

theme *(continued)*
  core conflictual relationship t.
  cultural t.
  death t.
  depressed mood t.
  deserved punishment t.
  disease t.
  grandiose t.
  guilt t.
  identity t.
  inflated worth t.
  t. interference
  knowledge t.
  manic mood t.
  mythological t.
  nihilism t.
  persecution t.
  personal inadequacy t.
  power t.
  recurring t.
  religious t.
  self-derogatory t.
  special relationship to deity t.
  special relationship to famous
    person t.
  typical t.
  violent t.
themomatic paralogia
theocracy
theologian
theologic
  t. issue
  t. matters
theologize
theology
  natural t.
theomania
theonomous
theophany
theorem
  central-limit t.
theoretical
  t. assumption
  t. implication
  t. orientation
  t. system
  t. understanding
theorist
  defect t.
theorize
theory
  abstract t.
  adaptation level t.
  Adler t.
  adlerian t.
  affective-arousal t.
  aggressive behavior t.
  aging t.

Allport group relations t.
Allport personality trait t.
t. of anxiety
anxiety sensitivity t.
arousal t.
attachment t.
attitude t.
attribution t.
balance t.
behavioral t.
behavior-constraint t.
biofeedback t.
biolinguistic language t.
biologic t.
biosocial t.
Burn and Rand t.
Cannon t.
Cannon-Bard t.
catastrophe t.
causal-attributional t.
classical psychoanalytical t.
clinical t.
cloacal t.
t. of cognition
cognitive dissonance t.
cognitive learning t.
color t.
communication t.
t. of constitutional bisexuality
constitutional bisexuality t.
continuum t.
crisis t.
cross-linkage t.
cybernetic t.
decay t.
decision t.
degeneracy t.
deontologic t.
developmental t.
dietary t.
ding-dong t.
double blind t.
drive reduction t.
dual-instinct t.
dual-process t.
ego alter t.
emergency t.
emotive t.
empiricist t.
environmental learning t.
environmental load t.
environmental stress t.
epigenetic t.
equity t.
etiology t.
evolution t.
exclamation t.

existence, relatedness, and growth t. (ERG)
existential-humanistic t.
expectancy t.
factor t.
family systems t.
field t.
Flourens t.
focal conflict t.
Freud t.
freudian t.
game t.
gate t.
gate-control t.
gating t.
general systems t.
genetic t.
gestalt t.
group relations t.
hearing t.
Hilgard neo-dissociation t.
humanistic t.
human-motivation t.
humoral t.
iceblock t.
immanence t.
implicit personality t.
incentive t.
information t.
innateness t.
interference t.
interpersonal t.
item response t. (IRT)
James-Lange-Sutherland t.
Jung t.
jungian t.
Klein suffocation alarm t.
labeling t.
language t.
leadership t.
learning t.
libido t.
life cycle t.
life-event stress t.
mass action t.
memory t.
Meyer t.
miasma t.
t. of mind
t. of mind task
mixture t.
mnemenic t.

mnemism t.
t. of mnemism
moral t.
nativist t.
object relations t.
observational learning t.
periodicity t.
personal construct t.
personality trait t.
person-centered t.
phonatory t.
place t.
psychoanalytical t.
psychodynamic t.
psycholinguistic t.
psychological t.
quantum t.
rankian t.
rapid-change t.
rapid-smoking t.
ratification t.
response t.
rival normative t.
rogerian t.
role-enactment t.
Semon-Hering t.
sensorimotor t.
social causation t.
social dominance t.
t. of social dominance
social learning t.
social selection t.
societal reaction t.
Spearman two-factor t.
steppingstone t.
stimulus-response t.
stuttering block t.
tension-reduction t.
thank-you t.
three-component t.
topographical t.
total composite t.
trace-decay t.
trait t.
understimulation t.
utilitarian t.
violence t.
vulnerability t.
watchspring t.
Wollaston t.
X-bar t.

theosophist

NOTES

681

theosophy
theoterrorism
theotherapy
therapeusis
therapeutic
    t. abortion (TAB)
    t. advantage
    t. agent
    t. alliance
    t. approach
    t. atmosphere
    t. blood level
    t. botulinum neurotoxin
clinical t.
    t. communication
    t. community (TC)
    t. connection
    t. contract
    t. contribution
    t. crisis
    t. dose
    t. dose dependence
    t. drug holiday
    t. effect
    t. efficacy
    t. electric stimulation
    t. environment
    t. exercise
    t. exploration
    t. failure
    t. gender neutrality
    t. goal
    t. group
    t. group analysis
    t. impasse
    t. index
    t. insight
    t. intervention
    t. malaria
    t. matrix
    t. measure
    t. milieu
    t. modality
    t. nihilism
    t. optimism
    t. option
    t. outcome
    t. pessimism
    t. play group (TPG)
    t. process
    t. profile
    t. program
    t. range
    t. reaction (TR)
    t. recreation
    t. relationship
    t. relaxation
    t. response

    t. role
    t. safety
    t. school placement
    t. strategy
    t. success
    t. target
    t. trial
    t. trial visit (TTV)
    t. vocational placement
    t. window
therapeutically justified
therapeutist
therapia (*var. of* therapy)
therapist
    active t.
    activities t.
    t. authentication
    auxiliary t.
    corrective t.
    educational t.
    female t.
    group t.
    individual t.
    language t.
    licensed marriage and family t.
    male t.
    monkey t.
    movement t.
    t. obligation
    occupational t. (OT)
    passive t.
    physical t.
    registered recreation t. (RRT)
therapist-guided therapy
therapist-patient relationship
therapy, therapia (Rx)
    aboriginal t.
    active t.
    activity group t. (AGT)
    activity play t.
    acute t.
    adaptation-promoting t.
    adjunctive t.
    adjustment t.
    adjuvant t.
    administrative t.
    adolescent group t.
    adult group t.
    agonist t.
    alternative t.
    American Association for Marriage and Family T. (AAMFT)
    anaclitic t.
    analytic t.
    analytical play t.
    animal-assisted t.
    antiandrogen t.
    antidepressant t.

antiinflammatory t.
antioxidant t.
antipsychotic drug t.
apotreptic t.
art t.
assertion structured t.
assignment t.
Association for Advancement of
  Behavior T. (AABT)
Association for the Advancement
  of Gestalt T.
atropine coma t.
attitude t.
aversive t.
avoidance t.
ballet t.
behavioral couples group t.
behavioral marital t. (BMT)
behavior modification t.
bioenergetic t.
biologic t.
biomedical t.
body t.
branching steps in t.
brief group t.
brief stimulus t. (BST)
carbon dioxide t.
chelation t.
chemical aversion t.
child group t.
child-guidance t.
cholinergic t.
clay-modeling t.
client-centered t.
cloaca t.
cognitive analytic t. (CAT)
cognitive behavior t. (CBT)
cognitive behavioral group t.
  (CBGT)
cognitive enhancement t.
cognitive-physiological t.
cognitive remediation t.
collaborative t.
color t.
coma t.
combined t.
common sense t.
communication t.
computer-aided t.
computer-guided t.
concurrent t.
conditioned reflex t.

conditioning t.
conjoint t.
contextual t.
continuation t.
continuous sleep t.
contract t.
convulsive shock t.
cooperative t.
COPE computer software program
  for depression t.
corrective t. (CT)
corticoid t.
counselor-centered t.
couples group t.
couples sex t.
crisis t.
dance t.
delay t.
delayed t.
deliberate t.
dependence on t.
depot medication injection t.
depth t.
deterrent t.
diagnostic t.
dialectical behavior t. (DBT)
directed group t.
diversional t.
divorce t.
drug t.
dual-sex t.
dual transference t.
ego-oriented individual t.
ego-state t.
elective t.
electric shock t.
electroconvulsive t. (ECT)
electroconvulsive shock t. (ECST)
electroshock t. (ECT, EST, est)
electrosleep t. (ETS)
electrotherapeutic sleep t.
emotional control t.
emotional release t.
emotive t.
endocrine t.
environmental t.
estrogen replacement t.
exercise t.
existential-humanistic t.
experiential t.
experimental t.
exploratory t.

NOTES

therapy *(continued)*

exposure-based cognitive behavior t.
expressive t.
extended family t. (EFT)
family group t.
family member t.
family unit t.
FearFighter computer program tailored for specific fear t.
filial t.
first-line t.
fluency shaping t.
focused expressive t.
food t.
gestalt t.
t. goal
goal-limited adjustment t.
graphic-arts t.
grief t.
group t.
group adjustment t. (GAT)
helper t.
heroin antagonist and learning t. (HALT)
humanistic t.
imagery t.
implosion t.
implosive t.
inadequate t.   .
indirect method of t.
individual t. (IT)
individual marital t.
industrial t.
insight t.
inspirational group t.
instigation t.
integrated psychological t.
interaction-oriented group t.
interpersonal t. (IPT)
interpretive t.
interview t.
irritation t.
language t.
language enrichment t. (LET)
leaderless group t.
light t.
long-term t.
magnetic seizure t.
maintenance drug t.
major role t. (MRT)
marital couples group t.
marriage t.
mass t.
megavitamin t.
Metrazol shock t.
milieu t.
minimum-change t.
modified ECT t.

Morita t.
morning bright light t.
motivational enhancement t.
movement t.
multidimensional family t.
multimodal behavior t.
multiple family t.
multisystemic t. (MST)
music t. (MT)
musical t.
narrative t.
network t.
nicotine replacement t.
nonconfrontive t.
nondirective t.
nonphobic anxiety behavior t.
nutritional t.
occupational t. (OT)
old-age t.
online t.
operant t.
organic t.
orgone t.
outcome-based t.
oxygen t.
paradoxical t.
paraverbal t.
parent-child group t.
passive immunization t.
persuasion t.
physical t.
pineal t.
plastic arts t.
play t.
play group t. (PGT)
positive reinforcement t.
postelectroconvulsive t.
precision t.
primal scream t.
programmed t.
prolonged sleep t.
psychedelic t.
psychiatric somatic t.
psychoanalytic t.
psychodrama group t.
psychoeducation group t.
psychological t.
psychologic programming t.
psychopharmacological t.
psychotherapeutic t.
quadrangular t.
radical t.
rational t. (RT)
rational emotive t. (RET)
reality oriented t.
reconditioning t.
reconstructive t.
recreational t. (RT)

reeducative t.
reflex t.
relationship t.
relaxation t.
release t.
reminiscence t.
replacement t.
restitutive t.
restraining t.
restricted environment stimulation t.
  (REST)
rhythmic sensory bombardment t.
  (RSBT)
rogerian group t.
role t.
sabotage of t.
second-line t.
self-control t.
self-exposure t.
semantic t.
sensate-focus-oriented t.
t. session
sex t.
sexuality conversion t.
shame-aversion t.
shock t. (ST)
short-term t.
simulated presence t.
situational t.
sleep t.
sleep-electroshock t.
social interaction t.
social learning group t.
social network t.
socioenvironmental t.
solution-focused t.
somatic t.
sound t.
spectator t.
speech t.
standard antipsychotic t.
stimulant t.
stimulus t.
strategic family t.
structural family t.
structural-strategic t.
subcoma t.
subshock t.
substitutive agent t.
suggestion t.
supportive group t.
suppressive t.

symptomatic t.
systematic family t.
systematized assertive t. (SAT)
systemic assertive t.
talk t.
task force on electroconvulsive t.
tension reduction t.
termination of t.
therapist-guided t.
theta-criterion t.
third-force t.
third-line t.
thought field t.
three-cornered t.
time-consuming t.
time-extended t.
time-line t.
total push t.
trauma-focused t.
triadic t.
understimulation t.
unmodified ECT t.
validation t.
verbal aversion t.
video t.
virtual reality t.
vitamin t.
weight loss t.
Weir Mitchell t.
will t.
work t.
Zen t.

there-and-then approach
theriomorphism
thermal
  t. anesthesia
  t. drive
  t. sense
  t. stimulus
thermalgesia, thermoalgesia
thermalgia
thermanalgesia, thermoanalgesia
thermanesthesia (*var. of*
  thermoanesthesia)
thermesthesia
thermesthesiometer (*var. of*
  thermoesthesiometer)
thermic sense
thermoalgesia (*var. of* thermalgesia)
thermoanalgesia (*var. of* thermanalgesia)
thermoanesthesia, thermanesthesia
thermocoagulation

NOTES

thermoeffector
    t. activity
    antagonistic t.
    t. function
    t. response
thermoesthesiometer, thermesthesiometer
thermogenesis
    catecholamine-induced t.
    nonshivering t.
    normal t.
    shivering t.
    sympathomimetic-induced t.
thermogenic
    t. action
    t. component
    t. effect
    t. mechanism
    t. tissue mass
thermohyperalgesia
thermohyperesthesia
thermohypesthesia, thermohypoesthesia
thermometer
    fear t.
thermoneurosis
thermoplastic
thermoreceptor
thermoregulation
thermoregulatory
    t. function
    ·t. property
    t. response
    t. system
thermosensory
    t. information
    t. property
theroid
theta
    t. criterion
    t. index
    t. level
    t. rhythm
    t. wave
    t. wave on EEG
theta-criterion therapy
theurgist
theurgy
thiamine, thiamin
    t. deficiency
    t. deficiency encephalopathy (TDE)
thickheaded
thick-skinned
thick-witted
thief
thigmesthesia
thin
    desire to be t.
thinking
    t. ability

abnormal t.
abstract t.
adolescent t.
allusive t.
animistic t.
archaic-paralogical t.
t. aside
associative t.
asyndetic t.
autistic t.
black-and-white t.
categorical t.
circular t.
clear t.
clinical t.
combinative t.
t. compulsion
conceptual t.
concrete t.
concretistic t.
convergent t.
creative t.
t. creatively with sounds and
    words (TCSW)
critical t.
delusional t.
dereistic t.
dichotomous t.
directed t.
t. disorder
disordered t.
disorganized t.
distorted inferential t.
distortion of inferential t.
t. disturbance factor (TDF)
disturbance in form of t.
divergent t.
eccentric t.
egocentric t.
either-or t.
erratic t.
externally oriented t. (EOT)
t. fear
fragmentation of t.
futuristic t.
hypothetical deductive t.
idiosyncratic t.
illogical t.
impoverishment in t.
incomprehensible t.
inferential t.
janusian t.
magic t.
magical t.
marginal t.
normal t.
numerical t.
obsessional t.

oppositional t.
paranoid t.
perverted t.
physiognomic t.
prearchaic t.
precausal t.
preconscious t.
predicate t.
prelogical t.
preoperational t.
primary process t.
process t.
productive t.
psychotic t.
realistic t.
ritualistic t.
secondary process t.
self-defeating t.
stress effect on adult t.
suicidal t.
symbolic t.
syncretic t.
tangential t.
tertiary-process t.
t. through
trouble t.
t. type
undirected t.
vague t.
wishful t.

think tank

thinner

paint t.

thin-skinned

thioxanthene

t. antipsychotic
t. derivative

third

t. degree
t. ear
t. nervous system
t. person attitude
t. sex

third-force therapy

thirdhand information

third-line therapy

third-person auditory hallucination

third-rate

thirst

t. drive
insensible t.
morbid t.

subliminal t.
twilight t.

Thorndike

T. law of effect
T. trial-and-error learning

Thorndike-Lorge criteria

thoroughness, reliability, efficiency, analytic ability (TREA)

thought

abstract logical t.
adaptive control of t. (ACT)
aggressive t.
alien t.
anxious t.
archaic t.
audible t.
automatic t.
blasphemous t.
t. blockade
t. blocking
t. broadcasting
t. broadcasting delusion
categorical t.
characteristic pattern of t.
children's development of moral t.
coherent stream of t.
compulsive t.
considered t.
t. constraint
constraint of t.
constriction of t.
content of t.
t. content
t. control
t. of death
t. deletion
delusional t.
t. deprivation
t. derailment
difficulty with t.
diminution of t.
disconnected t.
t. disorganization
t. disorientation
distress t.
distressing t.
t. disturbance
disturbance in content of t.
disturbing t.
t. echo
t. echoing
emotional t.

NOTES

thought (*continued*)
    errant t.
    evil t.'s
    t. fear
    fear-related t.
    t. field therapy
    fluency of t.
    focus of t.
    t. form
    free t.
    gambling t.
    t. hearing
    homicidal t.
    imageless t.
    impoverished t.
    inappropriate t.
    incomprehensible t.
    increased speed of t.
    increase speed of t.
    inelasticity of t.
    inner t.
    t. insertion
    t. insertion delusion
    interruption of t.
    intrusive t.
    latent t.
    logical analysis of automatic t.
    lost in t.
    maladaptive t.
    maladaptive pattern of t.
    moral t.
    motor theory of t.
    multifocal t.
    obsessional t.
    obsessive t.
    t. obstruction
    t. omnipotence
    omnipotence of t.
    operational t.
    painful t.
    t. pattern
    t. period
    persistent t.
    phenomenalistic t.
    phenomenistic t.
    poverty of content of t.
    preoccupation of t.
    preoperational t.
    pressing t.
    t. pressure
    t. process
    t. process disorder
    productivity of t.
    t. provoking
    psychopathological t.
    racing t.
    rambling flow of t.
    reactive t.

    t. reading
    recurrent t.
    reenforced t.
    t. reform
    t. rehearsal
    reinforced t.
    ruminative t.
    school of t.
    second t.
    self-deprecating t.
    self-related t.
    sexual t.
    sick t.
    slowness of t.
    speed of t.
    stimulus-independent t.
    t. stopping
    stream of t. (SOT)
    substituting t.
    suicidal t.
    t. of suicide
    supervalent t.
    t. suppression
    symbolic t.
    syncretic t.
    syntaxic t.
    t. system
    train of t.
    t. transfer
    t. transference
    t. transfer experience
    t. transfer phenomenon
    trend of t.
    unacceptable t.
    uncontrollable t.
    unemotional t.
    unrelated t.
    unsocialized disturbance of t.
    verbal t.
    violent t.
    wandering t.
    wide circles of t.
    t. wit
    t. withdrawal
thought-out
threadbare
thready
threat
    acute suicide t.
    t. of death
    death t.
    direct t.
    t. of imminent suicide
    t. of job loss
    t. to life
    suicide t.
    veiled t.

t. of violence
t. of war
threatened death
threatening
t. behavior
t. comment
t. hallucination
t. message
t. voice
threctia
three
t. dimensional
t. essays on the theory of sexuality
oriented and alert times t.
t. strikes law
t. times a day
three-component theory
three-cornered therapy
three-day schizophrenia
three-factor model of global rating
three-step task
threshold
absolute t.
acoustic reflex t.
auditory t.
awareness t.
blackout t.
brightness t.
t. of consciousness
convulsant t.
detectability t.
detection t.
t. differential
differential t.
t. of discomfort (TD)
discomfort t.
double-point t.
electroshock t. (EST, est)
false t.
intelligibility t.
low anger t.
motor t.
pain t.
pain intensity t.
reflex t.
relational t.
t. of responsiveness
sedation t.
seizure t.
sensory t.
t. shift-masking technique

speech reception t. (SRT)
t. stimulus
stimulus t.
t. symbolism
taste t.
vibrotactile t.
vulnerability t.
thriftless
thrive
failure to t. (FTT)
throat
lump in the t.
t. slashing
throaty
throbbing
through
carry t.
fall t.
muddle t.
thinking t.
working t.
throw
t. off
t. out
t. over
t. in the towel
t. up
throwback
thrust
extensor t.
thrusting
pelvic t.
thug
thumb
cerebral t.
rule of t.
t. sucking
thumbs-down
thumb-sucking
thumbs-up
thwart
thymonoic reaction
thyroid
t. augmentation
t. delirium
t. disorder
t. response element (TRE)
thyroid-stimulating hormone (TSH)
thyrotoxic
t. coma
t. encephalopathy

T

NOTES

thyrotropin-releasing
    t.-r. hormone (TRH)
    t.-r. hormone stimulation
thyrotropin-stimulating hormone (TSH)
tibiarum
    anxietas t.
tic
    articulatory t.
    attitude t.
    body t.
    breathing t.
    child problem t.
    chronic t.
    chronic motor t.
    chronic spasm t.
    comorbid t.
    complex motor t.
    complex vocal t.
    compulsive psychogenic t.
    compulsive spasms and t.'s
    convulsive t.
    t. convulsive with coprolalia
    current t.
    t. de Guinon
    t. de pensee
    t. de sommeil
    t. disorder
    t. disorder of organic origin
    facial t.
    glossopharyngeal t.
    habit t.
    lid t.
    local t.
    maladie des t.'s
    mimic t.
    motor t.
    motor-verbal t.
    occupational t.
    t. orbicularis
    past t.
    primary t.
    psychic t.
    psychogenic t.
    rotatory t.
    ruling in t.'s
    t. scriptorius
    simple motor t.
    simple vocal t.
    spasm t.
    spasm and t.
    spasmodic t.
    t. symptom
    tardive t.
    tonic t.
    Tourette t.
    vocal t.
tickle threshold

tickling
tic-like
    t.-l. behavior
    t.-l. facial grimace
tic-related obsessive-compulsive disorder
tidal air
ties
    incestuous t.
    reality t.
    t. with reality
tight-lipped
tight-mouthed
tightrope
tilt
    head t.
timbromania
time
    abuse of leave t.
    adaptation t.
    t. agnosia
    association reaction t.
    attention t.
    biologic t.
    central reflex t.
    t. confusion
    t. consciousness
    t. consuming
    t. context
    t. of death
    t. deixis
    t. disorientation
    t. distortion
    t. dominance
    dream t.
    t. error
    t. faction
    t. fear
    inertia t.
    t. interval
    t. killer
    leisure t.
    losing t.
    t. of maximum concentration
    t. and motion study
    one day at a t.
    oriented to person, place, and t.
    t. out
    t. out from reinforcement
    t. perception
    t. periods of satisfactory relating
    t., place, and person (TP&P)
    t. point
    t. pressure
    processing t.
    quality t.
    reaction t. (RT)
    recognition t.

reflex t.
relaxation t.
response processing t.
t. and rhythm disorder
t. sense
t. splitting
survival t.
total sleep t. (TST)
wake t.
t. zone
t. zone-change syndrome
time-consuming therapy
timed behavioral rating sheet (TBRS)
time-extended therapy
timeless
time-limited psychotherapy (TLP)
timeliness
time-line therapy
timely
t. death
time-motion study
time-out
involuntary t.-o.
t.-o. procedure
t.-o. technique
voluntary t.-o.
time-sample behavioral checklist (TSBC)
time-series design
time-specific event
timid
timidity
timing
circadian t.
timorous
tingling
t. sensation
tinnitus
tiotixene
tip of the iceberg
tip-off
tip-of-the-tongue (TOT)
t.-o.-t.-t. phenomenon
tipsy
tiqueur
tirade
tiredness
tireless
tissue
arachnoid t.
caudate t.
cingulate t.
gray matter t.

insular cortex t.
mammalian t.
occipital cortex t.
parietal t.
postmortem brain t.
t. respiration
splenium t.
temporal t.
thalamus t.
white matter t.
tissue-type metabolic response
titillate
titillating
titration
titubation
tizzy
TL
team leader
tolerance level
TLC
tender loving care
TLE
temporal lobe epilepsy
TLP
time-limited psychotherapy
TM
team member
transcendental meditation
TMH
trainable mentally handicapped
TMR
trainable mentally retarded
TMS
transcranial magnetic stimulation
to
face up to
to a fault
to the point
to-and-fro tremor
tobacco
t. abuse
t. addiction
t. amblyopia
t. dependence
t. smoker
t. use
t. use disorder
t. use reduction
t. withdrawal
tobaccoism
tobacism
tobacosis

NOTES

tobagism
tocomania
toddler
> t. negativism
> t. stage

Todeserwartung syndrome
toe
> t. clonus
> t. drop
> t. phenomenon

toe-walking
together
> fraternal twins raised t.
> hang t.
> live t.

togetherness need
toilet training
token economy reward
tolerability
tolerance
> acute t.
> alcohol dependence with t.
> ambiguity t.
> anxiety t.
> barbiturate t.
> benzodiazepine t.
> caffeine t.
> cross t.
> t. dose
> drug t.
> frustration t.
> t. level (TL)
> level of pain t.
> low frustration t.
> metabolic t.
> opioid t.
> pain t.
> pharmacodynamic t.
> t. potential
> t. range
> social t.
> substance t.
> t. test
> zero t.

tolerant
tolerate
toll
> psychological t.

Tolman purposive behaviorism
Tolosa-Hunt syndrome
toluene
Tom
> peeping T.

tomboy behavior
tomboyish
Tomism
> Uncle T.

tommy gun

tomomania
tonaphasia
tone
> affective t.
> belligerent t.
> biofeedback t.'s
> complex t.
> t. deafness
> depressed t.
> dopaminergic t.
> emotional t.
> episodic bilateral loss of muscle t.
> feeling t.
> t. of feeling
> fundamental t.
> hostile t.
> hyperattentiveness to voice t.
> inhibitory t.
> t. of voice

toner
> psychological t.

tonetic
tongue
> t. clucking
> forked t.
> t. kiss
> t. phenomenon

tongue-lash
tongue-tied
tonic
> t. convulsion
> t. epilepsy
> t. inhibitor control
> t. pupil
> t. seizure
> t. spasm
> t. tic

tonic-clonic
> t.-c. conversion
> t.-c. movement
> t.-c. seizure

tonicity
tonoclonic spasm
tonogenic
tonogeny
tonotopic
tonus
> plastic t.

tool
> communication t.
> genetic t.
> relationship t.

tool-using behavior
tooth, pl. teeth
> t. fear
> t. grinding
> t. spasm

TOP
temporal, occipital, parietal
test orientation procedure
topagnosia
topagnosis
topalgia
top dog
top-down
t.-d. organization of memory
t.-d. regulation
topesthesia
topic
change of t.
emotionally laden t.
t. shifting
topoanesthesia
topographagnosia
topographic
t. hypothesis
t. mapping
topographical
t. agnosia
t. disorientation
t. organization
t. psychology
t. theory
topography
mental t.
topological psychology
topology
toponarcosis
toponeurosis
toposcope
torment
tormented
being t.
tornado epilepsy
torpedoing
torpent
torpid
t. idiocy
t. idiot
torpillage
torpor
torrid
tort
torticollis
hysterical t.
psychogenic t.
tortuosity
tortuous
torture

TOT
tip-of-the-tongue
total
t. abstinence
t. AIMS score
t. aphasia
t. battery composite
t. brain volume
t. communication
t. composite theory
t. disability
t. emotional memory score
t. mergent
t. neuroleptic dosage
t. parenteral nutrition (TPN)
t. phobic anxiety (TPA)
t. push therapy
t. push treatment of schizophrenia
t. recall
t. response (lz R)
t. response index (TRI)
t. scale
t. sleep time (TST)
t. symptom
t. symptom score
t. weighted sum score
totalis
alopecia t.
totalism
totality of possible events
totally disabled
totemism
totemistic
toto
pars pro t.
touch
t. off
out of t.
t. perception
t. sensation
t. sense
soft t.
t. spot
toucher
delire de t.
toucherism
touching
t. communication pattern
genital t.
t. rituals
sexual t.
touch-me-not

T

NOTES

tough
  hang t.
  t. love
  t. poise
tough-minded tendency
Tourette
  T. disorder
  T. syndrome (TS)
  T. tic
towel
  throw in the t.
TOWER
  testing, orientation, and work evaluation
  for rehabilitation
tower
  ivory t.
town
  skip t.
toxic
  t. action
  t. amaurosis
  t. amblyopia
  t. cirrhosis
  t. confusional state
  t. convulsion
  t. delirium
  t. dementia
  t. disorder
  t. dose
  t. edema
  t. effects of alcohol
  t. encephalopathy
  t. hypoxia
  t. ingredient
  t. injury
  t. insanity
  t. level
  t. myocarditis
  t. neuritis
  t. nystagmus
  t. psychosis
  t. reaction
  t. schizophrenia
  t. side effect
  t. substance
  t. tetanus
toxica
  alopecia t.
toxic-infectious psychosis
toxicity
  acute drug t.
  alcohol t.
  behavioral t.
  caffeine t.
  drug t.
  social t.
toxicological analysis
toxicology screen

toxicomania
toxin
  dietary t.
  exposure to t.'s
  t. exposure
toxin-provoked amnesia
toy
  sex t.
TPA
  total phobic anxiety
TPG
  therapeutic play group
TPN
  total parenteral nutrition
TP&P
  time, place, and person
TPR
  temperature, pulse, respiration
TR
  therapeutic reaction
trace
  t. conditioning
  memory t.
  mnemonic t.
  perseverative t.
trace-decay theory
tracer
  flow t.
tracing
  abnormal EEG t.
  dipole t. (DT)
  EEG t.
  I t.
  interrupted t.
track
  fast t.
  needle t.
tracking
  eye t.
  saccadic t.
  speech t.
  visual t.
tract
  census t.
  cholinergic t.
  dopaminergic t.
  extrapyramidal t.
  mesolimbic-mesocortical t.
  serotonergic t.
tractable
traction alopecia
trading
  drug t.
  t. sex
tradition
  childhood t.
  cultural t.
  t. directed

meditative t.
religious t.

traditional

    t. antipsychotic
    t. belief
    t. counseling
    t. lifestyle
    t. limbic circuit
    t. marriage
    t. neuroleptic
    t. neuroleptic agent
    t. phonetic analysis
    t. psychoanalytic concept
    t. psychotherapy
    t. society
    t. treatment
    t. value

traditionalism
traditionalist
traditionalize
traffic

    t. court
    drug t.

trafficker
trafficking

    drug t.

Trager method
tragic
trailing

    t. image
    t. phenomenon

train

    t. fear
    orphan t.
    t. of thought

trainability
trainable

    t. mentally handicapped (TMH)
    t. mentally retarded (TMR)

trainer
training

    aggression replacement t.
    alpha wave t.
    American Association of Directors
    of Psychiatric Residency T.
    (AADPRT)
    t. analysis
    anxiety control t. (ACT)
    anxiety management t. (AMT)
    assertive t.
    assertiveness t.
    audiovisual t.

auditory t.
autogenic t.
aversive t.
avoidance t.
biofeedback t.
biologic t.
bladder t.
bowel t.
clinical t.
cognitive self-hypnosis t.
cooperative t.
cross t.
cultural t.
delayed toilet t.
t. discrimination
emotion regulation t.
Erhardt seminar t.
escape t.
evaluation of t.
general relaxation t.
t. group
habit t.
habit reversal t. (HRT)
human relations t.
hypnotic relaxation technique t.
improvement t.
inappropriate religious t.
interviewer t.
laboratory t.
leadership t.
memory t.
neurofeedback t. (NT)
occupational skill t.
parent effectiveness t.
perceptual t.
personnel t.
problem-solving skills t.
relaxation t.
relaxation technique t.
retention control t.
self-reliance t.
sensitivity t.
skill t.
social skills t. (SST)
spontaneity t.
stress inoculation t. (SIT)
toilet t.
trait factor t.
t. transfer
transfer of t.
t. unit

T

NOTES

training *(continued)*
    visual t.
    vocational t.
train-of-four stimulus
trait
    abnormal t.
    t. anxiety
    anxious-neurotic personality t.
    cardinal t.
    t. carrier
    central t.
    character t.
    t. characteristic
    cluster B t.
    cognitive personality t.
    common t.
    compensatory t.
    complex psychological t.
    culture t.
    dependence t.
    t. dependent
    dominant t.
    environmental mold t.
    t. factor
    t. factor training
    harm-avoidant t.
    identified t.
    impulsive-aggressive t.
    inflexible personality t.
    interpersonal personality t.
    intrapsychic personality t.
    introversive t.
    maladaptive personality t.
    novelty-seeking t.
    t. organization
    paranoid t.
    pathologic t.
    peculiar personality t.
    pervasive and persistent maladaptive
      personality t.'s
    polygenic t.
    premorbid personality t.
    primary personality t.
    t. profile
    psychological t.
    psychopathic t.
    t. rating
    recessive t.
    secondary personality t.
    self-defeating t.
    sensation-seeking t.
    temperament t.
    t. theory
    unique t.
    t. variability
trait-dependent psychopathology rating
  scale
trait-level region abnormalities

trait-like
    t.-l. feature
    t.-l. syndrome
trajectory
    behavioral t.
    cognitive t.
    emotional t.
trance
    amnesia after t.
    t. coma
    death t.
    deep t.
    dissociative t.
    ecstatic t.
    hypnotic t.
    hysterical t.
    induced t.
    involuntary state of t.
    light t.
    t. logic
    medium t.
    possession t.
    somnambulistic t.
    t. state
trancelike
    t. behavior
    t. state
trance-possession disorder
tranquilization
    rapid t.
tranquilizer
    t. abuse
    t. chair
    t. drug dependence
    major t.
    minor t.
transaction
    ulterior t.
transactional
    t. analysis (TA)
    t. evaluation
    t. psychotherapy
    t. theory of perception
transaminase
transcend
transcendence
    ego t.
    t. need
transcendental
    t. meditation (TM)
    t. state
transcendentalism
transcendent reality
transcerebral electrotherapy (TCET)
transcortical
    t. aphasia
    t. apraxia

t. motor
t. sensory
transcranial magnetic stimulation (TMS)
transcultural psychiatry
transderivational search
transdermal
t. absorption
t. patch
t. scopolamine
transduce
transduction
chemical-mechanical t.
postreceptor information t.
transfer
bilateral t.
correctional t. (CT)
t. of custody
custody t.
general t.
t. by generalization
interhemispheric t.
intersensory t.
t. of learning
memory t.
positive t.
t. of principle
secure file t.
thought t.
training t.
t. of training
transference
affectionate t.
aim t.
alter ego t.
analysis of t.
t. behavior
collective t.
counter t.
t. cure
t. dilution
erotic t.
extrasensory thought t.
t. feeling
floating t.
hostile t.
idealizing t.
identification t.
t. improvement
institutional t.
libidinal t.
t. love
mirror t.

mirroring the t.
narcissistic t.
negative t.
t. neurosis
t. paradigm
t. phenomenon
positive t.
t. reaction
t. relationship
t. remission
t. resistance
self-object t.
thought t.
traumatic t.
twinship t.
transference-countertransference
transferential
transferred
t. meaning
t. sensation
transformation
t. of affect
perceptual t.
t. theory of anxiety
Z score t.
transformational
T. Leadership Development
Program
t. related
t. rule
transformationally related
transforming agent
transfusion
blood t.
transgender
transgenderism
transgenerational role of giving
transgress
transgression
behavioral t.
transience
transient
t. amnesia
t. auditory hallucination
t. auditory illusion
t. blindness
t. channel activation
t. depressive reaction
t. distortion
t. ego ideal
t. emotional disturbance
t. emotional stress

NOTES

T

697

transient *(continued)*
    t. global amnesia (TGA)
    t. group
    t. hallucinatory experience
    t. hypersomnia
    t. ideas of reference
    t. image
    t. insomnia
    t. organic psychosis
    t. phenomenon
    t. postictal confusional state
    t. situational disturbance
    t. situational personality disorder
    t. spasm tic disorder of childhood
    t. state of anger
    t. stress-related paranoid ideation
    t. tactile hallucination
    t. tactile illusion
    t. tic disorder
    t. tremor
    t. visual hallucination
    t. visual illusion
transilluminate
transition
    age t.
    high-intensity t.
    life-cycle t.
    normal t.
    t. process
    role t.
    sleep-wake t.
    t. zone
transitional
    t. change
    t. employment workshop
    t. halfway house
    t. object
    t. probability
    t. program
    t. sleep (TS)
transitivism
transitivity
transitory
    t. mania
    t. psychosis
translation
translocation
    chromosomal t.
translucent
transmigrate
transmissible
    t. agent
    t. virus dementia (TVD)
transmission
    cholinergic t.
    cultural t.
    duplex t.
    familial t.

    genetic t.
    indirect genetic t.
    intergenerational t.
    neurohumoral t.
    parent-child t.
    synaptic t.
    vertical t.
transmitter
    chemical t.
    t. system
transmutation
transorbital
    t. lobectomy
    t. lobotomy
transosseous
transpersonal psychology
transpicuous
transplantation
    organ t.
    t. reaction
    t. shock
transport
    active t.
    passive t.
transporter
    dopamine t.
    drug t.
transposition of affect
transsexual (TS)
    nuclear t.
    t. voice
transsexualism
transsynaptic
transtentorial
transverse
    t. hermaphroditism
    t. orientation
transvestic
    t. fetishism (TF)
    t. phenomenon
transvestism paraphilia
transvestite
    marginal t.
    nuclear t.
transvestitism
Transylvania effect
trap
    death t.
    social t.
trash
    white t.
trauma, pl. **traumata**
    acoustic t.
    acute head t.
    aftermath of t.
    amnesia for t.
    birth t.
    brain t.

cerebral t.
t. characteristic
child-abuse-specific treatment of t.
  (CASST)
childhood t.
civilian t.
closed head t.
CNS t.
combat t.
t. cue
dementia due to head t.
disaster t.
effects of t.
emotional t.
exposure to t.
extreme t.
head t.
intensity of t.
intergenerational t.
late-age t.
long-term effects of t.
occult head t.
t. organic psychosis
original t.
physical t.
premorbid t.
primal t.
psychic t.
psychological t.
recollection of t.
reexperienced t.
self-inflicted t.
sexual t.
t. spectrum disorder
subsequent t.
t. survivor
type 1, 2 t.
trauma-focused therapy
trauma-induced delirium
trauma-related
  t.-r. repetition
  t.-r. stress
trauma-specific
  t.-s. anxiety
  t.-s. reenactment
traumasthenia
traumata (*pl. of* trauma)
traumatic
  t. alopecia
  t. amblyopia
  t. amnesia

t. anesthesia
t. anxiety
t. aphasia
t. asphyxia
t. bereavement
t. brain injury (TBI)
t. childhood abuse
t. death
t. defect state
t. delirium
t. dementia
t. epilepsy
t. experience
t. grief
t. headache
t. idiocy
t. life event
t. mutism
t. neurasthenia
t. neuritis
t. neurosis
t. progressive encephalopathy
t. pseudocatatonia
t. psychosis
t. scene
t. seizure
t. separation
t. stress
t. stressor
t. suffocation
t. transference
traumatica
  amnesia t.
traumatism
traumatization of the libido
traumatize
traumatized child
traumatology
traumatophilia
trauma-type symptom
travail
traverse jury
travesty in wit
TRE
  thyroid response element
TREA
  thoroughness, reliability, efficiency,
    analytic ability
treacherous
tread
treason

NOTES

T

treated
    ineffectively t.
    t. prevalence
treatise
treatment
    achievement through counseling and t. (ACT)
    acidification t.
    active t.
    acute t.
    acute intensive t. (AIT)
    acute-phase t.
    addiction t.
    adequate t.
    adjunct to t.
    adjunctive t.
    alternative t.
    amenable to t.
    analytic t.
    antidepressant t.
    antipsychotic drug t.
    appropriate t.
    t. authorization
    behavioral t.
    Center for Substance Abuse T. (CSAT)
    t. change
    t. choice
    coerced t.
    coercive t.
    cognitive-behavioral t.
    cognitive-linguistic t.
    cold-pack t.
    communication/cognition t.
    community-based mental health t.
    t. completion
    t. completion rate
    t. compliance
    comprehensive t.
    t. condition
    conservative t.
    t. consideration
    continuation t.
    continuous antipsychotic drug t.
    continuous bath t.
    conventional neuroleptic t.
    t. cost
    course of t.
    court-mandated t.
    court-ordered involuntary outpatient t.
    day care residential t.
    t. decision
    definitive t.
    depression t.
    Depression: Awareness, Recognition, and T. (D/ART)
    T. of Depression Collaborative Research Program
    diet t.
    direct t.
    disrespectful t.
    t. driven
    t. dropout
    drug-induced t.
    drug maintenance t.
    drug-responsive t.
    duration of t.
    t. duration
    early t.
    early and periodic screening, diagnosis, and t. (EPSDT)
    educational t.
    t. effect
    effective t.
    t. effectiveness
    electric shock t.
    electroconvulsive shock t. (ECST)
    electroshock t. (EST, est)
    emergency t.
    t. emergent
    empiric drug t.
    enforced t.
    enhanced methadone maintenance t.
    ethanol t.
    t. evaluation strategy
    evening t.
    exercise t.
    t. experience
    experimental t.
    t. facility
    family t.
    feasible alternative t.
    fluoxetine t.
    forced t.
    format t.
    former t.
    frequency of t.
    t. gap
    general medical t.
    group t.
    habit t.
    hazardous t.
    holistic t.
    hormone t.
    humane t.
    inadequate t.
    individual t.
    ineffective t.
    inhalation convulsive t.
    t. initiation
    initiation of t.
    inpatient drug t.
    insight-oriented t.
    insulin coma t.

insulin shock t.
t. intensity
t. intensity-by-time interaction
t. intensity parameter
t. interference
intravenous t.
intrusive t.
invasive t.
involuntary t.
t. issue
light t.
long-term maintenance t.
low-dose t.
lower-intensity t.
maintenance t.
mandatory t.
medical t.
medication t.
mental health t.
methadone maintenance t. (MMT)
Metrazol shock t.
Mitchell t.
t. modality
t. model
moral t.
multicomponent behavioral t.
multimonitored electroconvulsive t. (MMECT)
neuroleptic t.
new t.
noncompliance with medical t.
nutrition t.
obesity t.
ongoing neuroleptic t.
optimal t.
t. option
t. outcome
outpatient t.
overly stimulating t.
t. package strategy
t. period
pharmacologic t.
t. phase
t. philosophy
t. plan (TRPL)
t. planning
prefrontal sonic t. (PST)
prescribed t.
previous t.
t. program
t. progress
prolonged sleep t.

prophylactic t.
t. protocol
psychiatric t.
psychodynamic interpretation and t.
psychopharmacological t.
psychoprophylactic t.
psychosocial t.
psychotherapeutic t.
t. refractory
refusal of t.
t. refusal
t. regimen
regressive electroshock t. (REST)
rehabilitation t.
residential t.
t. resistant
t. response
t. response rate
t. responsive
t. responsivity
retention in t.
right to refuse t.
school-based child-and-parent focused psychosocial t.
scope of t.
t. services review
shock t.
short-term t.
silent t.
sleep t.
social support after t.
social support during t.
somatic antidepressant t.
somatized plea for t.
specialty mental health t.
t. specificity
stimulant t.
suboptimal t.
substance abuse t.
symptomatic t.
t. team
traditional t.
unilateral ECT t.
t. unit
Weir Mitchell t.
treatment-emergent
t.-e. adverse event
t.-e. akathisia
t.-e. asthenia
t.-e. extrapyramidal side effect
t.-e. hypertonia
t.-e. hypokinesia

NOTES

treatment-emergent *(continued)*
    t.-e. hypomania
    t.-e. somnolence
treatment-intolerant patient
treatment-refractory
    t.-r. catatonia
    t.-r. depression
    t.-r. patient
    t.-r. schizophrenia
treatment-relevant issue
treatment-resistant
    t.-r. depression
    t.-r. schizophrenia
    t.-r. schizophrenic
treble safeguard principle
tree
    decision t.
    family t.
    maidenhair t.
tremblant
    delire t.
trembling
    t. abasia
    t. palsy
    t. voice
tremens
    delirium t. (DT)
tremogram
tremograph
tremolo massage
tremor
    action t.
    acute cerebral t.
    alcoholic withdrawal t.
    alternating t.
    arsenical t.
    benign essential t.
    beta-adrenergic medication-induced
      postural t.
    cerebellar t.
    cerebral outflow t.
    coarse t.
    continuous t.
    counting money t.
    cycles per second t.
    dopaminergic medication-induced
      postural t.
    dystonic t.
    emotional stress precipitating t.
    end point t.
    essential t. (ET)
    facial t.
    fibrillary t.
    fine postural t.
    flapping t.
    flopping t.
    hand t.
    head and neck t.

    hepatic encephalopathy t.
    heredofamilial t.
    hysterical t.
    intention t.
    intentional t.
    kinetic t.
    medication-induced postural t.
    mercurial t.
    metabolic t.
    metallic t.
    neuroleptic-induced postural t.
    non-neuroleptic-induced t.
    no-no t.
    nonparkinsonian t.
    nonpharmacologically induced t.
    oscillating t.
    passive t.
    perioral t.
    persistent t.
    physiological t.
    pill-rolling t.
    positional t.
    postural t.
    precipitating t.
    preexisting t.
    progressive cerebellar t.
    psychologic t.
    rapid t.
    rest t.
    resting t.
    rhythmic t.
    senile t.
    shaking t.
    small-amplitude rapid t.
    static t.
    stimulant-induced postural t.
    stress precipitating t.
    striatocerebral t.
    substance withdrawal t.
    t. tendinum
    terminal t.
    to-and-fro t.
    transient t.
    volitional t.
    wing-beating t.
    withdrawal t.
    writing t.
    yes-yes t.
tremorgram
tremulous
    t. movement
    t. speech
tremulousness
    alcohol withdrawal t.
trench warfare
trend
    age-related t.
    amoral t.

death t.
diverging t.
global sociocultural t.
malignant t.
mortality t.
nonsignificant t.
paranoid t.
pernicious t.
phobic t.
psychiatric t.
secular t.
significant t.
sociocultural t.
statistical t.
t. of thought
trendsetter
trephination, trepanation
trephine, trepan
trepid
trepidans
abasia t.
trepidant
trepidation
TRH
thyrotropin-releasing hormone
TRI
total response index
triable
triad
Charcot t.
cognitive t.
oral t.
Sandler t.
triadic
t. symbiosis
t. therapy
triage situation
trial
t. analysis
clinical t.
competent to stand t.
controlled medication t.
t. court
t. and error
t. examiner
failure of drug t.
head-to-head clinical t.
t. home visit
t. identification
t. jury
t. lawyer
t. lesson

t. marriage
medication t.
murder t.
open-label t.
placebo-controlled t.
placebo medication t.
randomized clinical t. (RCT)
randomized controlled t. (RCT)
t. run
t. separation
therapeutic t.
t. visit
trial-and-error
t.-a.-e. learning
triangle
triazolopyridine antidepressant
tribade
tribadism
tribalism
tribe
tribesman
tribulation
tribunal
tribute
trichoesthesia
trichologia
trichology
trichomania
trichomoniasis
trichophagia
trichophagy
trichorrhexis nodosa with mental retardation
trichorrhexomania
trichosis sensitiva
trichotillomania (TTM)
trichotillomania-induced alopecia
trick
turn a t.
triclofos
tric scriptorius
tricyclic
t. antidepressant drug (TCAD)
t. antipsychotic (TCA)
t. drug
t. effect
t. secondary amine
t. tertiary amine
tridimensional
t. evaluational scale
t. theory of feeling

NOTES

trigeminal
 t. decompression
 t. nerve
 t. neuralgia
trigger
 active t.
 t. for anger
 anticipation of t.
 t. area
 exposure to t.
 t. finger
 t. point
 t. reaction
 situational t.
 t. zone
trigger-happy
triggering
 t. event
 t. mechanism
 t. situation
 t. stimulus
triggerman
trigram
triolist
triorchid
trip
 bad t.
 drug t.
 ego t.
triphosphate
 adenosine t. (ATP)
triple
 t. insanity
tripped out
trisexuality
trismic
trismoid
trisomy
 t. 13–15
 t. 17–18
 autosomal t.
 chromosome 13, 18, 21 t.
 E t.
 t. syndrome
triste
 post coitum t.
tristful
tristimania
trite
trivial act
triviality
trochaic stress
trois
 folie à t.
 menage a t.
tromomania
troops
 shock t.

trophesic
trophesy
trophic change
trophicity
trophism
trophoneurotic
trophopathy
tropism
trouble
 t. concentrating
 t. thinking
troubled
 t. adolescent
 t. child
 t. children
 t. marriage
 t. relationship
 t. teen
troublemaker
troubleshooter
troublesome
 t. adolescent
 t. symptom
troubling
 t. behavior
 t. experience
Trousseau
 T. point
 T. spot
trovato
 ben t.
TRPL
 treatment plan
truancy
 school t.
 socialized childhood t.
 unsocialized childhood t.
truant
truce
truculence
truculent
true
 t. addiction
 t. amnesia
 t. anosmia
 t. anxiety
 t. aphasia
 t. belief
 t. chancre
 t. communication stage
 t. component
 t. difference
 t. epilepsy
 t. hermaphroditism
 t. insight
 t. intersex
 t. motivation
 t. negative

t. perception
t. positive
t. self
t. symbolism
t. vertigo
trumped-up
trumpet
angel's t.
truncate
trunk ataxia
trust
atmosphere of t.
basic t.
blind t.
interpersonal t.
mutual t.
sense of t.
t. vs. mistrust
trusting physician-patient relationship
trustworthiness
doubts of t.
unjustified doubts of t.
trustworthy
truth
t. disclosure
moment of t.
obscuring fundamental t.
t. serum
support, empathy and t. (SET)
tryst
TS
Tourette syndrome
transitional sleep
transsexual
TSA
test of syntactic ability
TSBC
time-sample behavioral checklist
TSH
thyroid-stimulating hormone
thyrotropin-stimulating hormone
TST
total sleep time
TTM
trichotillomania
TTS
temporary threshold shift
TTV
therapeutic trial visit
tuberculomania
tuberosa
tubulization

tularemic chancre
tulipmania
tumefacient
tumefaction
tumescence
nocturnal penile t. (NPT)
penile t.
tumescent
tumultuous
t. growth
t. life
tunnel vision
turbulence
chronic psychosocial t.
family t.
marital t.
psychosocial t.
turbulent
turf
turgid
turkey
cold t.
turkomania
turmoil
adolescent t.
depressive t.
emotional t.
turn
t. around
t. away
t. back
t. in
t. a trick
turnabout
turned-on
turning
t. against self (TAS)
t. aggression against self
turpitude
moral t.
turricephaly
tussive
t. absence
TVD
transmissible virus dementia
twice-born
twice a day
twice-repeated multivariate analysis of variance
twilight
t. attack
t. confusional state

T

NOTES

twilight *(continued)*
    t. epilepsy
    t. sleep
    t. thirst
    t. vision
twin
    biovular t.'s
    t. concordance
    conjoined t.'s
    dizygotic t.'s
    fraternal t.'s
    identical t.'s
    t. language
    monozygotic t.'s (MZ)
    t. research
    same-sex t.'s
    t. separation
    Siamese t.'s
    t. studies
twinship transference
twirling of object
twisted mouth
twitch
    facial t.
    focal t.
    involuntary t.
    muscle t.
    rhythmical t.
two-dimensional proton echo-planar spectroscopic imaging
two-faced
two-factor theory of emotion
two-person interview team
two-sided message
two-timer
two-way
two-word messages stage
type
    t. A, B behavior
    t. A, B personality
    actively aggressive reaction t.
    adenoid t.
    affective reaction t.
    aggressive predatory t.
    t. I, II alcoholic
    apoplectic t.
    asthenic constitutional t.
    athletic constitutional t.
    attention deficit disorder, residual t.
    attention deficit hyperactivity disorder, combined t.
    attention deficit hyperactivity disorder, predominantly hyperactive-impulsive t.
    attitude t.
    attitudinal t.
    basic personality t.
    behavior t.

blood t.
blood-injection-injury t.
body t.
bulimia nervosa, nonpurging t.
bulimia nervosa, purging t.
character t.
choleric t.
chronic t.
circumplex of premorbid personality t.
complex t.
constitutional t.
conversion disorder, mixed t.
conversion disorder, motor t.
conversion disorder, seizure t.
conversion disorder, sensory t.
dementia of Alzheimer t. (DAT)
depressed t.
deterioration reaction t.
Don Juan t.
dysplastic constitutional t.
ectomorphic constitutional t.
eidetic t.
endomorphic constitutional t.
erotic t.
erotomanic t.
t. I, II error
explicit t.
exploiting t.
extroverted t.
family t.
functional t.
grandiose t.
hypochondriasis with poor insight t.
idiotropic t.
t. indicator
introverted t.
intuitive t.
irrational t.
jealous t.
Kretschmer t.
libidinal t.
linear t.
melancholic constitutional t.
mesomorphic constitutional t.
mixed t.
MMPI Code T.
noradrenaline dementia of Alzheimer t.
nosotropic drug dementia of Alzheimer t.
objective t.
obsessional t.
obsessive-compulsive disorder with poor insight t.
paranoid reaction t.
persecutory t.

personality change due to a
general medical condition,
aggressive t.
personality change due to a
general medical condition,
aphasic t.
personality change due to a
general medical condition,
disinhibited t.
personality change due to a
general medical condition,
labile t.
personality change due to a
general medical condition,
paranoid t.
phlegmatic constitutional t.
physique t.
primary degenerative dementia of
Alzheimer t. (PDDAT)
primary hypersomnia, recurrent t.
pyknic constitutional t.
reaction t.
reactive attachment disorder of
infancy or early childhood,
disinhibited t.
reactive attachment disorder of
infancy or early childhood,
inhibited t.
receiving t.
restricting t.
sanguine constitutional t.
schizoaffective disorder, bipolar t.
senile dementia of Alzheimer t.
(SDAT)
social t.
somatic t.
t. specifier

substitutive reaction t.
thinking t.
t. 1, 2 trauma
undersocialized conduct disorder,
aggressive t.
undersocialized conduct disorder,
nonaggressive t.
unspecified t.
working t.
typical
t. absence
t. absence seizure
t. age
t. antipsychotic
t. antipsychotic agent
t. behavior
t. neuroleptic
t. presentation
t. theme
typical-onset case
typify
typing
genetic t.
sex t.
typology
anxiety t.
personality disorder t.
typomania
tyramine-rich food
tyrannical
t. behavior
t. decision making
tyrannism
tyranny of silence
tyrant
evil t.

NOTES

UA
    unauthorized absence
ubiquitous
ubiquity
UCR
    unconditioned reflex
    unconditioned response
UCS
    unconditioned stimulus
ugliness
    imagined u.
Uhthoff sign
UL
    unauthorized leave
ulcer
    u. personality
    psychogenic duodenal u.
    psychogenic gastric u.
    psychogenic peptic u.
ulegyria
Ullmann line
ulterior
    u. motive
    u. transaction
ultradian rhythm
ultradistant
ultrafastidious
ultrafeminine
ultraism
ultraliberal
ultramarginal zone
ultramasculine
ultrashort-acting barbiturate
ultrastructural study
ultraviolent
ultromotivity
ululation
umbrage
umbrageous
unabashed
unable
    u. to follow instruction
    u. to listen
unacceptable
    u. behavior
    u. feeling
    u. impulse
    u. thought
unadulterated
unaffective
unaggressive
    u. conduct disorder
    u. undersocialized reaction
unaided augmentative communication
unaltered drug

unambiguous measure
unanalyzable
unanswered question
unanticipated crisis
unapproachable
unarmed
unarousable
unassertive
    u. aggression
    u. expression
unattached
unattained goal
unattractive
unauthorized
    u. absence (UA)
    u. leave (UL)
unavailable
    emotionally u.
unavoidable placement
unawareness of environment
unbearable
unbecoming
unbelievable
unbendable
unbiased
    u. evaluation
    u. information
unblinking
uncanny emotion
uncertain biological status
uncertainty
    u. factor
    u. level
uncertainty-arousal factor
uncharacteristic
    u. behavior
    u. outburst
uncharacteristically
uncinate
    u. attack
    u. convulsion
    u. epilepsy
    u. fit
    u. seizure
uncivil
uncleanliness
unclear
    u. diagnosis
    u. etiology
Uncle Tomism
unclothed
uncluttered
uncomplaining
uncomplicated
    u. alcohol withdrawal

U

uncomplicated *(continued)*
    u. arteriosclerotic dementia
    u. arteriosclerotic psychosis
    u. bereavement
    u. presenile dementia
    u. recovery
    u. sedative, hypnotic, or anxiolytic
      withdrawal
    u. senile dementia
uncomprehending
uncompromising
unconcernedness
unconditional
    u. positive regard
    u. reflex
unconditioned
    u. reflex (UCR)
    u. response (UCR)
    u. stimulus (UCS)
unconscionable
unconscious
    u. cerebration
    collective u.
    u. concern
    u. conflict
    u. distress
    u. emotion
    u. factor
    familial u.
    u. fantasy
    u. guilt
    u. homosexuality
    impersonal u.
    u. impulse
    u. memory
    u. motivation
    u. need for punishment
    personal u.
    u. process
    u. processing
    u. rage
    u. resistance
    superpersonal u.
unconsciousness
    absolute u.
    conversion u.
    u. conversion
unconsolable
unconsummated marriage
uncontrollability
    stressor u.
uncontrollable
    u. action
    u. anxiety
    u. crying
    u. laughter
    u. quality

    u. sleep attack
    u. thought
uncontrolled
    u. laughter
    u. worry
unconventional
uncooperative
uncoordinated
    u. gait
    u. motor skills
uncovering technique
uncriticalness
uncued
    u. behavior
    u. panic attack
undauntable
undeniable
under
    knuckle u.
    u. the skin
    snow u.
underachievement disorder
underachiever
underage gambling
underarousal
underclass
undercontrolled
undercover
undercurrent
undercutting
underdeveloped
underdiagnosed sequela
underdog
undereducated
underestimate
underestimating
    u. danger
    u. risk
underestimation
underfocused
undergo
underhanded
underinsured
underlie
underload
    information u.
underlying
    u. condition
    u. depression
    u. emotional issue
    u. medical illness
    u. psychological manifestations
    u. structure
undermine
undermining
undernourished
undernutrition
underpayment

underprepared
underprivileged
underproductive speech
underrate
underreact
underreporting
underrepresented minority
underscore
undersexed
undersocialized
 u., aggressive reaction
 u. conduct behavior
 u. conduct disorder, aggressive type
 u. conduct disorder, nonaggressive type
 u. disorder
 u. nonaggressive reaction
 u. runaway reaction
 u. socialized disturbance
understandable
understanding
 clinical u.
 consensual u.
 core consensual u.
 shared u.
 theoretical u.
 word u.
understatement
understimulation
 u. theory
 u. therapy
understood
understudy
undertake
under-the-counter
under-the-table
undertone
undertreated
underwrite
undesirable
 social u.
undetermined origin (UO)
undeviating
undifferentiated
 u. attention-deficit disorder
 chronic u.
 u. effect
 u. schizophrenia
 schizophrenic reaction, acute, u. (SR/AU)

schizophrenic reaction, chronic, u. (SR/CU)
 u. somatoform disorder
 u. wholeness
undifferentiated-type
 u.-t. conduct disorder
 u.-t. schizophrenia
 u.-t. schizophrenic disorder
undinism
undirected thinking
undisciplined self-conflict
undisturbed nocturnal sleep
undoing defense mechanism
undoubtedly
undressed
undressing
 paradoxical u.
undue social anxiety
unduly
unearned
unease
unemotional
 u. learning task
 u. thought
unemployable
unemployment insurance
unencapsulated joint receptor
unencumbered
unendurable psychological pain
unequal distribution
unequivocal change in functioning
unethical behavior
unexpected
 u. behavior
 u. panic attack
 u. response
unexplained
 u. absence from work
 u. pain
 u. tearfulness
unexpressive
unfaithful
unfaltering
unfamiliar
 u. face
 u. place
unfathered
unfathomable
unfavorable
unfazed
unfeeling
unfinished

NOTES

unfit
unflappable
unfocused delirium
unforgiving
unformed
 u. auditory hallucination
 u. image
 u. visual hallucination
unformism
unforthcomingness
unfounded complaint
unfriendly
ungiving parent
ungodly
ungrateful
unhappiness
 u. and misery disorder
 pattern of pervasive u.
 pervasive u.
unhappy
 u. facial expression
 u. love affair
 u. memory
unhealthy
unhinge
unifactorial
unifamilial
unification in wit
uniformly progressive deterioration
unifying force
unilateral
 u. abductor paralysis
 u. adductor paralysis
 u. anesthesia
 u. brief pulse ECT
 u. decision
 u. ECT treatment
 u. focus
 u. hermaphroditism
 u. migraine
 u. migraine headache
 u. nondominant-hemisphere ECT
 u. organic neglect
 u. seizure
 u. sine wave ECT
 u. spatial neglect
 u. visual neglect
unimaginable
unimportant
unimproved
uninhibited
 u. behavior
 u. motor planning
 u. neurogenic bladder
uninsured patient
unintelligible speech

unintended
 u. effect
 u. sleep
unintentional
 u. daytime sleep episode
 u. death
unintentionally produced symptom
uninterested
uninterrupted episode
unio mystica
union
 mystic u.
unipolar
 u. chronic depression
 u. disorder
 u. major depression
 u. mania
 u. manic-depressive psychosis
 u. patient
 u. recurrent depression
unique
 u. characteristic
 u. trait
unisex
unit
 acute adolescent inpatient u.
 acute care u. (ACU)
 addictive disease u. (ADU)
 adolescent inpatient u.
 adult u.
 child inpatient u.
 cognition of semantic u. (CSU)
 communication u.
 day treatment u.
 delirium u.
 emergency u. (EU)
 family u.
 inpatient u.
 intensive care u. (ICU)
 intensive treatment u. (ITU)
 life change u. (LCU)
 locked hospital u.
 maximum security u.
 memory for symbolic u. (MSU)
 polysensory u.
 psychiatric u.
 psychiatric intensive care u. (PICU)
 relational u.
 u. restriction
 u. secretary
 state hospital children's u. (SHCU)
 training u.
 treatment u.
 work-for-pay u.
unitary
 u. consciousness
 u. disorder

United
    U. States Pharmacopeia (USP)
    U. States Public Health Service
    (USPHS)
    U. States-United Kingdom Study
    U. States vs. Brawner
unitization
unity
    functional u.
    u. and fusion
universal
    u. symbol
universalis
    alopecia u.
universalism
universality
universalization
universals
    formal u.
    substantive u.
unjustified
    u. doubt of loyalty
    u. doubts of trustworthiness
unkempt
    u. appearance
    u. manner
unkindly
unknowing
unknown
    u. language
    u. meaning
    u. substance-induced mood disorder
unlawful behavior
unlearning
unlicensed handgun
unlocked seclusion
unmarried
unmedicated patient
unmentionable
unmerciful
unmet
    u. dependence
    u. dependency need
unmistakable
unmitigated echolalia
unmodified ECT therapy
unmotivated
unnatural cheerfulness
unnecessarily
unnecessary
    u. medication
    u. sedation

unnerve
unobtrusive measure
unorganized
unpalatable
unpardonable
unplanned pregnancy
unpleasant
    u. hallucination
    u. mood
unpleasantness
unpleasure
unpredictability
unpredictable
    u. act of violence
    u. agitation
    u. mood change
    u. parenting
unprepared
unpretentious
unprincipled
unproductive mania
unprofessional
unpromising
unprotected
    u. intercourse
    u. sex
unpunished
unpurposeful behavior
unquestionable
unquiet
unravel
unrealistic
    u. expectation
    u. worry
unreality
    feeling of u.
    idea of u.
unreasonable
    u. belief
    u. demand
    u. fear
    u. idea
unreasoning
unrecognized
unrefined motor skill
unrelated
    u. diagnosis
    u. thought
unrelenting
    u. pain
unreliability
unreliable

U

NOTES

unrelieved agitation
unremitting
unresolved
    u. bereavement
    u. conflict
    u. grief
    u. loss
unresponsive
    u. patient
    u. state
unrest
unrestricted diet
unruffled
unruly child
unsanctioned
    culturally u.
    u. response
unsanitary drug administration
unsatisfactory relationship
unsavory
unsayable
unscientific
unscrupulous
unseasonable
unseen reality
unselective observation
unselfish
unsettled
unsex
unshakable
    u. belief
    u. preoccupation
unsightly
unskilled
unsociable
unsocialized
    u. aggressive disorder
    u. aggressive reaction
    u. childhood truancy
    u. disturbance of thought
unsophisticated
unspeakable
unspecified
    bipolar I disorder, most recent
      episode u.
    u. depression
    u. mental disorder
    u. mental disorder, nonpsychotic
    u. mental retardation
    mental retardation, severity u.
    u. mood episode
    u. psychological factor
    u. schizophrenia
    u. substance dependence
    u. type
unspecified-type
    u.-t. delusion
    u.-t. dyssomnia

unstable
    u. affect
    u. attachment
    u. behavior
    emotionally u.
    u. interpersonal relationship
    u. lifestyle
    u. mood
    u. personality
    u. self-image
unsteadiness
    postural u.
unsteady gait
unstoppable flow of speech
unstructured
    u. interview
    u. verbal information
    u. verbal material
unsuccessful
unswerving
unsympathetic attitude
unsystematized delusion
untenable
unthinkable
untimely
    u. death
    u. demise
    u. pregnancy
untiring
untouchable
untouched
untoward
    u. cholinergic effect
    u. outcome
untreated
    u. episode
    u. psychiatric illness
    u. psychosis
    u. sequela
untriggered agitation
untroubled
untrue
untruthful
unusual
    u. behavior
    u. detail response (Dd)
    u. fatigue
    u. manner
    u. personality
    u. punishment
    u. rare detail response (dr)
    u. sleep posture
unveiling
unwanted
    u. child
    u. pregnancy
    u. sexual advance
unwarranted idea

unwieldy
unwilling
unwise dieting
unwitting
unwonted
unworldly
unworthiness
    feeling of u.
unworthy
unyielding
UO
    undetermined origin
up
    act up
    acting up
    ball up
    up in the clouds
    damming up
    ups and downs
    dream up
    drum up
    dry up
    face up
    fed up
    gang up
    knock up
    knocked up
    mixed up
    open up
    rub up
    send up
    shack up
    shoot up
    shore up
    shut up
    speak up
    talk up
    tear up
    throw up
    washed up
upbeat
upbringing
    religious u.
update
up-front
upheaval
    emotional u.
uphill
uphold
uplift
upper
    u. abdominal periosteal reflex

    u. bound
    u. crust
    u. hand
    u. motor neuron
upper-class
uppity
up-regulated
up-regulation
    u.-r./downregulation hypothesis
    receptor u.-r.
uproar
uproot
uprooted psychology
uprooting neurosis
upset
    emotional u.
    emotionally u.
    excessively u.
    gastrointestinal u.
    mental u.
upsetting
upstanding
upswap
uptake site
uptight
up-to-date medications
upward
    u. masking
    u. mobility
upwardly mobile
UR
    utilization review
uranism
uranoplasty
urban
    u. crisis
    u. psychiatry
urbanite
urbanization
urchin
ur-defense
uremia
uremic
    u. convulsion
    u. seizure
urethral
    u. anxiety
    u. erotism
    u. phase
    u. stage
urge
    anomalous sexual u.

U

NOTES

urge *(continued)*
> ego-syntonic gambling u.
> u. to gamble
> gambling u.
> inappropriate u.
> u. incontinence
> intense sexual u.
> intrusive u.
> involuntary premonitory u.
> masochistic sexual u.
> premonitory u.
> sexual u.

urgency
urinary
> u. continence
> u. incontinence

urinate
urine
> dirty u.
> drug-negative u.
> u. drug screen
> u. testing
> u. toxicology screen
> white turbid u.

uriposia
uroclepsia
urocrisia, urocrisis
urolagnia
urophilia
urticaria
> giant u.
> psychogenic u.

US
> Sex Information and Education
> Council of the US (SIECUS)

usage
> idiomatic u.

use
> adjunctive u.
> adolescent drug u.
> age at onset of u.
> alcohol u.
> caffeine u.
> chemical of u.
> chronic u.
> clinical u.
> compulsive substance u.
> employee drug u.
> excessive drug u.
> excessive laxative u.
> fatal complications of illicit
>   drug u.
> frequency of drug u.
> general medical u.
> history of tobacco u.
> illegal drug u.
> illicit drug u.
> illicit opiate u.

> intravenous drug u.
> I.V. drug u.
> long-term heavy u.
> medical u.
> neuroleptic u.
> nicotine u.
> nonpathological substance u.
> opioid u.
> opium u.
> past month alcohol u.
> pathologic substance u.
> potentially fatal complications of
>   illicit drug u.
> prenatal illicit drug u.
> psychoactive substance u. (PSUD)
> recreational drug u.
> routine u.
> substance u.
> tobacco u.

user
> caffeine u.
> chronic cocaine u.
> chronic ethanol u.
> cocaine u.
> drug u.
> ethanol u.
> heroin u.
> intravenous drug u.
> needle u.
> nicotine u.
> regular caffeine u.
> regular drug u.

USP
> United States Pharmacopeia
USPHS
> United States Public Health Service
usual
> u. behavior
> u. childhood illness
> u. mood

usurp
utilitarian
> u. principle
> u. theory
utilitarianism
> act u.
> hedonistic u.
> negative u.
> pluralism u.
> pluralistic u.
> rule u.
utility
> expected u. (EU)
utilization
> evaluation u.
> medical u.
> u. review (UR)

u. review committee
u. technique
utilizer
high u.
Utopia

utricular reflex
utterance
uxorial
uxoricide
uxorious

NOTES

U

V

V. code
V. factor

v, vs

versus

vacant

v. spell
v. stare

vaccination

vache

coitus a la v.

vacillate

vacuo

hydrocephalus ex v.

vacuous affect

vacuum

v. activity
existential v.
v. headache

vagabondage

vagabond neurosis

vagal attack

vagarious

vagina, pl. **vaginae**

v. dentata

vaginal

v. envy
v. father
v. hypesthesia
v. orgasm
v. plethysmograph

vaginam

per v.

vaginate

vaginism

vaginismus, vaginism

lifelong-type v.
psychic v.

vagolysis

vagolytic

vagomimetic

vagotomy

vagotonia

vagotropic

vagovagal

vagrancy

vagrant

vague

v. communication
v. complaint
nouvelle v.
v. perplexity
v. speech
v. thinking

vagueness

vagus

v. nerve
v. nerve stimulation (VAS, VNS)

vail

vain

vainglorious

vainglory

valence

emotional v.
normal v.
positive v.

valerate

ammonium v.
amyl v.

valerian

valetudinarian

valetudinary

valid

v. consent
v. diagnosis
v. information

validating variable

validation

v. communication pattern
consensual v.
cross v.
v. strategy
v. therapy

validity

clinical v.
v. coefficient
concergent and divergent v.
concurrent v.
construct v.
content v.
criterion v.
criterion-related v.
descriptive v.
discriminant v.
ecological v.
empirical v.
etiological v.
external v.
face v.
factorial v.
internal v.
internalized v.
intervening v.
item v.
known group v.
predictive v.
psychometric v.
v. scale

Valleix point

valor

V

valuable
value

acculturation problem with
expression of political v.
acculturation problem with
expression of religious v.
aesthetic v.
affective v.
Allport-Vernon-Linzey Study
of V.'s
being v.
confusion of v.'s
core v.'s
critical v.
cultural v.
educational v.
face v.
fluidity v.
foreign v.
idealized v.
internal v.
v.'s inventory
v. judgment
moral v.
nontrivial v.
p v.
parental v.
personal v.
political v.
predictive v.
prognostic v.
religious v.'s
self-reference v.
sentimental v.
sharing of v.'s
social v.
spiritual v.
status v.
Study of V.'s (SV)
symbolic v.
v. system
traditional v.
Wilder law of initial v.

valve

safety v.

vamp
vampirism

parasitic v.

vandal
vandalism

sexual v.

vandalize
van der Kolk law
vaniteuse

folie v.

vanity
vantage

variability

behavioral v.
metabolic v.
trait v.

variable

antecedent v.
antecedent-consequence v.
autochthonous v.
v. behavior
biopsychosocial v.
clinical v.
cognitive v.
continuous v.
criterion v.
demographic v.
dependent v.
dynamic v.
experimental v.
health-related v.
independent v.
index v.
v. interval (VI)
intervening v.
moderator v.
organic v.
organismic v.
outcome v.
predictor v.
psychiatric v.
quantitative v.
random v.
v. ratio (VR)
v. reinforcement
situational v.
sociodemographic v.
validating v.

variable-interval reinforcement schedule
variance

analysis of v. (ANOVA)
between-group v.
error v.
multivariate analysis of v.
(MANOVA)
twice-repeated multivariate analysis
of v.

variant

bizarre v.
epileptic v.

variate
variation

cerebral hemodynamic v.
chance v.
coefficient of v. (CV)
conative negative v. (CNV)
contingent negative v. (CNV)
cultural v.
diurnal mood v.
interindividual v.

negative v.
physiological functional v.
reverse diurnal v.
situational tic v.
variety of sexual behavior
varimax rotation
VAS
vagus nerve stimulation
vascular
v. dementia
v. dementia with delirium
v. dementia with delusions
v. dementia with depressed mood
v. depression
v. headache
v. muscle
v. neurosyphilis
v. territory
vasculogenic loss of erectile functioning
vase
Rubin v.
vasectomy
vasoactive
v. effective
v. intestinal peptide (VIP)
vasoconstriction
caffeine-induced v.
sympathetic-nervous-system-
medicated v.
vasoconstrictive action
vasogenic shock
vasomotor
v. absence
v. component
v. epilepsy
v. headache
v. imbalance
v. instability
v. spasm
v. syncope
vasoneurosis
vasopressor
v. syncope
vasoreflex
vasostimulant
vasovagal
v. attack
v. attack of Gowers
v. epilepsy
v. syncope
v. syndrome
vaunt

VBR
ventricle-to-brain ratio
VC
visual communication
VD
venereal disease
VDR
vitamin D receptor
VDT
visual distortion test
vecu
déjà v.
veganism
vegan vegetarian diet
vegetarian diet
vegetarianism
vegetate
vegetative
v. level
v. life
v. nervous system
v. neurosis
v. retreat
v. state
v. subscale
v. symptom
vehemence
vehement
vehicle
v. for communication
v. fear
veil
aqueduct v.
veiled threat
velar assimilation
velars
backing to v.
velleity
vellicate
vellication
velocity
nerve conduction v.
vendetta
venereal
v. bubo
v. disease (VD)
v. sore
veneris ardor
vengeance
vengeful
venial sin
venomous

V

NOTES

venter
  abactus v.
ventilate concern
ventilation of feeling
ventilatory
ventral
  v. amygdala fugal pathway
  v. amygdaloid fugal projection
  v. paralimbic region
ventricle
  lateral v.
  v. size
ventricle-to-brain ratio (VBR)
ventricular
  v. arrhythmia
  v. dysphonia
  v. system
ventriculi (*pl. of* ventriculus)
ventriculitis
ventriculography
ventriculoscopy
ventriculus, pl. ventriculi
  fomes ventriculi
ventromedial
  v. cortex
  v. hypothalamus
  v. prefrontal cortex of the brain
venturesome
VEP
  visual evoked potential
VER
  visual evoked response
vera
  melancholia v.
  neuralgia facialis v.
veracious
veracity
verbal
  v. abuse
  v. aggression
  v. agnosia
  v. agraphia
  v. alexia
  v. amnesia
  v. aphasia
  v. apraxia
  v. automatism
  v. aversion therapy
  v. behavior
  v. communication
  v. comprehension factor
  v. comprehension index
  v. conceptualization ability
  v. cue
  v. deficit
  v. expression
  v. fluency
  v. generalization

v. information
v. insult
v. intellectual functioning
v. intelligence
v. intervention
v. language quotient
v. leakage
v. learning
v. masochism
v. material
v. mediation
v. memory exercise
v. memory impairment
v., numerical, and reasoning (VNR)
v. outburst
v. paraphasia
v. perceptual speed
v. perseveration
v. play
v. reasoning
v. reinforcement
v. scale (VS)
v. slur
v. subtest
v. suggestion
v. technique
v. thought
v. weighted sum score
v. working memory
verbal-auditory agnosia
verbalis
  asemasia v.
verbalism
verbalization of feeling
verbalize
verbalizing
  inappropriate v.
verbal-visual agnosia
verbatim recall
verbiage
verbicide
verbigerate
verbigeration
  hallucinatory v.
verbochromia
verbomania
verborum
verbose
verboten
verbous
verdict
  guilty v.
veridical dream
verifiable
veritable
verity
vermicular movement
verminous

vermis
 anterior v.
vernacular
veroomania
versatile
versatility
verse
versenate
version
 episode v.
versus (v, vs)
vertebral
 v. cervical instability
vertebrobasilar insufficiency
vertical
 v. conflict
 v. mobility
 v. nystagmus
 v. transmission
 v. vertigo
vertiginosa
 epilepsia v.
vertiginosus
 status v.
vertiginous
 v. epilepsy
 v. seizure
vertigo
 Charcot v.
 chronic v.
 endemic paralytic v.
 epileptic v.
 essential v.
 galvanic v.
 height v.
 horizontal v.
 hysterical v.
 laryngeal v.
 lateral v.
 mechanical v.
 nocturnal v.
 objective v.
 organic v.
 paralyzing v.
 postural v.
 psychogenic v.
 rotary v.
 sham-movement v.
 subjective v.
 systematic v.
 true v.

 vertical v.
 voltaic v.
vesania
vesanique
 delire v.
vestibular
 v. hallucination
 v. migraine
 v. movement
 v. nerve
vestibuloequilibratory control
vestibulospinal
veteran
 combat v.
 Vietnam-era v.
vex
vexatious
VI
 variable interval
 visual imagery
viable
 v. alternative
 v. synapse
vial
vibrant
vibration
 forced v.
 v. syndrome
vibrator
vibratory
 v. massage
 v. sensibility
vibrotactile
 v. response
 v. threshold
VIBS, vibs
 vocabulary, information, block design,
  similarity
VIC
 visual communication
vicarious
 v. function
 v. learning
 v. liability
 v. living
 v. trial and error (VTE)
 v. violence
vice
vice-like pain
vicious
 v. circle
 v. cycle

NOTES

V

vicissitude
    instinctual v.
vicissitudes of life
victim
    v. abuse
    accident v.
    crime v.
    v. of criminal violence
    cyberstalking v.
    depressed suicide v.
    v. of domestic violence
    v. empathy
    female v.
    home invasion v.
    intended v.
    male v.
    potential suicide v.
    primary v.
    v. psychology
    rape v.
    v. recidivism
    v. role
    stalking v.
    suicide v.
    v. syndrome
victimization
    multiple v.
victimize
victimized teen
victimology
victorianism
victorious
video
    v. feedback
    v. game
    v. game violence
    v. lottery terminal (VLT)
    v. lottery terminal gambling
    v. therapy
videoconferencing
videotape
Vienna
    V. Psychoanalytic Society
Viet Cong
Vietnam
    V. syndrome
    V. war
Vietnam-era veteran
view
    point of v.
    Pollyanna-like v.
    stilted v.
viewing
viewless
viewpoint
    alternative v.
    biologic v.
    economic v.

    genetic v.
    health v.
vigil
    coma v.
    fatiguing v.
vigilambulism
vigilance
    v. deficit
    perceptual v.
    visuomotor v.
vigilant
vigilante
vigility of attention
vignette
vigor
vigorous
Vigotsky
vile
vilification
vilify
villainous
villa system
vincible
vindicate
vindictive
violate
violated
    sexually v.
violating behavior
violation
    boundary v.
    civil rights v.
    ethics v.
    nonsexual boundary v.
    probation v.
    restraining order v.
    v. of rules
    sexual boundary v.
violator
    norm v.
violence
    activity of v.
    acts of v.
    adolescent v.
    adolescents risk for v.
    alcohol-related risk for v.
    alleviating v.
    American Academy of Pediatrics
      Task Force on V.
    antecedents of v.
    community v.
    domestic v. (DV)
    drug-related v.
    exposure to v.
    extreme act of v.
    extreme level of v.
    family v.
    good kid v.

graphic v.
juvenile v.
manifestation of v.
media v.
motion picture v.
National Resource Center on
  Domestic V.
origin of v.
pathogen of v.
peer support for v.
perpetrator of v.
predatory v.
predisposing socioculture factors
  for v.
v. prevention
prior v.
random act of v.
repetitive v.
v. risk
risk factors for v.
sign of impending v.
v. in stalking
teen v.
teenage v.
television v.
terrorist v.
v. theory
threat of v.
unpredictable act of v.
vicarious v.
victim of criminal v.
victim of domestic v.
video game v.
witness to repetitive v.
workplace v.
youth v.
violence-promoting factor
violent
  v. act
  v. acting out
  v. acts on television
  v. adolescent
  v. agitation
  v. child
  v. command hallucination
  v. conduct disorder
  v. crime
  v. criminal behavior
  v. death
  v. delinquent
  v. fantasy
  v. figure

v. media
v. offender
v. offense
v. outburst
v. past
v. pediatric patient
v. personal assault
v. resistance
v. stalker
v. temper
v. theme
v. thought
VIP
  vasoactive intestinal peptide
  voluntary interruption of pregnancy
  VIP syndrome
virgin
  v. fear
  V. Mary vision
virginal anxiety
virginity
  v. scruple
  v. taboo
virgophrenia
virile
  molimen climactericum v.
virilescence
virilia
virilism
virility
virilization
virtuality
virtual reality therapy
virtue
  cardinal v.
  easy v.
  v. ethics
virtuous
virulence
virulent
virus
  Epstein-Barr v. (EBV)
  herpes simplex v.
  human immunodeficiency v. (HIV)
  slow v.
VIS
  vocational interest schedule
visage
  scanning v.
visceral
  v. anesthesia
  v. disorder

V

NOTES

visceral *(continued)*
    v. emotional state
    v. epilepsy
    v. learning
    v. nervous system
    v. neurosis
    v. sense
visceromotor
    v. pathway
viscerotonia
viscosity
    v. of libido
    v. personality
    social v.
visibility
visible
visile
vision
    altered v.
    beatific v.
    binocular v.
    blurred v.
    blurring of v.
    central v.
    darkening v.
    v. disparity
    double v.
    entopic v.
    field of v.
    foveal v.
    hemifield of v.
    hypnagogic v.
    impaired v.
    inner v.
    patterning v.
    phantom v.
    photopic v.
    stereoscopic v.
    subjective v.
    tunnel v.
    twilight v.
    Virgin Mary v.
visionary
visionism
visionless
visit
    baseline v.
    clinical v.
    conjugal v.
    followup v.
    home v.
    post baseline v.
    reason for v.
    therapeutic trial v. (TTV)
    trial v.
    trial home v.
    weekend v.
visitant

visitation
    conjugal v.
    v. rights
visiting nurse
vista response
visual
    v. accommodation
    v. acuity
    v. agnosia
    v. aid
    v. alertness
    v. alexia
    v. amnesia
    v. aphasia
    v. association cortex
    v. attention
    v. aura
    v. center
    v. choice reaction time test
    v. closure
    v. communication (VC, VIC)
    v. cortical area
    v. cue
    v. discrimination
    v. disorientation reaction
    v. distortion
    v. distortion test (VDT)
    v. epilepsy
    v. evoked potential (VEP)
    v. evoked response (VER)
    v. extinction
    v. field
    v. field construction
    v. field cut
    v. field defect
    v. field disturbance
    v. hallucination
    v. hallucination denial syndrome
    v. hearing
    v. illusion
    v. image
    v. imagery (VI)
    v. inattention
    v. letter dysgnosia
    v. literacy
    v. memory impairment
    v. memory span task
    v. neglect
    v. number dysgnosia
    v. obstruction
    v. pattern recognition
    v. perception
    v. perceptual deficit
    v. perceptual skill
    v. perceptual speed
    v. processing
    v. prodrome
    v. pursuit movement

v. radiation
v. region
v. representation strategy
v. reproduction
v. seizure
v. sensation
v. sensory modality
v. spatial memory
v. stimulation
v. stimulus
v. subtest
v. symptom
v. threat test
v. tracking
v. training
v. zone
visualization
visualize
visual-kinetic dissociation
visual-motor
v.-m. coordination
v.-m. impairment
v.-m. task
visual-spatial
v.-s. acalculia
v.-s. agnosia
v.-s. distortion
visuoauditory
visuoconstructional ability
visuognosis
visuomotor
v. ability
v. problem-solving skill
v. vigilance
visuoperceptive defect
visuopsychic
visuosensory
visuospatial
v. attention
v. disorder
v. disorientation
v. functioning
v. memory
v. problem solving
v. processing
v. scratch pad
v. stimulus
visuotopic
vita
dolce v.
vital
elan v.

v. energy
v. sign (VS)
v. statistics
vitality
vitalize
vitam
intra v.
vitamin
v. B12 neuropathy
v. deficiency
v. D receptor (VDR)
v. therapy
vituperate
vituperative
vivacious
vivid
v. dream
v. dream image
v. dream recall
v. hallucination
v. nightmare
vividness
vivify
vivo
ex v.
exposure in v.
in v.
vivos
inter v.
vixen
vizard
VLT
video lottery terminal
VNR
verbal, numerical, and reasoning
VNS
vagus nerve stimulation
vocabulary
active v.
v., information, block design, similarity (VIBS, vibs)
v. language quotient
passive v.
v. scale
v. skills
v. test
vocal
v. abuse
v. amusia
v. attack
v. band
v., chronic motor, or tic disorder

V

NOTES

vocal *(continued)*
    v. pitch abnormality
    v. tic
vocalization
    involuntary v.
    motor v.
    nonrhythmic v.
    rapid v.
    recurrent v.
    stereotyped v.
    sudden v.
vocalize
vocation
vocational
    v. achievement
    v. adjustment
    v. appraisal
    v. choice
    v. counseling
    v. evaluation
    v. functioning
    v. goal setting
    v. guidance
    v. identity
    v. interest schedule (VIS)
    v. maladjustment
    v. performance
    psychological, social, and v. (PSV)
    v. rehabilitation (VR)
    v. rehabilitation and education
      (VR&E)
    v. service
    v. strain
    v. training
vociferate
vociferous
Vogt-Spielmeyer idiocy
voguish
voice
    active v.
    adolescent v.
    altered v.
    breathy v.
    chest v.
    v. commenting
    condescending tone of v.
    conversational v.
    v. conversing
    disapproving v.
    discordance of v.
    v. disorder
    esophageal v.
    eunuchoid v.
    falsetto v.
    gravel v.
    hallucinated v.
    hearing v.'s
    high-pitched v.

    hysterical v.'s
    v. inside head
    v. intonation
    monotone v.
    monotonous v.
    muted v.'s
    negative v.
    v. outside head
    panicky v.
    pejorative v.
    quavering v.
    shaking v.
    soundless v.
    threatening v.
    tone of v.
    transsexual v.
    trembling v.
voiceless
voiceprint
void fear
voiding
    inappropriate v.
voilá
vol
    monomanie du v.
volatile
    v. disposition
    v. personality
    v. situation
    v. solvent
    v. solvent dependence
    v. temper
volition
    act and v.
    derailment of v.
    hedonic v.
volitional
    v. capacity
    v. drinking
    v. impairment
    v. movement
    v. tremor
volley
voltage-gated
voltaic vertigo
volte-face
volubility
    excessive v.
voluble
volume
    amygdala v.
    blood v.
    brain v.
    cortical v.
    frontal lobe v.
    hippocampal raw v.
    intracranial brain v.
    intracranial raw v.

mean intracranial raw v.
mean normalized whole brain v.
normalized whole brain v.
prefrontal cortical v.
raw v.
total brain v.
whole brain raw v.
volumetric loss
volumetry
    MRI v.
voluntarism
voluntary
    v. active imagining
    v. admission
    v. behavior
    v. commitment
    v. control
    v. dehydration
    v. euthanasia
    v. hospitalization
    v. hysterical overbreathing
    v. impulse
    v. interruption of pregnancy (VIP)
    v. motion
    v. motor functioning
    v. muscle movement
    v. mutism
    v. napping phenomenon
    v. retention
    v. sensory functioning
    v. time-out
voluptuous
volupty
vomiting
    cyclic v.
    cyclical psychogenic v.
    v. fear
    nausea and v. (N&V)
    nervous v.
    psychogenic cyclical v.
    v. reflex
    self-induced v.
vomitory
vomiturition
vomitus
von
    v. Domarus principle
    v. Graefe sign
    v. Hippel-Lindau disease
    v. Knorring criterion
    v. Zerssen circumplex model of premorbid personality

voodoo death
voodooism
voodooistic
voracious appetite
vorbeireden
votary
votive
voulu
    déjà v.
vow
    celibacy v.
    marriage v.'s
    solemn v.
vowel assimilation
voxel
    cerebral v.
    contiguous v.
voyeur
voyeurism
    adolescent v.
    v. paraphilia
voyeuristic
    v. activity
    v. sexual behavior
    v. sexually arousing fantasy
voyeuse
VR
    variable ratio
    vocational rehabilitation
VR&E
    vocational rehabilitation and education
VS
    verbal scale
    vital sign
VTE
    vicarious trial and error
vu
    déjà vu
    jamais vu
vulgar
    v. language
vulgaris
    Artemisia v.
vulgarism
vulgarity
vulgarize
vulnerability
    danger-laden schema v.
    emotional v.
    genetic v.
    narcissistic v.
    pretraumatic v.

V

NOTES

vulnerability *(continued)*
    putative adoptee v.
    suicide v.
    v. theory
    v. threshold
vulnerable
    v. child
    v. child syndrome

Vulpian effect
vulpine
vulturous
vulvismus

W

whole response

WA

Workaholics Anonymous

waddling gait

wage

w. earner

living w.

wager

waggish

wagon

fall off the w.

off the w.

on the w.

waif

wail

waiver

wakefulness

w. epochs

full w.

intermittent w.

midpontine w.

primary disorder of w.

w. quiet

w. resting

wakeful state

wake time

waking

w. EEG

w. frequency

w. hypnosis

w. numbness

wallerian

wallow

wan

wand

NCP programming w.

wander

wandering

aimless w.

w. attention

w. cell

w. impulse

w. mind

w. pain

w. thought

wanderlust

wane

wax and w.

wanton

war

w. baby

w. bride

consequences of w.

drug w.

w. footing

gang w.

w. gas

injury of w.

Korean W.

limited w.

w. of nerves

w. neurosis

not prisoner of w. (NPOW)

nuclear w.

w. on drug

w. power

prisoner of w. (POW)

threat of w.

Vietnam w.

world w.

World W. I (WWI)

World W. II (WWII)

w. zone

ward

disturbed w.

locked w.

long-stay w.

open w.

psychiatric w.

wardrobe

Wardrop method

warehousing

mental patient w.

warfare

ABC w.

atomic, biological, chemical w.

biologic w.

biologic and chemical w. (BCW)

chemical and biological w. (CBW)

chemical, radiological, and
biological w.

gang w.

guerrilla w.

psychological w. (PW)

trench w.

war-game player

warlike

warlock

warm

w. effector

failure to w.

w. sensitivity

warmhearted

warm-sensitive neuron

warmth

paradoxical w.

warn

duty to w.

failure to w.

W

warning
    black box w.
    Tarasoff w.
warp
warrant
    bench w.
    death w.
    search w.
war-related stress
warrior
wartime
wary
washed
    w. out
    w. up
washout
    drug w.
WASP
    World Association for Social Psychiatry
waspish
wastage
    air w.
wastebasket diagnosis
wasted
wasting
    w. palsy
    w. paralysis
watchful
watchfulness
    frozen w.
watching
    repetitive w.
watchspring theory
watchword
water
    w. balance
    w. balance in schizophrenia
    body w.
    w. deprivation
    w. drinking
    w. intoxication
    w. on the brain
water-seeking behavior
watershed
    w. area
    w. infarction
wave
    alpha w.
    w. analyzer
    aperiodic w.
    beta w.
    brain w.
    delta w.
    electromagnetic w.
    flat top w.
    gamma w.
    new w.
    random w.

    sine w.
    theta w.
waveform
    brief pulse w.
    early component w.
    pulse w.
waveshape
waving
    hand w.
waxen
wax and wane
waxy flexibility
way
    maladaptive w.
    parting of the w.'s
    set in one's w.'s
wayward
weak
    w. ego
    w. ego control
    w. parent
    w. sister
    w. stress
weak-hearted
weakling
weak-minded
weak-mindedness
weakness
    color w.
    ego w.
    w. fear
    localized w.
    psychological w.
    strengths and w.'s
weak-willed
wealth
    delusion of w.
wealthy
wean
weaning
weapon
    assault w.
    assault with a deadly w. (ADW)
    availability of w.'s
    biologic w.
    chemical w.
    w.'s hoard
weaponry
wear down
weariless
wearisome
weary
weasling
weathered
weatherworn
weaving
    head w.
Web counseling

Weber
    W. test
Weber-Fechner law
wedding
    w. night
    shotgun w.
Wedensky facilitation
wedlock
    out of w.
Wednesday Evening Society
weed
    loco w.
week
    drinking days per w.
weekend
    w. drinker
    w. drinking
    w. headache
    w. hospital
    w. hospitalization
    w. neurosis
    w. parent
    w. pass
    w. visit
weeping
    overt w.
weepy
we-group
weigh down
weight
    beta w.
    brain w.
    w. discrimination
    failure to gain w.
    w. gain
    w. gain potential
    ideal body w. (IBW)
    w. issue
    w. liability
    w. lifter
    w. loss
    w. loss maintenance
    w. loss therapy
    w. management
    w. perception
    w. regulation
    target w.
    W. Watchers diet
weight-control program
weighted-harm principle
weighted sum score

weighting
    item w.
weight-loss program
weight-neutral psychotic medication
Weir
    W. Mitchell therapy
    W. Mitchell treatment
weird
welfare
    w. emotion
    Health, Education, and W. (HEW)
    International Committee on
      Social W. (ICSW)
    live on w.
    w. organization
    social w.
    w. system
well
    w. adjusted for age
    w. groomed
    w. oriented
well-advised
well-articulated speech
well-being
    emotional w.-b.
    global w.-b.
    w.-b. scale
    sense of w.-b.
    subjective w.-b.
well-conditioned
well-defined
well-delineated psychiatric disorder
well-formed
    w.-f. delusion
    w.-f. outcome
well-groomed
well-motivated
wellness
    w. principle
    sense of w.
well-off
well-read
well-rounded
well-spoken
well-systematized delusional system
well-timed
well-to-do
welsh
welt
weltmerism
weltschmerz
wench

W

NOTES

Werdnig-Hoffmann disease
werewolf
Wernicke
    W. aphasia
    W. area
    W. 22, 39, 40 area
    W. center
    W. cramp
    W. dementia
    W. dysphasia
    W. fluent encephalopathy
    W. reaction
    W. syndrome
Wernicke-Korsakoff
    W.-K. encephalopathy
    W.-K. syndrome
Werther syndrome
Western
    W. blot test
    W. ethics
    W. medicine
    W. subtype
Westphal
    W. disease
    W. phenomenon
    W. pseudosclerosis
    W. sign
Westphal-Leyden syndrome
Westphal-Piltz phenomenon
wet
    w. behind the ears
    w. beriberi
    w. brain syndrome
    w. dream
Wever-Bray
    W.-B. effect
    W.-B. phenomenon
wheal
wheel
    activity w.
wheelchair sports
whereabouts
whiff
whimper
whine
whinge
whininess
whiplash injury
whipping
whirling
whisper
    forced w.
whispered speech
whispering
    involuntary w.
whispery
white
    w. Anglo-Saxon Protestant

    w. blood cell
    w. collar crime
    w. knuckling sobriety
    w. lie
    w. lightning
    w. matter
    w. matter change
    w. matter disease
    w. matter hyperintensity
    w. matter lactate
    w. matter lactate level
    w. matter pathology
    w. matter region
    w. matter structure
    w. matter tissue
    w. noise
    w. supremacist
    w. trash
    w. turbid urine
white-collar worker
white-headed
whitewash
WHO
    World Health Organization
    WHO instrument
whole
    w. brain atrophy
    w. brain blood flow
    w. brain boundary
    w. brain raw volume
    detail response elaborating the w. (DdW)
    w. focus orientation
    w. response (W, WR)
wholeness
    sense of w.
    undifferentiated w.
whore
    Wiccan w.
Wiccan whore
wide
    w. circles of thought
    w. range
wide-based gait
widowed status
widowhood
    w. crisis
wieldy
wife, pl. wives
    battered w.
wife-beating
wife-to-husband aggression
wihtiko
wild
    w. behavior
    w. psychoanalysis
Wilder law of initial value

NOTES

W

withdrawal *(continued)*
benzodiazepine w.
caffeine w.
cocaine w.
w. criteria
w. delirium
w. destructiveness
w. disorder
drug w.
w. dyskinesia
w. dystonia
w. effect
emotional w.
ethanol w.
w. from social affair
w. hallucinosis
heroin w.
hypnotic w.
infant narcotic w.
w. insomnia
interpersonal w.
w. method of contraception
morphine w.
w. movement
narcotic w.
newborn drug w.
nicotine w.
opioid w.
physical w.
w. process
psychoactive substance w.
w. reaction of adolescence
w. reaction of childhood
w. reflex
sedative w.
w. seizure
w. sign
social w.
w. state
substance-specific w.
sympathomimetic w.
w. symptom
w. syndrome
w. syndrome alcoholic psychosis
w. syndrome drug psychosis
thought w.
tobacco w.
w. tremor
uncomplicated alcohol w.
uncomplicated sedative, hypnotic, or
anxiolytic w.
withdrawal-based craving
withdrawal-related mood disorder
withdrawn
w. behavior
w. catatonic schizophrenia
withhold

within-family environmental factor
within normal limits (WNL)
withstand
witless
witness
w. to assault
character w.
w. credibility
w. to crime
expert w.
w. to murder
w. to repetitive violence
Wittigo psychosis
Wittmaak-Ekbom syndrome
witzelsucht
primary affective w.
wizardry
WNL
within normal limits
wolf-man
Wollaston theory
Woltman sign
woman, pl. **women**
women at risk
drug-using w.
medicine w.
non-drug-using w.
other w.
phallic w.
physiology of women
psychology of women
womanhood
woman's
w.'s liberation
w.'s liberation movement
w.'s role
womb
w. envy
w. fantasy
wonder drug
wont
woodbine
wool hwa-byung
woozy
word
w. approximation
w. association
w. association technique
w. attack
base w.
w. blindness
w. cathexis
w. center
class w.
w. coinage
coin new w.'s
w. configuration
w. deafness

w. debris
derogatory w.
dirty w.'s
w. discrimination score
w. dumbness
empty w.
feared w.'s
w. fluency
function w.
Jonah w.'s
last w.
microcosm of w.'s
phonetically balanced w.'s
phonologically irregular w.'s
phonologically regular w.'s
play on w.'s
w. processing
w. production
w. retrieval
w. rhyming
w. salad
w. search
stimulus w.
w. stimulus
thinking creatively with sounds
    and w.'s (TCSW)
w. understanding
w. wit
word-attack skill
word-building test
word-finding
w.-f. ability
w.-f. ability disturbance
w.-f. difficulty
w.-f. skill
word-recognition skill
work
w. addict
w. addiction
Bachelor of Social W. (BSW)
breath w.
case w.
circadian rhythm sleep disorder,
    shift w.
w. cure
w. decrement
w. disability
disaster w.
dream w.
w. dysfunction
w. ethic
family social w.

field w.
w. force
gratifying w.
grief w.
w. group
group w.
inability to finish w.
w. inhibition
Master of Social W. (MSW)
w. motivation
mourning w.
w. paralysis
w. performance
psychiatric social w.
w. schedule
social w.
testing, orientation, and w.
w. therapy
unexplained absence from w.
wit w.
workable
workaholic
W.'s Anonymous (WA)
worker
aftercare w.
blue-collar w.
certified social w. (CSW)
childcare w.
clinical social w.
disaster w.
indigenous w.
intake w.
linkage w.
mental health w.
National Association of
    Social W.'s
pink collar w.
psychiatric social w.
skilled w.
social w.
white-collar w.
work-for-pay unit
workhorse
working
w. alliance
w. community
w. diagnosis
w. environment
w. memory
w. memory function
w. mother
w. out

W

NOTES

working *(continued)*
  w. over
  w. relationship
  w. through
  w. type
work-limit test
workload
  mental w.
workmanship
workplace
  w. problem
  w. psychopath
  w. psychopathy
  w. safety
  w. violence
work-related task
work-release center
workshop
  career w.
  employment w.
  sheltered w.
  survival skills w.
  transitional employment w.
work-study program
world
  W. Association for Social Psychiatry (WASP)
  W. Congress of Psychiatry
  dream w.
  external w.
  W. Health Organization (WHO)
  inner w.
  intrapsychic w.
  make-believe w.
  on top of the w.
  W. Psychiatric Association (WPA)
  w. soul
  w. war
  W. War I (WWI)
  W. War II (WWII)
world-destruction fantasy
worriers
  born w.
worrisome
worry
  w. beads
  w. circuit
  constant w.
  w. control
  disabling w.
  duration of w.
  excessive w.
  severity of w.
  uncontrolled w.
  unrealistic w.
worrying symptom
worsening
  symptom w.

worse sleep continuity
worship
  ancestral w.
  devil w.
  hero w.
  Satan w.
  satanic w.
worth
  comparable w.
  inflated w.
worthless
worthlessness
  feeling of w.
  preoccupation with w.
  self-reported w.
wound
  gunshot w. (GSW)
  multiple stab w.'s (MSW)
  psychic w.
  self-inflicted w. (SIW)
  self-inflicted gunshot w.
  self-inflicted stab w.
wounded
  w. in action
  w. feeling
  w. victim syndrome
wounding
  narcissistic w.
  symbolic w.
WPA
  World Psychiatric Association
WR
  whole response
wraparound
wretched
wrist
  w. clonus
  w. cutting
  w. drop
  w. restraint
  w. skin cutting
wristed
writhe
writing
  w. ability
  w. assignment
  ataxic w.
  automatic w.
  compulsive w.
  developmental expressive w.
  w. disorder
  w. fear
  w. hand
  mirror w.
  pornographic w.
  self-directed w.
  spirit w.
  w. tremor

written
    w. communication
    w. expression
    w. language
    w. language quotient
wrongdoer
wrongdoing
    moral w.

wry neck
WWI
    World War I
WWII
    World War II
Wyburn-Mason syndrome

NOTES

W

X

X chromosome
X zone
X-bar theory
Xe clearance method
xenoglossophilia
xenon inhalation

xenorexia
xerophagia
xerostomia
X-linkage
X-linked dominance
xyrospasm

X

Y

Y chromosome

Yale
yan
yancy
yang

shuk y.
suo y.
yin and y.

yantra
yawning

psychogenic y.

yawn-sign approach
YBR

yellow brick road

year

y. of birth (YOB)
childhood y.'s
jail days per y.
quality-adjusted life y. (QALY)

yearbook
yearning
yellow brick road (YBR)
yen sleep
Yerkes-Dodson law
YES

Youth Enjoying Sobriety

yes-no

y.-n. answer
y.-n. question

yes-yes tremor
yin and yang
YOB

year of birth

yoga

Hatha y.
tantric y.

yohimbe

Pausinystalia y.

yohimbine
yoke
yoked control
yong

shook y.

York retreat
young

y. adulthood
y. adult psychiatry
Y. Adult self-report
developmentally appropriate self-
stimulatory behaviors in the y.

young-old patient
youngster

rebellious y.

youth

y. counselor
y. culture
delinquent y.
Y. Enjoying Sobriety (YES)
y. gambling
incarcerated y.
maladaptively aggressive y.
middle-class y.
Y. self-report
y. self support (YSR)
y. violence

youthful
YSR

youth self support

Y

Z

Z code
Z score transformation

z

z score
z score map

Zanarini concept
Zange-Kindler syndrome
zaniness
Zanoli-Vecchi syndrome
Zappert syndrome
Zarit burden interview
zazen
zealot
zealous
zealousness
Zeigarnik

Z. effect
Z. effect phenomenon

Zeitgeber

endogenous Z.
exogenous Z.

Zeitgebers

social Z.

Zeitgeist
zelotypia
Zen

Z. Buddhism
Z. therapy

zeppia
zero

z. family
z. population growth (ZPG)
z. tolerance

zero-order elimination kinetics
zest

loss of z.
reasonable z.

zimeldine
zoanthropic
zoanthropy

melancholia z.

zodiac
zoetic
zoic
Zollner illusion
zombie-like
zombiism
zonal
zona medullovasculosa
zone

analectrotonic z.
anelectrotonic z.
anterior speech z.
body buffer z.

chemoreceptor trigger z.
color z.
cortical z.
dolorogenic z.
epileptogenic z.
erogenous z.
erotogenic z.
genital z.
Head z.
hyperesthetic z.
hypnogenic z.
hysterogenic z.
intimate z.
language z.
latent z.
limbic z.
Marchant z.
motor z.
peripolar z.
personal distance z.
polar z.
posterior language z.
primary z.
reflexogenic z.
Rolando z.
social z.
subplate z.
tender z.
time z.
transition z.
trigger z.
ultramarginal z.
visual z.
war z.
X z.

zonesthesia
zonifugal
zonipetal
zooerastia
zooerasty
zoogenic
zoolagnia
zoolatry
zoomania
zoomorphism
zoon politikon
zoophagous
zoophile psychosis
zoophilia
zoophilic
zoophilism

erotic z.

zoopsia
zoosadism
zootic

Z

zoroastrianism
zoster
    herpes z.
zosteriform
zosteroid

ZPG
    zero population growth
Zung
zwischenstufe

Appendix 1
Alphabetical Listing of DSM-IV Diagnoses and Codes

Editor's Note: This listing is reprinted with permission from the *Diagnostic and Statistical Manual of Mental Disorders, Fourth Edition, Text Revision.* Copyright 2000, American Psychiatric Association. Please note that the terms in this listing follow APA style, which does not always conform with AAMT or AMA style. NOS = Not Otherwise Specified.

V62.3	Academic Problem	291.3	With Hallucinations
V62.4	Acculturation Problem	91.89	–Induced Sexual Dysfunction
308.3	Acute Stress Disorder		
	Adjustment Disorders	291.89	–Induced Sleep Disorder
309.9	Unspecified	303.00	Intoxication
309.24	With Anxiety	291.0	Intoxication Delirium
309.0	With Depressed Mood	291.9	-Related Disorder NOS
309.3	With Disturbance of Conduct	291.81	Withdrawal
		291.0	Withdrawal Delirium
309.28	With Mixed Anxiety and Depressed Mood	294.0	Amnestic Disorder Due to (indicate the General Medical Condition)
309.4	With Mixed Disturbance of Emotions and Conduct	294.8	Amnestic Disorder NOS
			Amphetamine (or Amphetamine-Like)
V71.01	Adult Antisocial Behavior	305.70	Abuse
995.2	Adverse Effects of Medication NOS	304.40	Dependence
		292.89	–Induced Anxiety Disorder
780.9	Age-Related Cognitive Decline	292.84	–Induced Mood Disorder
			–Induced Psychotic Disorder
300.22	Agoraphobia Without History of Panic Disorder	292.11	With Delusions
	Alcohol	292.12	With Hallucinations
305.00	Abuse	292.89	–Induced Sexual Dysfunction
303.90	Dependence		
291.89	–Induced Anxiety Disorder	292.89	–Induced Sleep Disorder
291.89	–Induced Mood Disorder	292.89	Intoxication
291.1	–Induced Persisting Amnestic Disorder	292.81	Intoxication Delirium
		292.9	–Related Disorder NOS
291.2	–Induced Persistent Dementia	292.0	Withdrawal
		307.1	Anorexia Nervosa
291.2	–Induced Psychotic Disorder	301.7	Antisocial Personality Disorder
291.5	With Delusions		

293.84	Anxiety Disorder Due to (indicate the General Medical Condition)		Bipolar I Disorder, Most Recent Episode Mixed
300.00	Anxiety Disorder NOS	296.66	In Full Remission
299.80	Asperger's Disorder	296.65	In Partial Remission
	Attention Deficit/Hyperactivity Disorder	296.61	Mild
		296.62	Moderate
314.01	Combined Type	296.63	Severe Without Psychotic Features
314.01	Predominantly Hyperactive-Impulsive Type	296.64	Severe With Psychotic Features
314.00	Predominantly Inattentive Type	296.60	Unspecified
		296.7	Bipolar I Disorder, Most Recent Episode Unspecified
314.9	Attention-Deficit/ Hyperactivity Disorder NOS		Bipolar I disorder, Single Manic Episode
299.00	Autistic Disorder	296.06	In Full Remission
301.82	Avoidant Personality Disorder	296.05	In Partial Remission
V62.82	Bereavement	296.01	Mild
296.80	Bipolar Disorder NOS	296.02	Moderate
	Bipolar I Disorder, Most Recent Episode Depressed	296.03	Severe Without Psychotic Features
296.56	In Full Remission	296.04	Severe With Psychotic Features
296.55	In Partial Remission	296.00	Unspecified
296.51	Mild	296.89	Bipolar II Disorder
296.52	Moderate	300.7	Body Dysmorphic Disorder
296.53	Severe Without Psychotic Features	V62.89	Borderline Intellectual Functioning
296.54	Severe With Psychotic Features	301.83	Borderline Personality Disorder
296.50	Unspecified	780.59	Breathing-Related Sleep Disorder
296.40	Bipolar I Disorder, Most Recent Episode Hypomanic	298.8	Brief Psychotic Disorder
	Bipolar I Disorder, Most Recent Episode Manic	307.51	Bulimia Nervosa
			Caffeine
296.46	In Full Remission	292.89	–Induced Anxiety Disorder
296.45	In Partial Remission	292.89	–Induced Sleep Disorder
296.41	Mild	305.09	Intoxication
296.42	Moderate	292.9	–Related Disorder NOS
296.43	Severe Without Psychotic Features		Cannabis
296.44	Severe With Psychotic Features	305.20	Abuse
		304.30	Dependence
296.40	Unspecified	292.89	–Induced Anxiety Disorder

300.12	Dissociative Amnesia
300.15	Dissociative Disorder NOS
300.13	Dissociative Fugue
300.14	Dissociative Identity Disorder
302.76	Dyspareunia (Not Due to a General Medical Condition)
307.47	Dyssomnia NOS
300.4	Dysthymic Disorder
307.50	Eating Disorder NOS
787.6	Encopresis, With Constipation and Overflow Incontinence
307.7	Encopresis, Without Constipation and Overflow Incontinence
307.6	Enuresis (Not Due to a General Medical Condition)
307.6	Exhibitionism
315.31	Expressive Language Disorder
Factitious Disorder	
300.19	With Combined Psychological and Physical Signs and Symptoms
300.19	With Predominantly Physical Signs and Symptoms
300.16	With Predominantly Psychological Signs and Symptoms
300.19	Factitious Disorder NOS
307.59	Feeding Disorder of Infancy or Early Childhood
625.0	Female Dyspareunia Due to (Indicate the General Medical Condition)
625.8	Female Hypoactive Sexual Desire Disorder Due to (Indicate the General Medical Condition)
302.73	Female Orgasmic Disorder
302.72	Female Sexual Arousal Disorder
302.81	Fetishism

302.89	Frotteurism
Gender Identity Disorder	
302.85	in Adolescents or Adults
302.86	in Children
392.6	Gender Identity Disorder NOS
300.02	Generalized Anxiety Disorder
Hallucination	
305.30	Abuse
304.50	Dependence
292.89	–Induced Anxiety Disorder
292.84	–Induced Mood Disorder
	–Induced Psychotic Disorder
292.11	With Delusions
292.12	With Hallucinations
292.89	Intoxication
292.81	Intoxication Delirium
292.89	Persisting Perception Disorder
292.9	–Related Disorder NOS
301.50	Histrionic Personality Disorder
307.44	Hypersomnia Related to (Indicate the Axis I or Axis II Disorder)
302.71	Hypoactive Sexual Desire Disorder
300.7	Hypochondriasis
313.82	Identity Problem
312.30	Impulse-Control Disorder NOS
Inhalant	
305.90	Abuse
304.60	Dependence
292.89	–Induced Anxiety Disorder
292.84	–Induced Mood Disorder
292.82	–Induced Persisting Dementia
	–Induced Psychotic Disorder
292.11	With Delusions
292.12	With Hallucinations
292.89	Intoxication
292.81	Intoxication Delirium
292.9	–Related Disorder NOS

307.42 Insomnia Related to (Indicate the Axis I or Axis II Disorder)
312.34 Intermittent Explosive Disorder
312.32 Kleptomania
315.9 Learning Disorder NOS

Major Depressive Disorder, Recurrent
296.36   In Full Remission
296.35   In Partial Remission
296.31   Mild
296.32   Moderate
296.33   Severe Without Psychotic Features
296.34   Severe With Psychotic Features
296.30   Unspecified

Major Depressive Disorder, Single Episode
296.26   In Full Remission
296.25   In Partial Remission
296.21   Mild
296.22   Moderate
296.23   Severe Without Psychotic Features
296.24   Severe With Psychotic Features
296.20   Unspecified
608.89 Male Dyspareunia Due to (Indicate the General Medical Condition)
302.72 Male Erectile Disorder
607.84 Male Erectile Disorder Due to (Indicate the General Medical Condition)
608.89 Male Hypoactive Sexual Desire Due to (Indicate the General Medical Condition)
302.74 Male Orgasmic Disorder
V65.2 Malingering
315.1 Mathematics Disorder
Medication-Induced

333.90 Movement Disorder NOS
333.1 Postural Tremor
293.9 Mental Disorder NOS Due to (Indicate the General Medical Condition)
319 Mental Retardation, Severity Unspecified
317 Mild Mental Retardation
315.32 Mixed Receptive-Expressive Language Disorder
318.0 Moderate Mental Retardation
293.83 Mood Disorder Due to (Indicate the General Medical Condition)
296.90 Mood Disorder NOS
301.81 Narcissistic Personality Disorder
347 Narcolepsy
V61.21 Neglect of Child
995.52 Neglect of Child (if focus of attention is on victim)
Neuroleptic-Induced
333.99   Acute Akathisia
333.7   Acute Dystonia
332.1   Parkinsonism
333.82   Tardive Dyskinesia
333.92 Neuroleptic Malignant Syndrome
Nicotine
305.10   Dependence
292.9   –Related Disorder NOS
292.0   Withdrawal
307.47 Nightmare Disorder
V71.09 No Diagnosis on Axis II
V71.09 No Diagnosis or Condition on Axis I
V15.81 Noncompliance With Treatment
300.3 Obsessive-Compulsive Disorder
301.4 Obsessive-Compulsive Personality Disorder
V62.2 Occupational Problem

Opioid
305.50   Abuse
304.00   Dependence
292.84   –Induced Mood Disorder
        –Induced Psychotic
        Disorder
292.11   With Delusions
292.12   With Hallucinations
292.89   –Induced Sexual
        Dysfunction
292.89   –Induced Sleep Disorder
292.89   Intoxication
292.81   Intoxication Delirium
292.9   –Related Disorder NOS
292.0   Withdrawal
313.81   Oppositional Defiant Disorder
625.8   Other Female Sexual
        Dysfunction Due to
        (Indicate the General
        Medical Condition)
608.89   Other Male Sexual
        Dysfunction Due to
        (Indicate the General
        Medical Condition) Other
        (or Unknown) Substance
305.90   Abuse
304.90   Dependence
292.89   –Induced Anxiety Disorder
292.81   –Induced Delirium
292.84   –Induced Mood Disorder
292.83   –Induced Persisting
        Amnestic Disorder
292.82   –Induced Persisting
        Dementia
-Induced Psychotic Disorder
292.11   With Delusions
292.12   With Hallucinations
292.89   –Induced Sexual
        Dysfunction
292.89   –Induced Sleep Disorder
292.89   Intoxication
292.9   –Related Disorder NOS
292.0   Withdrawal

Pain Disorder
307.89   Associated With Both
        Psychological Factors and
        a General Medical
        Condition
307.80   Associated With Psychological
        Factors
Panic Disorder
300.21   With Agoraphobia
300.01   Without Agoraphobia
301.0   Paranoid Personality Disorder
302.9   Paraphilia NOS
307.47   Parasomnia NOS
V61.20   Parent-Child Relational
        Problem
V61.10   Partner Relational Problem
312.31   Pathological Gambling
302.2   Pedophilia
310.1   Personality Change Due
        to. . . (Indicate the General
        Medical Condition)
301.9   Personality Disorder NOS
299.80   Pervasive Developmental
        Disorder NOS
V62.89   Phase of Life Problem
        Phencyclidine (or
        Phencyclidine-Like)
305.90   Abuse
304.60   Dependence
292.89   –Induced Anxiety Disorder
292.84   –Induced Mood Disorder
        –Induced Psychotic Disorder
291.11   With Delusions
291.12   With Hallucinations
292.89   Intoxication
292.81   Intoxication Delirium
292.9   –Related Disorder NOS
315.39   Phonological Disorder
V61.12   Physical Abuse of Adult (if by
        partner)
V62.83   Physical Abuse of Adult (if by
        person other than partner)
995.81   Physical Abuse of Adult (if

780.59	Mixed Type	302.3	Transvestic Fetishism
780.59	Parasomnia Type	312.39	Trichotillomania
307.46	Sleep Terror Disorder	300.82	Undifferentiated Somatoform
307.46	Sleepwalking Disorder		Disorder
300.23	Social Phobia	300.9	Unspecified Mental Disorder
300.81	Somatization Disorder		(nonpsychotic)
300.82	Somatoform Disorder NOS	306.51	Vaginismus (Not Due to a
300.29	Specific Phobia		General Medical Condition)
307.23	Stereotypic Movement	290.40	Uncomplicated
	Disorder	290.41	With Delirium
307.0	Stuttering	290.42	With Delusions
307.20	Tic Disorder NOS	290.43	With Depressed Mood
307.23	Tourette's Disorder	302.82	Voyeurism
307.21	Transient Tic Disorder		

Sample Reports and Dictation

BIPOLAR DISORDER TYPE II — CASE SUMMARY, DISCHARGE SUMMARY, AND AFTERCARE

RESULTS OF ASSESSMENTS AND SIGNIFICANT FINDINGS:

a. **History, Physical and Neurological Examinations:** Upon completion of the H&P and neurological examination, allergic rhinitis was diagnosed, and it was recommended to closely follow the patient. Psychological testing is not indicated.

b. **Laboratory Testing:** A urine drug screen is negative for all drugs tested. A blood chemistry profile shows a high phosphorous of 5.1. Thyroid testing is within normal limits. A complete blood count and differential are within normal limits. VDRL is nonreactive. Pregnancy test is negative.

c. **Activities:** The patient is to attend individual and group psychotherapy, school classes, and other age-appropriate milieu activities.

CLINICAL COURSE: This is the patient's first hospitalization and she is an 11-year-old preteen female who was brought to the hospital accompanied by her mother and stepfather. The patient wrote a suicide note and had a plan to overdose on drugs. She is depressed about, "school and stuff." The patient began writing suicide notes about a month ago. The mother has used the notes to find bits of information.

The mother feels that the father's death has something to do with the depression. The mother is unsure of other factors. She has recently been seeing an outpatient therapist and has no previous inpatient psychiatric history. Her father died in 1998. She is a student, making average grades and enrolled in regular education classes. She denies substance use or abuse. She reports no difficulty with her appetite. She does report difficulty falling and staying asleep, sleeping approximately 6-1/2 hours a night.

The patient does not report being on medication prior to admission. Vistaril 25 mg q4h p.r.n. was made available for severe agitation. This did not have to be utilized during the course of her hospitalization. Consent was obtained for Celexa, and Celexa was started at 10 mg q.a.m.

The patient reports continued feelings of sadness, anxiety, and low self-esteem. She reports that she is taking her medication, with no side effects reported. She does appear sad and preoccupied. The patient feels some support from the therapeutic program and is willing to approach the staff if suicidal ideations become apparent. At this time, the patient seems to require stabilization and medication to continue help manage her feelings of rejection.

As hospitalization continues, the patient admits to chronic depression since her father's death. Since April of this year, she feels her depression has become more acute. She continues to have no side effects from the medication, and they are helping her to deal with the early loss of her father. As hospitalization continues, the patient indicates that she is feeling much better. She indicates that she has no thoughts of hurting herself or others, and she feels more positive about the future. She is tolerating Celexa without any side effects. Celexa was is increased to 20 mg q.d. The patient is displaying an improved mood and improved interest in taking care of herself and working things out with her family.

RECOMMENDATIONS: The patient will be discharged, and it is recommended that she be seen at a local guidance clinic.

MEDICATIONS ON DISCHARGE: Celexa 20 mg q.d.

PROGNOSIS: Fair.

FINAL DIAGNOSES:

Axis I:	Bipolar disorder type II, rule out major depressive disorder single episode, rule out dysthymia.
Axis II:	None.
Axis III:	None.
Axis IV:	Severe
Axis V:	GAF upon Admission: 25.
	GAF on Discharge: 40.

DISCHARGE SUMMARY: RECURRENT DEPRESSION WITH SEVERE PSYCHOTIC FEATURES

ADMITTING DIAGNOSES

Axis I:	Major depressive disorder with psychotic features.
Axis II:	Deferred
Axis III:	Decreased visual acuity, secondary to cataract; status post detached retina.
Axis IV:	Stressors severe (loss of vision).
Axis V:	Current global assessment of functioning is 20.

DISCHARGE DIAGNOSES
Axis I: Major depression, recurrent, severe, with psychotic features.
Axis II: Deferred.
Axis III: Loss of visual acuity and malnutrition.
Axis IV: Severe.
Axis V: Current global assessment of functioning is 20.

CHIEF COMPLAINT: "I am depressed."

HISTORY OF PRESENT ILLNESS: This patient is well-known to this hospital, having been admitted here over the last two years for ECT treatment as an inpatient and subsequent followup for outpatient ECT once a week. She was admitted from the outpatient ECT service once it was determined that outpatient ECT was not sufficient to maintain a remission of her depressive symptomatology.

The patient is a 74-year-old woman who is married, lives with her husband, and has one daughter. On admission, the patient further complains, "I just want to sleep at night." She has had declining mini-mental status scores over the past several weeks, with increased agitation, decreased sleep, and decreased oral intake, refusing fluids as well as food and with an objective decrease in appetite. She has not been combative or delusional. She has been cooperative for the most part. With regard to her decreased appetite, she states, "nothing tastes good." She also has decreased energy, decreased interest, anhedonia, and decreased motivation and concentration. This patient did fairly well initially following ECT. However, she had a decline in her mental status over the past several weeks and has failed to maintain functional status and euthymic mood as an outpatient.

ALLERGIES: Demerol.

CURRENT MEDICATIONS: Ativan p.r.n., Ecotrin 50 mg q.h.s. and Mellaril 50 mg q.h.s.

POST PSYCHIATRIC HISTORY: The patient has a history of major depressive disorder in the past, dating back to the first episode shortly after her cardiac surgery. She was previously admitted to the hospital, presenting with depressed mood and decreased oral intake, refusing to eat and refusing fluids. She had a difficult course of hospitalization, frequently becoming combative and resisting treatments. However, she did receive sufficient ECT treatments that resulted in a remission of her symptoms, and she returned to a normal level of functioning.

She did well for several months following her discharge. However, she was admitted again, following increasing depressive symptomatology, with decreased appetite and oral intake, with concomitant weight loss. A nasogastric tube was placed in view of her poor nutritional status, and no organic etiology could be identified. She received a course of ECT, with remission of her symptoms, and she was discharged. She was to continue with outpatient maintenance ECT, which she did. In the past, she had a poor response to medications and has failed to attain euthymic mood on oral medication alone, but as indicated above she had a good response to electroconvulsive therapy.

LABORATORY DATA: At the time of admission, her electrolytes reflected a decreased potassium at 3.4, and two days following further decline to 3.3. Chloride was also low at 100. She also has elevated lipoproteins and cholesterol of 223. In addition, CBC with differential was within normal limits, as were thyroid function tests. These laboratories were repeated approximately three weeks following her admission, with electrolytes having normalized and with normal potassium at 4.0. Her CBC with differential showed a decreased RBC at 3.7, decreased hemoglobin 11.8, and decreased hematocrit at 35.0.

EKG was obtained on admission and showed normal sinus rhythm with right atrial enlargement and an ST and T wave abnormality, suggestive of possible inferior ischemias, as well as anterolateral ischemia. This was computer read, and on further evaluation it was felt to be nonpathological. Approximately three weeks following admission, in view of the patient's decreasing weight and declining nutritional status, the EKG was repeated and showed normal sinus rhythm with a rate of 60 beats per minute, which was decreased, with no further evidence of a T-wave inversion in inferior leads or in the anterolateral leads, which were present on admission.

PHYSICAL EXAMINATION: The patient was cooperative. She had no significant physical findings. Physical exam was essentially normal, with the exception of decreased visual acuity in that she was unable to detect movement. There was a prominent cataract in the left eye and a detached retina in the right eye. The funduscopic exam was incomplete in the right eye.

HOSPITAL COURSE: The patient voluntarily signed in to the inpatient unit at the hospital. She received ECT on the day of admission and again on the third, fifth, eighth, tenth, and twelfth day of her admission. She was required to sign informed consent for ECT treatment each day prior to treatment, and after treatment she became resistant to providing a signed informed consent, even at the strong urging of her husband. She also intermittently refused medication and refused oral intake, even at the urging of staff, refusing food and fluids. She would periodically pick at her meals but failed to maintain adequate nutritional intake as reflected by her decrease in weight from a 139 pounds on admission to 131 pounds at discharge. During the third week of admission, she refused ECT and began refusing medications. She stated that she just wanted to be "asleep in a coffin." She also stated, "Why don't you people just let me die; you don't know what it is like to live as a blind person. I would rather be dead because I have nothing to live for."

An order of protective custody was requested from mental illness court and was granted. She was held under an OPC. ECT treatment was terminated, and future ECT treatment was not offered. The decision was made to transfer the patient to the state hospital where she could receive treatment.

At the time of discharge, she was medically stable although severely depressed, with suicidal ideation and desire. She was ambulating unassisted. She was able to dress herself and was capable of feeding herself. Her family has been supportive of the treatment decisions that were made. She was in agreement with her husband and her daughter regarding the transfer to the state hospital. Her husband had visited here daily and has been very supportive regarding her care. Her daughter, who lives in Houston, has visited on two different occasions and met with the treatment team. Although her daughter was initially distressed regarding her mother's decision not to continue ECT, she was in agreement with the transfer plan as well as the OPC.

DISCHARGE PLAN: The patient is transferred to the state hospital by ambulance in the company of her husband.

DISCHARGE MEDICATIONS: Effexor 25 mg p.o. q.h.s.; zolpidem 10 mg p.o. q.h.s.; Risperdal 0.5 mg q.a.m. and 1 mg at h.s.; Mellaril 50 mg q.h.s.; KCl 20 mEq p.o. q.a.m.; and chloral hydrate 1 gram p.o. q.h.s.

INPATIENT NEUROPSYCHOLOGY CONSULTATION #1

REASON FOR REFERRAL: The patient is a 70-year-old male who was referred for neuropsychological consultation during his inpatient stay at an area specialty hospital to explore his current level of cognitive functioning.

PROCEDURES ADMINISTERED: The chart was reviewed. I interviewed his wife over the phone at length. I provided his wife with emotional support. I attempted to evaluate the patient, but his status is not currently elevated enough to tolerate formal neuropsychological testing or meaningful interview. I consulted with the patient's physician and provided feedback.

HISTORY OF PRESENT ILLNESS: The patient recently suffered a fall and had a headache after this fall but was generally able to continue about his daily life and ambulate, talk, etc. Two days later he became stuck in his shirt while attempting to get dressed, and he fell again, hitting his head again. He was admitted to the hospital on that day. CT brain scan demonstrated a right temporal intraparenchymal hematoma, and he underwent neurosurgical drainage. During the hospital course, the patient failed extubation several times and eventually underwent tracheostomy and feeding jejunostomy. The patient also experienced seizures during his hospitalization, which have been subsequently controlled with Dilantin. The patient was transferred to the specialty hospital for ongoing medical care and rehabilitation. Therapists report that he is not currently tolerating therapy due to noncompliance and combative behavior including verbal outbursts.

PAST MEDICAL HISTORY: Chronic obstructive pulmonary disease. The patient has smoked two packs of cigarettes a day for 40 years. His record notes a history of heavy alcohol use. His wife reports that she suspects he drank approximately three to four drinks per day, but it is difficult for her to ascertain the exact quantity as she works during the day, and prior to admission he was home alone, drinking. The patient suffered a fall in 1978 when he was working and fell head first into a grease pit. He suffered a shoulder injury, broken ribs, and a lesion of the C5 to C7 area. He suffered chronic neck pain and headaches after that incident. In 1982, the patient's legs were crushed by an 18-wheeler. He did not experience a head injury at that time. Eight years ago he was in a car accident and hit his head on the left side. He suffered no loss of consciousness but had a headache for several days.

FUNCTIONING PRIOR TO ADMISSION: The patient's wife states that his memory and thinking skills have been mildly declining in recent years, but the currently seen severe impairment is recent in origin. He drove a car and was fully functional in his ADLs activities of daily living prior to his fall, per his wife's report.

SOCIAL/EDUCATIONAL/OCCUPATIONAL HISTORY: The patient was born in Hungary, where he left at age 24. His wife is not sure of his highest level of education completed, but she is relatively certain he did not complete high school as she does not believe that this was offered to him at the time when he was in Hungary. However, she states that he was able to read and write Hungarian fluently and did not appear to have any learning problems. The patient's first language was Hungarian, but his wife is not Hungarian; they speak English together. The patient met his wife in 1968. They have no children, but he has two children from a previous marriage. His wife reports that these two children live in the state, but are not involved in his life and are not supportive. The patient previously worked as a truck mechanic. He ceased working in 1982 after a work-related accident. The patient's wife works during the day in a shop that they own that sells blinds. She is concerned about how she will be able to continue running the business and care for the patient following discharge. She wishes to avoid placing the patient in a nursing home.

PSYCHIATRIC ISSUES: The patient was in Hungary during the war and had many friends who were killed in front of him, according to his wife. He was forced to escape by crossing the border emergently and could not say goodbye to his mother. His wife suspects that he has had resultant lifelong issues with depression. His wife feels he is severely depressed right now and that this is interfering with his compliance.

BEHAVORIAL OBSERVATIONS: The patient is not yet able to tolerate formal testing at this time secondary to issues including vacillating arousal, poor attention, and inability to follow one-step commands. He answered some questions but did not respond to all questions. His speech was heavily accented, quite raspy, and poorly articulated, the combination of which rendered his speech poorly comprehensible. At times he was silent when questions were asked. At times he responded, and at times he appeared to be uttering profanities. Sometimes he appeared cooperative and at other times he showed vacillating attention and appeared to doze off during the interview. I understand from the patient's physician that he has been more clearly comprehensible and alert at other times in the day. His status appears quite variable. He was able to respond to the question, "What is your name," but could not respond accurately to any orientation questions. His apparent confusion and disorientation correspond to the report of his wife and therapist's notes. His wife noticed severe cognitive impairment after his fall, which improved over time (but did not approach baseline). However, she is concerned that he seems to have declined physically, cognitively, and emotionally over the past two weeks. She has noted the onset of visual hallucinations over the past two weeks. (He reports that there are flies on the ceiling and mentions objects in the room that are not there.)

IMPRESSION: This 70-year-old male, who is status post fall and drainage of right temporal IPH, is not yet tolerant of formal testing but clearly shows impaired mental status demonstrated by impaired attention, vacillating arousal levels, inability to respond to simple-step commands (close your eyes), and apparent confusion and disorientation. His cognitive impairment is likely of multiple etiologies. Severe impairment appeared with the onset of his IPH. However, there are likely other variables, such as pre-existing cognitive impairment secondary to chronic alcohol use. The additional possibility of a degenerative dementing process cannot be excluded. Therapists have noted that he is combative and noncompliant; his wife notes that he is depressed and has visual hallucinations of recent onset.

RECOMMENDATIONS
1. Antidepressants to help the patient's mood and hopefully improve his interest in complying with therapies as his noncompliance may be at least partially rooted in depression.
2. I am concerned by reports that the patient's status may be declining in recent weeks, which is not the course I would expect with improvement from his IPH. Input from neurology may be helpful.
3. While I hope for and expect improvement, I am concerned that the patient could still be quite impaired at discharge. I discussed this with case management who will pursue long-term care so the patient may be able to have in-house caregivers while his wife is at work.
4. When and if the patient is able to tolerate therapies, he could benefit from intensive inpatient neurorehabilitation.

5. I will continue to follow the patient. Neuropsychological examination will be provided if appropriate in the future, pending significantly improved status. Due to the fact that he has limited education, English is his second language, and he may have had premorbid neuropsychological deficits secondary to alcohol use, it is possible that formal psychometric testing will not be extremely meaningful, even when his tolerance improves. I will monitor this issue and follow him for informal assessment, psychotherapeutic support, and behavioral management.

6. The patient should receive assistance in making any significant decisions regarding his care, pending cognitive improvement.

INPATIENT NEUROPSYCHOLOGY CONSULTATION #2

HISTORY OF PRESENTING ILLNESS: The patient is a 36-year-old, right-handed man with a history of seizures for the past three years, characterized by loss of awareness, problems with expressive speech, and occasional secondary generalization. These events occur generally when falling asleep or upon awakening. He was assessed during an inpatient stay in the epilepsy monitoring unit of another facility. He was referred for evaluation of his current cognitive and emotional functioning as part of an evaluation for epilepsy surgery.

PAST MEDICAL HISTORY: Left shoulder surgery in 1988 and right knee surgery in 1996. He reported he is otherwise healthy.

SOCIAL HISTORY: He denied birth or developmental problems, but stated he has mild problems with reading in school. He is currently taking classes towards an undergraduate degree. He denied experiencing any problems with his classes. He works as a supervisor for an insurance company; he stated that he has had mild problems with his memory and word retrieval. He is married and has three teenage stepchildren. He denied any past treatment for psychiatric illness.

PROCEDURES ADMINISTERED: Chart review, clinical interview, Wechsler Adult Intelligence Scale-III (selected subtests), Trial Making Test, California Verbal Learning Test, Brief Visuospatial Memory Test, Controlled Oral Word Association Test, Animal Naming, Finger Tapping Test, Beck Depression Inventory-II, Minnesota Multiphasic Personality Inventory-II.

EXAMINATION FINDINGS: He was evaluated as an inpatient. He was alert and oriented. Speech was normal in rate, rhythm, and prosody. No word finding difficulties were observed on clinical interview or during testing. Thought content was goal oriented and appropriate. He had no problems understanding task directions. Affect was appropriate to the testing session. He showed good cooperation; therefore this evaluation is judged to accurately reflect his current level of cognitive functioning.

He was administered measures of intellectual functioning. He obtained a core verbal intellect index score of 96; that falls in the average range, and he obtained a core visuospatial intellect index score of 118, which falls in the high-average range. This 22-point difference between index scores was significant, favoring visuospatial abilities. Performance on verbal subtests was variable; verbal abstraction was in the high-average range and consistent with his performance on measures of visuospatial reasoning. Vocabulary and general knowledge were relative weaknesses, falling in the low-average range. From his academic history, the relative weaknesses on these measures may represent long-standing weaknesses rather than a recent change in intellectual functioning.

Verbal memory was assessed with a word list learning test. He learned 8, 8, 9, 10, 10 words of a possible 16 words per trial. This performance falls in the mildly impaired range (T = 34). Recall after a delay was 11 of 16 words, which is in the low-average to average range (T = 41). Learning on a Visuospatial Memory Test was in the high-average range. He learned 8, 10, 11 details of a possible 12 details (T = 56). Performance after a delay was also in the high-average range (11 of 12 details; T = 57).

Basic attention was in the average range (7 digits forward); however, auditory concentration was mildly impaired (4 digits in reverse order). Complex concentration was in the average range. Performance on the Trail Making Test, Part A, a measure of processing speed and visual tracking, was 27 seconds, 0 errors. Performance on Part B, which also requires conceptual sequencing, was 63 seconds, 1 error. This performance was in the average range. Verbal fluency was impaired. Word generation according to first letter was mildly impaired (29 words in three minutes) and word generation according to category was severely impaired (13 words in one minute).

Fine motor functioning was intact bilaterally.

Emotional functioning was assessed by clinical interview and self-report. On the Beck Depression Inventory-II, he endorsed mild problems with feeling discouraged and low self-confidence. He also endorsed mild problems with fatigue, concentration, and decision-making. The BDI-II score of 10 was in the mildly depressed range. The valid MMPI-II profile showed no evidence of personality problems.

IMPRESSIONS AND RECOMMENDATIONS: This is a 36-year-old, right-handed man with a three-year history of seizures. Neuropsychological evaluation showed moderate problems with verbal fluency and word retrieval and mild problems with new verbal learning within the context of otherwise intact cognitive functioning in average to above-average intellectual functioning. He endorsed a mild degree of depression at the current time. These findings are suggestive of mild impairment in left temporal lobe functioning. Given that a recent MRI showed intact hippocampi, and he showed only mild memory problems, he may experience a decline in verbal memory ability following left temporal lobectomy, if this is medically indicated to treat his seizures.

Neuropsychological Consultation #1

History of Present Illness: The patient is a 53-year-old female with a history of double vision and occasional dizziness for several months. She was found to have a contrast-enhancing, tentorial-based left cerebellopontine angle tumor, with associated edema and displaced fourth ventricle.

She recently underwent left lateral supracerebellar intratentorial image-guided resection. Pathology findings were consistent with a ganglioglioma. Followup neuroradiological images indicated worsening hydrocephalus, and she subsequently underwent right frontal ventriculostomy. Head CT indicated improving hydrocephalus.

This patient was evaluated for inpatient neurorehabilitation by her doctor. She believed that the patient would benefit most from an outpatient program. She referred the patient for a neuropsychological evaluation to document her current level of functioning and aid in rehabilitation and discharge planning.

Procedures: Records were reviewed, and the patient was interviewed. She was administered the BNI Screen for Higher Cerebral Functions, the Controlled Oral Word Association Subtest of the Multilingual Aphasia Examination, the Trailmaking Test, the Wechsler Adult Intelligence Scale-Third Edition, Selected Subtest of the Wechsler Memory Scale, Revised, the Rey Auditory Verbal Learning Test, the Brief Visuospatial Memory Test-Revised, the Halstead Finger Tapping Test, and the Wisconsin Card Sorting Test.

Past Medical History: The patient has cutaneous neurofibromatosis, type 1. She has undergone right nephrectomy secondary to renal cell carcinoma. Per records, she has been followed and there is no evidence of local or systemic recurrence of carcinoma. She is currently on low-dose hormone replacement therapy and will occasionally take Ambien for sleep.

Social History: The patient is single and is the main caretaker of her 92-year-old mother. There is a woman from Assistance for Independent Living that helps care for her mother, and should be able to assist the patient to some degree when she returns home.

The patient works part-time and is going to school for her masters in health profession education. She reduced her work hours in October to pursue school full time. The patient also has a master's degree in genetics. She has currently taken medical leave from her program and hopes to be well enough to return to school in March.

The patient reported that she does not use tobacco or alcohol.

EXAMINATION FINDINGS: This patient was very pleasant and cooperative with all evaluation procedures. She reported that she still experiencing double vision when she looks up, and it takes awhile for her eyes to focus. Her balance is a bit unsteady, but she feels this is getting progressively better. She has noticed some difficulty with concentration.

She reports that she has some difficulty falling asleep because she cannot get comfortable. Once she is asleep, she sleeps well and feels rested in the mornings. Her appetite is good. She has noticed some echoing in her ears at times and has not noticed any changes in her sense of smell or taste.

The patient was asked to rate, on a scale from 0–10 (with 0 meaning no difficulty and 10 meaning a severe problem), her ability to remember important things or things that she wishes to recall. She rates this difficulty at a 3. Concentration difficulties are rated at 4. Word-finding difficulties are rated at 5–6. Irritability is rated at 6. Anxiety is rated at 8–9. Depression is rated at 3. Problems with energy level are rated at 6. In general, she was somewhat anxious regarding the evaluation. She reported that she has had negative experiences with testing in the past.

On examination, her speech was very rapid at times, and she tended to be hyperverbal. She displayed mild impulsive and disinhibited tendencies. At times, she would interrupt instructions to ask for clarification and need information repeated.

The patient's speech was fluent, without obvious paraphasic errors or dysarthria. Mild word-finding difficulties were noticed. She was oriented to situation, place, and date.

On the BNI Screen, the patient completed brief tasks of basic language functioning without error. She had no difficulty on tasks involving constructional praxis, mental and written arithmetic, visual scanning, visual sequencing, pattern copying, and pattern recognition. She could repeat five digits forward but not in reverse.

On a task of Basic Visual Associative Learning, she learned only two out of four number/symbol associations. She could recall two out of three words following a brief delay.

She could adequately generate affect in her voice and perceive facial affect. She displayed appropriate spontaneous affect.

Her total score on the BNI Screen was 44 out of 50 (T score equalled 47). While this performance is in the average range, her performance is notable for difficulties with complex attention, learning, and recall, consistent with her medical history.

On the Wechsler Adult Intelligence Scale-Third Edition, she obtained a verbal IQ of 99 (average range) and a performance IQ of 87 (low-average range), yielding a full scale IQ of 94 (average range). Age-adjusted scale scores are as follows: Vocabulary equals 12; Similarities equals 12; Arithmetic equals 8; Digit Span equals 7; Information equals 11; Picture Completion equals 11; Digit Symbol-Coding equals 8; Block Design equals 8; Picture Arrangement equals 6; and Symbol Search equals 8. Her pattern of performance, as well as her professional accomplishments, suggests that her estimated premorbid intellectual abilities were most likely in the high average to superior range prior to her neurological problems. She is demonstrating weaknesses in speed of information processing, complex attention/working memory, and sequencing of visual information.

On the Controlled Oral Word Association Subtest of the multilingual aphasia examination, she generates a total of 28 words, which is in the low-average range.

She completes the Trailmaking Test, Part A, in 35 seconds without errors (T score equals 37). She completes Part B in 92 seconds, with one set-shifting error (T score equals 28), which is in the impaired range.

On the Rey Auditory Verbal Learning Test, she fails to demonstrate an adequate learning curve. She recalls 4, 7, 6, 7 and 10 words respectively across trials. The total number of words recalled was 34, which is in the mild to moderately impaired range. After a brief distraction, she can recall only 6 out of 15 words, which is impaired. Twenty minutes later, she recalls only 7 out of 15 words.

On the Brief Visuospatial Memory Test-Revised, her initial recall of visuospatial designs was in the low-average range, and she gains little information with repeated trials (T scores equalled 41, 39, and 42 respectively across three trials). Her overall learning is in the low-average range (T score equals 39). Following a 25-minute delay, she does recall all of the information she learned.

On the Wechsler Memory Scale, Revised form, her recall of short stories is at the 41st percentile for immediate recall and at the 31st percentile for delayed recall. Recall of visuospatial information is at the 17th percentile for immediate recall and the 5th percentile for delayed recall. She appears to have more difficulty with visual learning and memory when information is complex and presented without repetition.

Speed of finger tapping was measured at 48.33 taps in her right hand (T score equals 50) and 38.17 taps in her left hand (T score equals 43). While these scores are both in the average range, her speed of tapping with her left hand is significantly lower than her right hand. In addition, her tapping with both hands was very variable, ranging from 41–57 taps in her right hand, and 29–48 taps in her left hand.

On the Wisconsin Card Sorting Test, she completes 6 out of 6 categories. While her performance is within normal limits, her error and perseverative response rates are somewhat below expectations given the patient's estimated premorbid level. In addition, she did have initial difficulty learning the task (trials to complete first category, 6th-10th percentile).

IMPRESSIONS/RECOMMENDATIONS: This 53-year-old, right-handed female, 10-days status post resection of a left cerebellopontine angle ganglioglioma, is currently demonstrating cognitive difficulties on formal testing.

As mentioned above, this patient has had negative experiences with testing in the past and has understandable concerns about the validity of results from this type of evaluation, as well as any restrictions that could be placed on her due to these results.

The doctor discussed the results of this evaluation with the patient. She indicated that she never did well on these types of tasks. Therefore, it is unclear how much these results indicate true decline from estimated premorbid levels.

However, she does appear to have difficulties on tasks involving complex attention, speed of processing, learning and recall verbal and visual information, and subtle motor difficulties with her left hand, which would be consistent with her known medical history.

We agree with the doctor that this patient would be an excellent candidate for a comprehensive rehabilitation program. The services provided by these types of programs were briefly discussed with this patient, and she was very interested in their services. It is our understanding that case management is assisting this patient in contacting these programs.

In addition, case management has arranged for Home Health Services, including physical, occupational, and speech therapy until she can transition into a comprehensive rehabilitation program.

This is an intelligent woman with very good judgment; therefore, options for rehabilitation services should be fully discussed with her to help determine what services would best fit her lifestyle.

The patient is aware that she will require some assistance at home and with the responsibilities of caring for her mother during her recovery. She has arranged for different family members and friends to stay with her at least for the next couple of weeks.

DIAGNOSES
1. Left cerebellopontine angle ganglioglioma – ICD-9 code 191.6.
2. Cognitive difficulties associated with the above – ICD-9 code 310.8.

NEUROPSYCHOLOGICAL CONSULTATION #2

HISTORY OF PRESENTING ILLNESS: The patient is a 64-year-old, right-handed man who was diagnosed with lung cancer two years ago. He had left lower lobe resection and underwent postoperative chemotherapy and radiation. In the past, he developed headaches and was found to have meningeal carcinomatosis. An MRI scan of the brain was read as showing worsening hydrocephalus. A neuropsychological evaluation was requested to document his current cognitive status and to make recommendations concerning his care.

PAST MEDICAL HISTORY: Deferred.

PSYCHOSOCIAL HISTORY: The patient has a bachelor's degree. He worked up until six months ago. He is married and has four children.

TESTS AND PROCEDURES: The chart was reviewed, and the patient was interviewed. The patient was administered the BNI Screen for Higher Cerebral Functions, the Trail Making Test, the Patient Distress Scale for Neurorehabilitation (Patient Form) and the Patient Competency Rating Scale for Neurorehabilitation (Patient Form).

EXAMINATION FINDINGS: On examination, the patient was alert and cooperative. He was observed to have a steady left-hand tremor, which he stated began approximately one year ago. He also had notable gait disturbance and became dizzy toward the end of testing.

On the BNI Screen for Higher Cerebral Functions, his speech is fluent. There is no evidence of paraphasic errors or dysarthria. On speech and language tasks, he is able to do brief tasks of comprehension, naming, repetition, reading, writing and spelling, with no difficulty. He showed no right-left orientation confusion and was oriented to person, place and time. He showed no right- or left-hand constructional dyspraxia. He could do a written arithmetic task but had difficulty with a mental arithmetic task. He could recite five digits in the forward and reverse order. He could do tasks of visual scanning but had difficulty with visual sequencing, pattern copying and pattern recognition. He could generate affect in his tone of voice and perceive facial affect. With regard to memory, he could recall 0/3 words following a brief distraction and 2/4 number-symbol associations.

His total score on the BNI Screen is 40/50 points, which produced a T score value of 41; this is in the lower end of the average range.

Trail A was completed in 74 seconds, with no errors. This produced a T score value of 27, which is in the moderately impaired range. Trail B was completed in 203 seconds, with 1 error. This produced a T score value of 31, which is in the mildly to moderately impaired range.

On the Patient Distress Scale for Neurorehabilitation (Patient Form), the patient reported moderate difficulties with feeling frustrated, self-confidence and discouragement.

On the Patient Competency Rating Scale, he reported moderate difficulties with memory and activities of daily living (ADL).

IMPRESSIONS AND RECOMMENDATIONS: The results of this brief evaluation revealed moderate deficits in basic memory, visual processing/problem-solving, visuospatial organization and speed of information processing. He also showed impaired awareness of his cognitive deficits. Emotionally, he reported moderate dysphoria, difficulty adjusting to unexpected changes and difficulty controlling his temper when he is upset.

Continued rehabilitation services and 24-hour supervision are recommended.

He will require assistance in the management of his finances in order to reduce the risk of error.

A neuropsychological reevaluation is recommended in approximately three months postdischarge. The results of this evaluation were given to the patient.

PARANOID SCHIZOPHRENIA: CASE SUMMARY, DISCHARGE SUMMARY, AND AFTERCARE

IDENTIFYING DATA AND REASONS FOR ADMISSION: The patient is a 14-year-old female and she was admitted because of problems at school.

HISTORY OF PRESENT ILLNESS: The patient has difficulty elaborating on the reason of her admission. On the other hand, her mother said that she was depressed, had made several suicidal statements over the previous couple of weeks, tried to drown herself in the bathtub 2 days prior to the assessment, and believed people were coming, "to get" her. Her mother also said that the patient was unable to sleep, has not been eating, and thought that she was pregnant. History indicated that this past year that the patient was abducted for 3 days and raped numerous times. The patient was seen last year at a rape counseling center and is currently seeing a therapist. She is not on any psychotropic medications.

During the assessment, the patient denied the misuse of drugs, alcohol, or any other substance. She acknowledged having sleep difficulties. She acknowledged not eating. She has a police record for shoplifting. In the past, she has done average work in school.

The patient's developmental history, according to the mother, was within normal limits except that she suffered from bronchial asthma and had to use an Albuterol inhaler on a p.r.n. basis.

The patient lives with both parents.

RESULTS OF ASSESSMENTS AND SIGNIFICANT FINDINGS:

a. **Mental Status Examination:** On admission, she was observed to be a poorly groomed, well-developed, young woman with no eye contact and difficulty answering even simple questions. Psychomotor activity was normal. Level of anxiety was minimal. Speech was just a few monosyllables. Mood was mildly depressed. Affect was flat. Thinking was laborious. She did say that she would like to become a lawyer. I couldn't tell whether she was orientated or not. Intellectual capacity from history appeared to be within normal limits. Again, her memory, which I attempted to test by digits and knowledge of events, was difficult to assess. Judgment appeared non-reality orientated. Patient had no insight into condition.

b. **Physical and Neurological Evaluation:** The physical and neurological examinations was were conducted by our consulting pediatrician, and the findings were within normal limits, except for the presence of bronchia asthma.

c. **Psychological Testing:** Full psychological testing was not deemed to be necessary.

d. **Laboratory Testing:** Laboratory examination consisted of blood count with differential, urinalysis, and basic metabolic panel. All findings were within normal limits. VDRL was nonreactive. Pregnancy test was negative.

CLINICAL COURSE: On admission, the identified problems were that this youngster's altered thought process as manifested by poor judgment, confused thinking, delusions, and quite likely auditory hallucinations.

The discharge goal was help with reality orientation and to establish interpersonal relationship with peers and the staff at least 50% of the time.

Intervention strategy, frequency, and services provided were to monitor this youngster for safety through the day, as well as to assist her in initiating conversation and expressing her feelings.

The patient was also going to participate in the level privilege system to assist her in improving and strengthening her problem solving skills. Further, the staff was to provide group and reality orientation therapy daily, as well as family therapy twice a week to reinforce positive behavior and to provide opportunities for appropriate interactions.

I was to see the patient in individual psychotherapy no less than five times a week to help her build a trusting relationship, to encourage her to ventilate her feelings, and to assist her in developing more adaptive coping mechanisms. Because of the obvious evidence of an asthenic disorder, I began her on Risperdal 1 mg in the morning and 2 mg at bedtime. Elavil 50 mg was prescribed twice a day to avoid side effects and Celexa 20 mg a day for what appears to be an underlying depression.

Within 24 hours the patient was consciously cloudy and had major difficulty understanding and articulating thoughts, so the Risperdal was increased to 2 mg twice a day.

At the end of the first week in the hospital, the patient still appeared to be depressed, and was isolative and withdrawn. In response to questions, she did say that she was eating and sleeping well. There were no psychotic symptoms but she seemed to be obsessed with her past rape. Because of the staff reporting some difficulty sleeping, I added Remeron 10 mg at bedtime to her regimen, for both the hypnotic and antidepressant actions.

By the end of this admission, the patient was in good contact with reality. Her thinking was intact. There was no significant mood disorder, but she is still obsessing over the rape. It was felt at that point that this youngster was not a danger to herself or others, and that treatment could continue on an outpatient basis.

The patient was discharged improved to her parents.

RECOMMENDATIONS: Return home, return to school, and continue treatment with her therapist.

MEDICATIONS ON DISCHARGE: Benadryl 15 mg twice a day, Celexa 20 mg a day, Remeron 15 mg at bedtime, and Risperdal 2 mg twice a day.

EMPLOYABILITY: Does not apply.

PROGNOSIS: Fair.

FINAL DIAGNOSES:

AXIS I: Paranoid schizophrenia.
AXIS II: None.
AXIS III: Bronchial asthma.

AXIS IV: Severe.
AXIS V: GAF on Discharge: 45.

PSYCHOLOGICAL EVALUATION: ASSESSMENT FOR GLOBAL DELAY AND FAILURE TO THRIVE/PEDIATRIC UNDERNUTRITION

REFERRAL AND BACKGROUND INFORMATION: The patient was referred for assessment through the state early intervention program due to concern regarding global delay as well as failure to thrive/pediatric undernutrition. She was referred by her pediatrician and is undergoing neurological and genetic assessment to rule out Angelman syndrome.

A copy of the initial genetic consultation report was available for review. The patient was initially referred for genetics assessment at the county medical center due to poor growth and developmental delay. Her mother first became concerned about her development at when the child was 4 months of age, although referral for evaluation was not made until 11 months of age, when she was seen in the emergency room for diarrhea and dehydration. She was subsequently seen in the neurology and gastroenterology clinics. The patient has been diagnosed with dysphagia and gastroesophageal reflux. Neurological assessment is ongoing. Followup genetics evaluation is scheduled in 1 month.

The patient was born at the gestational age of 40 weeks and weighed 6 pounds 2 ounces. Her mother indicated that she had fever and a bladder infection during the fifth month of pregnancy; she also noted decreased fetal movement. The patient had an uneventful neonatal course and was discharged from the hospital after 24 hours. She was hospitalized at approximately 1 month of age for treatment of difficulties described as intussusception ("she had a tube twisted in her stomach"). She remained in the hospital for a total of 8 days.

The doctor noted microcephaly, significant developmental delay, and constant movement, with symmetrical small growth parameters. High-resolution chromosome analysis was recommended, as well as metabolic testing and magnetic resonance imaging of the brain to rule out a structural abnormality.

There is no family history of developmental disorder, congenital defects or pregnancy losses. The patient's development has been significantly delayed; she began smiling at 5 months of age and rolled over at 13 months. She does not coo, babble, or use any words. The patient's family speaks Spanish. She lives with her parents and older brother. The brother has not had any developmental difficulties.

TESTING AND OBSERVATIONS: The patient was accompanied by her mother, and translation was provided by a medical assistant. The patient sat on her mother's lap throughout the assessment and appeared alert and responsive.

Cognitive assessment was completed with the Mental Scale of the Bayley Scales of Infant Development, Second Edition. This is a general measure, which is comprised of verbal and nonverbal tasks. Results are expressed in terms of the Mental Development Index (mean = 100; standard deviation = 15). The higher the score, the better the child's performance compared to others the same age.

The patient scored a Mental Development Index of less than 50, with a performance that corresponds to the developmental age of 5 months. She was able to grasp toys and transfer them from one hand to the other, although she frequently lost her grasp and objects simply fell to the ground. She did not look for fallen objects as they fell. She did not bang objects against a hard surface and does not bring her hands together to bang objects and does not yet clap. She did respond playfully to her mirror image, smiling and showing increased motor movement. She was able to pick up two 1-inch blocks, one in each hand and could hold them at the same time. She tended to mouth items. She did manipulate a bell, briefly rang the bell in what appeared to be a purposeful attempt, and she played with a rattle. She did not appear to attend to specific pictures in a book and did not vocalize.

Further assessment was done via parent interview using the Vineland Adaptive Behavior Scales. This covers major areas of functioning and yields standard scores (mean = 100; standard deviation = 15). Global delay is represented, with particular delay in language skills and significant feeding difficulties. Results are as follows:

DOMAIN	STANDARD SCORE	PERCENTILE RANK	AGE EQUIVALENT
Communication	69	2	1 month
Daily Living Skills	78	7	8 months
Socialization	76	5	6 months
Motor Skills	68	2	5 months
Adaptive Behavior Composite	67	1	—

The patient attends to sounds but does not seem to enjoy music or other auditory stimuli. Her mother reports that she does raise her arms to anticipate being picked up, yet does not gesture to indicate her needs or desires. She does not consistently smile in response to family members, does not coo or imitate sounds. Her diet is supplemented with PediaSure although she chokes on this at times. She is able to take very little solid food. She gags at the sight of her bottle and did this today, although she subsequently drank without difficulty. She is able to hold the bottle by herself. The patient does show some anxiety and protest when she is separated from her mother and cared for by another family member. She will reach for her mother. She plays with some simple toys for brief periods, although she is not able to maintain a grasp on objects. Her mother noted that she also tends to keep her head in a downward position. She can sit supported for a short period of time, with pillows propped around her. She does not yet have a pincer grasp (she was unable to pick up a Cheerio today).

SUMMARY: The patient demonstrates significant global delay, with likely moderate to severe mental retardation. She is eligible for therapy and educational services through the state early intervention program. A feeding evaluation is recommended, along with physical therapy and occupational therapy evaluations, and she would benefit from a comprehensive program.

Evaluation is recommended again in 1 year to track her progress and confirm her level of cognitive functioning.

PSYCHOLOGICAL EVALUATION: DEVELOPMENTAL ASSESSMENT #1

REFERRAL AND BACKGROUND INFORMATION: The patient was seen for the first time at the developmental clinic through the newborn followup program. His mother contacted the clinic due to concerns that his functioning in a general preschool program does not appear to be age appropriate. His preschool teacher reports that he does not speak in class, although he has attended this preschool for 6 months. He has difficulty remembering names and calls all of the children the same name. In addition, concern about his motor skills is reported; he cannot pedal a tricycle or catch a ball and has a hard time holding a pencil or crayon and steering a motorized truck. When he puts sentences together, it is difficult to understand what he says.

The patient was born at the gestational age of 32 weeks and weighed 1900 gm. Pregnancy was complicated by pregnancy-induced hypertension. His mother received ampicillin and Celestone prior to delivery. The patient's Apgar scores were 9 and 9 at one and five minutes respectively. He experienced transitory respiratory distress at delivery and required blow-by oxygen for two minutes. Respiratory problems resolved on the first day of life.

The patient has been healthy except for ear infections, and he was treated for respiratory syncytial virus (RSV) in the past. Hearing testing done three months ago was normal; followup is scheduled for next month. He takes Zyrtec as needed for allergies. He has complained about headaches as well as neck and facial pains. He recently had an MRI; the results of this are not yet available.

Measurements taken today are as follows: Weight 15 kg; height 99.5 cm; head circumference 51.4 cm. No prior measurements are available for comparison.

The patient walked at the age of 14 months; he said "mama" and "dada" at 10 months, and said the word "ball" at 13 to 14 months. At this point, he speaks in sentences. He eats regular table foods, with no history of eating problems reported. He sleeps through the night for 9 to 10 hours.

The patient has 2 younger brothers. There is no reported family history of development difficulties. His mother is a homemaker. His father is a mail carrier. English is the only language spoken at home.

TESTING AND OBSERVATIONS: The patient was accompanied by his mother and was friendly, cooperative and talkative. He was easily engaged in test activities and displayed a generally high activity level, with some impulsivity and distractibility. He commented about his activities as he played, e.g., after a tower of blocks fell down with a loud clatter, he commented, "I don't want that to happen. That scared me."

Cognitive testing was done with the Mental Scale of the Bayley Scales of Infant Development, Second Edition. This is a general cognitive measure, which comprises verbal and nonverbal tasks. Results are reported in terms of the Mental Development Index (mean = 100; standard deviation = 15). The higher the score, the better the child's performance compared to others the same age.

The patient obtained a Mental Development Index of 72, a score that is more than one-and-a-half standard deviations below the mean. His performance corresponds to a developmental age of 33 months and is indicative of moderate delay. He was able to name colors, demonstrate an understanding of prepositions and identified himself by gender. He also replicated simple block constructions. He had difficulty on items dependent upon immediate visual and auditory memory, e.g., remembering pictures and repeating sequences of three numbers. He did not use past tense to describe his experiences, and he showed incomplete mastery of comparative concepts (more, heavy). He had difficulty with a fine motor planning task that consisted of placing a string of beads in a narrow tube. Overall, no particular areas of strength or weakness are depicted.

Further information was obtained via parent interview, using the Vineland Adaptive Behavior Scales. These are standardized measures (mean = 100; standard deviation = 15), which depict major areas of ability. The patient obtained a low-average score for general communication skills, with scores in the moderately delayed (well below average or borderline) range on measures of self-care skills, play, social skills and motor abilities. His results are as follows:

DOMAIN	STANDARD SCORE	PERCENTILE RANK	AGE EQUIVALENT
Communication	82	12	31 months
Daily Living Skills	71	3	27 months
Socialization	72	3	23 months
Motor Skills	71	3	31 months
Adaptive Behavior Composite	68	2	— — — —

The patient is not able to give his own first and last name on request. When he is asked his age, he typically responds with his first name. He does not yet point to all major body parts and does not relate his experiences in detail. He has difficulty listening in school and does not respond to his teacher's questions.

The patient is toilet trained during the day, although he still requires a diaper at times at night. He does not yet dress himself. He recently put boots on the correct feet on one occasion for the first time. He will try to put on his underwear, although he puts this on backwards and is not able to put on other clothing. He becomes fussy when his clothes are wet or messy, and he dislikes being messy. He does not yet answer the phone appropriately or maintain a conversation on the telephone.

He engages in general play and simple representational play with small vehicles and figures. He shows a preference for one friend in particular at preschool, yet tends to refer to all the other children with the name of his favorite friend. It is not known if he is able to participate in organized games, such as duck-duck-goose or hokey-pokey.

The patient was observed today while he walked up and down stairs, holding onto a railing; he does not yet alternate his feet when walking down stairs. He reportedly is afraid of high play equipment and does not climb on tall slides or other objects. He cannot pedal, and he was over three years of age before he was able to scoot on a small vehicle. When he scribbles, he uses a fisted grasp and does not draw any recognizable forms. He is able to cut across a piece of paper with scissors, although he is not adept with this.

SUMMARY: The patient was seen for psychological evaluation that demonstrates moderate cognitive delay and delays in adaptive abilities. Since he demonstrates delays across two or more areas of functioning, it is recommended that the results of this evaluation be shared with his school district for consideration of enrollment in a special education preschool program. He would benefit from an individualized program, which offers educational activities, guidance in adaptive skills and play and social skills. Physical therapy evaluation is recommended.

Based on indications of distractibility and impulsivity, it is recommended that his behavior be monitored, especially in the context of a preschool program, to ensure that he is able to follow along with small group activities and participate without continual guidance. Given persistent behavioral concerns, further assessment would be warranted and may be available through the family's insurance plan. The patient could see a psychologist with who has experience in working with preschool children for diagnostic assessment, to rule out the diagnosis of attention deficit hyperactivity disorder.

Complete psychological evaluation is recommended at the age 5 to track the patient's progress and assist in determination of eligibility for special education in kindergarten. This evaluation is typically done in the school district, although it may be done on a private basis.

PSYCHOLOGICAL EVALUATION: DEVELOPMENTAL ASSESSMENT #2

REFERRAL AND BACKGROUND INFORMATION: This is the patient's first visit to the developmental clinic through the newborn followup program. Referral was arranged through the division of developmental disabilities, where the patient's younger brother receives services. Screening with the Ages and Stages Questionnaire reflected significant concerns across general areas of development, with raw scores of 3Ero in the area of communication and problem solving. His mother indicates that he does not yet talk and is unable to follow directions. He has not previously received developmental assessment.

Born at the gestational age of approximately 34 weeks, the patient was delivered by C-section secondary to double-footling breech presentation. Poor respiratory effort was noted with Apgar scores at 5 and 6 at one and five minutes, respectively. He was monitored in the intensive care unit, with nasal continuous positive air pressure for approximately 9 hours, then hood oxygen for a day. He was discharged from the hospital and was doing very well at that time. He has not had any significant medical problems.

The patient's mother reports that his general development has been delayed. He walked at 16 months of age and started using one word at 12 months of age. He mumbles and vocalizes, yet cannot be understood. He does not yet point to body parts and cannot follow one-step directions. He is cared for at home, along with his two sisters and twin brothers. One sister has severe developmental delay, is physically compromised, and receives services through the division of developmental disabilities. The other sister is in a special education program due to severe learning disabilities. She failed one grade in school and is reportedly working at the kindergarten level.

The family is Hispanic and both English and Spanish are spoken at home. It is the impression of this evaluator that Spanish is spoken more than English. The patient's mother received special education through the 10th grade and the father received a 9th grade education.

Measurements taken today reflect growth parameters within normal limits, as follows: Weight 14.1 kg; height 91 cm; head circumference 50 cm. The patient eats regular table foods and uses a spoon to feed himself. He sleeps through the night without any problems. He is generally described as happy and content.

Hearing screening was attempted today, but he became very fussy with this and was not able to be tested. He passed a general vision screening.

The patient's mother is on disability through Social Security. His father has reportedly been incarcerated on a parole violation, and his mother has been working to have him released. Approximately 3 days ago, Child Protective Services placed the patient and his siblings with their maternal grandmother. His grandmother accompanied his mother and the children to the clinic today. The reason for removal from their mother's home is not known. The mother related this to a dispute with her landlord.

TESTING AND OBSERVATIONS: The patient was accompanied by his mother, with other family members remaining in the waiting area during his assessment. He readily imitated vocalizations and used approximately three words: ball, uh-oh, and bye-bye. His mother is concerned that he is "tongue tied" and but has not sought medical advice for this. The patient did not open his mouth today to allow a general examination. The assessment was conducted in English, with the patient's mother repeating directions in Spanish and offering much encouragement. The patient was smiling, friendly, and was easily engaged in test activities.

Cognitive assessment was completed with the Mental Scale of the Bayley Scales of Infant Development, Second Edition. This is a general cognitive measure that is comprised of verbal and nonverbal learning and problem solving. Results are expressed in terms of the Mental Development Index (mean = 100; standard deviation = 15). The higher the score, the better the child's performance compared to others who are the same age.

The patient obtained a Mental Development Index of less than 50, a score that is more than three standard deviations below the mean. His score corresponds to a developmental age of 16 months. He passed three items beyond the formal test ceiling, with the difficulty of these items corresponding to the developmental age of 18 months, which shows slight scatter in his abilities. He was able to complete a three-piece form board consisting of basic geometric shapes, and he quickly completed a small pegboard. The patient imitated a crayon stroke and stacked a tower of four small blocks. He was unsuccessful with items involving immediate visual memory. He did not point to pictures on request other than pointing to a picture of a dog, and he was not able to follow one-step directions or show his shoes or other clothing on request. These results reflect general cognitive delay.

Further assessment of his language abilities using the Vineland Adaptive Behavior Scales reflects significant language delay, with general communication abilities at the 12-month level. His standard score on the Communication Domain is 63, a score that is more than two standard deviations below the mean. It is reported that he will listen to a story for several minutes at a time and that he attends to television programs. He attempts to say the name of one of his sisters but does not use any other names. As previously indicated, he does not yet point to body parts and is unable to follow verbal directions.

SUMMARY: The patient was seen for psychological assessment that reflects moderately severe cognitive and language delays. A comprehensive intervention program is recommended for him, and this report will be forwarded to the division of developmental disabilities for consideration. It is recommended that he receive a speech and language evaluation and a motor screening as needed. At the age of three, he will likely be eligible for a special education preschool program in the public school system.

This family is severely challenged by developmental and learning disabilities, in addition to the special medical care required for the patient's brother. It is strongly recommended that parent aid services be considered and test overall family functioning be reviewed by representatives of the division of developmental disabilities, Child Protective Services and Adult Protective Services, with coordination of care.

Appendix 3
Common Terms by Procedure

Bipolar Disorder Type II: Case Summary, Discharge Summary, and Aftercare
age-appropriate milieu
Celexa
chronic depression
individual and group psychotherapy
outpatient therapist
psychiatric history
suicidal ideation
Venereal Disease Research Laboratory
  (VDRL)

Discharge Summary: Recurrent Depression with Severe Psychotic Features
Ativan
complete blood (cell) count (CBC)
Ecotrin
euthymic mood
functional status
major depressive mood
Mellaril
mental status
nutritional intake
Risperdal

Inpatient Neuropsychology Consultation #1
case management
chronic obstructive pulmonary disease
  (COPD)
cognitive functioning
cognitive impairment
combative behavior
degenerative dementing process
depression
feeding jejunostomy
formal testing
impaired mental status

inability to follow
intraparenchymal hematoma (IPH)
memory and thinking skills
neuropsychological consultation
neuropsychological deficits
neurorehabilitation
neurosurgical drainage
psychometric testing
tracheostomy
vacillating attention
visual hallucinations

Inpatient Neuropsychology Consultation #2
Animal Naming Test
Beck Depression Inventory—II (BDI-II)
Brief Visuospatial Memory Test
California Verbal Learning Test
cognitive and emotional functioning
cognitive functioning
Controlled Oral Word Association Test
emotional functioning
fine motor functioning
Finger Tapping Test
index score
intact hippocampi
intellectual functioning
Minnesota Multiphasic Personality
  Inventory-II (MMPI-II)
Trial Making Test
verbal fluency
Wechsler Adult Intelligence Scale-III
word retrieval

Neuropsychological Consultation #1
Basic Visual Associative Learning
BNI Screen for Higher Cerebral
  Functions
Brief Visuospatial Memory Test, Revised

complex attention
Controlled Oral Word Association
    Subset of the Multilingual Aphasia
    Examination
cutaneous neurofibromatosis
displaced fourth ventricle
double vision
edema
energy level
ganglioglioma
Halstead Finger Tapping Test
hydrocephalus
image-guided resection
language functioning
left cerebellopontine angle tumor
neuropsychological evaluation
premorbid level
recall
renal cell carcinoma
Rey Auditory Verbal Learning Test
right frontal ventriculostomy
right nephrectomy
Selected Subset of the Wechsler
    Memory Scale, Revised
speed of processing
Trailmaking Test
Wisconsin Card Sorting Test
word-finding

Neuropsychological Consultation #2

BNI Screen for Higher Cerebral
    Functions
chemotherapy and radiation
cognitive deficits
cognitive status
constructional dyspraxia
dysphoria
facial affect
gait disturbance
hydrocephalus
information processing
left hand tremor

meningeal carcinomatosis
neuropsychological evaluation
Patient Competency Rating Scale for
    Neurorehabilitation
Patient Distress Scale for
    Neurorehabilitation
pattern copying
pattern recognition
problem-solving
rehabilitation
Trail Making Test
visual processing
visual scanning
visual sequencing
visuospatial organization

Paranoid Schizophrenia: Case Summary, Discharge Summary, and Aftercare

Albuterol inhaler
auditory hallucinations
Benadryl
Celexa
Elavil
level privilege system
non-reality oriented
paranoid schizophrenia
psychomotor activity
Remeron
Risperdal
Venereal Disease Research Laboratory
    (VDRL)

Psychological Evaluation: Assessment for Global Delay and Failure to Thrive/Pediatric Undernutrition

Angelman syndrome
auditory stimuli
chromosome analysis
cognitive assessment
developmental delay
dysphagia

gastroesophageal reflux
genetic assessment
global delay
intussusception
language skills
magnetic resonance imaging
Mental Development Index
mental retardation
Mental Scale of the Bayley Scales of
    Infant Development, Second Edition
metabolic testing
microcephaly
motor movement
poor growth

motor abilities
motor skills
nonverbal tasks
parent interview
pregnancy-induced hypertension
psychological evaluation
respiratory syncytial
self-care skills
special education preschool program
transitory respiratory distress
verbal tasks
Vineland Adaptive Behavior Scales
visual and auditory memory
Zyrtec

Psychological Evaluation: Developmental Assessment #1

age appropriate
alternate feet
ampicillin
Apgar scores
behavioral concerns
Celestone
cognitive measure
cognitive testing
comparative concepts
delays in adaptive abilities
diagnostic assessment
difficulty remembering names
distractibility
fine motor planning task
general play
high activity level
impulsivity
Mental Development Index
moderate cognitive delay

Psychological Evaluation: Developmental Assessment #2

Ages and Stages Questionnaire
Apgar scores
Bayley Scales of Infant Development,
    Second Edition
cognitive delay
Communication Domain
developmental age
developmental assessment
developmental delay
general development
intervention program
language delay
Mental Development Index
Mental Scale
motor screening
speech and language evaluation
standard deviation
Vineland Adaptive Behavior Scales
visual memory

Appendix 4
Slang Terms

A Bean	ecstasy
Abe	$5 worth of drugs
Abe's cabe	$5 bill
151	crack cocaine
2-for-1 sale	crack sales promotion
24–7	crack cocaine
2CB	nexus
3750	marijuana and crack rolled into a joint
420	a marijuana user
45-minute psychosis	dimethyltryptamine
714s, 7–14s	methaqualone
10¢ bag	$10 drug supply
10¢ pistol	$10 bag of poisoned heroin that is sold to an informer
25	LSD
49er	a cocaine user
A	
a-bomb, atom bomb	marijuana joint, with heroin or opium
a-boot	under the influence of drugs
a-head	an amphetamine user
AC/DC	cough syrup with codeine
Acapulco gold	gold-colored Mexican marijuana
Acapulco red	Mexican marijuana
ace	marijuana joint; PCP
acid	LSD
acid cube	LSD on a sugar cube
acid freak	a heavy user of LSD
acid head	LSD user
acid rock	a style of rock music that has a repetitive beat and lyrics suggestive of psychedelic experiences
action	gambling activity; sexual activity
ad	an addict; PCP
Adam	ecstasy
Adam and Eve	MDMA, MDEA combination
Afghani or Afgani indica	marijuana
Afghanistan black	hashish
African black	marijuana
African bush	marijuana
African woodbine	marijuana cigarette

age out	to reach an age where drugs no longer have the effect they once had
ager	a senior citizen
agonies	withdrawal symptoms
ah-pen-yen	opium
AIP	heroin from Afghanistan, Iran, and Pakistan
air blast	inhalant
airhead	marijuana user
airplane	marijuana
a la canona	abrupt (cold turkey) withdrawal from heroin
alamout black hash	hash, belladonna
Al Capone	heroin
alcopops	flavored alcohol-containing drinks
Alice	LSD or mushrooms
Alice B. Toklas	marijuana brownie
alien sex fiend	strong, powdered PCP with heroin
alki, alky	alcohol
all day and night	a life sentence to prison
all lit up	under the influence of drugs
all star	a user of multiple drugs
all-American drug	cocaine
alley cat	a sexually promiscuous woman
alley juice	methyl alcohol
alligator	a physically attractive male
alpha-ET	alpha-ethyltryptamine
ambition	amphetamine
ames, aimes	amphetamine; amyl nitrite
amidone	methadone
ammo	amobarbital
amoeba	PCP
amp	ampule; amphetamine; marijuana cigarette dipped in formaldehyde or embalming fluid, sometimes laced with PCP
amp head	an LSD user
amp joint	a marijuana cigarette laced with a narcotic
amped	under the influence of drugs
amped-out	fatigue after using amphetamines
amping	an accelerated heartbeat after drug use
AMT	dimethyltryptamine
amys	amyl nitrite
anavar	an oral steroid

angel	PCP
angel dust	PCP
angel hair	PCP
angel mist	PCP
angel poke	PCP
angels in a sky	LSD
angel tears	liquid LSD
Angie	cocaine
angola	marijuana
animal	LSD
animal trank/tranq	PCP
animal tranquilizer	PCP
antifreeze	heroin
Anything going on?	Do you have drugs to sell?
Apache	fentanyl
apple jacks	crack
apples	fellow addicts
Archie Bunker	a bigoted person
Are you anywhere?	Do you use marijuana?
Are you holding?	Do you have any drugs?
Aries	heroin
arm	a police officer
aroma of men	isobutyl nitrite
around the turn	has gone through withdrawal
artillery	equipment for injecting drugs
ashes	marijuana
Asian white	cocaine
assassin of youth	marijuana
astro turf	marijuana
ate up	one who is always under the influence of drugs
at liberty	unemployed
atom bomb	(see a-bomb)
atshitshi	marijuana
attitude	a sudden hostile feeling
Aunt Hazel	heroin
Aunti, auntie	opium
Aunti, Auntie Emma	opium
Aunt Mary	marijuana
Aunt Nora	cocaine
aurora borealis	PCP
Australian	1 ounce/ozzy

B	amount of marijuana to fill a matchbox
B-40	cigar laced with marijuana and dipped in malt liquor
babe	drug used for detoxification; a sexually attractive woman
baby	marijuana; minor heroin habit; one who is just getting started on drugs
baby bhang	marijuana
baby habit	occasional use of drugs
baby boomers	generation of people born immediately following World War II
baby boomlets	generation of people born in the 1980s and 1990s
baby-sitter	one who guides an individual through the first drug experience
baby slits	ecstasy
baby T	crack cocaine
backbreakers	LSD and strychnine
back dex	amphetamine
back door	residue left in a pipe
backjack	to inject a drug
back to back	smoking crack after injecting heroin or heroin used after smoking crack
backtrack	to gradually inject a drug by pulling back and reinjecting it repeatedly to increase the drug's effect
backup	to prepare a vein for injection
backwards	depressant; to get a habit again
bad	crack cocaine; good
bad bundle	inferior quality heroin
bad go	a bad reaction to a drug
bad paper	a worthless check
bad pizza	PCP
bad rock	crack cocaine
bad scene	uncomfortable or unfriendly surroundings; an unpleasant experience or situation; ugly reverberation
bad seed	peyote; heroin; marijuana; mescaline
bad trip	a frightening reaction after use of a hallucinogen
baddie	a criminal
badge bandit	a police officer
badger game	a method of extortion

bag	a drug container (usually 1 ounce); an unattractive woman; to kill
bag; baggage	measurement of marijuana or heroin; condom(s)
bag boy	one who sells dope for someone else
bag bride	crack-smoking prostitute
bag lady	a female street person
bag man	a person who transports money; one who has a small habit; a drug dealer
bagging	using an inhalant
bake	to smoke marijuana
baked	under the influence of drugs or alcohol
baker (the)	the electric chair
bale	one pound of marijuana
ball	crack cocaine; a testicle
balling	vaginally implanted cocaine
balloon	heroin supplier; a balloon that contains drugs
ballot	heroin
bam, bamb	depressant; amphetamine
bambalacha	marijuana
bambita, bombita	Desoxyn or amphetamine derivative
bammies, bammer	inferior-quality marijuana
bammy	marijuana
banano	marijuana or tobacco cigarette laced with cocaine
bang	to inject a drug; inhalant; sexual intercourse
bangin' it in	shooting heroin via needle
banging	under the influence of drugs; engaging in sexual intercourse
bank	cash flow for buying drugs
bank bandit pills	depressant
bar	marijuana
Barbara Jean	marijuana
Barbies	depressants
barbs	barbiturates; jagged edges on a used hypodermic needle
barr	codeine cough syrup
bareback rider	a man who has sex without using a condom
barf tea	peyote
barfly	a heavy drinker
bark at the moon	under the influence of drugs or alcohol
barrels	LSD

basket case	one who is distraught
Bart Simpson	LSD
base	to free-base cocaine; crack
baseball	crack cocaine
base crazies	searching on hands and knees for crack
base head	person who free-bases
base house	place for smoking freebase cocaine or crack cocaine
based out	one who has lost control over free-basing
bash	marijuana; party
baste (to)	to beat
basuco (Spanish)	cocaine; coca paste residue sprinkled on marijuana or tobacco cigarette
bat	marijuana pipe, easily disguised as a cigarette
bathtub crank	poor quality methamphetamine
bathtub speed	methcathinone
batt	IV needle
batted out	to be arrested
battery acid	LSD
batu	smokable methamphetamine
bazooka	cocaine; crack; crack and tobacco
bazulco	cocaine
BC Budd	high-grade marijuana from British Columbia
BD	belladonna
BDMPEA	nexus
beagle	a detective or investigator
beam me up Scottie	crack dipped in PCP
beamers, beemers	crack users
bean	Benzedrine
beaners	drugs
beans	amphetamine; depressant; mescaline
bear	a capsule that contains a narcotic
bear in the air	a police officer in a helicopter
bear trap	a police radar trap
beast	LSD; a prostitute; an unattractive woman
beat	a counterfeit drug
beat artist	person selling bogus drugs
beat generation	young people of the 1950s and 1960s, known for rejecting conventional social values
beat it	to leave in a hurry
beat off	to masturbate (male)

beat the bricks	to get out of jail or prison
beat the gong	to smoke opium
beat the rap	to go unpunished or be acquitted
beat vials	vials containing sham crack
beautiful boulders	crack
beautiful people (the)	individuals who are stylish and wealthy
Beavis & Butthead	crack cocaine
bebe	crack cocaine
bedazzled	under the influence of drugs
bedbugs	fellow addicts
bee	bong hits
beedies	East Indian cigarettes, resemble joints
been had	arrested; to have had sexual intercourse
beemers	(see beamers)
beetle crusher	a police officer
behind the iron house	in jail or prison
behind the scale	to weigh and sell cocaine
beiging	cocaine chemically altered to make it appear to be a higher purity
belch	to inform
belly habit	to take a drug orally
belongs	uses drugs
belt	a marijuana cigarette; an alcoholic drink
belted	under the influence of drugs; to rapidly consume an alcoholic drink
Belushi; Belushi cocktail	cocaine and heroin mixture
belyando spruce	marijuana
bender	drug party; rave
benny, bennie(s)	Benzedrine
benz	Benzedrine
Bernice	cocaine
Bernie	cocaine
Bernie's flakes	cocaine
Bernie's gold dust	cocaine
Betsy, betsy, Betsie	a gun
bhang	marijuana, East Indian term
big 8	1/8 kilogram
big bag	heroin
big bloke	cocaine
big C	cocaine
big chief	peyote; mescaline
big D	LSD
biggy	marijuana

big H	heroin
big Harry	heroin
big house	prison
big John	a police officer
big flake	cocaine
big man	drug supplier
big O	opium
big one	a $1,000 bet
big rush	cocaine
big-timer	a gambler or risk taker
bike	a motorcycle police officer
biker's coffee	methamphetamine and coffee
biker's speed	methamphetamine
bill	a $100 bill
Bill Blass	cocaine
billie hoke	cocaine
bimbo	an immature woman; a prostitute
bindle	small packet of drug powder; heroin
bing	enough of a drug for one injection
bingers	crack addicts
bingler	one who sells narcotics
bingo	to inject a drug
bingo houses	where addicts go to buy and use drugs
bird cage hype	addicts who have trouble supporting their habits
birdhead	LSD
birdie powder	heroin; cocaine
birds	marijuana
bird's eye	extremely small quantity of narcotics
biscuit	50 rocks of crack
bitch	a malicious woman; to complain
bitchy	malicious or arrogant behavior
bite	arrest
bite one's lips	to smoke marijuana
biz	equipment for injecting drugs
BJs	crack cocaine
black	tar heroin
black acid	LSD; LSD and PCP mixture
black and white	amphetamine; a patrol car
Black Bart	marijuana
black beauties	depressants; amphetamine
blackbird	type of LSD
black bombers	amphetamine

black button	dried button of peyote
black Cadillacs	amphetamines
black dust	PCP
black ganga	marijuana resin
black gold	high quality marijuana
black gungi	marijuana from India
black gunion	marijuana
black H	potent Mexican heroin with the consistency of tar
black hash	opium and heroin
black hole	depression associated with ketamine use
black Maria	highly potent marijuana
black mo; black moat; black mote	marijuana that has been cured in sugar or honey, then buried for some time
black Mollies	amphetamines; diet pills
black mote	(see black mo)
black pearl	heroin
black pill	opium pill
black powder	black hash ground into powder
black rock	crack cocaine
black Russian	hashish mixed with opium
black star	LSD
black stuff	heroin; black tar opium
black sundae	brown heroin cut with cocoa
black sunshine	LSD
black tabs	LSD
black tar	potent heroin
black tootsie roll	black tar heroin
black whack	PCP
blacks	amphetamine
blade	a knife
Blade Queen	a girl that is obsessed with doing blades
blades	after heating 2 knives on an element, one picks up a desired drug with the hot knives and inhales it
Blanca (Spanish)	cocaine; heroin
blank	container of nonnarcotic powder that is sold as heroin or cocaine
blanket	marijuana cigarette
blanks	inferior quality drugs
blast	to smoke marijuana; to smoke crack; a party; a rave; to shoot with a firearm
blast a joint	to smoke marijuana

blast a roach	to smoke marijuana
blast a stick	to smoke marijuana
blasted	under the influence of drugs or alcohol
blaster	a gunman
blaze	to smoke marijuana
blind munchies	an overwhelming desire for something to eat, usually after smoking marijuana
blind squid	ketamine, belladonna, LSD
bliss out	the mystic daze one is in while under the influence of a guru
blitzed	under the influence of drugs or alcohol
blizzard	white cloud in a pipe used to smoke cocaine
block	marijuana
blockbusters	depressants
blond hash	hashish that is gold in color
blonde	marijuana
Bloods	the name of a well-known gang
blotter	LSD; cocaine; the daily arrest record kept in a police station
blotter acid	LSD
blotter cube	LSD
blow	cocaine or crystal amphetamine; to inhale cocaine; to smoke marijuana
blow a fix	(see blow the vein)
blow a shot	to miss a target one is shooting at
blow job	fellatio
blow the joint	to leave a place
blow the vein	to use too much pressure on a weak or sclerosed vein, causing it to rupture
blow a stick	to smoke marijuana
blow away	to overcome emotionally; to kill with a firearm
blow blue	to inhale cocaine
blowcaine	crack diluted with cocaine
blow Charley	to sniff cocaine
blow grass	to smoke marijuana
blow horse	to sniff heroin
blow coke	to inhale cocaine
blow off	to dismiss or avoid
blow one's roof	to smoke marijuana
blow up	crack cut with lidocaine to increase size, weight, and street value; to lose one's temper

blow one's mind	to soar beyond reality while under the influence of drugs
blow smoke	to inhale cocaine; to exaggerate
blowing smoke	marijuana
blow snow	to sniff cocaine
blown	high on marijuana
blowout	crack; a rave; a party at which drugs and alcohol are used to excess
blue	depressant; crack cocaine
blue acid	LSD
blue and red	secobarbital
blue angels	amobarbital
blue bag	heroin
blue barrels	LSD
bluebirds	amobarbital
blue boy	amphetamine
blue bullets	depressant
blue caps	LSD
blue cheer	LSD
blue de Hue	marijuana from Vietnam
blue devils	amobarbital
blue dolls	amobarbital
blue flags	LSD
blue flick	a pornographic movie
blue fly	LSD
blue hair	a senior citizen
blue heaven	LSD
blue heavens	amobarbital
blue hero	heroin
blue kisses	ecstasy (MDMA)
blue lips	ecstasy (MDMA)
blue madman	PCP
blue meth	methamphetamine
blue microdot	LSD
blue mist	LSD
blue moons	LSD
blue morph	Numorphan (oxymorphone), a narcotic used in maintenance programs
Blue Nitro Vitality	GBL-containing product
blue sage	marijuana
blue sky	heroin
blue sky blond	high potency Colombian marijuana
blue star	LSD/PCP

blue tips	depressant
blue velvet	paregoric and amphetamine mixture
blue vials	LSD
blued	tattooed
blues	amobarbital; melancholia; police officers
blunt	marijuana inside a cigar or a large rolled joint
blunted out	smoked many blunts of marijuana
bo	marijuana
boat	marijuana laced with PCP
Bob	marijuana
bobo	crack
bobo bush	marijuana
body packer	person who ingests drug vials to transport them or to avoid prosecution
body shake	a skin search for needle marks
body stuffer	person who ingests drug vials to transport them or to avoid prosecution
Bogart	keeping marijuana to oneself
Bogart a joint	to salivate on a marijuana cigarette
bohd	marijuana; PCP
bolasterone	injectable steroid
Bolivian marching powder	cocaine
bollo	crack
bolo	crack
bolt	isobutyl nitrite
bomb	crack; heroin; large marijuana cigarette; high potency heroin
bomb squad	crack-selling crew
bombed out	intoxicated by narcotics
bomber	a large marijuana cigarette
bombido, bombito, bombita	injectable amphetamines and cocaine
bombs away	heroin
bone	marijuana; $50 piece of crack
bone crusher	crack
bones	crack
bone shaker	a gambler or risk taker
bong	a device used to smoke marijuana or hashish
Bonita	heroin
boo	marijuana
boo boo bama	100 dose units of LSD
booger	cocaine (in the Florida Keys)
boogered up	high on cocaine (in the Florida Keys)
boofing	expelling concealed drugs from your body

book	a one-year prison sentence
book (the)	the maximum prison sentence allowed by law
bookie	an individual who handles bets
boom	marijuana
boom boom	sexual activity
boom-boom girl	a prostitute
boom-boom house	a whorehouse
boomers	psilocybin/psilocin
boonies	rural area; away from a populated area
boost	to inject a drug; to shoplift
boost and shoot	steal to support a habit
booster	to inhale cocaine
boot	to inject a drug gradually by pulling back and reinjecting repeatedly to increase the drug's effect
boot the gong	to smoke marijuana
booted	under the influence of drugs
booty juice	MDMA dissolved in liquid
boppers	amyl nitrite
boss	excellent quality drug
BOT	balance of time (remaining time of a prison sentence)
both hands	a 10-year prison sentence
botray	crack
bottles	crack vials; injectable amphetamines
boubou	crack
boulder	$20 worth of crack
boulya	crack
bouncing powder	cocaine
bouncy bouncy	sexual intercourse
bowl	between 1/32 and 1/16 ounce of marijuana or a small pipe used to smoke marijuana
bowling	smoking several bowls in a row
boxed	in jail or prison
box man	an expert in breaking into safes
boxcars	sixes on dice
boy	heroin
boys uptown (the)	a group of influential criminals
bozo	heroin; an unpleasant, unattractive, or insignificant person
brain bucket	a helmet
brain damage	heroin

brain dead	one who has used drugs for an extended period of time and who has difficulty functioning normally
brain pills	amphetamines
brain ticklers	amphetamines
brand X	inferior quality marijuana
brass (the)	upper ranks of the armed forces
bread	money
breakdowns	$40 crack rock sold for $20
breakfast of champions	crack
break loose	to escape from jail or prison
break night	staying up all night until day break
brew	beer
brewery	place where drugs are made
brick	1 kilo of a drug
brick agent	an FBI agent
brick gum	heroin
bridge up or bring up	ready a vein for injection
bring down	something or someone unpleasant; to cause the downfall of another
Bristol Brown	bad marijuana
britton	peyote
broccoli	marijuana
brodie, Brodie	suicide committed by jumping from a high place
bromo	nexus
brother	heroin
broker	go-between in a drug deal
brown	Mexican heroin, usually light brown
brown bagger	a physically unattractive person
brown bombers	LSD
brown crystal	heroin
brown dots	LSD
brown horse	Mexican heroin
brown noser	a person who flatters in order to gain approval or advantage
brown rhine	heroin
brown sugar	heroin
brown tape	heroin
brownies	brownies laced with marijuana
browns	long-lasting amphetamines
bruiser	a physically fit male
bubble gum	cocaine; crack

buck	a physically fit male; one dollar; a $100 bet
bud(s)	marijuana
Buddha, buda, budda	high-grade marijuana joint laced with opium
buffer	crack smoker; a woman who exchanges oral sex for crack
bufo	5-hydroxy-N,N-dimethyltryptamine, a hallucinogenic drug
bugged	annoyed; to be covered with sores and abscesses from repeated use of dirty needles
build a collar	to gather evidence in order to make an arrest
bull	a federal narcotics agent; a police officer; a prison guard
bullet	isobutyl nitrite
bullet bolt	an inhalant
bullion	crack
bullpen	a holding cell in a jail or prison
bumblebees	amphetamine
bummer trip	unsettling and threatening experience from drug intoxication
bump	crack; fake crack; boost a high; small dose of crystal meth
bundle	twenty-five $5 bags of heroin
bunk	counterfeit drugs
burnese	cocaine
burn	to take money for heroin with no plan to deliver, or by delivering counterfeit bags; to inform on another; to put someone to death in the electric chair; to kill; ex-addict who lectures on the dangers of drug abuse
burn bag	counterfeit drugs
burned	to purchase counterfeit drugs
burned out	to be physically and mentally debilitated from prolonged drug use or prolonged stress
burner	the electric chair
burnie	marijuana
burning logs	smoking a joint
burn one	to smoke marijuana
burnout	heavy abuser of drugs
burnt	one who has smoked too much marijuana
burn the main line	to inject a drug

burrito	marijuana
bush	cocaine; marijuana; female genitalia
businessman's high	psilocin/psilocybin mushrooms
businessman's LSD	dimethyltryptamine (DMT)
businessman's special	dimethyltryptamine (DMT)
busted	arrested
busters	depressant
bust out	to escape from jail or prison
busy bee	PCP
butler	crack
butt	inferior quality marijuana
butt naked	PCP
butter	marijuana; crack
butter flower	marijuana
buttons	sections of peyote cactus
butu	heroin or crack
buzzed	slightly under the influence of drugs or alcohol
buzz bomb	nitrous oxide
C	cocaine
CA	cocaine addict
caballo	heroin
cabbage	money
caca	inferior or adulterated heroin, cocaine, or marijuana
cache	a hidden supply of drugs or money
Cacti Joint	a joint of dried and ground up peyote
cactus	mescaline; peyote
cactus buttons	mescaline; peyote
cactus head	mescaline; peyote
cadet	a new addict
Cad	1 ounce
Cadillac	PCP
Cadillac express	methcathinone
cafeteria	use of various drugs simultaneously
cage	jail or prison cell
caine	cocaine
calbo	heroin
cake	drugs that are smuggled into a jail, prison or hospital
cakes	round discs of crack
caine	cocaine; crack
California cornflakes	cocaine

California sunshine	LSD
California turnarounds	amphetamines
call girl	a prostitute
calling card	needle marks
cam trip	high potency marijuana
Cambodian red/Cam red	reddish-brown Cambodian marijuana
Cambodian trip weed	potent Cambodian marijuana
came	cocaine
campfire boy	an opium addict
can	1 ounce of marijuana
Can you do me good?	Do you have drugs I can buy?
Canadian black	Canadian marijuana
Canadian blues	methaqualone
Canadian quail	methaqualone
canamo	marijuana
canappa	marijuana
canary	Nembutal capsule (bright yellow color); an informer
cancelled stick	marijuana cigarette
cancer stick	a cigarette
candied	a cocaine addict
candy	any drug
candy blunt	blunt cigarettes or cigars dipped in cough syrup
candy C	cocaine
candy flip	1 hit ecstasy per three hit(s) LSD
candy a J	to add another drug to a marijuana cigarette
candy canes and gumdrops	LSD
candy man	a drug supplier or seller
candy raver	a person who attends raves
canned goods	cans containing drugs
cannon	a huge marijuana cigarette; a gun; a pickpocket
cannon ball	an injection of mixed drugs
canoe	a marijuana cigarette with a hole in its side that looks like a canoe
canvas back	a street person
cap	capsule of drugs; gelatin capsule used to package drugs; packet of heroin
caps	crack
captain	an influential drug distributor
cap up	to transfer drugs from bulk to capsules
capital H	heroin

caps	heroin; psilocybin/psilocin mushrooms
carburetor	drug paraphernalia that mixes smoke with air
card	a prepared ration of cocaine which is weighed on a card
card shark	a card-playing gambler
carga	heroin
carmabis	marijuana
carnie	cocaine
carpet patrol	smokers searching the floor for crack
Carrie, Carrie Nation	cocaine
carrier	one who sells drugs as part of a distribution chain
carry, carrying, carry weights	to have drugs in one's possession
cartucho	package of marijuana cigarettes
cartoon acid	LSD
cartwheels	amphetamines
cascade	to move to stronger drugs
cashed	a container of marijuana that has been completely used
cashing a script	getting forged or bogus prescription orders dispensed
Casper the ghost	crack
cast iron horrors	delirium tremens (DTs)
cat	methcathinone
cat's pee	crack
cat valium	ketamine
catnip	marijuana cigarette
catch up	withdrawal process
catcher's mitt	a diaphragm
Catholic aspirin	cross-scored amphetamine tablets
cattail	a marijuana cigarette
cattle rustler	one who steals meat and sells it for drug money
caught in a snowstorm	under the influence of cocaine
cave	an abscessed or collapsed portion of a vein
cave digging	searching for a suitable site in which to inject drugs
caviar	combination of cocaine, crack, and marijuana
cavite all star	marijuana
cavities	needle marks
CD	glutethimide

C dust	cocaine
cereal	marijuana smoked in a bowl
Cecil	morphine
Cecil Jones	a morphine addict
cement	a large quantity of wholesale drugs
cement arm	an addict's heavily scarred arm
cent	one dollar
cess	marijuana
C game	cocaine
C & H	cocaine and heroin mixture
cha cha	an opium pipe
chalk	methamphetamine; amphetamine tablets that crumble easily
chalked up	under the influence of cocaine
chalking	chemically altering the color of cocaine so it is white
chamber pipe	a pipe designed to hold a large amount of marijuana
champagne	marijuana and cocaine mixture
chandoo/chandu	Chinese opium
channel	a drug source; the favored vein for injection of drugs
channel swimmer	an addict who takes drugs by injecting into a vein
charas, charash, charras	pure resin of Indian hemp, sometimes mixed with opium
charge	a drug portion
charged up	under the influence of drugs
Charles, Charlie, Charley	cocaine; one dollar
Charley Cotton	cotton that is used to strain a drug before an injection
Charley goon	a police officer
chase	to smoke cocaine or marijuana
chaser	compulsive crack user
chase the bag	to shop for the best quality of drug
chasing the dragon	inhaling the fumes from heroin or opium through a tube
chasing the nurse	regularly using morphine
chasing the tiger	smoking heroin
chaze	to christen a new bowl or pipe
C head	a cocaine user
cheap basing	crack
cheaters	marked playing cards

check	one's personal supply of drugs
cheeba	marijuana
cheeo	chewable marijuana seeds
cheese	heroin
chef	one who cooks and prepares opium
chemical	crack
cherry meth	gamma hydroxybutyrate (GHB)
cherry top	LSD
chestbonz	one taking the biggest bong hit
chewed	severely stoned
chewies	crack; blunt with powdered cocaine inside
chewing the gum	chewing opium
chiba chiba	potent Colombian marijuana
Chicago black	a dark variety of marijuana grown in the Chicago area
Chicago green	a dark green variety of marijuana cured in opium, grown in the Chicago area
Chicago leprosy	scars caused by multiple venous injections
chicharra	mixture of tobacco and marijuana
chick	heroin; an attractive female
chicken feed	a small amount of money
chicken hawk	a child molester
chicken head	cocaine addict
chicken powder	powdered amphetamines
chicken scratch	searching floor on hands and knees for crack
chicken-shit habit	a small drug habit
chicle	heroin
chicory	inferior quality opium
chief	peyote; mescaline
chieva	heroin
Chillie Willies	snorting vodka or gin out of a bottle cap
chill	to ignore or refuse to sell drugs to one suspected of being an informer; to relax; to kill
chill out	relax
chill pill	a depressant
chillum	equipment used for smoking marijuana
chillun	pipe used to smoke hashish
China	opium
China cat	high potency opium
China girl	fentanyl
China town	fentanyl

China White, Chinese	superior quality Asian heroin
Chinaman on one's back	withdrawal symptoms
Chinese connection	Chinese drug smugglers
Chinese cure	gradual drug withdrawal
Chinese molasses	opium in its raw state
Chinese red	heroin
Chinese saxophone	an opium pipe
Chinese tobacco	opium
Chino	a Chinese drug dealer
chip	drug dose taken in a small enough amount to avoid addiction
chipper	occasional drug user
chipping	using small amounts of drugs on an irregular basis
chippie, chippy	one who takes small amounts of drugs irregularly; a prostitute
chips	marijuana or tobacco cigarettes laced with PCP
chira	marijuana
chiva	heroin
chlorals	chloral hydrate
chocolate	opium; amphetamine
chocolate chip cookies	MDMA (ecstasy), heroin or methadone mixture
chocolate chips	MDMA (ecstasy); LSD
chocolate powder	mescaline
chocolate rock	crack and heroin mixture
chocolate rocket	crack made brown in color by adding powdered chocolate milk during processing
chocolate Thai	marijuana
choke	to dilute drugs
choker	large or powerful hit of crack cocaine
cholly	cocaine
chop	to process heroin or marijuana
Christians	cross-scored amphetamine tablets
Christina	amphetamines
Christine	crystal methamphetamine
Christmas rolls, Christmas trees	different colored barbiturate capsules; amphetamines; dextroamphetamines
chronic	marijuana and crack mixture
chuck a Charley, chuck a dummy	to fake a withdrawal spasm in an attempt to get drugs from a medical practitioner

chuck horrors	voracious craving for food during withdrawal
chucks	hunger following withdrawal from heroin
chuck the habit	to break a drug addiction
chug, chug-a-lug	to quickly drink alcohol
chunky	marijuana
church	LSD paper with cross on it
church key	an opener used to open cans or bottles that contain alcohol
churus	marijuana
cibas (CIBAs)	Doriden
cid	LSD
cigarette papers	packets of heroin
cigarrode crystal	PCP
circles	Rohypnol
circus	faking a withdrawal spasm in an attempt to get drugs from a medical practitioner
citizen	nonuser of drugs
citrol	high potency Nepal marijuana
CJ, KJ	PCP in crystalline form
C joint	a place where cocaine can be purchased; place where cocaine is sold
clanks	delirium tremens
clarity	MDMA (ecstasy)
clay	hashish
clean	one who has ceased using drugs; an addict's arm which is free of needle marks; not in possession of drugs
clean and manicured	marijuana that is free of stems and seeds
clear light	superior quality LSD in gelatin capsule form
clear up	to cease using drugs
clickem, clickum	a marijuana cigarette that has been dipped in embalming fluid and laced with PCP
clicker	crack and PCP mixture
cliffhanger	PCP
climax	butyl nitrite
climb	to ascend to a high from smoking a marijuana cigarette
clink	jail or prison
clip	holder for a marijuana cigarette; to rob
clipped one's wings	arrested
clips	rows of vials heat-sealed together
clocker	an entry-level drug dealer who sells 24 hours a day

clocking paper	money made from selling drugs
closed	a drug source who is not selling because of law enforcement suspicion
closet baser	a free-base cocaine user who prefers anonymity
cloud	smoke created by using pipes
cloud nine	euphoria felt from smoking drugs
clouted	arrested
club	a place to smoke marijuana
cluck	crack smoker
clucker	cocaine addict
Clydesdale	a physically fit or handsome male
C & M	cocaine and morphine mixture
coasting	under the influence of drugs
coast to coast	long-acting amphetamines
coca	cocaine
coca paste	a potent form of cocaine
cocaine blues	depression after extended cocaine use
cochornis	marijuana
cock	a male; penis
cock pipe	drug paraphernalia that is shaped like a penis and is used to smoke marijuana
cockle burrs	amphetamines
cocktail	tobacco cigarette mixed with marijuana or dipped in hashish oil
cocoa puff	to smoke cocaine and marijuana
coconut	cocaine
coco rocks	crack cocaine that is made dark brown crack made by adding chocolate pudding during production
cod cock	cough syrup containing codeine
coffee	LSD
coffee cups	bags that hold marijuana
coffee dodger	a chain smoker
coffin nail	a cigarette
coke	cocaine; crack
coke bar	a bar where cocaine is openly used
coke blower	one who sniffs powdered cocaine
coke break	a break one takes to use cocaine
coke bugs	sensation that bugs are crawling under the skin after using cocaine
coke crash	severe anxiety or depression following heavy cocaine use

coke freak	a regular cocaine user
coke oven	a place where cocaine is used or sold
coke party, coke time	a gathering in which participants use cocaine
coke whore	one who performs sexual favors in exchange for cocaine
coked up	under the influence of cocaine
cokehead	a habitual cocaine user
cokeroaches	imaginary bugs crawling on one who is high on cocaine
cokie	a cocaine user
cola	cocaine
cold and hot	mixture of cocaine and heroin
cold turkey	an abrupt and complete withdrawal from a habit
coli	marijuana
coliflor tostao	marijuana
collar	a narrow strip of paper that secures a needle to an eyedropper; to make a drug bust; to arrest
collard greens	marijuana
Colorado	cocaine
Colorado Kool-Aid	Coor's beer
Colorado Rockies	crack cocaine
Colombian connection	Colombian drug smugglers
Colombian gold	potent Colombian marijuana
Colombian green	superior quality Colombian marijuana
Colombian roulette	smuggling drugs from Colombia by swallowing packets and excreting them on delivery
Columbo	PCP
Columbus black	marijuana grown in the Columbus, Ohio area
Columbus black tea	marijuana
come back	cocaine that has been adulterated for conversation to crack
come home	to return to reality after an LSD trip
come up	to increase profit made in drug sales
communist M & Ms	red Seconal capsules
comp man	a drug dealer
con	to manipulate by using applied psychology; a convict
conductor	one who guides others through LSD trips
Congo brown	a brown-colored variety of African marijuana

Congo dirt	superior quality African marijuana
connect	to purchase illegal drugs
connection, contact	one who sells or supplies illegal drugs
constitutional	an addict's first injection of the day
contact high	psychological feeling of being high merely from being around a person who is under the influence of drugs or alcohol
contact lens	LSD
convert	one who is recently addicted to drugs
cook	an opium den attendant who prepares opium; to smoke marijuana or hashish
cook down	process in which users liquify drugs
cooking up	to process cocaine into crack cocaine
cook up a pill	to prepare a drug for smoking
cooker	a container that is used for heating and dissolving heroin, amphetamines, or cocaine
cookin'	having a good time; process in manufacturing methamphetamines
cool	very good; composed; in a mellow state
coolie	cigarette laced with opium
coolie mud	inferior quality opium
cooler	cigarette laced with a drug
coop	jail or prison
coozie, cozy, couzie, couzy stash	a condom or other parcel of drugs concealed in the vagina
cop	to get anything; to buy dope; a police officer
cop a buzz	to smoke marijuana
cop a deuceway	to purchase a $2 package of narcotics
cop a drag	to draw smoke from a cigarette
cop a feel	to fondle
cop a fix	to obtain a dose of drugs
cop a match	to purchase a matchbox of marijuana
cop a pill	to smoke an opium pellet
cop a sneak	to leave a place
cop and blow	to purchase drugs and quickly leave the scene
co-pilot	amphetamine; sober companion for one who is under the influence of drugs or alcohol
cop man	a police officer
cop out	to back out; to inform
cop-out	an excuse for changing one's mind
copper	a police officer

copycat crime	a crime that is committed in imitation of another crime
copping zones	areas where drugs can be purchased
corals	chloral hydrate
coriander seeds	money
cork the air	to inhale cocaine
corn	marijuana
corn dog	a marijuana cigarette laced with cocaine
cornstalk	marijuana cigarette rolled in the shuck of a corn cob, then sealed with honey
Corinne, Corine	cocaine
cosmic, cozmic	experience on drugs
cosmos, cosmos	PCP
cotics	narcotics
cotton	paper money
cotton brothers	the cotton used with drugs requiring use of a cotton strainer
cotton catcher, cotton top	an addict who begs for used straining cotton
cotton fever	fever from infection, allergic reaction, blood poisoning, or other illness contracted after using contaminated straining cotton
cotton freak	one who inhales from straining cotton
cotton shooter	addict who injects residue from straining cotton
cotton shot	water added to cotton in an attempt to get whatever drug is left on straining cotton
cottonhead	one who uses previously used straining cotton as a drug source
cottons	pieces of cotton used to strain dissolved, heated drugs before injecting them
couch doctor	a psychiatrist
count	the purity level of a drug
courage pills	heroin or barbiturates
course note	any bill larger than $2
cowboy	an independent drug seller
crack	a purer, more potent form of cocaine, usually mixed with ammonia or baking soda and formed into crystals
crack attack	to crave crack cocaine
crack back	crack and marijuana
crack cooler	crack soaked in a wine cooler
crack gallery	a place where cocaine is sold and used

crack house	a gathering place where participants use cocaine
crack kit	glass pipe and copper mesh for use by cocaine users
crack pipe	a pipe used for smoking crack
cracker	one to uses crack cocaine
cracker jacks	crack smokers
crackers	animal crackers laced with LSD; mixture of Talwin and Ritalin
crackhead	one who uses crack cocaine
crack spot	an area where people can purchase or use crack
crack star	a frequent user of crack
crack weed	marijuana laced with crack
cracking	gesturing as if cracking a whip, used to advertise crack
crank	methamphetamines in powdered form
crank bugs	feeling that bugs are crawling under the skin after heavy amphetamine use
crank freak	one who alternates between amphetamines and barbiturates and tranquilizers
crankster	one who uses and/or manufactures crank
cranking up	to inject a drug
crap	inferior quality heroin; nonsense
crapper	toilet
crapper dick	a law enforcement agent who patrols public toilets looking for illicit sexual activity and drug deals
crappy	markedly inferior quality
crash	to sleep or lose consciousness after drug use; to spend the night
crash pad	a place to recover from a drug trip
crashed	raided by law enforcement agents
crater	a scar of indentation left at a healed abscess site from an injection
crazy coke	PCP
crazy Eddie	a marijuana or tobacco cigarette dipped in embalming fluid and laced with PCP
crazy weed	marijuana
creamed	alcohol or drug intoxicated
credit card	crack stem
creeper	slow-acting marijuana
creeps	delirium tremens

crib	an addict's dwelling; residence
criddy	methamphetamines
crill	a marijuana cigarette laced with cocaine
crimmie	a tobacco cigarette laced with crack
crink	methamphetamines; amphetamines
Crips	the name of a well-known gang
cripple	a marijuana cigarette laced with a drug
cris	methamphetamine in powdered form
crisco	crystal methamphetamine
crisp	under the influence of drugs
crispo	one who is mentally, socially, and physically burned out from drug use
crispy critter	under the influence of marijuana
crisscrossing	snorting heroin in one nostril and cocaine in the other nostril simultaneously from parallel lines
crissy	crystal methamphetamine
Cristina	methamphetamine
Cristy	smokable methamphetamine
croak	crack and methamphetamine; to die
croaker	a physician
croaker joint	a hospital
crock	an opium pipe; a lie
crocked	intoxicated from alcohol intake
cross tops	cross-scored amphetamine tablets
cross-country hype	an addict who goes from place to place in search of drugs from medical practitioners
crosses	cross-scored amphetamine tablets
crossroads	cross-scored amphetamine tablets
crow	cocaine
crown crap	heroin
crumbs	tiny pieces of crack
crumb snatcher	an addict who steals tiny pieces of crack
cruise	to drive slowly back and forth along a designated route
crumbs	small rock cocaine particles
crunch & munch	crack
crusher	a police officer
crusty treats	crack
crutch	a device used to hold a marijuana cigarette butt
crying weed	marijuana

crypto	methamphetamine
crystal	crystallized methamphetamine
crystal doe	crystallized methamphetamine
crystal joint	PCP
crystal meth	crystallized methamphetamine
crystal pop	cocaine and PCP
crystal ship	a syringe containing a dissolved crystallized drug
crystal tea/T	LSD
cube	approximately 1 ounce of morphine; LSD on a sugar cube; a person who does not use drugs or alcohol
cube juice	morphine
cubehead	a user who prefers to take LSD in the form of a sugar cube
cubes	sugar cubes that have been laced with LSD
cupcakes	LSD
curbstones	cigarette butts retrieved from gutters
cushion	vein site for injecting a drug
cut	to dilute a drug by adding some other substance, such as milk, sugar, quinine; to stab someone
cut deck	heroin or morphine diluted with powdered milk
cut loose	to escape from jail or prison
C.W.	completely wrecked (stoned or high on drugs)
cyclones	PCP
D	Dilaudid; LSD; dust
DA	a drug addict
dabble	to use drugs occasionally
dabbler	an occasional drug user
daddy	a pimp
dagga	South African marijuana
dagga rooker	a smoker of South African marijuana
daisy chaining	injecting and withdrawing a drug back into a needle for injection by the next user; sexual coupling involving three or more
dai-yen	opium that is prepared for smoking
dals	Dalmane
dama blanca	cocaine
Dame DuPaw	marijuana

damps	barbiturates
dance fever	fentanyl
dance hall	chamber in which prisoners are executed
dank	marijuana
dans	oxycodone
date	sex between a John and a hoe (whore)
dawamesk	marijuana
DD	a deadly dose of drugs
D & D	drunk and disorderly
dead	out of drug money; out of drugs
dead on arrival	heroin
deadly nightshade	belladonna
deadwood	an undercover law enforcement agent who is working to trap those involved in drug deals
dealer	one who sells or supplies drugs
deans	codeine
death trips	LSD mixed with another drug
death wish	PCP
death's head	the Amanita muscaria mushroom
death's herb	belladonna
deazingus	a hypodermic syringe or medicine dropper with a needle attached
debs	MDMA (ecstasy); barbiturates
decadence	MDMA (ecstasy)
deck	folded paper containing heroin
deck up	to fill a packet or envelope with a dose of powdered drugs
deeda	LSD
deens, deines, denes	codeine
dees, Ds	Dilaudid
Delilah	a prostitute
demis, dems, demies	Demerol
demo	a sample-size quantity of crack
demolish	crack
desert horse	a Camel cigarette
designer drugs	variations of amphetamines, methamphetamines, and heroin
desire	PCP and cocaine mixture
destroyed	heavily drug intoxicated
DET	diethyltryptamine, a hallucinogen
Detroit punk	PCP
deuce	$2 worth of drugs

devil	Seconal
devil dust	PCP
devil's apple	jimsonweed
devil's dandruff	powdered cocaine
devil's dick	crack pipe
devil's smoke	crack cocaine
dew	marijuana; hashish
dews	$10 worth of drugs
dex	Dexedrine (dextroamphetamine)
dexies	dextroamphetamine
diablo	LSD paper with a devil on it
diambista	marijuana
diamonds	amphetamines; ecstasy
Diane	meperidine
dib &dab	to use drugs intermittently
dice	methamphetamines
dick	a police officer; penis
diddleums	delirium tremens
dids	Dilaudid
dies	Valium
diesel	heroin
digatee	the rush one feels following an injection of a drug
digger	a pickpocket
digging the bowls	smoking marijuana from a pipe
digie	scales used to weigh drugs
diggidy	a good herb
diggity	heroin
dill	Placidyl
dillie, dillies, dilies, dilly	Dilaudid
dimba	marijuana from West Africa
dime	a ten-year prison sentence; a $1000 bet
dime bag	a $10 drug purchase
dime special	crack
dime-store high	glue sniffing
dime-dropper	an informer
dime's worth	amount of heroin to cause death
dinosaurs	LSD
ding	marijuana
dingbats	delirium tremens
dingers	equipment for injecting drugs
dinghizen	a medicine dropper with a needle attached
dingus	a medicine dropper with a needle attached

dinky dow	marijuana
dinosaurs	baby boomer population who still use illegal drugs
dip	to immerse cigarettes in embalming fluid
dipped	addicted to narcotics
dipper	an opium pipe
dipping out	to take a portion of crack from vials
dirt	marijuana
dirt grass	inferior quality marijuana
dirty arm	scarred arms from needle marks
dirty deed	to inject drugs
dirty joint	marijuana cigarettes laced with another drug
dirty laundry/linen	private matters that have been publicly exposed
disco biscuits	MDMA (ecstasy); Quaaludes
disco drug	the vapors from butyl nitrite used by some dancers
discorama	inhalants
dispatcher	a killer
disease	drug of choice
dissing	showing disrespect
ditch	the best vein site for drug injection, usually the inside of the elbow; to get rid of
ditch digger	one who injects drugs
ditch weed	inferior quality marijuana
dithers	delirium tremens
divider	sharing a joint with someone
dizz	a feeling of dizziness following marijuana use
djamba	marijuana
D-man	a federal drug enforcement officer
DMT	N-dimethyltryptamine; a short-duration, fast-acting hallucinogen
DMZ	benactyzine
DOA	PCP; dead on arrival
Do a Brodie/Brody	to commit suicide
do a joint	to smoke marijuana
do a line	to snort a drug from a line
do a number	to smoke a marijuana cigarette
doctor	MDMA (ecstasy)
dodo	a drug addict
do drugs	to use illegal drugs
does	methamphetamines

dog	weak opium residue
dog biscuits	peyote
dog food	heroin
doggie, dojee, doojee	heroin
do it Jack	to use PCP
doja	strong marijuana
dollar	$100 worth of drugs
dolls, dollies	depressants; amphetamines; MDMA
dolo	methadone
domes	ecstasy; LSD
domestic	marijuana grown in the United States
dominoes	black and white capsules that contain an amphetamine and a barbiturate
donjem	marijuana
Dona Juana, Juanita	marijuana
doobie, dubbe, duby	a marijuana cigarette
doobie/dubbe/duby	marijuana
doogie/doojee/dugie	heroin
dool, dooley	an addict
doormat	a person who is regularly exploited by others
doors and 4s	combination of Doriden and Tylenol 4
dope	habit-forming narcotics
dope daddy	a drug supplier or seller
dope den	a place where users gather to use drugs
dope fiend	a person who is drug-dependent
dope gun	a hypodermic needle
dope sick	an addict who is in need of drugs
dope smoke	to smoke marijuana
doped up	under the influence of drugs
doper	a drug user or addict
dopium	opium
doradilla	marijuana
dork	an unpleasant, unattractive, or insignificant person
dose(s)	specific amount of a drug
dossing	sleeping after using drugs
dots	mescaline; peyote
doub	$20 rock or crack
double blue	a capsule of Amytal
double breasted dealing	simultaneous dealing of cocaine and heroin
double bubble	cocaine
double crosses	cross-scored amphetamine tablets

double deed	injecting drugs and taking pills
double dome	LSD
double header	two marijuana smoked at the same time
double narky	a double dose of narcotics
double rock	crack diluted with procaine
double trouble	barbiturates
double up	when a dealer delivers extra drugs as a marketing scheme
double ups	a $20 rock that can be broken into two $20 rocks
double yoke	crack
douche	to inject a drug
douche bag	a sleazy person
do up	to shoot or inject a drug; to smoke marijuana; to place a tourniquet around the arm in preparation for an injection
douse the lamp	to ejaculate during a sexual dream while in a stupor from opium use
dove	base cocaine rock
dover's deck	opium
Dover's powder	opium
downs, downers	sedatives, barbiturates, alcohol, tranquilizers, and narcotics
downtown	heroin
downtown Brown	inferior quality marijuana
dozer	marijuana; depressants
DPT	dipropylphyptamine; a hallucinogen
Dr. Bananas	amyl nitrite
Dr. Feelgood	a physician who will prescribe or sell drugs on request
Dr. White	cocaine
draf weed	marijuana
drag	an unpleasant experience of any kind; puff from a cigarette
drag weed	marijuana
dragged	an anxious state induced by smoking marijuana
draw up	to inject a drug
dread weed	marijuana
dream beads	opium pellets
dream boat	a drug dealer's establishment
dream gum	opium
dream pipe	an opium pipe

dream stick	an opium pipe; a marijuana cigarette
dream, dreamer	morphine; opium; depressants
dreams	opium
dreck	heroin
drink	PCP
drink Texas tea	to smoke marijuana
dripper	equipment for injecting drugs, usually an eye dropper
dripping bum	one returning from a cocaine high
drive	a euphoric rush one feels following a drug injection
drivers	amphetamines
droopy	feeling the effects of sedative drugs
drop	to take drugs or pills by mouth
drop a bop	to take drugs in pill form
drop a roll	to take a variety of 3 to 5 pills at once
drop man	one who makes deliveries of substantial amounts of drugs; usually not a user
dropper	to inject a drug
drops	a place to leave drugs after a purchase; point of pick up for drugs
drought	a shortage of drugs
drowsy high	feeling the effects of sedative drugs
drug deal	the exchange of money for drugs
drug store heroin	Dilaudid
drug	to take a large quantity of drugs
druggie	a drug user
drugstore Johnson	addiction to drugs usually used as medication
dry high	marijuana
dry out	to stop using drugs for a while
dry spell	when drugs are unavailable; abstinence from drug use
dry up	to stop using drugs for a while
DTs	delirium tremens
dube	marijuana
dubie, duby	marijuana
dub sack	$20 worth of drugs
duct	cocaine
due	residue of oils remaining in a pipe after smoking base
dugout	veins that are pitted and scarred from multiple injections

duji	heroin
dummies	propoxyphene
dummy	bogus heroin
dummy dust	bogus PCP
dust	heroin; cocaine; PCP mixed with various chemicals
dust a joint	to lace a cigarette with PCP
dust blunt	marijuana and PCP mixture
dust of angels	PCP
dust of Morpheus	morphine
dusted	drug intoxicated
dusted parsley	PCP
duster	heroin and tobacco mixed in a cigarette
dusthead	PCP user
dusting	adding a drug to marijuana
dusty roads	mixture of cocaine and PCP for smoking
dweeb	an unpleasant, unattractive, or insignificant person
dyls	Placidyl
dynamite	heroin and cocaine mixture
dyno	heroin
dyno-pure	heroin
E	ecstasy
earth	a marijuana cigarette
ease on in	to move slowly so no one knows what you are doing
easing powder	opium; morphine
east side player	crack user
easy lay	one who takes GHB; Rohypnol
easy score	obtaining drugs or sex easily
eat	to take acid or mushrooms
eater	a user who takes drugs orally
eating	taking a drug orally
E-ball	a type of ecstasy with an eightball on it
E-Bomb	ecstasy
echoes	LSD trip flashbacks
ecstasy	MDMA
Edge City	where an addict is when contemplating withdrawal
egg	crack
Egyptian driver	a drug dealer
eight	heroin
eightball	3.5 grams of cocaine or methamphetamine

eighth, eighth piece	1/8 ounce of a drug
eighty-six	to kill
ekies	Mandrax
Elaine	ecstasy
elbow	one pound of marijuana
El Cid	LSD
Eleanor	a narcotic antagonist
electric	hallucinogenic matter
electric butter	marijuana leaves saut,ed in butter
electric Kool Aid	LSD
electric wine	wine laced with LSD
elephant, elephant tranquilizer	PCP
elephant flipping	back-and-forth use of ecstasy and PCP
elephant trank	PCP
elephant tranquilizer	PCP
elevator	a regularly used preparation of opium
eleventh finger	penis
els, l's	Elavil
Ellis Day	LSD
Elvis	LSD
embalming fluid	PCP
emergency gun	a safety pin or sewing machine needle used as a substitute for a hypodermic needle
empties	recycled gelatin capsules that are returned to a drug dealer for a discount on a purchase
emsel	morphine
endo	marijuana
ends	money used for drugs
energizer	PCP
enforcer	a strongman for a drug dealer
eng shee	an alcohol extraction of opium residue used for injections
engine	an opium smoking outfit
enhanced	under the influence of drugs
erase	to kill
essence	a variation of amphetamine or methamphetamine; ecstasy
Eve	a variation of amphetamine or methamphetamine; MDEA
enoltestovis	injectable steroid
ephedrone	methcathinone
E-puddle	sleeping after taking ecstasy or exhaustion after attending a rave

ex	ecstasy
extasy	ecstasy
erth	PCP
esra	marijuana
estuffa	heroin
ET	alpha-ethyltryptamine
E-tard	person under the influence of ecstasy
euphoria	MDMA, mescaline, and crystal meth
experience	an LSD trip
explorers? club	a group of LSD users
exposures	marijuana cigarettes
eyelid movies	images seen during an LSD trip
everclear	GHB; Rohypnol
eye opener	first narcotcs injection of the day; amphetamines
fachiva	heroin
factory	place where drugs are packaged, diluted, or manufactured
faded	under the influence of marijuana
fair share	the amount of a drug one individual shares with another
fairy	an opium smoker's lamp
fairy dust	PCP
fairy powder	a powdered narcotic
fake	substitute for a hypodermic needle
fake a blast	to pretend to be under the influence of drugs
fake STP	PCP
fall	arrested
fall guy	one who takes the blame for another's mistakes
Fallbrook redhair	marijuana, term from Fallbrook, CA
famine	to be out of drugs
famous dimes	crack
fang	a hypodermic needle
fantasy, fantasia	GHB; Rohypnol
farm-to-arm	referring to individuals who grow, process, and sell drugs
farmer	one who grows marijuana at home
fart	a foolish or contemptible person
fat bags	bags full of drugs
fat jay	a thick marijuana cigarette
fat pappy	a thick marijuana cigarette

fatty	a thick marijuana cigarette
feathered	under the influence of drugs
fed	a federal law enforcement agent
feebie	an FBI agent
feeblo	a drug addict
feed	drugs; to use drugs
feed and grain man	a drug supplier or seller
feed bag	a package of drugs
feed one's head	to take drugs by mouth
feed store	a place to buy and sell drugs
feeder	a hypodermic needle
feeling high	alcohol or drug intoxicated
feeling no pain	alcohol or drug intoxicated
Felix the Cat	LSD
fen	fentanyl citrate
fender bender	barbiturate
F-forties, F40s	Seconal tablets that bear the Identi-Code symbol F40
fi-do-nie	opium
fields	LSD
fiend	a drug addict
fifteen cents, 15¢	$15 worth of drugs
fifty, 50	LSD
fifty-one, 51	crack; a cigarette laced with crack
figure-8	an addict who feigns a withdrawal spasm in an attempt to get drugs
film can	a container for marijuana
fine stuff	high quality drugs
finger	a condom or finger cot that is filled with drugs, then swallowed or concealed in the rectum or vagina
finger lid	marijuana
finger wave	digital exam of the rectum or vagina for concealed drugs
fir	marijuana
fire	to inject a drug; crack and methamphetamine
firecracker	a marijuana cigarette
fire it up	to smoke marijuana
fired	marijuana ashes with no active ingredient remaining
firewater	GBL-containing product
firing the antiaircraft gun	smoking a cigarette that has been laced with heroin

firing up the ack ack gun	smoking a cigarette that has been dipped in heroin
first line	morphine
fish	one who has been arrested
fishbowl	a jail's holding area
fish scales	crack
fish slip	the charge brought against an individual who has been arrested
fit	equipment used for preparation or use of drugs
five-cent bag	$5 worth of drugs
five-cent paper	$5 worth of powdered drug folded in paper
five-C note	$500 bill
five dollar bag	$50 worth of drugs
five-O	the police
fives	amphetamines
fix	a ration of drugs
fixed up	provided with a ration of drugs
fixer	a drug dealer
fizzies	methadone
flag	appearance of blood in a syringe or medicine dropper, indicating that a needle has entered a vein
flake	cocaine; an eccentric person
flake acid	diluted solution of LSD placed on blotter paper and cut into small servings
flaky	an addict; acting in an eccentric manner
flame cooking	smoking cocaine base with a pipe over a stove flame
flamethrowers	cigarette laced with cocaine and heroin
Flannigan	marijuana
flash	a drug rush; hallucination
flash house	where users congregate to use drugs
flash in the pan	a brief rush after taking heroin cut with quinine
flash out	momentary unconsciousness caused from sniffing an inhalant
flashback	a recurrent hallucination experienced long after an LSD trip
flasher	an exhibitionist
flat blues	LSD
flat chunks	crack cut with benzocaine

flatfoot	a police officer
flats	LSD
flatten the poker	impotence caused from drug use
flattened	alcohol or drug intoxicated
flea powder	drugs of inferior quality
flesh peddler	a pimp; a person who solicits clients for a prostitute
flex	counterfeit crack
flier	a drug user who is always high
flip out	to lose control of oneself as a result of using drugs
flip over	to stop taking drugs temporarily; to become infatuated with a person
flipped	stupefied as a result of drug use
floater	a bit of congealed blood clogging a hypodermic needle; a corpse that is found floating in water
floating	alcohol or drug intoxicated
flogged	alcohol or drug intoxicated
floozy	a prostitute
flophouse	a cheap hotel or rooming house
Florida snow	white powdered drugs
flossin'	showing off
flow	to experience euphoria after taking a hallucinogenic drug
flowers	morning glory and poppy seeds
flower child	a person (also known as a hippie) who was part of a movement of the 1960s and 1970s that advocated love, beauty, and peace
flower power	morning glory and poppy seeds; peace
flower tops	morning glory and poppy seeds
fluff	to clean marijuana; to run powdered drugs through a nylon stocking; to chop up dope to make it bulkier and more even in consistency; nonsense
flunk out	to move from occasional drug use to addiction
flunky, flunkey	one who delivers drugs; one who takes foolish risks to obtain drugs; one who is used to perform menial tasks
flush and mush	to flush drugs down the toilet or swallow them so they cannot be found

flushing	injecting and withdrawing a drug back into a needle for injection by the next user
fly	to be intoxicated on drugs
fly high	to experience euphoria after drug use
fly Mexican airlines	to smoke marijuana
fly swatter	the muscle man for a drug dealer
fly the coop	to escape from jail or prison
flying	under the influence of drugs
flying saucers	PCP; morning glory seeds
flying triangle	LSD
focus	liquid narcotics
fold up	to become unconscious after alcohol or drug use; to stop selling or taking drugs
following the cloud	searching for drugs
foil	heroin
foilers	smoking cocaine on tin foil
foo foo stuff	heroin; cocaine
foo-foo dust	powdered drugs
foolish powder	powdered drugs
foon	a pellet of roasted opium
footballs	mixture of amphetamines and dextroamphetamine
foreign mud	opium
foreign smoke	opium
forget-me drug	Rohypnol
forget-me pill	Rohypnol
forties, 40s	Seconal
fortnighter	one who uses drugs occasionally
forwards	amphetamines
four twenty	marijuana
four ways	LSD, methamphetamine, strychnine, and STP mixture
fours	painkillers with codeine in tablets or capsules marked with a 4
fours and doors	Tylenol 4 and Doriden
fourteen	narcotics
fourth degree	withdrawal sickness
four-way hits	cross-scored amphetamine tablets
four-way star	LSD combined with 3 other substances
foxy	looking good
fraho/frajo	marijuana
frame a twister	feign a withdrawal spasm in an attempt to get drugs

frantic	in need of drugs
freak	a bizarre-acting person; to experience a bad drug trip; to be afraid
freak house	commune where individuals gather to use drugs
freak out	to have a panic reaction to a drug
freaked out	disturbed or psychotic as a result of previous LSD use
Freddy, Freddie	a stimulant
free trip	a flashback as a result of previous LSD use
freebase	cocaine that has been purified by dissolving it in a heated solvent, such as ether, then separating and drying until it produces vapors for inhalation
freebase rocks	pure form of cocaine
freebie	something for nothing
freeze	refuse to sell drugs to certain individuals; renege on a drug deal
French blues	amphetamines
french fried	under the influence of drugs
french fries	crack
Freon freak	one who inhales Freon gas
fresh	PCP
fresh and sweet	recently released from prison; new prostitute; new drug user
fresh kill	to steal someone's drugs
freshman	new drug user or addict
fried	alcohol or drug intoxicated
friend	fentanyl
fries	crack
frios	marijuana laced with crack
Frisco special	cocaine, heroin, and LSD mixture
Frisco speedball	cocaine, heroin, and LSD mixture
frisky, frisky powder	cocaine
frog	one who "hops" from place to place in pursuit of drugs
front	to pay money prior to receiving goods or services
frosty	under the influence of cocaine
frozen	under the influence of cocaine
fry stick	a marijuana cigarette laced with embalming fluid or LSD; to be executed in the electric chair

Fu, Fu Manchu	marijuana
fucked up	alcohol or drug intoxicated
fuel	marijuana mixed with insecticides; PCP
full moon	a large portion or the top of peyote cactus
fun joint	a place where individuals gather to use drugs
funny paper	marijuana concealed in a newspaper
funny stuff	marijuana
fur	law enforcement agents
future	crystal methamphetamine
fuzz	law enforcement agents
G	a portion of a dollar bill that seals a hypodermic needle onto a medicine dropper; a dollar bill that is rolled up and used for sniffing powdered drugs; $1000; 1 gram of drugs; term for an unfamiliar male; GHB
gacked	under the influence of amphetamines
gaffel	counterfeit cocaine
gaffled	arrested
gaffus	an improvised hypodermic needle
gag	heroin
gage/gauge	marijuana
gage butt	a marijuana cigarette
gagers	methcathinone
gaggers	methcathinone
gaggler	amphetamines; ecstasy
Gainesville green	marijuana presumably grown near Gainesville, Florida
gak	line of meth or coke
galhead	a drug addict
gallery	a place that sells drugs and equipment for drug users
gallon distemper	delirium tremens
galloping horse	heroin
gallop	heroin
Gamma O	GHB
gammon	1 microgram of LSD
gamot	heroin; morphine
gange	marijuana
gang bang	rape by a group or a gang
gangster	marijuana
gangster pills	barbiturates

ganja, ganga	potent marijuana
gank	counterfeit crack; to steal
gap	yawning and drooling, symptoms of early drug craving
gapper	one who shows early stages of withdrawal
gar	marijuana rolled in cigar paper
garbage	inferior quality or adulterated drugs; food or meals
garbage freak	a person who will take any kind of drug
garbage head	a person who will take any kind of drug
garbage rock	crack
Garden of Eden	female genitalia
garden variety	middle class citizens
gargoyle	a drug user or addict
garr	large marijuana cigarette
gas	to sniff gasoline fumes; to use nitrous oxide
gash	marijuana; sex
gasket	whatever is used to seal a hypodermic needle onto a syringe
gasper	a marijuana cigarette
gasper stick	a marijuana cigarette
gassing	inhaling through a drug-saturated cloth
gate	the vein used to inject drugs
gato	heroin
gauge butt	marijuana
gazer	a federal law enforcement agent
G.B.	depressants
GBH	gamma hydroxybutyrate; date rape drug
GBL	gamma butyrolactone, used in making GBH
gear	equipment used to inject drugs; drugs in general
gee	opium
gee fat	residue of smoked opium pellet which lines an opium bowl
gee gee	an opium pipe
gee head	a paregoric user
gee rag	materials that are used to hold parts of an opium pipe together
gee stick	an opium pipe
gee yen	opium residue
geed up	under the influence of opium
geek	a person who does not fit into the group; marijuana and crack mixture

geek joints	cigarettes filled with marijuana and crack mixture
geeker	a crack user
geeze, geez	to inject drugs
geezer	one who injects drugs
geezin' a bit of dee gee	injecting a drug
gel caps	form of acid
gel tabs	acid
gelatin	blotter paper soaked in a dilute solution of LSD
generation X	generation following baby boomers, people born in the early 1960s to the late 1970s
generation Y	generation following generation X, people born in early 1980s to the late 1990s
George	heroin
George smack	potent heroin
Georgia home boy	GHB
Geronimo	mixture of alcohol and barbiturates
gestapo	police officers; IRS agents; any oppressive group of people
get a fix	to get drugs
get a gage up	to smoke marijuana
get a gift	receive drugs
get a hit	to take a drug
get behind it	to enjoy or appreciate something
get busy	to rob
get down	to take a drug; to have fun
get high	to be under the influence of drugs
get in the groove	to take a drug
get it on	to take a drug; to engage in sexual activity
get lifted	to be under the influence of drugs
get off	to experience an orgasmic rush after injecting a drug; to come down from a drug trip; to copulate or ejaculate
get off on	to be stimulated by something
get one's nose cold	to snort cocaine
get straight	to relieve a drug craving by taking a dose of a drug; to shake a drug habit
get up	first drug dose of the day
get the wind	to smoke marijuana
get through	obtain drugs
get with it	to inject a drug; to get tasks completed
Ghana	marijuana

GHB	gamma hydroxy butyrate
ghost	an opium addict
ghost busting	smoking cocaine; searching for white particles that may be crack
GI gin	terpin hydrate cough medicine mixed with alcohol
gick monster	crack smoker
gift of the sun	cocaine
gift of the sun god	cocaine
gig	a drug high
giggle smoke	marijuana
giggle weed	marijuana
gigolo	a man who is supported by a woman in return for his attention
gimmicks	equipment used for preparing and injecting drugs
gimmie	crack and marijuana mixture
gin	cocaine
gin mill	a bar
girl, girly	cocaine; crack; heroin
girlfriend	cocaine
gismo	equipment used for injecting drugs
give birth	to defecate hard feces after constipation from prolonged opium use
Give me five.	Put your hand on mine palm to palm.
give someone the go-by	to refuse to sell drugs to an untrustworthy or undesirable buyer
give wings	inject someone or teach someone to inject heroin
give up	to inform someone; to stop looking; to let anything go
gizzy	marijuana
glacines	heroin
glad stuff	addictive drugs
gladiator school	maximum security prison or penitentiary
glading	using inhalant
glass	hypodermic needle; crystal methamphetamine
glass gun	hypodermic syringe
glasses	a glass pipe
glassy eyes	eyes that resemble glass as a result of being intoxicated from alcohol or drugs
glo	crack

globetrotter	one who moves from place to place in pursuit of drugs; a homeless person who wanders from place to place
glom	to steal drugs
glooch	one whose senses are diminished from prolonged drug use
glory hole	a hole between stalls in a toilet
glory seeds	morning glory seeds
glove	a condom
glued	to be arrested
gluey	a person who sniffs glue
glue stick	a marijuana cigarette that has been dipped in hashish oil
go	amphetamines; ecstasy
go fast	methcathinone; methamphetamines
go faster	amphetamines
go into the sewer	to inject a drug into a vein
go loco	to smoke marijuana
go on a sleigh ride	to use cocaine
go on the boot	a way to inject drugs that allows the user to prolong the rush
go on the wagon	to stop drinking alcohol
go pills	amphetamines; ecstasy
go talk to Al and Herbie	to drink alcohol and smoke marijuana
go to the cathedral	to smoke hashish
go up	to be under the influence of drugs
go with the flow	to deal with adversity
godfather	a marijuana cigarette or cigar that is laced with a drug
God's flesh	psilocybin/psilocin mushrooms
God's medicine	opium
God's drug	morphine
going 90 mph	the peak of a trip
going to the dentist	nitrous oxide
gold	marijuana
gold bud	marijuana, presumably grown in Colombia
gold dust	cocaine
gold duster	one who uses cocaine
gold leaf special	a potent marijuana cigarette
gold star	marijuana
golden dragon	LSD
golden eagle	methamphetamines
golden girl	superior quality cocaine

golden grain	Lebanese hashish
golden leaf	superior quality marijuana
golden spike	a hypodermic needle
golden triangle	boundary areas of Burma, Laos, and Thailand where opium is grown
goldfinger	synthetic heroin
golf balls	crack
golpe	heroin
goma	opium; black tar heroin
gondola	opium
gong	opium
gong beater	one who uses opium
gong ringer	one who uses opium
gonga smudge	a marijuana cigarette
gongola	an opium pipe
goob	methcathinone
good	PCP
good and plenty	heroin
good butt	a marijuana cigarette
good giggles	marijuana
good go	drugs that are good for the amount paid
good H	heroin
good horse	heroin
good lick	good drugs
good fella	fentanyl and heroin mixture
good stuff	potent drugs
good time man	a drug dealer
good trip	a pleasant experience with hallucinogens
goods	addicting drugs; stolen property
goody-goody	marijuana
goof artist	one who takes unusual drugs
goof butt	a marijuana cigarette
goof balls	barbiturates; amphetamines
goofers	barbiturates
goofing	to be under the influence of a barbiturate; just hanging out
goofy	LSD
goon	PCP
gooney birds	LSD
goon dust	PCP
goop	GHB
gopher	a person who is paid to pick up drugs
goric	paregoric

gorilla	powerfully addicted
gorilla biscuits	PCP
gorilla pills	barbiturates
gorilla tabs	barbiturates
Got any zings?	Do you have amphetamines?
got it going on	a fast sale of drugs
gouch off	to lose consciousness while using drugs
gouger	a marijuana smoker
gow cellar	a place to buy and use opium
gow, ghow	opium
gowhead	an opium user
gowster	an opium user
gozniks	drugs that are addicting
GQ	good quality
grads	amphetamines
graduate	to completely stop using drugs, or to progress to stronger drugs
granulated orange	methamphetamine
gram	hashish
granny	to become addicted
grape parfait	LSD
grapes of wrath	a wine hangover
grass	marijuana
grass brownies	marijuana
grass mask	a mask with a hose attached to a marijuana pipe
grata	marijuana
gravel	crack
gravy	mixture of heroin and coagulated blood in a hypodermic syringe
gray dust	stale PCP
grease	money
great bear	fentanyl
grease pit	a dealer's place of business
greasy	a destitute addict; a severely addicted person; one who is unkempt
greasy bag	a bag in which heroin is kept
great Scott	an opium pipe
great tobacco	opium
greefa, greefo	marijuana
greefer	one who smokes marijuana
green	marijuana that has a low resin content; ketamine

green acorn salad	LSD
green and blacks	Librium
green and clears	Dexamyl
green angelfish	LSD on a blotter stamped with an angelfish
green ashes	usable opium residue from an opium pipe
green beauty	Dexamyl
green bud	home-grown marijuana
green button	a fresh button of peyote
green caps	green LSD capsules
green cigarette	a marijuana cigarette
green dots	LSD
green double domes	LSD
green dragons	LSD on a blotter stamped with a green dragon; LSD combined with another drug
green frog	barbiturates
green goddess	marijuana
green gold	cocaine
green goods	paper money
green hornets	Dexamyl
green hype	a new addict
green leaves	PCP
green meanies	amphetamines
green Moroccan	marijuana grown in Morocco
green mud	usable opium residue from an opium pipe
green paint	marijuana
green rot	inferior quality opium
green single domes	LSD
green swirls	LSD combined with another drug
green tea	PCP
green wedge	LSD
greens	Dexamyl
green stuff	paper money
greenies	Dexedrine and amobarbital combination; ecstasy
greeter	marijuana
Greta	marijuana
grey shields	LSD
griefs	marijuana
grievous bodily harm	GHB
griff, griffa, griffo	marijuana
G-riffic	GHB
grimmy	a marijuana cigarette laced with methamphetamine or crank

grit	crack
groceries	crack
grocery boy	an addict in need of food
G-rock	one gram of rock cocaine
grogged	under the influence of drugs
groover	a drug user
grooving	alcohol or drug intoxicated; getting to know someone
groovy	anything one likes
groovy lemon	a yellow LSD tablet
gross out	to totally repulse
ground control	one who guides a user through a hallucinogenic experience
groupie	a person who follows famous people from appearance to appearance, offering assistance or sexual favors
grower	one who grows marijuana
G-shot	a small amount of liquefied narcotic
G-spot tornado	equal parts of rum and Nyquil
guide	one who guides an LSD user through a trip
gulf	Persian Gulf heroin
gum	opium
gumball	a potent form of heroin; the light bar on top of a police car
gumdrop	Seconal
guma, gumma	opium
gun	a hypodermic needle
gungeon	a potent type of marijuana
gunja	marijuana
gungun	marijuana
gunk	morphine
gunny	a potent type of marijuana
gunpowder	raw opium
guns	equipment used for injecting drugs
Gunther	a neighborhood drug dealer
guru	one who has experienced an LSD trip and coaches another through it
gutter	the vein inside the elbow used for injecting drugs
gutter hype	a destitute addict
gutter junkie/junky	a destitute addict
guttersnipe	a child who lives on the streets
guy	marijuana

gweebo	an unpleasant, unattractive, or insignificant person
gyve	a marijuana cigarette
gyve stick	a marijuana cigarette
H	heroin
habit	an addiction
hache	heroin
hail	crack
hair of the dog	a drink of liquor taken in an attempt to cure a hangover
haircut	marijuana
hairy	heroin
half	¹⁄₂ ounce
half a C	$50 bill
half a football field	50 rocks of crack
half a G	$500
half ass	worthless or near worthless heroin
half bundle	twelve $5 bags of heroin
half kee	fraction of a kilogram
half load	fifteen $3 bags (decks) of heroin
half moons	hashish that is molded into the shape of a half moon; peyote
half piece	one-half ounce of powdered drugs
half spoon	one-half spoon of cocaine
half track	crack
half and half	oral and straight sex
halva	illicit drugs
halves	one-half ounce of heroin
hamburger helper	crack
hand-to-hand	delivery that is made by handing drugs to the buyer
hang-up	anything that takes time; a bother; a personal problem
hanhich	marijuana
hanyak	smokable methamphetamine
happy cigarette	a marijuana cigarette
happy dust	powdered drugs
happy grass	marijuana
happy hour	a specified time to gather for drinks and companionship
happy medicine	morphine
happy pills	barbiturates
happy powder	powdered drugs

happy sticks	marijuana cigarettes that are dusted with powdered drugs
happy-time weed	marijuana
happy trails	cocaine
hard candy	heroin
hardcore	heavy drug user
hard hat	a bigoted person
hard line	crack
hard nail	a hypodermic needle
hard rock	crack
hard stuff	morphine; heroin; cocaine; opium; other opiates
hard time	a sentence without parole
hardware	isobutyl nitrite; inhalants
harm reducer	marijuana
harness bulls	uniformed police officers
harpoon	a hypodermic needle
Harry	heroin; morphine
Harry Jones	heroin
harsh	hashish; marijuana
Harvey Wallbanger	STP-LSD combination
hats	LSD
hash	hashish
hash cannon	a device used to smoke hashish
hash house	a place where hashish is sold or used
hash oil	oil residue from hashish
hashhead	one who smokes hashish
hatchet man	a killer
have a Chinaman on one's back	to experience withdrawal symptoms; to have a heroin or opium habit
have a dust	cocaine
haven dust	cocaine
Hawaiian	potent marijuana
Hawaiian black	marijuana
Hawaiian grass	marijuana, presumably grown in Hawaii
Hawaiian hay	marijuana
Hawaiian pods	a potent hallucinogenic drug
Hawaiian sunshine	LSD
hawk	LSD
hay	inferior quality marijuana
hay burner	a marijuana smoker
hay butt	a marijuana cigarette
hay head	a marijuana smoker

hay puffer	a marijuana smoker
haze	LSD
Hazel	heroin
H & C	heroin and cocaine combination
H caps	powdered heroin in gelatin capsules
he-man	fentanyl
head	someone who uses drugs; a person who is high much of the time; toilet
head bob	a personal blunt of marijuana
head drugs	drugs that affect the mind
head kit	equipment used for smoking or injecting drugs
head rush	the dizziness one experiences after taking a drug
head shop	a shop that specializes in drug paraphernalia
headlights	LSD
head shrinker	a psychiatrist
heaped	alcohol or drug intoxicated
hearts	heart-shaped amphetamine tablets
heat	the police; pressure from law enforcement agents
heater	a gun
heaven	cocaine
heaven and hell	PCP
heaven dust	powdered drugs
heavenly blue	LSD; morning glory seeds
heavies	addictive drugs
heavy	an altered state of consciousness after drug use; serious
heavy artillery	equipment used for preparing or injecting drugs
heavy joint	a marijuana cigarette that is laced with PCP
heavy metal	a style of loud music that is characterized by shouted, violent lyrics
heebie jeebies	delirium tremens
heeled	having plenty of money
Helen	heroin
hell	crack
hell dust	powdered heroin or morphine
he-man	fentanyl
helpers	amphetamines
hemp	marijuana
hemp humper	a marijuana smoker

hemp roller	a marijuana smoker
henpecking	searching on hands and knees for crack
Henry	heroin
Henry VIII	1/8 ounce of cocaine
her	cocaine
Herb	marijuana
Herb and Al	marijuana and alcohol
Hercules	superior quality PCP
herms	PCP
hero, heroina	heroin
hero of the underworld	heroin
hessle	heroin
heavy biter	one who needs to take more than the usual amount of drugs to feel the effect
hi-fi	mixture of morphine and cocaine
high	intoxicated, excited, euphoric, or stupefied after the use of drugs or alcohol
high as a kite	alcohol or drug intoxicated
high hat	a prepared opium pellet
high kick	a drug rush
high roller	one who spends money or gambles freely and recklessly
high speed	amphetamines
high tea	a marijuana smoking party
highball	inhalants
highbeams	the wide eyes seen on a person who is on crack
hikori, hikuli	peyote; mescaline
hillbilly heroin	OxyContin
him	heroin
Hinkley	PCP
hip	keenly informed and aware
hip layer	an opium smoker
hippie, hippy	a person who rejects the mores of an established society
hippie crack	inhalants
hippieflip	use of ecstasy and hallucinogenic mushrooms
hired gun	a killer
hiropon, hironpon	methamphetamines
hit	to purchase drugs; to take a drug by snorting, sniffing, injecting, or smoking; an arrest; a dose of drugs

hit on	to purchase drugs; to flirt with a person of the opposite sex
hit spike	a substitute for a hypodermic needle
hit the flute	to smoke opium
hit the hay	to smoke marijuana
hit the mainline	to inject drugs into a vein
hit the pipe	to smoke opium
hit man	a killer
hit the needle	to inject drugs into a vein
hit the pit	to inject drugs into a vein
hitch	prison sentence; time in military service
hitch up the reindeer	to prepare to inject or inhale cocaine
hitter	a pipe that is designed for one hit
hitting up	injecting drugs into a vein
ho	a whore
HO	one-half ounce of marijuana
hocus	liquor that has been laced with drugs; morphine
hoe	a whore or prostitute
Hoffman's bicycle	LSD
hog	PCP; one who requires large doses of drugs to sustain a habit; a motorcycle
hog leg	a fat marijuana cigarette
holding	in possession of illicit drugs
hole in one	a bullet wound in a body orifice
holy week	menstrual period
hombre	heroin
home	the vein that is the target for an injection
homegrown	marijuana
honey	money
honey blunts	marijuana cigars sealed with honey
honey oil	hashish extract
honeymoon	the stage of drug use before addiction or dependence occurs
hong-yen	heroin in a red pill form
hooch	alcohol; marijuana
hoochie-mamma	a two-paper marijuana cigarette
hood	neighborhood
hook	an improvised injection device
hookah	a device used to cool smoke by filtering it through liquid
hooked	addicted or dependent on drugs
hooker	a prostitute

hook up	to put an individual in contact with a dealer
hoosegow	jail or prison
hooter	cocaine; marijuana
hootchie	a prostitute
hop/hops	opium
hophead	a drug addict
hopped up	under the influence of drugs
horn	to inhale, snort, or sniff a drug; crack pipe
horning	heroin; to inhale cocaine
horny	sexually aroused
horror drug	belladonna
horrors	delirium tremens
hors d'oeuvres	Seconal
horse	heroin
horse and buggy	a hypodermic needle and medicine dropper used for injecting drugs
horse bite	heroin
horse heads	amphetamines
horse hearts	Dexedrine
horse tracks	PCP
horsed	under the influence of heroin
horseradish	heroin
hospital heroin	Dilaudid
hot	wanted by the police; stolen items; sexually aroused
hot and cold	mixture of heroin and cocaine
hot box	to fill up a closed area with second-hand marijuana smoke
hot dope	heroin
hot heroin	heroin that has been poisoned with the intent of giving it to a police informant
hot ice	methamphetamine that can be smoked
hot load	lethal injection of a drug
hot rolling	inhaling liquefied methamphetamine from an eye dropper
hot shot	fatal dose; an injection of poison instead of drugs
hot stick	a marijuana cigarette
hotcakes	crack
house fee	money paid to enter a house where drugs are being used
housewife's delight	tranquilizers

How do you like me now?	crack
How does your garden grow?	Are you growing marijuana?
hows	morphine
H & R	hit and run (quick drug purchase and exit)
HRN	heroin
huatari	peyote; mescaline
hubba	crack
hubba pigeon	a user looking for crack on the floor after a police raid
huff	an inhalant
huffer	an inhalant abuser
huffing	using an inhalant
hug drug	ecstasy; GHB; Rohypnol
hulling	using others to get drugs
Humboldt Green	marijuana, presumably grown in Humboldt County, CA
humming	alcohol or drug intoxicated
hungry croaker	a physician who accepts a bribe for prescription drugs
hunk	a small amount of hashish; a physically fit or handsome male
hunter	cocaine
hustle	to make money by drug dealing, gambling, stealing, or prostitution
hustler	a person who solicits clients for a prostitute; a prostitute
hydro	a water-cooled marijuana pipe
hygelo	an addict
hyke	cough syrup that contains codeine
hype	heroin addict; an addict
hype stick	hypodermic syringe and needle
I am back	crack
iboga	amphetamines; ecstasy
ice	cocaine; methamphetamine; smokeable amphetamines; ecstasy; diamonds; to kill someone
ice cream	drugs in crystallized form
ice cream habit	an occasional use of drugs
ice cream man	a drug supplier or dealer
ice cube	crack
ice pack	marijuana packed in dry ice to make it more potent

ice tong doc	a physician who will prescribe or sell drugs on request
ice tray	to smoke marijuana from an ice tray covered with foil
ice water doc	a physician who refuses to give drugs to an addict
icicles	crystallized cocaine
icing	cocaine
idiot pills	barbiturates
illies	marijuana cigarettes dipped in PCP
Illinois	marijuana, presumably grown in Illinois
I'm looking.	Do you have drugs you will sell me?
I'm way down.	I need drugs.
in	connected with drug suppliers
in betweens	a mixture of barbiturates and amphetamines
in flight	under the influence of drugs
in orbit	under the influence of drugs
in transit	on an LSD trip
incense	opium
Inca message	cocaine
Indian boy	marijuana
Indian hay	marijuana
Indian hemp	marijuana
Indiana hay	marijuana
Indiana ditch weed	inferior quality marijuana, grown from seeds meant to produce hemp for rope
Indians	mescaline; peyote
indica	species of cannabis, found in hot climates, grows 3.5 to 4 feet
indo	marijuana
Indonesian bud	marijuana; opium
infinity	long-acting drugs
instant Zen	LSD
interplanetary mission	travel from one crack house to another in search of crack
iron cure	withdrawal from drugs while imprisoned
isda	heroin
issues	crack
itching	sexually aroused
IZM	marijuana
J	marijuana
jab/job	to inject drugs
jab artist	one who takes drugs by injection

jab joint	where to buy and use drugs
jab stick	a hypodermic needle
jabber	a hypodermic needle
jack	steal someone else's drugs
Jack Ketch	a killer
Jack off	to masturbate
jack up	to inject a drug; barbiturate
jackpot	fentanyl
jackal	an undercover narcotics agent
jacked up	to be under the influence of drugs
jacking off the spike	to release pressure on a syringe before all the liquid has gone into the vein, allowing blood to re-enter the hypodermic syringe
jag	a gathering where drugs are used; a prolonged period of drug or alcohol use
jail bait	a female below the legal age of sexual consent
jailbird	a prisoner
jam	amphetamines; cocaine
Jamaican gold	Jamaican marijuana, gold in color
Jamaican red	Jamaican marijuana, reddish in color
jam Cecil	amphetamines
jammed up	an overdose
Jane	marijuana
jar wars	drug testing controversy
jay smoke	marijuana
jay	marijuana cigarette
jazz	heroin
J. Edgar Hoover	police officers; federal agents
jee gee	heroin
Jeff	methcathinone
Jefferson airplane	a device used to hold a partially smoked marijuana cigarette
jejo	a cigarette
jell	heroin which gels instead of dissolving when heated in water
jellies	barbiturates; ecstasy in gel capsules
jelly	cocaine
jelly babies	amphetamines
jelly beans	amphetamines
jelly roll	sexual intercourse; penis
jerk off	to masturbate
jerks	delirium tremens

Jerry Springer	heroin
Jersey green	marijuana thought to grow in New Jersey
jet	ketamine; amphetamines; methamphetamines; dextroamphetamines
jet fuel	PCP
Jezebel	a prostitute
Jim Jones	marijuana cigarettes laced with PCP
jim-jams	delirium tremens
jimmies	delirium tremens
Jimmy	a subcutaneous injection of drugs; amphetamines; a condom
Jimmy Valentine	a thief or robber
jib	crystal methamphetamine; GHB
jib head	crystal methamphetamine addict
Jim Jones	marijuana laced with cocaine and PCP
jimson	a weed containing hallucinogenic substances
jingo	marijuana
jive	marijuana; dishonest; not trustworthy
jive doo jee	heroin
jive stick	a marijuana cigarette
job pop	to inject drugs
Job's antidote	a hypodermic needle
jockey	an addictive drug
Joe Blakes	delirium tremens
john	a prostitute's client; a toilet
Johnny be good	a police officer
Johnny go fast	amphetamines
Johnny law	a police officer
Johnson	marijuana
Johnson grass	inferior quality marijuana
join the stream	to inject drugs
joint	a marijuana cigarette
joint stick	a marijuana cigarette
jojee	heroin
jolly beans	amphetamines
jolly green	marijuana
jolly pop	casual user of heroin
jolt	to inject a drug; strong reaction to drugs
Jones	a heroin habit
Jonesing	having a need for more drugs
joy dust	Vietnamese heroin
joy flakes	heroin
joy juice	chloral hydrate

joy plant	opium
joy pop	to inject a drug
joy popping	occasional use of drugs
joy powder	powdered drugs
joy prick	an injection of drugs
joyride	going out and getting high
joy smoke	marijuana
joy stick	a marijuana cigarette
J pipe	a pipe used to smoke marijuana
Js	joints
ju-ju	a marijuana cigarette
Juan Gomez	cocaine-laced marijuana
Juan Valdez	marijuana
Juanita	marijuana
Judas	heroin (a friend who turns on you)
juggle	to sell drugs to another addict to support a habit
juggler	a teen-age street dealer
jugs	injectable amphetamines; breasts
juice	steroids; alcohol; respect; power; illegally obtained money; gasoline
juiced	intoxicated from alcohol
juicehead	an alcoholic
juice joint	a bar; a marijuana cigarette laced with another drug
juju	marijuana
jum	sealed plastic bag containing crack
jumbos	large vials of crack
jump bail	failure to appear in a criminal trial after posting bail, causing forfeiture of bail
jumpy Stevie	one who is jumpy from using drugs
junk	narcotics
junk picker	a street person
junk pusher	a drug supplier or seller
junk squad	narcotics agents
junk tank	a jail cell in which addicts are held
junkie	an addict
junkie pro	a prostitute who sells drugs, or is addicted
juvie	juvenile hall
juvies	law enforcement agents and social workers who deal with juveniles
K	ketamine
kabayo	heroin

kabuki	a crack pipe made from a plastic bottle and a rubber spark plug cover
kaksonjae	smokable methamphetamine
kali	marijuana
kaleidoscope	LSD
katzenjammer	delirium tremens
kangaroo	crack
Kansas grass	inferior quality marijuana
kaps	PCP
Karachi	heroin
Kate bush	marijuana
kaya	marijuana
KB	potent marijuana
K blast	PCP
Kentucky blue	marijuana
kee, key	kilogram
keesh	a fat bag
keef, keif	inferior quality drugs
keeler	chloral hydrate drops
keister plant	drugs that are concealed in the rectum or vagina
Keller	ketamine
Kelly's day	ketamine
Ken dolls	barbiturates
Kentucky blue	marijuana thought to be grown in Kentucky
Kentucky fried	alcohol or drug intoxicated
ket	ketamine
key, kee	kilogram
keyed	high on drugs
keys to the kingdom	LSD
KGB (killer green bud)	marijuana
khat	milder than amphetamines
K-Hole, keyhole	ketamine-induced confusion
ki	marijuana
Kibbles & Bits	Ritalin and Talwin mixture; crumbs of crack
kick	getting off a drug habit; inhalant
kick back	relax
kicked	to pass out or about to pass out
kick stick	a marijuana cigarette
kick the clouds	to be under the influence of drugs
kick the engine around	to smoke opium
kick the habit	to discontinue drug use
kicked by a horse	addicted to heroin

kicked out in the snow	drug intoxicated
kicking it	withdrawing from drug use
kiddie dope	prescription medication
kiff, kif	marijuana
killer weed	potent marijuana
kilo	kilogram
kilo brick	marijuana packed into a brick shape that weights approximately 1 kilogram
kilter	a marijuana cigarette
kind bud	marijuana
king	cocaine
king ivory	fentanyl
King Kong	$200 or more a day drug habit
King Kong pills	barbiturates
king's habit	cocaine
king of the road	a homeless person who wanders from place to place
Kipper Lane	urban opium district
kiss ass	to be excessively attentive in order to gain favor
kiss Mary	to smoke marijuana
kiss the fish	to smoke marijuana
kissing	mouth-to-mouth exchange of plastic-wrapped crack rocks
kit	equipment used to prepare or use drugs
kit kat	ketamine
kite	1 ounce of drugs
kitty flipping	to use ketamine and ecstasy back and forth
KJ	PCP
Kleenex	ecstasy
klingons	crack addicts
knock off	to kill
knock up	to impregnate
knocked out	alcohol or drug intoxicated
knocked up	pregnant
knockout drops	chloral hydrate and alcohol
Kokomo	cocaine addict or user
koller joints	PCP
kools	PCP
Kona gold	Hawaiian marijuana
kook	an eccentric person
kools	PCP
kram	to pack a bowl tight with marijuana

kryptonite	crack
krystal	crystal methamphetamine; PCP
krystal joint	a marijuana cigarette laced with PCP
krippies	moist marijuana that is smoked out of a bowl or bong
kumba	marijuana
kushempeng	marijuana
kutchie	marijuana
KW	PCP
L	LSD
LA	long-acting amphetamine
lace	to add a drug or alcohol to ordinary food or drink
lactone	GBL
lady	cocaine
lady in white	powdered drugs
lady of the evening	a prostitute
lady caine	cocaine
lady snow	cocaine
lady white	powdered drugs
ladyfinger	a marijuana cigarette
lady killer	a gigolo
lag	a prisoner
LA glass	smokable methamphetamine
LA ice	smokable methamphetamine
lakbay diva	marijuana
Lamborghini	a pipe that is made of a plastic bottle and a rubber spark plug cover
lamb's bread	marijuana
lame	appearing foolish or weak
lamp habit	addicted to opium
Latin lettuce	marijuana
LA turnabouts	amphetamines
laugh and scratch	to inject a drug
laughing gas	nitrous oxide
laughing grass	marijuana
laughing weed	marijuana
lay	a sex partner; to have sexual intercourse
lay back	barbiturates
layout	equipment used for injecting drugs
lay out	to kill
lay up	to stay off the streets after a large drug supply has been obtained

LBJ, LBL	JB-336-N-methyl-3-piperidyl benzilate HCl; a hallucinogen
leaf	marijuana
leak	marijuana and PCP mixture
leaky bolla	PCP
leaky leak	PCP
lean	codeine cough syrup
leap over the wall	escape from jail or prison
leapers	amphetamines
leaping	under the influence of drugs
Leary's	LSD
legal speed	Mini thin, an over-the-counter asthma medication
lemon 714	PCP
lemonade	inferior quality heroin
lemon bowl	an opium pipe that has a lemon rind covering the bowel
lemon drop	methamphetamines of a dull yellow color
lemons	methaqualone
lens	LSD
leper grass	potent Colombian marijuana
Let me hold something.	An inquiry from one seeking to buy drugs
let sunshine do	LSD
lethal weapon	PCP
letter biscuits	ecstasy
lettuce	money
libs	Librium
lick up a tab	to swallow a tablet or capsule
licorice	opium
lid	approximately 1 ounce of marijuana
lid poppers	amphetamines
lie in state with the girls	to smoke marijuana
lifer	lifetime addict; one serving a lifetime prison sentence
lift pills	amphetamines
light artillery	equipment used for preparing or injecting drugs
light green	inferior quality marijuana
lightning	amphetamines
light somebody	to introduce someone to marijuana
light stuff	marijuana; nonaddictive drugs
lightweight	one who is minimally addicted
lima	marijuana

limbo	Colombian marijuana
lime acid	LSD
line	a vein in the arm; line formed by powdered drugs
liner	one who injects drugs
line shot	an injection of drugs
lint	morphine in fibrous or cotton form
lip	to test whether a drug apparatus is airtight by sucking the air out of it
Lipton Tea	inferior quality drugs
liquid bam	injectable amphetamines
liquid E	ecstasy
liquid lady	liquid cocaine that is used as a nasal spray
liquid X	ecstasy
lit, lit up	under the influence of drugs or alcohol
little bomb	amphetamines; heroin; barbiturates
little boy blue	a police officer
little bowl of Buddha	10-gram bowl of marijuana buds or hashish
little D	Dilaudid
little green friend	marijuana
little ones	PCP
little smoke	marijuana; psilocybin/psilocin
live in grass huts	to smoke marijuana
live ones	PCP
live, spit, and die	LSD
load	an injection of drugs; a drug supply; a large drug purchase; bulk sale of heroin
loaded	alcohol or drug intoxicated
loaded for bear	ready for a fight
loads	glutethimide mixed with codeine
loaf	marijuana
lobo	marijuana
locker room	isobutyl nitrite; inhalants
locoweed	marijuana
locust point	a place from which to buy drugs
log	a marijuana cigarette; an opium pipe
logor	LSD
long draw	a long pull on an opium or marijuana pipe
Looney Toons	LSD
loose	relaxed; sexually promiscuous
loose cannon	a dangerously irresponsible person
loose joint	a single marijuana cigarette
lords	hydromorphone

lorphs	hydromorphone
lotes	butabarbital
loused	covered by sores and abscesses from repeated use of unsterile needles
love	crack
love affair	cocaine and heroin mixture
love blow	marijuana
love boat	marijuana dipped in formaldehyde; PCP
love doctor	ecstasy; GHB; Rohypnol
love drug	ecstasy; GHB; Rohypnol
love nuggets	marijuana
love pearls	alpha-ethyltyptamine
love potion # 9	ecstasy
love pills	alpha-ethyltyptamine
love trip	ecstasy and mescaline
love weed	marijuana
lovelies	marijuana laced with PCP
lovely	PCP
lover's speed	ecstasy; GHB; Rohypnol
low	in a depressed mood
low rider	a drug addict who is on the skids
lowlife	an unpleasant, unattractive, or insignificant person
LSD	lysergic acid diethylamide
LT	living together
lubage	marijuana
Lucas	marijuana
Lucy in the sky with diamonds	LSD
Lucky Charms	ecstasy
ludes	Quaaludes
lude out	to take methaqualone and alcohol
luggage	LSD
lumber	marijuana stems and waste
lunch box	kids who do drugs
lunch head	alcoholic
lunch-hour trip	DMT taken on one's lunch break
lunch money drug	Rohypnol
lung duster	a cigarette
lush	an alcoholic
M	marijuana; morphine
ma'a	Samoan marijuana
machinery	equipment used to prepare and use drug
Machu Picchu	potent Peruvian marijuana

macon	marijuana
madman	PCP
mad dog	PCP
mad scientist	someone who makes crank
Maggie	marijuana
maggot	a cigarette butt
magic	PCP
magic dust	powdered drugs
magic flake	cocaine
magic mushrooms	hallucinogenic mushrooms
magic pumpkin	mescaline
magic smoke	marijuana
main line	to inject drugs through a vein, usually the median cephalic vein
mainliner	an addict whose habit is to inject drugs
maintain	to keep a certain level of drug effect
make	a person regarded as a sex partner
make a buy	to purchase drugs
make a croaker for a reader	to obtain a prescription drug from a physician
make a spread	to set up equipment for drug use
make it	to have sexual intercourse
make tracks	to leave needle marks on the arm from injecting drugs; to run away
make up	need to find more drugs
mama coca	cocaine
mama's mellow	the effect of taking sedatives
man	one's connection; a police officer
man about town	a gigolo
Manhattan silver	marijuana
manicure	to prepare marijuana for use
marathons	amphetamines
marbles	Placidyl
marching dust	powdered drugs
marching powder	powdered drugs
Margie wanna	marijuana
mariholic	a marijuana addict
Marley	marijuana
marimba	marijuana
marshmallow reds	barbiturates
Mary	marijuana
Mary and Johnny	marijuana
Mary Ann	marijuana
Mary Jane	marijuana

Mary Jonas	marijuana
Mary Warner	marijuana
Mary Weaver	marijuana
Mash Allah	opium
matchbox	one-fourth ounce of marijuana or 6 marijuana cigarettes
Maui wowie	Hawaiian marijuana
Max	GHB dissolved in water and mixed with amphetamines
maxibolin	oral steroids
mayo	cocaine; heroin
M&C	morphine and codeine combination
McCoy	pure drugs or alcohol
MDA	methyl diamphetamine
MDM, MDMA	ecstasy
Mean	high or superior quality; low or inferior quality drugs
mean green	PCP
meat market	a primarily singles bar where one may look for a sex partner
medical hype	one who is addicted to prescription drugs as a result of legitimate medical care
Medusa	inhalants
Meg, Megg, Meggie	marijuana
mellow	alcohol or drug intoxicated; relaxed
mellow out	to be under the influence of drugs or alcohol
mellow yellows	tranquilizers
melt wax	to smoke opium
melter	morphine
men in blue	male police officers
mepro	meprobamate
merchandise	drugs
Merck, Merk	cocaine
mesc	mescaline
mescal	mescaline
mescal beans	mescaline
mescy	mescaline
mess	mescaline
messed	alcohol or drug intoxicated
messorole	marijuana
metal	a metal pipe
meth	methamphetamine as liquid or in crystalline form

meth freak	a person who uses methamphetamines
meth head	regular user of methamphetamine
meth monster	person who has a violent reaction to methamphetamine
meth speed bass	methamphetamine and heroin mixture
Methlies Quik	methamphetamine
method	marijuana
metros	police officers
Mexican brown	potent marijuana in Mexico, with high resin content
Mexican crack	methamphetamine with the appearance of crack
Mexican green	marijuana grown in Mexico, less potent than Mexican brown
Mexican horse	heroin
Mexican jumping beans	barbiturates manufactured in Mexico
Mexican mud	heroin
Mexican mushrooms	hallucinogenic mushrooms that are grown in Mexico
Mexican red	reddish-brown Mexican marijuana
Mexican reds	secobarbital
Mexican speedballs	crack and amphetamines
Mexican valium	Rohypnol
mezc	mescaline
Michael	chloral hydrate
Michoacan, Mishwacan	potent marijuana, grown in Michoacan, Mexico
Mickey Finn	chloral hydrate and alcohol
Mickey's	barbiturates
Mickey Mouse	blotter impregnated with LSD and stamped with Mickey Mouse as the sorcerer's apprentice
Mickey Mouse ears	the lights and siren on top of a police car
microdot	one microgram of LSD on a tablet or on blotting paper
midget	a young child who is used to run drugs
midnight oil	opium
midnight toker	one who smokes marijuana before bed
Mighty Quinn	LSD
Mighty Joe Young	big heroin habit
mighty mezz	marijuana cigarette
Mighty Mite	breed of marijuana plant with huge buds
mike, mic	one microgram (usually refers to LSD dose)

milk	a marijuana cigarette dipped in embalming fluid and laced with PCP
milk a rush	to inject a drug, then draw blood back into the syringe and dilute it
mind bender	a hallucinogenic drug
mind detergent	LSD
mind spacer	a hallucinogenic drug
ming	a marijuana cigarette made from leftover butts
mingle wood	hashish and kind bud-filled marijuana cigarette or cigar
mini beans	amphetamines
mini bennies	amphetamines
mini white	amphetamines in tablet form
minstrels	amphetamine and barbiturate combination
mint leaf	mint leaves or parsley laced with PCP
mint weed	mint leaves or parsley laced with PCP
mired in the mud	addicted to opium
miser	a device for holding a marijuana cigarette butt
miss	to miss a vein while attempting to inject drugs, resulting in a subcutaneous or intramuscular injection
Miss Carrie	a stash of drugs carried on one's person
Miss Emma	morphine
Miss Emma Jones	a morphine addict
missile basing	crack liquid and PCP mixture
mission	to go shopping for drugs
missionary	one who attempts to create new addicts
Mississippi marbles	dice
mist	PCP; crack smoke
Mister Blue	hydromorphone
Mister Brownstone	hashish; brown heroin
Mister Natural	LSD
Mitsubishi	ecstasy with the Mitsubishi emblem on it
M.J.	marijuana
M&Ms	barbiturates
M.O.	marijuana
mohasky	marijuana
mojo	hard drugs; powdered narcotics
Molly	ecstasy
Molotov cocktail	an explosive made by pouring gasoline into a bottle and adding a cloth wick

monkey	a drug habit in which physical dependence is present; morphine; a small heroin habit
monkey bait	a free sample of an addictive drug
monkey drill	a hypodermic needle
monkey dust	powdered drugs
monkey jumps	the disoriented motions and staggering gait of a drug addict
monkey meat	a drug addict
monkey medicine	morphine
monkey on one's back	to be addicted to drugs
monkey pump	a hypodermic needle
monkey talk	the distorted speech of one who is intoxicated
monkey tranquilizer	PCP
monkey wagon	to be addicted to drugs
monolithic	heavily intoxicated by drugs
monos	a cigarette made from cocaine paste and tobacco
Monroe in a Cadillac	mixture of morphine and cocaine
monster	drugs that are powerful enough to affect the central nervous system
monster weed	potent marijuana
monte	marijuana
mooca/moocah	marijuana
mooch joint	a place where drugs are sold
moocher	a drug addict
mood elevators	antidepressants
moody blues	pentazocine mixed with tripelennamine
moon	mescaline; peyote; to show one's bare butt
moonbeams	PCP
moon gas	inhalants
moon rock	crack and heroin mixture
moonshine	illicit liquor
mooster	marijuana
moota, mutah	marijuana
mooters	a marijuana cigarette
mootie	marijuana
mootos	marijuana
mor a grifa	marijuana
morals	Demerol
more	PCP
morf tab	morphine
morning glory	the first injection of an addict's day

morning glory seeds	contain lysergic acid amide, related to LSD but only one-tenth as potent
morning shot	the first injection of an addict's day
morning wake-up	the first drug of the day
morotgara	heroin
morph, morf, morpho, morphie	morphine
morpho moron	a morphine addict
mortal combat	potent heroin
moscop	morphine and scopolamine combination
mosquito	cocaine
mota, moto	marijuana
mother	a drug dealer
mother dear	methadone
mother nature	marijuana
Mother's Day	the day one receives a welfare check
Mother of God	LSD paper with naked woman on it
mother's little helpers	tranquilizers
motorcycle crack	methamphetamine
mountain dew	illicit liquor
mouth habit	addiction to drugs taken orally
mouth worker	addiction to drugs taken orally
movie star drug	cocaine
mow the grass	to smoke marijuana
mowing the lawn	smoking marijuana
MPPP	synthetic meperidine
MPTP	synthetic drug derived from Demerol
Mr. Lovely	marijuana laced with PCP
Mr. Twenty-Six	26-gauge hypodermic needle
Mr. Warner	a marijuana smoker
Mr. Whiskers	a federal narcotics agent
Mrs. Warren	a prostitute
Mrs. White	a supplier or seller of white powdered drugs
M.S.	morphine
M.U.	marijuana
mu	marijuana
mud	unprocessed opium; heroin
mud wiggler	an opium addict
muff	female genitalia
mugger	one who attacks and robs a person; a comedian
muggie	marijuana
muggles	marijuana
mugglehead	a marijuana smoker

mule	marijuana soaked in whiskey; one who smuggles or carries drugs for a distributor
mule skinner	the person who recruits and supervises people who smuggle or carry drugs
munchies	craving for food after drug use
murder one	heroin and cocaine
murder 8	fentanyl
mushrooms	innocent bystanders who are wounded or killed in the crossfire of gun battles
musk	psilocybin/psilocin mushrooms
muscle pop	to inject a drug intramuscularly because there is not a good vein
muta, mutah, moota	marijuana
muzzle	heroin
my friend	menstrual period
my man	an addict's drug supplier
nail	a tobacco or marijuana cigarette; to catch
nailed	arrested
nail in the coffin	to smoke a tobacco or marijuana cigarette
Nam black	potent black marijuana that is grown in Vietnam or southeast Asia
nanny goat sweat	illicit liquor
nanoo	heroin
narc, nark, narco	an undercover narcotics agent; an informer
narco card	a registration card carried by addicts in order for them to obtain methadone
narcotic bull	a federal narcotics agent
Nazi vitamins	crystal meth
nebbies	pentobarbital
necessities	drug supplies
needle candy	drugs taken by injection
needle flash	a short high that might come between the time the needle enters the tissue and the drug enters the blood
needle freak	one who enjoys injecting; to get sexual pleasure from injecting
needle park	a public park where users and addicts gather to deal or inject drugs
nembies, nemmies	Nembutal
nemish	Nembutal
Nepalese hash	potent hashish from Nepal
nerd, nurd	an unpleasant, unattractive, or insignificant person

new acid	PCP
new magic	PCP
New Jack Swing	heroin and morphine
newspapers	LSD
nexus	4-bromo-2,5 diethoxy-phenyethylamine
nice and easy	heroin
nick	one-half gram
nicked	arrested
nickel	$5 supply of drugs; a 5-year prison sentence
nickel bag	$5 supply of drugs; heroin
nickel deck	$5 supply of drugs; heroin
nickel note	$5 bill
nickelodeons	crack addicts
night on the rainbow	a night spent under the influence of drugs
nightingale	an informer
nightshade	belladonna
night time	heroin withdrawal
nimbly, nimble, nimby	Nembutal
nineteen	ecstasy
nitro	speed or nitrous oxide
nix	stranger among the group
Nixon	inferior quality drugs
noble princess of the waters	hallucinogenic mushrooms
nod	to fall asleep for a short period immediately after drug use
nodded out	under the influence of drugs
nods	cough syrup with codeine
noise	heroin
nontoucher	user who does not want to be touched during or after using drugs
noodlelars	methyprylon
nooky, nookie	sexual intercourse
Northern Lights	potent marijuana
nose	any drug that is taken through the nose
nose candy	any drug that is taken through the nose
nose drops	any drug that is taken through the nose
nose stuff	any drug that is taken through the nose
nose powder	any powdered drug that is taken through the nose
noss	nitrous oxide
nox	nitrous oxide
Ns	Darvocet-N
nubs	peyote; mescaline

nuggets	crack
number	a marijuana cigarette
number 1	liquid hashish
number 3	cocaine, heroin
number 4	heroin
number 8	heroin
number 9	ecstasy
number 13	morphine
nurse	powdered drugs
O	opium
oboy	marijuana
octane	inhale gasoline
off	withdrawn from drugs
ogoy	heroin
oil	hashish oil
oil burner	an expensive drug habit
oiled	alcohol or drug intoxicated; to be injected with drugs
oink	a police officer
OJ	a marijuana cigarette dipped in opium
old lady White	powdered drugs
old Madge	powdered drugs
old Smoky	the electric chair
old Steve	powdered drugs
olive	cotton used to strain a drug solution as it is pulled into a syringe
on a mission	searching for drugs
on a trip	under the influence of drugs
on ice	in jail
on the bricks	walking the streets; a homeless person
on the lam	to escape from jail or prison
on the nod	under the influence of drugs
on the street	out of jail; public knowledge; a street person; a prostitute
on the stuff	a regular user of drugs; an addict
on top of it	in control
on the wire	using amphetamines
one and one	to use both nostrils when snorting a powdered drug
one hitter	a pipe that is big enough for one use
one-hit grass	DMT smoked with tobacco, marijuana, or parsley

one-night stand	a casual sexual encounter
one-on-one	Talwin and Pyribenzamine combination
one-toke weed	potent marijuana
one way	LSD
OP	opium
ope	opium
operator	a drug supplier or seller
OPP	PCP
optical illusions	LSD
orange barrels	LSD
orange bowl	an opium pipe which is fitted with an orange rind
Orange County	Quaaludes
orange crystal	PCP
orange cube	LSD
orange cupcakes	LSD, usually added to other drugs
orange haze	LSD
orange micro	LSD
orange mushrooms	a tablet or blotter impregnated with LSD in the image of a mushroom
orange sunshine	LSD
orange wedges	LSD
oranges	amphetamines
oregano	hashish; marijuana
organic Quaalude	GHB
ounce man	a drug dealer who sells small quantities of drugs
outer limits	crack and LSD
outfit	equipment used for preparing and using drugs
out in left field	under the influence of drugs
out of body	a feeling of separation of the mind from the body one experiences while under the influence of hallucinogens
out of it	alcohol or drug intoxicated; out of touch with reality
out of sight	a pleasurable experience
outside of myself	a feeling of separation of the mind from the body one experiences while under the influence of hallucinogens
overcharged	semiconscious state resulting from too much of a drug

overs and unders	amphetamines and barbiturates
owl	a narcotics agent who works at night
Owsley	LSD
Owsley's acid	LSD
oxy	OxyContin
oxy 80's	a semisynthetic opiate
oxycet	a semisynthetic opiate
oxycotton	OxyContin
oyster stew	cocaine
ozone	PCP
OZ	amyl nitrite
Ozzie, Ozzy	LSD
Ozzie's stuff	LSD
P	peyote; PCP; pure heroin
pacifier	a homemade hypodermic needle
pack	heroin; marijuana
pack it in	to commit suicide; to give up; to quit
pack of rockets	package of marijuana cigarettes
pack of rocks	crack
paca lolo, pakalolo	marijuana
pack one's coozie	to place a parcel of drugs into the vagina
pack one's keister	to place a parcel of drugs into the vagina or rectum
pack one's nose	to snort cocaine
packed up	under the influence of drugs
pad	where one resides; where people gather to use drugs
pad money	admission fee to a site where drugs are used
padded	to have drugs concealed on one's body
paid torch	a hired arsonist
painted woman	a prostitute
paisley caps	capsules or pills laced with LSD
Pakistani black	Pakistani marijuana
Panama cut	Panamanian marijuana
Panama gold	gold-color Panamanian marijuana
Panama red	reddish-color Panamanian marijuana
panatela	large marijuana cigarette
pancakes and syrup	combination of glutethimide and codeine cough syrup
pan up	to prepare a drug for injection
pane	LSD
panic	anxiety caused from a shortage of drugs
panic man	an addict who cannot obtain drugs

panic trip	a bad LSD trip
panther piss	raw and inferior quality liquor
paper	paper folded to conceal drugs; a prescription for drugs; paper that is saturated with drugs; money; counterfeit bills
paper acid	LSD consumed from a blotter
paper bag	container for drugs
paper blunts	marijuana within a paper casing rather than a tobacco leaf casing
paper boy	heroin peddler
paper fiend	a drug user who uses amphetamine-soaked paper strips from an amphetamine inhaler
paper hanger	a person who writes worthless checks or passes counterfeit money
parackie	paraldehyde
paradise	cocaine
paradise white	cocaine
parakeet	paraldehyde
paraphernalia	items involved in drug use
Park Lane No. 2	a type of marijuana sold and used during the Vietnam War
parlay	crack
parsley	marijuana; PCP
pass	a successful drug exchange
paste	to beat
pat	marijuana
pattern	a drug-induced hallucination
pavement princess	a prostitute
pay street	an expensive drug habit
paz	PCP
PCE	synthetic PCP
PCP	phencyclidine
PDAs	public display of affection
P-dope	20–30% pure heroin
peace	LSD, PCP
peace pills	PCP, LSD
peace weed	PCP
peaches	orange-colored amphetamines
peanuts	barbiturates
peanut butter	heroin
pearl	cocaine
pearls	amyl nitrite
pearly gates	LSD; morning glory seeds

pears	amyl nitrite
pebbles	crack
pecker	penis
peddler	a drug dealer
pee wee	a thin marijuana cigarette
peep	PCP
Peg	heroin
pekoe	high quality opium
pellets	LSD
pen shot	injection of drugs
pen yan	opium
penitentiary highball	a drink made from strained shellac and milk
penitentiary shot	an injection of drugs given from a pin and a medicine dropper
people (the)	influential heroin distributor
pep pills	amphetamines
peppermint swirl	LSD combined with another drug
pepper-uppers	amphetamines
Pepsi habit	occasional use of drugs
per	a prescription for drugs
perfect high	heroin
perform	to have sexual intercourse
period hitter	an occasional drug user
perkers, perkies, perks	oxycodone; Percodan
perp	counterfeit crack, made from candle wax and baking soda
Persian brown	brownish-colored heroin from the Middle East
peruvian flake	high-quality cocaine from Peru
peruvian rock	cocaine
peter	penis
Peter	chloral hydrate
Peter Jay	a police officer
Peter Pan	PCP
Peter, Paul, and Mary	menage a trois
permafried	an addict
peyote	the cactus from which mescaline is derived
P-funk	synthetic heroin
PG	tincture of opium; paregoric; pregnant
pharming	consuming a mixture of prescription drugs
phat rails	lines of powdered drugs
P-head	a phenobarbital user

phennies, phenies, phenos	phenobarbital
Phillies blunt	a cigar hollowed out and filled with marijuana
pianoing	using the fingers to find lost powdered drugs
picking	searching on hands and knees for crack
picking the poppies	an opium addict
pickup	an injection
piece	a gun; one ounce of a drug; the female partner in sexual intercourse
pig	a police officer
pig killer	one who kills a police officer
piggie	opium made into pellets for smoking
piggybacking	the simultaneous injection of two drugs
Pikachu	pills containing ecstasy and PCP
pile high and deep	to brag or exaggerate
piles	crack
pill cooker	one who is addicted to opium
pill freak	a user of dangerous drugs; someone who likes to take pills
pill head	a user of dangerous drugs; someone who likes to take pills
pill peddler	a physician
pill popper	a drug user who prefers pills
pill pusher	a physician
pillows	knockout drops; opium; methaqualone; a bag containing pills
pimp	a person who solicits clients for a prostitute
pimp dust	powdered drugs
pimp your pipe	to lend or rent one's crack pipe
pimpmobile	a customized luxury car that is used by a pimp
pin	a hypodermic needle or pin and medicine dropper used to inject drugs; a very thin marijuana cigarette
pin gun	equipment for injecting drugs, made from a pin and a medicine dropper
pin joint	a very thin marijuana cigarette
pinch	to arrest; a small amount of marijuana
pinch hitter	one who is hired to inject drugs
pine	marijuana
pineapple	a grenade or small bomb
ping a pill	to remove a bit of a pill for a small dose

ping in the wing	an injection of a drug into the arm
pinhead	one who injects drugs with the aid of a pin; an unpleasant, unattractive, or insignificant person
pinner	small joint of marijuana
pin gon	opium
pin yen	opium
pink, pinks	Seconal; morphine
pink blotters	LSD
pink elephants	delirium tremens
pink hearts	amphetamines
pink ladies	barbiturates
Pink Panther	LSD
pink robots	LSD
pink spiders	delirium tremens
pink swirl	LSD
pink wedges	LSD
pink witches	LSD
pinks and greens	amphetamines
pinned eyes	pinpoint pupils
pins and needles	morphine
pipe	a large vein; a device used for smoking marijuana or opium
pipe dream	a dream while under the influence of opium
piped	alcohol or drug intoxication
piper	one who snorts powdered drugs
piss off	to anger or disgust someone
pissed	angry; disgusted
pit	the crease on the inside of the elbow
pixies	amphetamines
pizza toppings	psilocybin/psilocin mushrooms
plant	to hide drugs upon an unsuspecting person; where opium is prepared
play around	to use drugs now and then
playing the harmonica	inhaling smoke from heated heroin through the rectangular cover of a matchbox
pleasure user	one who uses drugs for pleasure and who is not addicted
plow	marijuana
PMA	synthetic amphetamine/ methamphetamine
PO	paregoric
pocket rocket	a marijuana cigarette
pod	marijuana

pogo	cocaine
point	a needle
point shot	a shot made with the broken point of a needle or sewing machine needle
poison	heroin; fentanyl
poison people	heroin addict
poke	marijuana
pokey	jail or prison
pollutants	drug smoke; cigarette smoke
pony	crack
poof	smoking ice
poor man's heroin	Talwin and Ritalin combination
poor man's pot	inhalants
poor man's speedball	heroin and methamphetamine combination
pop	to inject drugs simultaneous
popcorn machine	the lights bar on a police car
poppers	isobutyl nitrite; amyl nitrite
poppy	opium
poppy alley	where opium dens are located
poppy grove	an opium den
poppy puffer	an opium addict
popstick	an opium pipe
pork	police officers
positive	positive attitude before and after drug use
pot	marijuana
pothead	a marijuana user
potato	LSD
potato chips	crack cut with benzocaine
potten bush	marijuana
powder	drugs in powdered form
powdered diamonds	cocaine
powder monkey	a supplier or seller of drugs
power puller	rubber piece attached to crack stem
powder room	a room where drugs are bought or sold
powdered joy	powdered narcotics
power hitter	a device used to concentrate marijuana
pox	opium
PR	Panama Red marijuana
preacher	an informer
predator	heroin
pregnant	a lump in the middle of a marijuana cigarette
press	cocaine; crack
prick	a contemptible person; penis

prime time	crack
primo	crack; marijuana mixed with crack
primos	cigarettes laced with cocaine and heroin
prod	a hypodermic needle
product	oral steroids; LSD that is combined with another drug
Prudential	crack user
prunes	testicles
P-stuff	PCP
psyched up	excited
psychedelic drug	a hallucinogen that produces abnormal psychic effects
puff	to smoke marijuana
puff the dragon	to smoke marijuana
puffer	crack smoker
puffy	PCP
pull a fast one	to rob; to deceive
pump full of lead	to shoot
pumping	selling crack
pumpkin seed	mescaline
puna butter	a variety of Hawaiian marijuana
punchboard	a promiscuous female
puppy	a gun
pure	pure heroin
pure love	pure heroin
purple	LSD
purple barrels	LSD
purple haze	LSD
purple hearts	LSD; amphetamines; phenobarbital
purple flats	LSD
purple microdot	LSD
purple ozoline	LSD
purple passion	combination stimulant and depressant
purple rain	PCP
push	to sell drugs
pusher	one who sells or deals drugs; a connection; metal hanger or umbrella rod used to scrape residue from crack stems
push shorts	to cheat or sell short amounts
pussy	female partner in sexual intercourse; female genitalia; a weak or timid person
put away	to kill
put it on paper	to saturate a paper with drugs

put on	to intentionally deceive or confuse
put on a circus	to fake withdrawal in an attempt to get drugs
QP	one-quarter pound of marijuana
Qs	Quaaludes
quack	methaqualone
quads	barbiturates
quarter	one-quarter ounce; $25 drug supply
quarter bag	$25 drug supply
quarter moon	hashish
quarter piece	a fraction of a kilogram
quartermaster	one who sells quarter bag of bags
quartz	smokable speed
quas	barbiturates
Queen Anne's lace	marijuana
quicksilver	isobutyl nitrite
quill	a matchbook cover used for sniffing cocaine or heroin
R-2	Rohypnol
racehorse Charlie	cocaine
radical chic	socially prominent people who associate with radicals or minority groups
rag and bones man	a street person
rag picker	a street person
Raggedy Ann	blotter paper stamped with LSD in the character of Raggedy Ann
ragman	a street person
ragweed	inferior quality marijuana
rail	a line of powdered drug
railroad tracks	needle marks along the veins of drug users
railroad weed	inferior quality marijuana
railroader	one who injects drugs intravenously
rainbow roll	various colored barbiturates
rainbows	various colored barbiturates
raincoat	condom
rainy day woman	marijuana
ram	a male
Rambo	heroin
rane	cocaine; heroin
ran good	marijuana that grows wild
rap	a conversation; to converse; rhythmic vocal expression; arrest or arraignment for a crime

raspberry	female who trades sex for drug money; an injection site that has abscessed
rasta weed	marijuana
rat	an informer
ration	a drug dose or stash
rat pack	a small gang that terrorizes others and vandalizes property
raw	crack
raw fusion	heroin
rawhide	heroin
rave	party designed to enhance a hallucinogenic experience through music and behavior
razed	under the influence of drugs
RB	resin bud (marijuana)
RDs	red devils (Seconal)
reader	a prescription
reader with tail	a forged prescription
ready rock	crack
Reagans	amobarbital
recycle	LSD
red	under the influence of drugs
red and blues	Tuinal
red angelfish	blotter paper saturated with LSD in the character of a red angelfish
red birds	barbiturates
red bullets	barbiturates
red caps	crack
red cross	cross-scored amphetamine tablets
red chicken	heroin
red devils	Seconal
red dimple	LSD combined with another drug
red dirt	marijuana
red dolls	barbiturates
red dot	LSD tablet with a red dot
red dragon	blotter paper saturated with LSD in the character of a red dragon
red eagle	heroin
red flag	something that incites anger
red hots	barbiturates
red jackets	barbiturates
red lilies	barbiturates
red lips	LSD
red phosphorus	smokable speed

red pipe	an artery
red rock	heroin
reds	barbiturates
red-light district	a district in which houses of prostitution are numerous
redneck	a bigoted and ultraconservative person
reefer	a marijuana cigarette
register	pulling blood into a syringe or medicine dropper to confirm entry into a vein
reindeer dust	powdered drugs
reekstick	tobacco laced with cocaine
reefer	marijuana
regs	marijuana
register	to allow blood to flow back into needle just prior to injecting heroin
Regular P	crack
reindeer dust	heroin
res	potent residue which is scraped from the pipe and smoked
rest in peace	crack
rhapsody	variation of amphetamine, methamphetamine
rhine	heroin
rhythms	amphetamines
rib	Rohypnol
Rice Krispies	amyl nitrite
rich man's aspirin	cocaine
riding the poppy train	to smoke opium
riding a white horse	using powdered heroin
riding a witch's broom	using powdered drugs
riding the thorn	injecting drugs
riding the train	using cocaine
riding the wave	under the influence of drugs
rifle range	where drugs are purchased and injected
rig	equipment used in preparing and using drugs
right croaker	a physician who provides drugs or sells prescriptions to addicts
righteous	superior quality drugs
righteous bush	marijuana
ringer	potent crack
rip off	to steal
ripped	alcohol or drug intoxicated
rippers	amphetamines
rits	Ritalin

Ritz and T	Ritalin and Talwin mixture injected
roach	butt of a marijuana cigarette; a police officer
roach bender	one who smokes marijuana
roach clip	a metal clip used to hold the butt of a marijuana cigarette
roach pin	a metal pin used to hold the butt of a marijuana cigarette
road dope	amphetamines
Road Runner	a type of ecstasy with the Road Runner's face emblem on it
road rage	a driver's anger that results in aggressive behavior on the road
roasting	smoking marijuana
rob the cradle	to date or marry someone much younger than yourself
Robbie, Robby	cough medicine with codeine
robin eggs	blue capsules of LSD
robotripping	drinking Robitussin
roche	Rohypnol
rock(s)	crystallized form of cocaine or heroin
rock attack	crack
rocket caps	dome-shaped caps on crack vials
rocket fuel	PCP
rockets	marijuana cigarettes
rockette	female who uses crack
rock fiend	crack addict
rock house	place where crack is sold and used
rocks of hell	crack
rock star	female who trades sex for crack or money to buy crack; someone addicted to crack cocaine
Rocky III	crack
rod	a gun
rogues gallery	a collection of photos of criminals
roll	ecstasy
roller	to inject a drug
rollers	law enforcement agents; veins that move during the process of injection
rolling	ecstasy
roll of reds	barbiturates
roll the boy	to smoke opium
rolling buzz	a drug high of a moderate length of time
rolling stone	a person who wanders from place to place

roofies	Rohypnol, date rape drug
rook	person who can't hang. . . . .can't handle their drugs
rooms	psilocin/psilocybin mushrooms
rooster	crack
root	marijuana
rope	marijuana
rophies, ropies	Rohypnol, date rape drug
Rose Marie	marijuana
roses	amphetamines
roto rooter	penis
rough stuff	marijuana
row of coke	an elongated line of cocaine
row-shay	Rohypnol, date rate drug
rox	crack
Roxanne	cocaine; crack
royal blues	LSD
Royal Temple Ball	resin mixed with LSD then rolled into a ball
Roz	crack
RPMs	amphetamines; dextroamphetamines
rub out	to kill
Ruffles, ruffies	Rohypnol, date rate drug
rumble	police in the neighborhood; a shakedown or search; a fight
run	the time during which a drug is continuously injected
runners	people who sell or get drugs for dealers
running	ecstasy
rupture	PCP
rush	the initial feeling of exhilaration from a drug dose
rush snappers	isobutyl nitrite
Russian sickles	LSD
sack	a person who distributes narcotics to the small-time dealers
sacrament	LSD that is placed on the tongue in communion wafer form
sacred mushroom	psilocybin/psilocin mushrooms
saidie-maisie	sadomasochism
safety pin mechanic	one who uses a safety pin and medicine dropper to inject drugs
sagebrush whacker	one who smokes marijuana
sak	bag of marijuana

Salmon River Quiver	marijuana
salt	heroin
salt and pepper	inferior quality marijuana; black and white police car
salty water	marijuana
Sam	federal narcotic agent; GHB
Sam and Dave	police officers
San Francisco bomb	mixture of cocaine, heroin, and LSD
San Quentin quail	a female below the legal age of sexual consent
sandbag	to beat; to assault some; to check a bet, then raise it
sandoz, sandos	LSD
sandwich	two lines of cocaine with a layer of heroin in the middle
sandwich bag	$40 bag of marijuana
San Pedro	mescaline; peyote
Santa Marta gold	Colombian marijuana
sassafras	marijuana
Satan's secret	inhalants
satch	paper or clothing that is saturated with a drug and smuggled into a hospital or prison
satch cotton	fabric used to filter a solution of narcotics before an injection
satellite	an empty paper towel roll used as a pipe to smoke numerous joints
sativa	marijuana
Saturday night special	a small-caliber revolver; a cheap handgun
sauced	alcohol intoxicated
saxophone	an opium pipe
scaffle	PCP
scab	heroin
scag, skag	heroin
scagged, skagged	addicted to heroin
scarf a joint	to swallow a marijuana cigarette in order to avoid getting caught
scat	heroin
scate	heroin
scattered	alcohol or drug intoxicated
schlock	drugs; junk
schmack	drugs
schmeek	heroin

schnozzler	a cocaine user
school boy	paregoric; codeine; a cocaine user
school craft	crack
schwillins	alcohol
scissors	marijuana
Scooby snacks	ecstasy
scoop	a folded matchbook cover used to snort powdered drugs; GHB
scootie	methamphetamines
score	to obtain something, usually drugs or sex; when blood appears in an eyedropper
scorpion	cocaine
Scott	heroin
Scottie, Scotty	cocaine; crack; the high from crack
Scrabble	crack
scramble	worthless or near-worthless heroin
scrape and snort	to share crack by scraping off small pieces to snort
scratch	money
screaming meemies	delirium tremens
screw	sexual intercourse; to cheat someone; a prison guard
scribe	one who can write acceptable forged prescriptions
script	a prescription
script doc	a physician who writes ethically questionable prescriptions
script writer	a sympathetic physician; someone who forges prescriptions
scroll	paper used to roll marijuana cigarettes
scrubwoman's kick	naphtha that is inhaled
scruples	crack
scuffle	PCP
sealed stuff	a can or bottle of opium
sec, seccy, seggy	Seconal
seco-8	secobarbital
second to none	heroin
second-story man	a thief or burglar
seconds	second inhalation of a drug from a pipe
seeds	morning glory seeds
selling rocks	selling crack cocaine
sen	marijuana
send it home	to inject a drug

seni	peyote; mescaline
serenity	chemically related to mescaline and amphetamines
serial speedballing	sequencing cough syrup with codeine and heroin over a one- to two-day period
sernyl	PCP
serpent	a hypodermic needle
Serpico 21	cocaine
server	crack dealer
ses, sess, sezz	sinsemilla (grade of marijuana)
set	amphetamine and barbiturate mixture
set up	to arrange for someone to be arrested or caught
Seven Up	cocaine; crack
sewer	the median cephalic vein
Shabu	methamphetamines
shakes	drug or alcohol withdrawal
sharps	needles
sharpshooter	one who most always hits the vein
shank	a small quantity of marijuana
shaman	peyote; mescaline
she	cocaine
shebanging	mixing cocaine with water and squirting it up the nose
sheets	PCP
sheet rocking	crack and LSD
Sherlock Holmes	a police officer
sherm	a cigarette that has been dipped in embalming fluid
shermans	PCP; PCP laced cigarette
shight or shighty	amphetamines
shit	heroin
shit-faced	alcohol or drug intoxicated
shmagma	marijuana
shmeck, schmeek	heroin
shoot, shoot up	to inject a drug
shoot below the belt	to inject into a vein in the lower part of the body
shoot gravy	to inject a mixture of cooked blood and a dissolved drug
shoot shit	to inject heroin
shoot skin	to miss a vein and inject into the skin
shoot the breeze	nitrous oxide

shoot up	to inject drugs
shoot Yancy	to inject opium
shooting gallery	where addicts gather to inject drugs
shooting up	to inject drugs
shot	to inject a drug
shot down	under the influence of drugs
shot to the curb	a person who has lost everything due to drug use
shotgun	someone puts the joint or blunt in their mouth backwards and blows the smoke into someones mouth
shovel	equipment used to prepare and use powdered drugs
shrooms	psilocybin/psilocin mushrooms
shrimp	marijuana
shrink	a psychiatrist
shwag	low grade marijuana
sick dizzies	a reaction to hallucinogenic experience
siddi	marijuana
Sidney	LSD
sightball	crack
silk and satin	amphetamines and barbiturates
Silly Putty	psilocybin/psilocin mushrooms
silo	psilocybin/psilocin mushrooms
Simple Simon	psilocybin/psilocin
sinse	marijuana
sinsemilla	potent marijuana
sip	a puff from a marijuana cigarette
sitter	one who coaches another during an LSD trip
sitting well	intoxicated on drugs
Skag Jones	a heroin addict
skag, scag	heroin
skagged out	alcohol or drug intoxicated
Skagtown	a neighborhood inhabited by addicts
sixty-two	$2\frac{1}{2}$ ounces of crack
skee	opium
skeegers/skeezers	crack smoking prostitute
sketch	a bad reaction to LSD or marijuana
sketching	coming down from a speed induced high
skid	heroin; someone who looks and dresses dirty because of smoking dope
skies	refers to scales used to weigh drugs
skied	under the influence of drugs

skin	paper used for rolling cigarettes
skin flick	a pornographic movie
skin popping	injecting drugs subcutaneously
skin pumping	a subcutaneous or intramuscular injection of drugs
skin search	to examine the skin of a suspected user for needle track marks
skin shooter	a subcutaneous injection of drugs
skin shot	a subcutaneous injection of drugs
skinhead	a person with a shaved head who participates in militant group activities
skinner	a subcutaneous injection of drugs
skirt	a female who trades sex for money and/or drugs
skuffle	PCP
skull buster	a police officer's night stick
skunk	marijuana said to be grown in California
sky river	LSD that is mixed with another drug
skyrockets	amphetamines
slab	a large piece of crack cocaine
slack	a very small amount of drugs
slam	to inject a drug
slammed	to be arrested
slammer	jail or prison
slanging	selling drugs
slanguage	the language of the street
slave	a drug addict
sleep 500	GHB
sleepers	barbiturates; heroin
sleepwalker	an addict
sleet	crack
sleigh ride	a cocaine party
sleigh rider	cocaine user
slick superspeed	methcathinone
slime	heroin
slinging	dealing drugs
slip the collar	to escape from jail or prison
slits	ecstasy
slow boat	a marijuana cigarette
slum	to use narcotics
slum dump	an opium den
slumber party	a gathering to use drugs
slut	a prostitute

S&M	sadomasochism
smack	heroin
smack freak	a heroin addict
smackhead	a heroin addict
smash	acetone extracts of marijuana that are added to hashish, rolled in little balls, and smoked
smashed	alcohol or drug intoxicated
smears	LSD
smell it up	to snort powdered drugs
smell the reindeer dust	to snort powdered drugs
smell the stuff	to snort powdered drugs
smizz	heroin
smoke	to smoke drugs that can be smoked
smoke a bowl	to smoke hashish or marijuana
smoke a joint	to smoke a marijuana cigarette
smoke house	a place where one can buy or smoke drugs
smoke joint	a place where one can buy or smoke drugs
smoked	alcohol or drug intoxicated; killed
smoke-out	a party where attendees smoke drugs
smoke you out	smoke marijuana with you
smoking gun	a marijuana or tobacco cigarette that has been laced with heroin and cocaine
smoothie	an undercover agent who is able to pull off a sale from an unsuspecting drug dealer
smudge	a small amount of heroin
Smurf	a cigar dipped in embalming fluid
snakes	delirium tremens
snapped up	intoxicated by drugs
snaps	amphetamines
snappers	isobutyl nitrite
snatcher	a police officer
sniff	to sniff powdered drugs through the nose
sniffer	one who habitually snorts powdered drugs
sniffer bag	$5 bag of powdered drugs
sniffing squad	undercover narcotics agents
snipe	a marijuana cigarette butt
snitch	an informer
snite	a lighter used to smoke drugs
snooze	to sleep following drug use
snop	marijuana
snort	to sniff powdered drugs
snort a line	to snort cocaine

snot	residue produced from smoking amphetamines
snot balls	rubber cement rolled into balls that are burned and the fumes inhaled
snow	powdered drugs
snowball	powdered drugs
snow bird	powdered drugs
snow cones	powdered drugs
snow drifter	one who sells powdered drugs
snow eagle	a primary figure in a drug ring
snow flower	a female user of powdered drugs
snowmobiling	using powdered drugs
snow pallets	amphetamines
snow seals	cocaine and amphetamines
snowstorm	a large amount of powdered drugs
snozzle	to snort powdered drugs
soapers	methaqualone
spliffy	a marijuana cigarette
social junker	one who uses drugs only in a social setting
social sniffer	one who uses powdered drugs only in a social setting
society high	one who uses cocaine in a social setting
softballs	barbiturates
soles	hashish
soma	PCP
songbird	an informer
soot the chimney	to snort powdered drugs
sophisticated lady	cocaine
soul searching	looking for a vein in which to inject drugs
soup	water bong
source	a drug supplier or wholesaler
space blasting	smoking cocaine and PCP together
space cadet	one who is intoxicated by drugs
space base	cocaine and PCP
space dust	crack dipped in PCP
spaced out	altered state of consciousness secondary to prolonged drug use
space ship	glass pipe used to smoke crack
spangles	Librium
spare time	possessing marijuana
spark an owl	smoke a gigantic joint
sparking an owl	lighting a joint
spark it up	to smoke marijuana

Sparkle Plenty	amphetamines
sparklers	amphetamines; ketamine
Sparky	the electric chair
splaff	marijuana cigarette laced with acid
spear	a hypodermic needle
special	superior quality drugs
special K	ketamine
speckled eggs	amphetamines
specks	LSD
spectrum	nexus
speed	methamphetamines; amphetamines
speed boat	marijuana, PCP, crack
speed demon	amphetamines; methamphetamines
speed freak	habitual user of methamphetamines
speed for lovers	ecstasy
speedball	two drugs injected together
speedster	an amphetamine user
spider blue	heroin
spike	a hypodermic needle
spit ball	a mouthful of free-base vapors puffed into someone else's mouth
splash	amphetamines
splash house	a place where amphetamines or methamphetamines are sold or used
splay	marijuana
spliff	a marijuana cigarette wrapped in newspaper
splim	marijuana
split	to leave
splits	tranquilizers
splivins	amphetamines
spoc	police officers (cops spelled backwards)
spook	a long-time narcotics user
spoon	a utensil used in preparing narcotics for injection; 2 grams of heroin
spores	psilocin/psilocybin mushrooms
sporting	to use drugs
sport of the gods	cocaine use
spray	inhalants
spread the good news	to share one's drug supply
spring	to post bail for someone who is in jail
sprouting	injecting drugs from one syringe to another syringe
sprung	a person who has just starting to use drugs

spur	one gram of a powdered drug
square	a person who uses neither alcohol nor drugs
square John	a person who uses neither alcohol nor drugs
square dancing tickets	LSD
square mackerel	marijuana
squat	an abandoned house that has been taken over by homeless people
squealer	an informer
squirrel	LSD combined with another drug
stack	a pack of marijuana cigarettes
stacking	taking steroids with a prescription
stackola	stacking money
stall	a finger cot or condom used as a package for powdered drugs
Stanley's stuff	LSD
star	methcathinone
stardust	heroin with cocaine
star-spangled powder	cocaine
star stuff	cocaine
start cooking	to begin injecting drugs into the veins
stash	a supply of concealed drugs
stash bag	a container in which drugs are stored
stash man	a drug dealer or drug runner
stale weed	prison tobacco
stat	methcathinone
steamboat	a device for smoking marijuana
steamroller	pipe used to smoke marijuana
steel and concrete cure	total abstinence from drugs while in prison
steerer	a person who recommends a heroin dealer in return for money or drugs
Stella	paper used to roll marijuana cigarettes
stem	a cylinder used to smoke crack; an opium pipe
stems	marijuana
step on	to dilute drugs
stepping high	alcohol or drug intoxicated
Steve's mission	a place to buy or use drugs
Stevie	a drug-induced hallucination
stick	a marijuana cigarette
stimey	a dime bag of drugs
stinger	a hypodermic needle
stinky	marijuana
stink weed	marijuana

stoms	barbiturates
stoned	under the influence of drugs
stoned to the eyes	very intoxicated
stoned to the gills	very intoxicated
stoner	someone who stays under the influence of marijuana
stones	crack
stone wall horrors	delirium tremens
stony bush	marijuana
stool pigeon	an informer
stoolie	an informer
stoppers	barbiturates
STP	serenity; tranquility; peace; a hallucinogen
straddle the pike	to inject drugs
straight	in possession of narcotics; a person who is not a drug user
straw	a marijuana cigarette
strawberries	barbiturates
strawberry	female who trades sex for drugs or money to buy drugs
strawberry fields	LSD
strawberry hill	LSD
strawberry shortcake	methamphetamine
street drugs	illicit drugs that are sold casually
street ounce	an ounce of diluted heroin for sale on the street
street pusher	one who deals drugs on the street
street value	the retail price of drugs that are illegally sold
streetwalker	a prostitute
stretch	to dilute a drug
strike	a dose of drugs
strung out	heavily addicted to drugs
stub	a marijuana cigarette butt
stud	a young man, especially one who is promiscuous
stud muffin	a physically fit or handsome male
student	one who is newly addicted to drugs
studio fuel	cocaine
stuff	heroin
stum	marijuana
stumblers	barbiturates
stumbles	inability to walk appropriately as a result of prolonged alcohol or drug use

stung by a viper	addicted to marijuana
stung by the hop	addicted to opium
stung by the white nurse	addicted to morphine
stung by white mosquitoes	addicted to cocaine
submarine	a large marijuana cigarette
suck up	to be excessively attentive in order to gain favor
sucks (it)	something that is extremely objectionable or inadequate
suds	beer
sugar	powdered drugs; LSD
sugar block	crack; LSD
sugar cubes	LSD
sugar daddies	amphetamines
sugar daddy	a man who supports a woman in return for sex; a physician who sells drugs to addicts
sugar down	to dilute powdered drugs with sugar
sugar lumps	LSD
sugar weed	marijuana that has been compressed into a brick with sugar
summer sky	morning glory seeds
sunrise	yellow or orange LSD tablet
sunshine	yellow or orange LSD tablet
super	one person puts the joint in his/her mouth and blows the smoke out for someone else to inhale; PCP
super acid	LSD
super C	cocaine; crack
supercharged	intoxicated by drugs
super flu	withdrawal symptoms
super grass	high-grade or superior quality marijuana
super ice	smokable methamphetamine
super-jaded	under the influence of drugs
super joint	high-grade or superior quality marijuana
super kools	PCP
super weed	marijuana or parsley treated with LSD; superior quality marijuana
supplier	drug source
surfer	PCP
swag	inferior quality marijuana
sweatin' me	pressuring me
sweet dreams	morphine
Sweet Jesus	morphine

Sweet Lucy	marijuana
sweet lunch	marijuana
sweet Mary	marijuana
sweet Morpheus	morphine
sweet stuff	heroin
sweet tooth	a desire for drugs
sweeties	amphetamines; ecstasy
sweets	amphetamines
swell up	crack cocaine
swilly	under the influence of alcohol
swing both ways	to have sex with either men or women
swinger	one who uses a variety of drugs in all forms; one who is sexually promiscuous
swisher	a cigar that has been emptied and filled with marijuana
Swiss purple	LSD
switched on	to be introduced to hallucinogenic drugs
syndicate acid	LSD; PCP
syrup	dark brown Mexican heroin
syrup head	a drug user who uses cough syrup with codeine and a barbiturate
T	PCP
tabs	a tablet or pill form of a drug
tac	PCP
tacky	shabby; seedy
tag	a euphoric sensation experienced after drug use
take	equipment for injecting drugs, usually an eyedropper; money obtained in a robbery; money obtained by selling drugs
take a Brody	to fake drug withdrawal
take a dive	to commit suicide
take a Duffy	to fake drug withdrawal
take a fall	to be arrested on drug-related charges
take a powder	to leave; to commit suicide
take a sweep	to snort cocaine
take a trip	to use a hallucinogen
take for a ride	to kill; to cheat
take it in line	to inject drugs into the median cephalic vein
take off	to begin a drug high
take-a-too	equipment for injecting drugs, usually an eyedropper
take off artists	addicts who rob other addicts

A139

taking a cruise	PCP
taking care of business	addicts' lives and actions on the street
tail lights	LSD
taima	marijuana
taking a cruise	PCP
takkouri	marijuana
talcum powder	a bogus powdered drug
tall	under the influence of drugs
tals	Talwin
tamale	a marijuana cigarette that resembles a tamale
tampon	a fat marijuana cigarette
tang	drug addiction
Tango & Cash	heroin laced with methyl fentanyl
tanks	PCP
tapping the bags	removing small amounts of drugs from bags before selling it, thus shorting the buyer
tar	opium; heroin
tar dust	cocaine
tarred and feathered	addicted to opium
taste	a small sample of drugs
tattoos	needle track marks
taxing	price paid to enter a crack house; charging more per vial if not a regular customer
T buzz	PCP
tea	marijuana; PCP
tea party	a gathering to smoke marijuana
team meeting	a gathering to smoke marijuana
teardrops	dosage units of crack packaged in the cut-off corners of plastic bags
Teddies and Betties	a mixture of Talwin and pyribenzamine
teddy bears	LSD
teenage	1/16 ounce of methamphetamine
teener	1/16 ounce of crack rock
teeth	bullets
ten cent pistol	heroin laced with poison
ten sack	$10 worth marijuana
tens, 10s	10-mg amphetamine tablets
tension	crack
tester	one who is able to judge the strength of diluted heroin
tex-mex	marijuana
Texas leaguer	a marijuana smoker
Texas pot	marijuana

Texas shoe shine	inhalants
Texas tea	marijuana
Thai sticks	bundles of marijuana soaked in hashish oil; marijuana buds bound on short sections of bamboo
the animal	LSD
the bad seed	peyote; mescaline
the beast	heroin
the C	methcathinone
the curse	menstrual period
the curse of Eve	menstrual period
the great white hope	crack
the devil	crack
the ghost	powdered drugs
the hawk	LSD
the heat	the police
the hole	solitary confinement
the witch	heroin
thing	a marijuana cigarette; heroin; main drug interest at the moment
thirst monsters	heavy crack smokers
thirteen	marijuana
thirty-eight	crack sprinkled on marijuana
thorn	a hypodermic needle
thoroughbred	drug dealer who sells pure narcotics; a prostitute; a prisoner
threes	a painkiller that contains 30 mg of codeine
thrill pills	barbiturates
thriller	a marijuana cigarette
thrust	isobutyl nitrite
thrusters	amphetamines
thumb	marijuana
thunder cookie	marijuana
thunder weed	marijuana
tia	marijuana leaf
tic	PCP in powder form
tic tac	PCP in powder form
ticket	a hallucinogen
ticket agent	a drug supplier or seller
tie	to inject a drug
tie off	to apply pressure on a vein with a tourniquet
tight	being clean in appearance

tighten up	to give drugs to an individual
tin	container for marijuana; a marijuana pipe made out of aluminum foil
tish	PCP
tissue	crack
titch	PCP
tits	black tar heroin
T man	a federal narcotics or treasury agent; a marijuana smoker
together	one who appears to live in an organized fashion
toke	a pull from a marijuana cigarette
toke pipes	pipes used to smoke marijuana
toke up	to light a marijuana cigarette
tom cat	a sewing machine needle that is used to open a vein for drug use
Tom Mix	an injection of drugs
tomcat	a sexually promiscuous male
toncho	octane booster which is inhaled
tongue	to inject drugs into a vein beneath the tongue
tooies	Tuinal capsules
tooles	depressant
tools	equipment used for injecting drugs; guns
toot	to snort or sniff cocaine
tooter	a tube used for snorting cocaine
tootsie	Tuinal
tootsie roll	a marijuana cigarette rolled in brown paper; potent heroin
top gun	crack
topi	mescaline; peyote
tops	peyote; marijuana
tops and bottoms	mixture of Talwin and pyribenzamine
torch	a marijuana cigarette; to deliberately set a fire
torch cooking	smoking cocaine base by using a propane or butane torch as a source of flame
torch up	to smoke marijuana
torn up	alcohol or drug intoxicated
tornado	crack cocaine
torpedo	a hired killer; a drink containing chloral hydrate
torture chamber	a place of incarceration where drugs are not available

toss up	female who trades sex for drugs or money to buy drugs
tossed	to be bodily searched for drugs by law enforcement agents
totalled	to be intoxicated by drugs
totally spent	to have a hangover
toucher	drug user who wants affection before, during, or after using drugs
tough	to inject a drug in a vein beneath the tongue
tour guide	one who guides an LSD user through a trip
tout	person who introduces buyers to sellers
toy	a small tin box of prepared opium; equipment used for injecting drugs
TR-6s	amphetamines
tracers	visual effects of hallucinogenics
Track One	area in which houses of prostitution are numerous
Track Two	area in which homosexual houses of prostitution are numerous
tracks	needle marks and abscess scars
tracked up	covered with needle and abscess scars
tracking	repeating a drug-induced hallucination; to repeat words or phrases while under the influence of drugs
trade	a sex partner
tragic magic	crack dipped in PCP
trail	needle marks
trails	LSD-induced perception that moving objects leave multiple images, or trails, behind them
train	gang rape
trained nurse	one who smuggles narcotics into a hospital or nurse
tranks, tranx	tranquilizers
tranq	depressant
tranquility	a hallucinogenic drug; mescaline; depressants
trap	hiding place for drugs
trash	methamphetamine
trash picker	a street person
trashed	alcohol or drug intoxicated
travel agent	one who guides an LSD user through a trip
tray	a $3 bag of marijuana
trays	vials

travel agent	one who guides an LSD user through a trip
tree jumper	a rapist
tree of knowledge	marijuana
trees	drugs in pill and capsule form
triangles	delirium tremens
trick	an act of prostitution or theft
trick track	a prostitute who is addicted to injectable drugs
tricycles and bicycles	mixture of Talwin and pyribenzamine
trip	what a person experiences after using a hallucinogenic drug
trip grass	marijuana mixed with an amphetamine
trip out	to become intoxicated by drugs
triple line	superior quality marijuana that is laced with heroin
tripper	a drug user; a person who takes hallucinogens
trippin'	to be intoxicated on psychedelic drugs
trips	amitriptyline; LSD
Trojan horse	one who smuggles drugs into a hospital or prison
troop	crack
truck drivers	amphetamines
Ts and blues	mixture of Talwin and pyribenzamine
TT1	PCP
TT2	PCP
TT3	PCP
tubes	water pipes or bongs
tuies	Tuinal
tune in	to experience the effects of a hallucinogenic drug
tuning in	to be under the influence of a hallucinogenic drug
turbo	a potent form of ecstasy
turd	drugs concealed in a condom in the rectum
turf	the territory gangs consider to be in their control
turkey trots	needle marks from drug injections
turn a cartwheel	to fake a drug withdrawal in an attempt to get drugs
turn a trick	to earn money by theft or prostitution
turn on	to use drugs; to excite sexually
turn out	to introduce someone to drugs or prostitution
turnabout	amphetamine
turned off	withdrawn from drugs

turned on	under the influence of drugs; sexually aroused
turnip greens	marijuana
turps	elixir of terpin hydrate with codeine
tutor (or tooter)	a straw or something similar to aid in snorting coke
tutti-frutti	flavored cocaine
tweak mission	on a mission to find leftover crack
tweaker	crack user looking for rocks on the floor after a police raid
tweeds	marijuana
twenty	a $20 rock of crack
twenty-five	LSD
twig	a marijuana cigarette
twins	two smaller particles of rock cocaine that equals a two-O
twirl	to sell drugs
twist	a marijuana cigarette
twisted	intoxication bordering on unconsciousness
twisty	a marijuana cigarette
twistum	a marijuana cigarette
twit	an unpleasant, unattractive, or insignificant person
two for nine	two $5 vials or bags of crack for $9
two-O	$20 piece of rock cocaine weight about 1.8 grams gross weight
U boat	a portion of a sealed rubber tube that is filled with drugs and concealed in the rectum
uglies	delirium tremens
ultimate	crack
umbilical cord	methadone
uncle	federal agents
Uncle Fester	a glass pipe
Uncle Milty	barbiturates
Uncle Sid	LSD
under the white cross	under the influence of cocaine
unkie	morphine
up against the stem	addicted to smoking marijuana
uppers, uppies	amphetamines
up and down	to inject drugs and take pills
up the creek	in trouble
ups and downs	amphetamines and barbiturates
uptight	worried; anxious; angry
uptown	cocaine

utopiates	hallucinogens
uzi	crack; crack pipe
V	Valium
valley	the inside crease of the elbow where drugs are injected
valley dolls	LSD
vals	Valium
Vatican roulette	the rhythm method of birth control
vegetarian	one who smokes marijuana
venom	PCP
vipe	marijuana
viper	one who smokes marijuana
vita G	GHB
vitamin E	ecstasy
vitamins	amphetamines
viper's weed	marijuana
vivor	a street person who survives
vodka acid	LSD
void	to be under the influence of drugs
volcano 5	red LSD paper
vons	Darvon
vroomed	to be under the influence of drugs
wac, wack	PCP; marijuana or tobacco cigarette dipped in embalming fluid
wacky backy	marijuana
wacky weed	marijuana
wafers	ecstasy; cookies laced with LSD
waffles	hits of LSD
Wake 'N' Bake	to use drugs first thing in the morning
wake-ups	the first drug of the day
wakowi	mescaline
Waldorf Astoria	solitary confinement in jail or prison
wall bangers	Quaaludes
warped	intoxicated on drugs
washed up	withdrawn from drugs; one who is no longer successful or needed
waste	to kill
wasted	alcohol or drug intoxicated; exhausted; killed
water	injectable amphetamines
watering hole	a bar where liquor is sold
water-water	marijuana cigarettes dipped in embalming fluid, sometimes laced with PCP

wave	crack
weasel	an informer
wedding bells	LSD; morning glory seeds
wedge series	LSD-STP combination
wedges	LSD-STP combination
weed	marijuana
weed head	a marijuana user
weed out	weed for sale
weed tea	marijuana
weekend warrior	one who uses drugs on weekends only
weight	the amount of narcotics an addict needs for one week
weightless	under the influence of drugs
weirded out	one who is disturbed by events which occur while under the influence of drugs
weirdo	an extraordinary eccentric person
west coast	Preludin; Ritalin
West Coast turnarounds	amphetamines
wet	PCP
wet daddy	a marijuana or tobacco cigarette dipped in embalming fluid and laced with PCP
wet dog shakes	delirium tremens
wet-wet	a marijuana or tobacco cigarette dipped in embalming fluid and laced with PCP
whack	to dilute a narcotic; to kill
whacked	intoxicated from drugs; killed
wheat	marijuana
wheels	ecstasy
when-shee	opium
whiff	cocaine
whiffle dust	powdered drugs
whippets	nitrous oxide
whistle blower	an informer
white	cocaine
white angel	a healthcare worker who smuggles drugs to patients or prisoners
white ball	crack
white boy	heroin
white cloud	vapors from drugs that are smoked
white cross	cross-scored amphetamine tablets
white domes	LSD
white dove	ecstasy

white dragon	opium
white dust	powdered drugs
white fluff	LSD
white ghost	crack
white girl	cocaine; heroin
white goddess	morphine
white-haired lady	heroin
white horizon	PCP
white horse	heroin
white junk	heroin
white lady	heroin
white lightning	LSD mixed with another drug; raw liquor
white merchandise	powdered drugs
white mosquito	cocaine
white nurse	powdered drugs
white Owsley's	LSD
white powder	cocaine; PCP
white silk	morphine crystals
white stuff	heroin
white sugar	crack
white tornado	free-base cocaine
whiteout	isobutyl nitrite
whites, whities	amphetamines
whiz bang	an injected mixture of drugs
whizz	amphetamines
whoops and jangles	symptoms of withdrawal
wicked	potent heroin
wide	under the influence of drugs
widows	amphetamines
wiggin'	an addict in need of drugs
wig out	to become psychotic during drug use
wig picker	a psychiatrist
wild cat	methcathinone and cocaine mixture
wild Geronimo	barbiturates mixed with alcohol
wimp	a weak or ineffectual person
window glass	LSD
window panes	LSD on clear plastic, cellophane, or sheets of gelatin
wings	powdered drugs
wiped out	alcohol or drug intoxicated; exhausted
wired	under the influence of drugs; having a recording device on one's person

wisdom weed	marijuana
witch	powdered drugs
witch Hazel	heroin
witch's brew	LSD mixed with datura
wizard	an ounce of marijuana
wizard of oz	an ounce of marijuana
wobble weed	marijuana
wokowi	peyote; mescaline
wolf	PCP
wollie	rocks of crack rolled into a marijuana cigarette
wonder star	methcathinone
woodpecker of Mars	Amanita muscaria mushroom
woolah	a hollowed out cigar refilled with marijuana and crack
woolas	a tobacco cigarette laced with cocaine; a marijuana cigarette sprinkled with crack
woolies	marijuana and crack or PCP mixture
wooly	a cocaine and marijuana cigarette
wooly blunts	marijuana cigarettes laced with crack or PCP
working	selling crack
working girl	a prostitute
working half	crack rock weighing one-half gram or more
working man's cocaine	methamphetamine
works	equipment for injecting drugs
world traveler	a homeless person who wanders from place to place
wrangled	to stop using drugs
wrecked	extremely intoxicated from using drugs
wrecking crew	crack
X	ecstasy
X-ing	using ecstasy
Xmas	to be euphoric from drug use
XTC	ecstasy
yahoo/yeaho	crack
yale	crack
yam yam	opium
yanked	arrested
yeh	marijuana
yellow	LSD; barbiturates
yellow bam	methamphetamine
yellow birds	pentobarbital

yellow bullets	pentobarbital
yellow dimples	LSD
yellow dolls	pentobarbital
yellow fever	PCP
yellow jack speed	amphetamines
yellow jackets	depressant
yellow submarines	pentobarbital
yellow sunshine	LSD
yen	desire for drugs
yen shee	opium ash
yen shee suey	opium wine
yen sleep	restless, drowsy state after LSD use
Yerba	marijuana
yesca	marijuana
yesco	marijuana
yimyom	crack
ying yang	LSD
yuppie	a young, upwardly mobile professional person
yuppie flu	the ongoing effects of a cocaine-snorting habit
Z	1 ounce of heroin
Zacatecas purple	potent marijuana grown in the Mexican state of Zacatecas
zambi	marijuana
zap	to kill; to berate an individual
Zen	LSD
zero	opium
zig zag man	LSD; marijuana; marijuana rolling papers
zings	amphetamines
zip	cocaine
zip gun	a homemade gun
zips	oz of any type drug
zol	a marijuana cigarette
zombie	PCP; an addict
zombie weed	PCP
zombie buzz	alcohol or drug intoxicated
zonked	under the influence of drugs
zooie	a device that is used to hold the butt of a marijuana cigarette
zoom	ecstasy
zoomers	amphetamines; individuals who sell counterfeit drug, then flee

Psychiatric and Psychological Tests

A Comprehensive Custody Evaluation Standard System (ACCESS)

A Measure of How You Think and Make Decisions

A Structured Addictions Assessment Interview for Selecting Treatment (ASIST)

Abbreviated Conners Rating Scale

Abbreviated Conners Teacher Questionnaire

Abbreviated Conners Teacher Rating Scale (ACTRS)

Abbreviated Life Event Questionnaire

ABC Inventory to Determine Kindergarten and School Readiness

Aberrant Behavior Checklist (ABC)

Ability-to-Benefit Admissions Test

Abnormal Involuntary Movements Scale (AIMS)

Abuse Risk Inventory for Women, Experimental Edition

Academic Advising Inventory

Academic Alertness Test

Academic Aptitude Test (AAT)

Academic Instruction Measurement System

Academic Orientation Scale

Academic Readiness Scale (ARS)

Acceptance of Disability Scale

Accounting Program Admission Test (APAT)

ACCUPLACER: Computerized Placement Tests

ACER Advanced Test B40

ACER Advanced Test B90

ACER Applied Reading Test

ACER Test of Basic Skills—Blue Series

ACER Test of Basic Skills—Green Series

ACER Test of Reasoning Ability

ACER Word Knowledge Test

Achenbach Child Behavior Checklist

Achenbach Child Behavior Test

Achievement Identification Measure Teacher

Achievement Motivation Profile

Achieving Behavioral Competencies

Ackerman-Schoendorf Scales for Parent Evaluation of Custody (ASPECT)

ACQ Behavior Checklist

ACT Study Power Assessment and Inventory

Activity Pattern Indicator (API)

Acuity of Psychiatric Illness Scale (APIS)

Acute Panic InventoryAdaptability Test

Adaptation of the Wechsler Preschool and Primary Scale of Intelligence for Deaf Children

Adapted Sequenced Inventory of Communication Development (A-SICD)

Adaptive Behavior Evaluation Scale (ABES)

Adaptive Behavior Evaluation Scale, Revised

Adaptive Behavior Inventory

Adaptive Behavior Inventory for Children (ABIC)

Adaptive Behavior Scale (ABS)

Adaptive Behavior: Street Survival Skills Questionnaire

Adaptive Functioning Index

Adaptive Style Inventory

ADD-H Comprehensive Teacher's Rating Scale

ADD-H: Comprehensive Teacher's Rating Scale, Second Edition (ACTeRS)

Addiction Research Center Inventory

Addiction Severity Index (ASI)
Additional Personality Factor Inventory
ADHD Behavior Checklist for Adults
Adjustment Scales for Children and
Adolescents
Adolescent Alienation Index (AAI)
Adolescent and Adult
Psychoeducational Profile
Adolescent Apperception Cards
Adolescent Coping Scale
Adolescent Diagnostic Interview (ADI)
Adolescent Dissociative Experiences
Scale
Adolescent Drinking Index (ADI)
Adolescent Drug and Alcohol
Diagnostic Assessment (ADAD)
Adolescent Language Screening Test
Adolescent Life Change Event
Questionnaire (ALCEQ)
Adolescent Multiphasic Personality
Inventory
Adolescent Problem Severity Index
(ASPI)
Adolescent Psychopathology Scale
Adolescent Risk Behavior
Questionnaire
Adolescent Self-Report Trauma
Questionnaire
Adolescent Separation Anxiety Test
Adolescent Symptom Inventory-4 (ASI)
Adolescent-Coping Orientation for
Problem Experiences
Adolescent-Family Inventory of Life
Events and Changes
Adult Attachment Interview
Adult Attention Deficit Disorder
Behavior Rating Scale
Adult Attention Deficit Disorder
Evaluation Scale
Adult Basic Learning Examination-
Level I (ABLE-I)
Adult Basic Learning Examination-
Level II (ABLE-II)

Adult Career Concerns Inventory
(ACCI)
Adult Growth Examination
Adult Language Assessment Scales
Adult Neuropsychological
Questionnaire (ANQ)
Adult Performance Level Survey
(APLS)
Adult Personal Adjustment and Role
Skills
Adult Personal Data Inventory (APDI)
Adult Personality Inventory (API)
Adult Personality Inventory, Revised
Adult Rating of Oral English
Adult Self-Expression Scale (ASES)
Adult Suicidal Ideation Questionnaire
(ASIQ)
Advanced Measures of Music
Audiation
Advanced Placement Examination (APE)
Advanced Placement Program (APP)
Advanced Progressive Matrices
Affect Balance Scale
Affect Grid Study
Affective Perception Inventory
Affective Perception Inventory-College
Level
Affective Style Index
Age Projection Test (APT)
Ages and Stages Questionnaire
Aggregate Neurobehavioral Student
Health and Educational Review
(ANSER)
Agoraphobic Cognitions Questionnaire
AGS Early Screening Profile
AH4 Group Intelligence Test
AH5 Group Test of High Grade
Intelligence
AH6 Group Tests of High Level
Intelligence
Ahr's Individual Development Survey
Ainsworth Strange Situation Test
Akerfeldt Test

Albany Panic and Phobia Questionnaire
Alberta Essay Scales: Models
Alcadd Test
Alcadd Test, Revised Edition
Alcohol Assessment and Treatment
  Profile
Alcohol Clinical Index
Alcohol Dependence Scale
Alcohol Usage Questionnaire (AUQ)
Alcohol Use Disorders Identification
  Test (AUDIT)
Alcohol Use Inventory (AUI)
Alliance for Mentally Ill Chemical
  Abusers
Alphabet Mastery
Alternative Lifestyle Checklist (ALC)
Alzheimer Disease Assessment Scale
  (ADAS)
American Association of Mental
  Retardation Adaptive Behavior Scale
  Residential and Community, Second
  Edition
American Drug and Alcohol Survey
American Law Institute Test
American Law Institute/Model Penal
  Code test
American Psychiatric Association Index
Amphetamine Interview Rating Scale
  (AIRS)
Analysis of Readiness Skills
Analytic Learning Disability
  Assessment
Analytical Reading Inventory
Analyzing the Communication
  Environment
Andreasen Six-Basic-Factors-Model
  Questionnaire (A-SBFM)
Animal and Opposite Drawing
  Technique (AODT)
Animal Naming Test
Ann Arbor Learning Inventory
Ann Arbor Learning Inventory and
  Remediation Program

Annett hand preference scale
Anomalous Sentences Repetition
Anorectic Attitude Questionnaire
Anorexic Behavior Observation Scale
  (ABOS)
Anorexic Behavior Scale
Antidepressant Treatment History
  Form
Anton Brenner Developmental Gestalt
  Test of School Readiness
Anxiety Disorders Association of
  America (ADAA)
Anxiety Disorders Interview Schedule
Anxiety Scale for the Blind (ASB)
Anxiety Scale Questionnaire (ASQ)
Anxiety Scales for Children and Adults
  (ASCA)
Anxiety Sensitivity Index (ASI)
Anxiety States Inventory
Aphasia Clinical Battery
Aphasia Diagnostic Profile
Aphasia Language Performance Scale
  (ALPS)
Applied Knowledge Test
Appraisal of Language Disturbances
  (ALD)
Apraxia Battery for Adults (ABA)
Apraxia Profile: A Descriptive
  Assessment Tool for Children
APT Inventory
Aptitude Interest Inventory
Aptitude Interest Measurement
Aptitude Survey and Interest Schedule-
  Interest Survey
Aptitude Test for School Beginners
  (ASB)
Aptitude-Intelligence Test Series
Arithmetic Grade Rating
Arithmetic Skills Assessment Test
Arizona Articulation Proficiency Scale
  (AAPS)
Arizona Articulation Proficiency Scale,
  Second Edition

Arizona Battery for Communication Disorders of Dementia (ABCD)
Arizona Sexual Experience Scale
Arlin Test of Formal Reasoning
Armed Services Civilian Vocational Interest Survey
Armed Services Vocational Aptitude Battery
Army Alpha Examination Revised
Army Beta tests
Army mental tests
Army General Classification Test
Arousal Seeking Tendency Scale
Arthritis Pain Formula
Arthur Adaptation of the Leiter International Performance Scale
Arthur Point Scale of Performance Test
Ashland Interest Assessment
ASSESS Personality Battery [Expert System Version 5.X]
Assessing and Teaching Phonological Knowledge
Assessing Linguistic Behaviors: Assessing Prelinguistic and Early Linguistic Behaviors in Developmentally Young Children
Assessing Motivation to Communicate
Assessing Reading Difficulties: A Diagnostic and Remedial Approach
Assessing Specific Competencies
Assessing Specific Employment Skill Competencies
Assessment for Persons Profoundly or Severely Impaired
Assessment in Infancy: Ordinal Scales of Psychological Development
Assessment Link Between Phonology and Articulation
Assessment of Adaptive Areas
Assessment of Aphasia and Related Disorders, Second Edition
Assessment of Basic Competencies (ABC)

Assessment of Career Decision Making (ACDM)
Assessment of Career Development (ACD)
Assessment of Chemical Health Inventory
Assessment of Children's Language Comprehension (ACLC)
Assessment of Conceptual Organization (ACO)
Assessment of Conceptual Organization (ACO): Improving Writing, Thinking, and Reading Skills
Assessment of Core Goals (ACG)
Assessment of Fluency in School-Age Children
Assessment of Individual Learning Style: The Perceptual Memory Task
Assessment of Intelligibility of Dysarthric Speech
Assessment of Interpersonal relations
Assessment of Living Skills and Resources
Assessment of Parenting Skills: Infant and Preschooler
Assessment of Phonological Processes, Revised
Assessment of Positive Symptoms
Assessment of Qualitative and Structural Dimensions of Object Representations, Revised Edition
Assessment Program of Early Learning Levels (APELL)
Assessment of School Needs for Low-Achieving Students: Staff Survey
Assigning Structure Stages Test
Assessment of Suicide Potential
Association Adjustment Inventory
Association of Mental Health Administrators (AMHA)
Athletic Motivation Inventory (AMI)
Attention Deficit Disorder Behavior Rating Scale (ADDBRS)

Attention Deficit Disorder Comprehensive Teacher Rating Scale

Attention Deficit Disorder Evaluation Scale Secondary-Age Student

Attention Deficit Disorder Evaluation Scale (ADDES)

Attention Deficit Disorder Evaluation Scale, Second Edition

Attention Deficit Scales for Adults

Attention Deficit/Hyperactivity Disorder Test

Attentional and Interpersonal Style Inventory

Attitude Survey Program for Business and Industry

Attitude to School Questionnaire (ASQ)

Attitudes Toward Disabled Persons (ATDP)

Attitudes Toward Mainstreaming Scale

Attitudes Toward Working Mothers Scale

Attributional Style Questionnaire

Atypical Depression Index (ADI)

Auditory Apperception Test (AAT)

Auditory Continuous Performance Test

Auditory Discrimination and Attention Test

Auditory Discrimination Test (ADT)

Auditory Selective Attention Test

Autism Behavior Checklist

Autism Diagnostic Interview

Autism Screening Instrument for Educational Planning

Autism Screening Instrument for Educational Planning, Second Edition

Autism Society of America

Autistic Behavior Composite Checklist and Profile

Automated Child/Adolescent Social History

Automated Multitest Laboratory (AML)

Automated Neuropsychological Assessment Metric Battery (ANAM)

Automated Office Battery

Bader Reading and Language Inventory

Balanced Emotional Empathy Scale

Ball Aptitude Battery

Balthazar Scales for Adaptive Behavior I: Scales of Functional Independence

Balthazar Scales for Adaptive Behavior II: Scales of Social Adaptation

Balthazar Scales for Adaptive Behavior (BSAB)

Bangs Receptive Vocabulary Checklist

Bankson Language Screening Test (BLST)

Bankson Language Test-2 (BLT-2)

Bankson-Bernthal Test of Phonology (BBTOP)

Barber Scales of Self-Regard for Preschool Children

Barclay Classroom Assessment System

Barclay Classroom Climate Inventory (BCCI)

Barclay Early Childhood Skill Assessment Guide

Barclay Learning Needs Assessment Inventory (BLNAI)

Barnes Akathisia Scale

BarOn Emotional Quotient Inventory

Barranquilla Rapid Survey Intelligence Test (BARSIT)

Barratt scale

Barron-Welsh Art Scale (BWAS)

Barry Five Slate System

Basic Achievement Skills Individual

Basic Concept Inventory

Basic Educational Skills Test

Basic English Skills Test

Basic Inventory of Natural Language

Basic Language Concepts Test

Basic Living Skills Scale

Basic Number Diagnostic Test

Basic Occupational Literacy Test (BOLT)

Basic Personality Inventory (BPI)

Basic Reading Inventory (BRI)
Basic Reading Inventory, Seventh
Edition
Basic School Skills Inventory—
Diagnostic
Basic School Skills Inventory (BSSI)
Basic School Skills Inventory Battery
Test
Basic School Skills Inventory-Screen
Basic Skills Assessment Program
Basic Skills Inventory
Basic Visual-Motor Association Test
BASIS-A Inventory
Bateria Woodcock-Munoz, Revisada
Battelle Developmental Inventory
(BDI)
Battelle Developmental Inventory
Screening Test
Battery for Health Improvement
Bauer Self-Rated Internal State Scale
Bay Area Functional Performance
Evaluation
Bay Area Functional Performance
Evaluation, Second Edition
Baycrest Neurocognitive Assessment
(BNA)
Bayer Select Pain Relief Formula
Bayley II Developmental Assessment
Bayley Scales of Infant Development
(BSID)
Beck Anxiety Inventory
Beck Anxiety Inventory [1993 Edition]
Beck Depression Inventory (BDI)
Beck Depression Inventory [1993
Revised]
Beck Depression Inventory score
Beck Depression Inventory-II
Beck Depression Scale
Beck Hopelessness Scale (BHS)
Beck Hopelessness Scale [Revised]
Beck Questionnaire
Beck Scale for Suicide Ideation
Beck Suicide Intent Scale

Beck Suicide Lethality Scale
Becker Work Adjustment Profile
Bedford Life Events and Difficulties
Scale
Bedside Evaluation and Screening
Bedside Evaluation and Screening Test
of Aphasia
Bedside Evaluation Screening Test,
Second Edition
Beery Picture Vocabulary Screening
(PVS)
Beery Test of Visual Motor Integration
Beery Visual Motor Test
Beery-Buktinica Developmental Test
Beery-Buktinica Developmental Test of
Visual Motor Integration
BEHAVE-AD Rating Scale
Behavior Activity Profile (BAP)
Behavior Analysis Forms for Clinical
Intervention
Behavior Analysis Language Instrument
Behavior Assessment Battery, 2nd
edition
Behavior Assessment System for
Children
Behavior Assessment System for
Children, Revised
Behavior Change Inventory
Behavior Dimensions Scale
Behavior Disorders Identification Scale
(BDIS)
Behavior Evaluation Scale
Behavior Evaluation Scale-2 (BES-2)
Behavior Pathology in Alzheimer's
Disease Rating Scale
Behavior Problem Checklist (BPC)
Behavior Problems: A System of
Management
Behavioral Problems Scale
Behavior Rating Instrument for Autistic
and Other Atypical Children
Behavior Rating Profile, Second Edition
(BRP-2)

Behavior Rating Scale
Behavior Status Inventory (BSI)
Behavior Style Questionnaire (BSQ)
Behavioral Academic Self-Esteem
Behavioral and Emotional Rating Scale:
    A Strength-Based Approach to
    Assessment
Behavioral Assessment of Pain (BAP)
Behavioral Assessment Test
Behavioral Characteristics Progression
Behavioral Deviancy Profile
Behavioral Health Systems (BHS)
Behavioral Inattention Test (BIT)
Behavioral Observation Scale for
    Autism
Behavioral Pathology in Alzheimer
    Disease Rating Scale
Behavioral Performance Situation
Behavioral Problems Scale
Behavioral Scale for Developmentally
    Deviant Preschoolers
Behavioural Assessment of the
    Dysexecutive Syndrome
Behn-Rorschach Test
Bekesy Functionality Detection Test
    (BFDT)
Belbin Team Roles Self-Perception
    Inventory
Bell Object Relations and Reality
    Testing Inventory
Bellevue Index of Depression
Bem Sex Role Inventory (BSRI)
Bender Visual Retention Test
Bender Visual-Motor Gestalt Test
    (BVMGT)
Bender-Gestalt hexagon
Bender-Gestalt Test (BGT)
Bender-Gestalt Visual Motor Test
Bender Visual Gestalt Drawing
Bennett Mechanical Comprehension
    Test
Benton Controlled Oral Word
    Association

Benton Revised Visual Retention Test
Benton Visual Retention Test (BVRT)
Benton Visual Retention Test-Revised
    (BVRT)
Bernreuter Personality Inventory
Bessell Measurement of Emotional
    Maturity Scales
Bexley-Maudsley Automated
    Psychological Screening
Bilingual Home Inventory
Bilingual Syntax Measure II Test
    (BSM)
Bilingual Verbal Ability Tests
Binet Scale
Binet-Simon Scale
Binet-Simon test
Binet test
Bingham Button Test (BBT)
Biographical and Personality Inventory,
    Series II
Biographical Inventory Form U
Bipolar Psychological Inventory (BPI)
Birth to Three Developmental Scale
Birth-to-Three Assessment and
    Intervention System
Black Intelligence Test of Culture
    Homogeneity (BITCH)
Blessed Behavior Scale
Blessed Dementia Rating Scale (BDRS)
Blessed Information and Concentration
    Test
Blessed Information-Memory-
    Concentration Test
Blind Learning Aptitude Test
Block Survey and SLIDE
Bloom Analogies Test
Bloom Sentence Completion Test
Bloomer Learning Test
Boder Test of Reading-Spelling
    Patterns
Body Image and Eating Questionnaire
Body Sensations Questionnaire
Body Shape Questionnaire

Boehm Test of Basic Concepts
Boehm Test of Basic Concepts,
    Preschool Version
Boehm Test of Basic Concepts, Revised
Bolam Test
Bolgar-Fischer Word Test
Booker Profiles in Mathematics:
    Numeration and Computation
Booklet Category Test, Second Edition
Boston Assessment of Severe Aphasia
    (BASA)
Boston Classification System
Boston Diagnostic Aphasia
    Examination (BDAE)
Boston Naming Test (BNT)
Botel Reading Inventory
Bowel Family Systems
Bracken Basic Concept Scale
Bracken Basic Concept Scale, Revised
Braille Assessment Inventory
Brazelton Neonatal Behavioral
    Assessment Scale
Bricklin Perceptual Scales
Brief Alcoholism Screening Test
Brief Aphasia Screening Examination
    (BASE)
Brief Cognitive Rating Scale (BCRS)
Brief Disability Questionnaire
Brief Drinker Profile
Brief Life History Inventory (BLHI)
Brief Neuropsychological Cognitive
    Examination
Brief Neuropsychological Mental Status
    Examination (BNMSE)
Brief Outpatient Psychopathology Scale
Brief Pain Inventory
Brief Psychiatric Rating Scale (BPRS)
Brief Psychiatric Rating Scale for
    Children (BPRS-C)
Brief Screening Tool and Problem List
Brief Symptom Inventory (BSI)
Brief Test of Attention (BTA)
Brief Test of Head Injury

Brief Visuospatial Memory Test (BVMT)
Brigance Diagnostic Comprehensive
    Inventory of Basic Skills
Brigance Diagnostic Comprehensive
    Inventory of Basic Skills, Revised
Brigance Diagnostic Employability
    Skills Inventory
Brigance Diagnostic Inventory of Basic
    Skills
Brigance Diagnostic Inventory of Early
    Development
Brigance Diagnostic Inventory of
    Essential Skills
Brigance Diagnostic Life Skills
    Inventory
Brigance Early Preschool Screen for
    Two-Year-Old and Two-and-a-Half-
    Year-Old Children
Brigance K & 1 Screen for
    Kindergarten and First-Grade
    Children
Brigance Preschool Screen
Brigance Screen
Bristol Achievement Tests
Bristol Language Development Scale
    (BLADES)
Bristol Social Adjustment Guides
British Ability Scale (BAS)
British Ability Scales: Spelling Scale
Brook Reaction Test (BRT)
Brown and Harris Life Event and
    Difficulty Schedule
Brown Assessment of Beliefs Scale
    (BABS)
Brown Attention Deficit Disorder Scale
Brown-Goodwin scale
Bruininks-Oseretsky Standardized Test
Bruininks-Oseretsky Test
Bruininks-Oseretsky Test of Motor
    Proficiency
Bryant-Schwan Design Test (BSDT)
Bulimic Investigatory Test, Edinburgh
    (BITE)

Bunney-Hamburg Rating Scale
Burks Behavior Rating Scale (BBRS)
Burns Brief Inventory of
  Communication and Cognition
Burns-Roe Informal Reading Inventory
Buschke Selective Reminding Test
Buschke Short-Term Recall Test
Buss-Durkee Hostility Inventory
Buswell-John Diagnostic Test for
  Fundamental Processes in Arithmetic
Butcher Treatment Planning Inventory
Bzoch-League Receptive-Expressive
  Emergent Language Scale
CAGE alcohol use questionnaire
CAGE screening
Cain-Levine Social Competency Scale
Calendar of Premenstrual Experiences
  (COPE)
Calev Recognition/Recall Test
Calgary Depression Scale for
  Schizophrenia
California Achievement Test (CAT)
California Achievement Test, Fifth
  Edition (CAT/5)
California Achievement Tests Writing
  Assessment System
California Computerized Assessment
  Package
California Critical Thinking
  Dispositions Inventory (CCTDI)
California Critical Thinking Skills Test
  (CCTST)
California Diagnostic Mathematics Test
California Diagnostic Reading Test
California F Scale
California Infant Scale for Motor
  Development (CISMD)
California Life Goals Evaluation
  Schedule
California Motor Accuracy Test,
  Southern Revised
California Occupational Preference
  Survey

California Personality Inventory (CPI)
California Preschool Social
  Competency Scale (CPSCS)
California Psychological Inventory Test
  (CPIT)
California Psychological Inventory,
  Revised
California Q-Sort (Revised Adult Set)
California Short-Form Test of Mental
  Maturity (CTMM-SF)
California Test of Basic Skills (CTBS)
California Test of Mental Maturity
  (CTMM)
California Test of Mental Maturity,
  Short Form
California Test of Personality (CTP)
California Verbal Learning Test
California Verbal Learning Test,
  Research Edition, Adult Version
California Verbal Learning Test,
  Children's Version
Callahan Anxiety Pictures
Callier-Azusa Scale
Campbell Interest and Skill Survey
Camberwell Family Interview (CFI)
Cambridge Mental Disorders in Elderly
  Examination
Campbell Organizational Survey
Cambridge Test Battery
Camelot Behavioral Checklist (CBC)
Campbell Leadership Index (CLI)
Canadian Achievement Survey Tests
  for Adults
Canadian Achievement Tests, Second
  Edition
Canadian Cognitive Abilities Test
  (CCAT)
Canadian Cognitive Abilities Test,
  Form 7
Canadian Occupational Interest
  Inventory
Canadian Test of Basic Skills, Forms 7
  and 8

Canadian Test of Cognitive Skills
Canadian Tests of Basic Skills (CTBS)
Candidate Profile Record
Canfield Instructional Styles Inventory
Canfield Learning Styles Inventory
Canter Background Interference
    Procedure for the Bender Gestalt Test
CAP Assessment of Writing
Card-sorting test
Career Anchors: Discovering Your Real
    Values, Revised Edition
Career Assessment Inventories for the
    Learning Disabled
Career Assessment Inventory (CAI)
Career Assessment Inventory, Second
    Edition
Career Assessment Inventory, The
    Enhanced Version
Career Attitudes and Strategies
    Inventory: An Inventory for
    Understanding Adult
Careers
Career Beliefs Inventory (CBI)
Career Decision-Making (CDM)
Career Decision Scale
Career Decision-Making Self-Efficacy
    Scale
Career Development Inventory
Career Directions Inventory
Career Exploration Inventory
Career Exploration Series, 1992
    Revised
Career Factors Inventory
Career Guidance Inventory
Career Interest Inventory
Career Interest Test
Career IQ Test
Career Problem Check List
Career Profile System, Second Edition
Career Thoughts Inventory
Career Values Card Sort
Caregiver Strain Index
Caregiver-Teacher Report Form

Carey Temperament Scales
Caring Relationship Inventory (CRI)
Carlson Psychological Survey
Carnegie Interest Inventory (CII)
Carrell Discrimination Test
Carroll Depression Scale (CDS)
Carroll Rating Scale for Depression
Carrow Auditory-Visual Abilities Test
Carrow Elicited Language Inventory
    (CELI)
Carrow Receptive Language Test
CAT/5 Listening and Speaking
    Checklist
Category Test (CT)
Cattell Infant Scale
Cattell Infant Intelligence Scale
Cattell Infant Scale for Intelligence
    (CISI)
Cattell Infant Scale Inventory (CISI)
Cattell Personality Factor Questionnaire
Cayuga-Onondaga Assessment for
    Children with Handicaps, Version 7.0
    (COACH)
Center for Epidemiologic Studies-
    Depression Scale (CES-D Scale)
CERAD Assessment Battery
CES-D Scale
CGI Scale
Change Agent Questionnaire (CAQ)
Chart of Initiative and Independence
Charteris Reading Test
Checklist for Child Abuse Evaluation
    (CCAE)
Checklist of Adaptive Living Skills
    (CALS)
Chestnut Lodge Prognostic Scale for
    Chronic Schizophrenia
Chicago Area Survey
Chicago Early Assessment and
    Remediation Laboratory
Chicago Word Fluency Test
Child Abuse Potential Inventory
Child Abuse Potential Inventory, Form VI

Child and Adolescent Adjustment Profile
Child Anxiety Scale
Child Assessment Schedule (CAS)
Child at Risk for Drug Abuse Rating Scale
Child Behavior Checklist (CBCL)
Child Care Inventory
Child Development Inventory
Child Development Rating
Child Development Review
Child Health Self-Concept Scale
Child Neuropsychological Questionnaire (CNQ)
Child Personality Scale (CPS)
Child Sexual Behavior Inventory
Child Symptom Inventory-4 (CSI)
Childhood Antecedents Questionnaire
Childhood Autism Rating Scale (CARS)
Children at Risk Screen: Kindergarten and Preschool
Children of Alcoholics Screening Test
Children of Alcoholism Screening Test (CAST)
Children's Academic Intrinsic Motivation Inventory
Children's Adaptive Behavior Scale, Revised
Children's Affective Rating Scale (CARS)
Children's Apperception Test (CAT)
Children's Apperception Test-Human (CAT-H)
Children's Apperceptive Story-Telling Test (CAST)
Children's Articulation Test (CAT)
Children's Attention and Adjustment Survey (CAAS)
Children's Auditory Verbal Learning Test-2 (CAVLT-2)
Children's Coma Score
Children's Depression Inventory (CDI)
Children's Depression Rating Scale-Revised (CDRS-R)

Children's Depression Scale (CDS)
Children's Diagnostic Inventory (CDI)
Children's Embedded Figures Test (CEFT)
Children's Global Assessment Scale (CGAS)
Children's Hypnotic Susceptibility Scale
Children's Inventory of Self-Esteem (CISE)
Children's Language Battery
Children's Manifest Anxiety Scale (CMAS)
Children's Memory Scale
Children's Perception of Support Inventory (CPSI)
Children's Personality Questionnaire (CPQ)
Children's Problems Checklist
Children's Psychiatric Rating Scale (CPRS)
Children's Role Inventory
Children's Self-Concept Scale (CSCS)
Children's Version of the Family Environment Scale
Children's Yale-Brown Obsessive Compulsive Scale (CY-BOCS)
Chinese Polarity Inventory
Christensen Dietary Distress Inventory
Chronic Disease Score
Chronicle Career Quest
CID Phonetic Inventory
CID Picture Spine
CID Preschool Performance Scale
City University Colour Vision Test, Second Edition
Clarke Reading Self-Assessment Survey
Clark-Madison Test of Oral Language
Classroom Atmosphere Questionnaire (CAQ)
Classroom Communication Skills Inventory: Listening and Speaking Checklist

Classroom Environment Index

Classroom Environment Scale, Second Edition

Classroom Environmental Scale (CES)

Classroom Reading Inventory, Seventh Edition

Claybury Selection Battery

Clerical Speed and Accuracy Test

Clifton Assessment Procedures for the Elderly

Clinical Adaptive Test

Clinical Analysis Questionnaire (CAQ)

Clinical Dementia Rating (CDR)

Clinical Evaluation of Language Fundamentals, 3 Screening Test

Clinical Evaluation of Language Fundamentals, Preschool

Clinical Evaluation of Language Fundamentals, Third Edition

Clinical Evaluation of Language Fundamentals-Revised

Clinical Global Impression of Change (CGIC)

Clinical Global Impression-Improvement

Clinical Global Impressions (CGI)

Clinical Global Impressions Scale

Clinical Global Impressions-Improved (CGI-I)

Clinical Global Improvement (CGI)

Clinical Linguistic Auditory Milestone Scale

Clinical Observations of Motor and Postural Skills

Clinical Rating of Drinking Scale (CRDS)

Clinical Rating Scale (CRS)

Clinical Support System Battery

Clinician Global Rating Scale

Clinician Rated Anxiety Scale (CRAS)

Clinician Rated Overall Life Impairment

Clinician Rated Overall Life Impairment Scale

Clinician-Administered PTSD Scale (CAPS)

Clinician's Global Rating Scale (CGRS)

Clinician's Interview Based Impression of Change (CIBIC)

Clinician's Interview-Based Impression of Change-Plus scale

Clock Test

Close Persons Questionnaire

Closed Head Injury Screener

Closed High School Placement Test

Cloze Reading Tests

Clyde Mood Scale (CMS)

Clymer-Barrett Readiness Test

Clymer-Barrett Readiness Test, Revised

Coaching Process Questionnaire

Coalition for the Family (CF)

Cocaine Selective Severity Assessment

Cochrane Collaboration

Cognistat (The Neurobehavioral Cognitive Status Examination)

Cognitive Abilities Scale

Cognitive Abilities Test (CAT)

Cognitive Abilities Test, Form 5

Cognitive Behavior Rating Scales

Cognitive Control Battery

Cognitive Diagnostic Battery

Cognitive Observation Guide (COG)

Cognitive Process Profile

Cognitive Skills Assessment (CSA)

Cognitive Skills Assessment Battery

Cognitive Skills Assessment Battery, Second Edition

Cognitive Symptom Checklist

CogScreen Aeromedical Edition

Cohen-Mansfield Agitation Inventory (CMAI)

Collaborative Study of the Psychobiology of Depression

Collaborative Study Psychotherapy Rating Scale

College Ability Test (CAT)

College Adjustment Scales

College and University Environment Scales (CUES)
College Basic Academic Subjects Examination
College Characteristics Index (CCI)
College English Placement Test
College Entrance Examination Board (CEEB)
College Major Interest Inventory
College Qualifications Tests
College Student Experiences Questionnaire
College Student Questionnaire (CSQ)
College Student Satisfaction Questionnaire (CSSQ)
College-Level Examination Program General Examination
Collegiate Assessment of Academic Proficiency
Collis-Romberg Mathematical Problem Solving Profile
Colorado Educational Interest Battery
Coloured Progressive Matrices
Columbia Mental Maturity Scale (CMMS)
Combat Exposure Scale
Committee of International Medical Graduates
Committee on Family Violence and Sexual Abuse
Committee on Psychiatric Diagnosis and Assessment
Committee on Quality Assurance and Improvement
Common-Metric Questionnaire
Communication Abilities Diagnostic Test (CADT)
Communication Abilities Diagnostic Test and Screen
Communication Activities of Daily Living
Communication and Symbolic Behavior Scales

Communication Knowledge Inventory
Communication Profile: A Functional Skills Survey
Communication Response Style: Assessment
Communication Sensitivity Inventory
Communication Skills Profile
Communications Profile Questionnaire
Communicative Abilities in Daily Living (CADL)
Community College Goals Inventory
Community College Student Experiences Questionnaire
Community College Student Experiences Questionnaire, Second Edition
Community Mental Health Centers Act
Complex Figure Test (CFT)
Composite International Diagnostic Interview (CIDI)
Composite International Diagnostic Interview-Substance Abuse Module (CIDI-SAM)
Composite Psycholinguistic Age
Composite Risk Index (CRI)
Comprehension of Oral Language
Comprehensive Ability Battery (CAB)
Comprehensive Adult Student Assessment System
Comprehensive Assessment of School Environment
Comprehensive Assessment of School Environment Information Management System
Comprehensive Assessment of Symptoms and History (CASH)
Comprehensive Assessment Program: Achievement Series
Comprehensive Behavior Rating Scale for Children
Comprehensive Career Assessment Scale (CCAS)
Comprehensive Developmental Evaluation Chart

Comprehensive Drinker Profile

Comprehensive Identification Process, Revised

Comprehensive Personality Profile

Comprehensive Psychiatric Rating Scale (CPRS)

Comprehensive Psychopathological Rating Scale

Comprehensive Qualifying Examination (CQE)

Comprehensive Receptive and Expressive Vocabulary Test

Comprehensive Scales of Student Abilities: Quantifying Academic Skills and School-Related Behavior Through the Use of Teacher Judgments

Comprehensive Screening Tool for Determining Optimal Communication Mode

Comprehensive Test of Adaptive Behavior

Comprehensive Test of Basic Skills, Forms U and V

Comprehensive Test of Nonverbal Intelligence (CTONI)

Comprehensive Test of Visual Functioning (CTVF)

Comprehensive Testing Program III

Comprehensive Tests of Basic Skills, Fourth Edition

Compulsive Sexual Disorders Interview

Computer Anxiety Index

Computer Literacy and Computer Science Tests

Computer Programmer Aptitude Battery (CPAB)

Comrey Personality Scale (CPS)

Concentration Performance Test (CPT)

Concept Mastery Test (CMT)

Concept-Specific Anxiety Scale (CAS)

Conceptual Systems Test (CST)

Conflict Management Survey (CMS)

Conflict in Marriage Scale (CIMS)

Conflict Resolution Inventory

Conflict Style Inventory

Conflict Tactics Scale (CTS)

Conners Abbreviated Symptom Questionnaire

Conners Continuous Performance Test

Conners Hyperkinesis Index, Parent Form

Conners Hyperkinesis Index, Teacher Form

Conners Parent and Teacher Symptom Questionnaire

Conners Parent Questionnaire (CPQ)

Conners Parent Rating Scale

Conners Parent-Teacher Rating Scale

Conners Preliminary Parent Report

Conners Rating Scale

Conners Rating Scale, Revised

Conners Teacher Preliminary School Report

Conners Teacher Questionnaire (CTQ)

Conners Teacher Rating Scale (CTRS-28)

Contextual Memory Test

Continuous Performance Task

Continuous Performance Test (CPT)

Continuous Visual Memory Test (CVMT)

Continuous Visual Memory Test, Revised

Controlled Oral Word Association test (COWA)

Controlled Substances Act (CSA)

Controlled Word Association Test

Conversational Skills Rating Scale

Cook-Medley Hostility Scale

Coolidge Axis II Inventory

Coolidge Personality and Neuropsychology Inventory for Children

Cooper Assessment for Stuttering Syndromes

Cooperative Primary Test (CPT)

Cooper-Farran Behavioral Rating Scale (CFBRS)
Cooper-MacGuire Diagnostic Word Analysis Test
Coopersmith Self-Esteem Inventories
Coping Inventory for Stressful Situations
Coping Orientations to Problems Experienced (COPE)
Coping Resources Inventory (CRI)
Coping Resources Inventory-Adult and Youth
Coping Resources Inventory for Stress
Coping with Stress Test
COPSystem Interest Inventory
Copy Drawings with Landmarks (CDL)
Corder-Haizlip Child Suicide Checklist
Cornell Critical Thinking Tests
Cornell Critical Thinking Tests, Level X and Level Z
Cornell Depression Scale
Cornell Dysthymia Rating Scale
Cornell Learning and Study Skills Inventory (CLASSI)
Cornell Medical Index
Cornell Scale for Depression in Dementia
Cornell Word Form (CWF)
Correctional Institutions Environment Scale (CIES)
Correctional Institutions Environment Scale, Second Edition
Correctional Officers' Interest Blank
Council for Exceptional Children
Council on Children, Adolescents, and Their Families
Couples Pre-Counseling Inventory
Couples Pre-Counseling Inventory, Revised Edition
Courtship Analysis
Covi Anxiety Scale
Craving Analog Scale
Creative Behavior Inventory
Creative Reasoning Test

Creative Styles Inventory
Creativity Assessment Packet
Creativity Attitude Survey (CAS)
Creativity Checklist
Creativity Tests for Children (CTC)
Cree Questionnaire
Criterion Test of Basic Skills
Critical Reasoning Test (CRT)
Croft Readiness Assessment in Comprehension Kit
Cross-Cultural Adaptability Inventory
Crowley Occupational Interests Blank (COIB)
Crown-Crisp Experiential Index
Crown-Crisp Experiential Inventory
Cues Checklist (CCL)
Cultural Attitude Inventory (CAI)
Cultural Attitude Scale (CAS)
Cultural Literacy Test
Culture Fair Intelligence Test (CFIT)
Culture Shock Inventory
Culture-Free Intelligence Test (CFIT)
Culture-Free Self-Esteem Inventories for Children and Adults
Culture-Free Self-Esteem Inventories, Second Edition (CFSEI-2)
Culture-Free Test
Cumulative Illness Rating Scale
Cumulative Illness Rating Scale-Geriatric
Current and Past Psychopathology Scale (CAPPS)
Curtis Completion Form
Curtis Interest Scale
Cybersex Addition List
D/ART Campaign
DABERON-2: Screening for School Readiness (DABERON-2)
Daily Rating Form (DRF)
Daily Rating Scale (DRS)
Daily Stress Inventory
Dallas Pre-School Screening Test
Dartmouth Assessment of Lifestyle Instrument (DALI)

Das-Naglieri Cognitive Assessment System
Dating Problems Checklist
Davidson Trauma Scale (DTS)
Death Anxiety Scale (DAS)
Death Personification Exercise (DPE)
Decision Making Inventory
Decoding Skills Test
Deductive Reasoning Test
Defense Mechanism Inventory (DMI)
Defense Mechanism Inventory, Revised
Defense Style Questionnaire
Defensive Functioning Scale (DFS)
Defining Issues Test
DeGangi-Berk Test of Sensory Integration
Degrees of Reading Power, Revised
Degrees of Word Meaning
Del Rio Language Screening Test (DRLST)
DeLong Interest Inventory
Dementia Behavior Disturbance Scale
Dementia Mood Assessment Scale (DMAS)
Dementia Rating Scale
Demographic Psychosocial Inventory (DPSI)
Dennis Test of Child Development (DCD)
Denver Articulation Screening Evaluation (DASE)
Denver Articulation Screening Examination Test II
Denver Community Mental Health Questionnaire, Revised
Denver Developmental Screening Test (DDST)
Denver II test
Depression Adjective Checklist (DACL)
Depression and Anxiety in Youth Scale
Depression Questionnaire for Children
Depression Rating Scale

Depression Status Inventory (DSI)
Depressive Experiences Questionnaire (DEQ)
Derogatis Affects Balance Scale, Revised
Derogatis Psychiatric Rating Scale
Derogatis Sexual Functioning Inventory
Derogatis Stress Profile
Description of Body Scale
Descriptive Tests of Language Skills
Descriptive Tests of Mathematics Skills
Desert Storm Trauma Questionnaire
Design Fluency Test
Design Judgment Test
Desire for Death Rating Scale
Detroit Test of Learning Aptitude — Primary, Second Edition (DTLA-P:2)
Detroit Test of Learning Aptitude (DTLA)
Detroit Test of Learning Aptitude, Third Edition (DTLA-3)
Detroit Test of Learning Aptitude, Fourth Edition (DTLA-4)
Detroit Test of Learning Aptitude-Adult (DTLA-A)
Developing Cognitive Abilities Test, Second Edition
Developing Skills Checklist (DSC)
Developmental Activities Screening
Developmental Activities Screening Inventory (DASI)
Developmental Articulation Test (DAT)
Developmental Assessment of Life Experiences (DALE)
Developmental Assessment of Life Experiences [1986 Edition]
Developmental Assessment of the Severely Handicapped
Developmental Assessment of Young Children
Developmental Indicators for Assessment of Learning (DIAL)

Developmental Indicators for Assessment of Learning, Revised/AGS Edition (DIAL-R)

Developmental Indicators for Assessment of Learning, Third Edition

Developmental Observation Checklist System

Developmental Profile II

Developmental Sentence Analysis

Developmental Sentence Scoring Test

Developmental Teaching Objectives and Rating Form, Revised

Developmental Test of Visual Motor Integration (DVMI)

Developmental Test of Visual Perception (DTVP)

Developmental Test of Visual Perception, Second Edition (DTVP-2)

Developmental Test of Visual-Motor Integration, 4th Edition, Revised

Developmental Test of Visual-Motor Integration, Third Edition

Devereux Adolescent Behavior Rating Scale

Devereux Behavior Rating Scale School Form

Devereux Elementary School Behavior Rating Scale II (DESBRS-II)

Devereux Scales of Mental Disorders

Devine Inventory

Diagnostic Achievement Battery, Second Edition (DAB-2)

Diagnostic Achievement Test for Adolescents

Diagnostic Achievement Test for Adolescents, Second Edition

Diagnostic Achievement Test in Spelling

Diagnostic and Statistical Manual of Mental Disorders (DSM)

Diagnostic and Statistical Manual of Mental Disorders-4th Edition (DSM-IV)

Diagnostic and Therapeutic Technology Assessment (DATTA)

Diagnostic Assessment of Reading (DAR)

Diagnostic Checklist for Behavior-Disturbed Children Form E-2

Diagnostic Employability Profile

Diagnostic Interview for Borderline Patients

Diagnostic Interview for Borderlines (DIB)

Diagnostic Interview for Children and Adolescents

Diagnostic Interview for Children and Adolescents, computer version (DICA-IV)

Diagnostic Interview for Children and Adolescents-Child Version (DICA-C)

Diagnostic Interview for Children and Adolescents-Parent Version (DICA-P)

Diagnostic Interview for Children and Adolescents-Revised (DICA-R)

Diagnostic Interview for Genetic Studies (DIGS)

Diagnostic Interview Schedule (DIS)

Diagnostic Interview Schedule for Children

Diagnostic Interview Schedule III

Diagnostic Inventory for Screening Children

Diagnostic Mathematics Inventory (DMI)

Diagnostic Mathematics Profile

Diagnostic Questions for Early or Advanced Alcoholism

Diagnostic Screening Batteries

Diagnostic Skills Battery

Diagnostic Spelling Potential Test

Diagnostic Symptom Questionnaire

Diagnostic Test of Arithmetic Strategies

Diagnostic Tests and Self-Helps in Arithmetic

Dichotomized MMPI Subscale

Differential Ability Scale

Differential Aptitude Tests (DAT)

Differential Aptitude Test for Personnel and Career Assessment

Differential Aptitude Tests, Computerized Adaptive Edition

Differential Aptitude Tests, Fourth Edition

Differential Aptitude Tests, Fifth Edition

Differential Diagnostic Technique

Differential Test of Conduct and Emotional Problems (DT/CEP)

Digit Span Distractibility Test

Digit Symbol Substitution Test (DSST)

Digit Vigilance Test

Digital Finger Tapping Test (DFTT)

Dimensional Assessment of Personality Pathology-Basic Questionnaire (DAPP-BQ)

Dimensions of Delusional Experience Scale

Dimensions of Excellence Scales [1991 Edition]

Dimensions of Self-Concept

Direct Assessment of Functional Status Scale

Directions for Mental Health

Disabled Peoples International

Discourse Comprehension Test

Dissociation Content Scale

Dissociative Disorders Interview Scale

Dissociative Disorders Interview Schedule

Dissociative Experience Scale

Diversity Awareness Profile (DAP)

Diversity Management Survey

Division of Developmental Disabilities (DDD)

Dodd Test of Time Estimation

Dole Vocational Sentence Completion Blank

Domestic Violence Inventory

Doron Driver Analyzer

Dos Amigos Verbal Language Scales

Draw A Person Screening Procedure for Emotional Disturbance (DAP:SPED)

Draw-A-Bicycle Test

Draw-A-Clock-Face Test

Draw-A-Family Test

Draw-A-Flower Test

Draw-A-House Test

Draw-A-Man Test

Draw a Person: A Quantitative Scoring System

Draw-a-Person (DAP)

Draw-A-Person Test

Draw-A-Picture-From-Memory Test

Draw-a-Story: Screening for Depression and Age or Gender Differences, Revised

Driver Risk Inventory (DRI)

Drug Abuse Control Amendments (DACA)

Drug Abuse Resistance Education (DARE)

Drug Enforcement Administration (DEA)

Drug Induced Rape Prevention and Punishment Act

Drug Risk Index

Drug Use Index

Drug Use Questionnaire

Drug-Taking Confidence Questionnaire

Drumcondra Verbal Reasoning Test 1

Duke Religion Index

Duke Severity of Illness Scale

Durrell Analysis of Reading Difficulty: Third Edition

Dyadic Adjustment Scale

Dynamic Personality Inventory (DPI)

Dysfunctional Attitudes Scale (DAS)

Dyslexia Determination Test

Dyslexia Screening Instrument
Dyslexia Screening Survey
Dysphagia Evaluation Protocol
Early Child Development Inventory
Early Childhood Attention Deficit
  Disorders Evaluation Scale
Early Childhood Behavior Scale
Early Childhood Environment Rating
  Scale
Early Childhood Environment Rating
  Scale, Revised Edition
Early Childhood Physical Environment
  Observation Schedules and Rating
  Scales
Early Coping Inventory
Early Development Scale for Preschool
  Children
Early Intervention Developmental Profile
Early Language Milestone Scale
Early Language Milestone Scale,
  Second Edition
Early Language: Assessment and
  Development
Early Mathematics Diagnostic Kit
Early Memories Procedure
Early School Assessment (ESA)
Early School Inventory
Early School Personality Questionnaire
  (ESPQ)
Early Screening Inventory
Early Screening Inventory, Revised
Early Screening Project
Early Social Communication Scale (ESCS)
Early Speech Perception Test (ESP)
Early Years Easy Screen (EYES)
Eating Attitudes Test (EAT)
Eating Disorder Evaluation Scale (EDES)
Eating Disorder Inventory (EDI)
Eating Disorder Inventory for Children
Eating Disorder Inventory, 2nd edition
  (EDI-2)
Eating Disorders Examination (EDE)
Eating Inventory

Ebbinghaus curve of retention test
Ebbinghaus test
Eby Elementary Identification Instrument
Eby Gifted Behavior Index
Edinburgh Articulation Test (EAT)
Edinburgh Handedness Inventory
Edinburgh Picture Test
Edinburgh Postnatal Depression Scale
Edinburgh Questionnaire
Edinburgh Reading Tests
Edinburgh Rehabilitation Status Scale
Educational Administrator
  Effectiveness Profile
Education and Career Exploration
  System (ECES)
Education Apperception Test (EAT)
Educational Development Series [1992
  Edition]
Educational Interest Inventory
Educational Leadership Practices
  Inventory
Educational Process Questionnaire
Educational Testing Service (ETS)
Edwards Personal Preference Schedule
  (EPPS)
Effective Reading Test
Effective School Battery (ESB)
Egan Bus Puzzle Test
Ego Development Scale (EDS)
Ego Function Assessment
Ego State Inventory (ESI)
Ego Strength Test
Egocentricity Index
Ego-Ideal and Conscience Development
  Test (EICDT)
Eidetic Parents Test (EPT)
Eight State Questionnaire
Einstein Assessment of School-Related
  Skills
Ekwall/Shanker Reading Inventory,
  Third Edition
El Senoussi Multiphasic Marital
  Inventory

Elicited Articulatory System Evaluation
Elihorn Maze Test
Elizur Test of Psycho-Organicity: Children and Adults
Embedded Figures Test (EFT)
Emotional and Behavioral Problem Scale
Emotional and Behavioral Checklist
Emotional or Behavior Disorder Scale
Emotional Problems Scales
Emotions Profile Index
Employability Inventory
Employability Maturity Interview
Employee Assistance Program Inventory
Employee Aptitude Survey
Employee Attitude Inventory
Employee Effectiveness Profile
Employee Reliability Inventory (ERI)
Employment Screening Test and Standardization Manual
Employment Values Inventory
Empowerment Inventory
Endeavor Instructional Rating System
Endicott Work Productivity Scale
Endler Multidimensional Anxiety Scale (EMAS)
Engineering and Physical Science Aptitude Test
English as a Second Language Oral Assessment, Revised
English Language Skills Assessment in a Reading Context
English Skills Assessment
Enhanced ACT Assessment
Ennis-Weir Critical Thinking Essay Test
Entrepreneurial Style and Success Indicator
Environment Scale
Environmental Language Inventory (ELI)
Environmental Pre-Language Battery

Environmental Response Inventory (ERI)
EPS Sentence Completion Technique
Epworth Sleepiness Scale
ERB Writing Assessment
Erhardt Developmental Prehension Assessment (EDPA)
Erhardt Developmental Vision Assessment (EDVA)
ETS Tests of Applied Literacy Skills
EuroQol visual analog scale
Evaluating Educational Programs for Intellectually Gifted Students
Evaluating Movement and Posture Disorganization in Dyspraxic Children
Evaluation Disposition Environment
Evaluation of Basic Skills
Everyday Memory Questionnaire
Everyday Worries Scale
Ewing and Roos four-question alcohol screening: cut down, annoyed, guilt, eye-opener (CAGE)
Examining for Aphasia Test
Executive Profile Survey
Exner Comprehensive System
Exner Scoring System
Experiences scale
Experiential World Inventory (EWI)
Expert Consensus Guidelines
Expressive One-Word Picture Vocabulary Tests (EOWPVT)
Expressive One-Word Picture Vocabulary Tests, Revised (EOWPVT-R)
Expressive One-Word Picture Vocabulary Tests, Upper Extension
Expressive & Receptive One-Word Picture Vocabulary Tests, 2000 Edition
Expressive Vocabulary Test
Extended Merrill-Palmer Scale
Extended Personal Attributes Questionnaire (EPAQ)

Extrapyramidal Symptom Rating Scale
Eyberg Child Behavior Inventory
Eysenck Personality Inventory (EPI)
Eysenck Personality Questionnaire (EPQ)
Facial Interpersonal Perception Inventory
Facial Recognition Test
Fagerstrom Nicotine Addiction Scale
Fagerstrom Tolerance Questionnaire
Fairview Language Evaluation Test (FLET)
Family Adaptability and Cohesion Evaluation Scale III (FACES III)
Family Apperception Test (FAT)
Family Aptitudes Questionnaire (FAQ)
Family Assessment Device (FAD)
Family Assessment Form: A Practice-Based Approach to Assessing Family Functioning
Family Assessment Measure Version III
Family Attitudes Questionnaire (FAQ)
Family Attitudes Test (FAT)
Family Day Care Rating Scale
Family Drawing Depression Scale (FDDS)
Family Environment Scale (FES)
Family Environment Scale, Second Edition
Family Environment Scale, Third Edition Manual
Family Evaluation Form (FEF)
Family History Assessment Module
Family History Research Diagnostic Criteria (FH-RDC)
Family Inventory of Life Events and Changes (FILE)
Family Psychosocial Screening
Family Relations Test (FRT)
Family Relations Test, Children's Version
Family Relationship Inventory
Family Risk Scale
Family Satisfaction Scale
Family Tracking System

Famous Sayings Test
Famous Writers Aptitude Test
Fast Health Knowledge Test, 1986 Revision
Fatigue Questionnaire
Fazekas Scale
Fear Questionnaire
Fear Questionnaire of Marks and Matthews
Fear Survey Schedule (FSS)
Federation of Families for Children's Mental Health
Feeding and Eating Disorders of Infancy or Early Childhood
Feelings, Attitudes, and Behaviors Scale for Children
Fels Parent Behavior Rating Scale
Fer-Will Object Kit
Figurative Language Interpretation Test (FLIT)
Filipino Work Values Scale
Filtered Audiometer Speech Test (FAST)
Finckh test
Finger Localization Test
Finger Oscillation Test
Firestone Assessment of Self-Destructive Thoughts
FIRO (Fundamental Interpersonal Relations Orientation) Awareness Scale
FirstSTEP: Screening Test for Evaluating Preschoolers
First Words and First Sentences Test
Fisher-Logemann Test of Articulation Competence (FLTAC)
Five-Minute Speech Sample (FMSS)
Five-Minute Verbal Sampling Test
Five Ps: Parent Professional Preschool Performance Profile
Five Ps: Parent Professional Preschool Performance Profile, Revised
Fixity of Beliefs Scale

Flanagan Aptitude Classification Test (FACT)

Flanagan Industrial Test (FIT)

Fleishman Job Analysis Survey (F-JAS)

Flight Aptitude Rating (FAR)

Flint Infant Security Scale (FISS)

Florida Kindergarten Screening Battery

Flowers Auditory Test of Selective Attention (FATSA)

Fluharty Preschool Speech and Language Screening Test

Follow-up Drinker Profile

Folstein Mini-Mental Scale

Folstein Mini-Mental Status Examination

Food Choice Inventory

Forer Structured Sentence Completion Test

Forms for Behavior Analysis with Children

Foster Mazes

Four Factor Index

Four Picture Test

Four Factor Theory of Etiology

Fournier test

Franck Drawing Completion Test (FDCT)

Frankfurt Complaint Questionnaire (FCQ)

Freedom from Distractibility Deviation Quotient (FDDQ)

Freeman Anxiety Neurosis and Psychosomatic Test (FANPT)

Freiburger Personality Inventory (FPI)

Frenchay Activities Index

Frenchay Aphasia Screening Test (FAST)

Frenchay Dysarthria Assessment

Friedman Well-Being Scale

Frost Self-Description Questionnaire (FSDQ)

Frostig Developmental Test of Visual Perception (FDTVP)

Frostig Movement Skills Test Battery (FMSTB)

Fuld Object Memory Test

Fuld Object-Memory Evaluation

Full Range Picture Vocabulary Test

Full Scale Broad Cognitive Ability

Full-Scale intelligence quotient (FIQ, FSIQ)

Fullerton Language Test for Adolescents

Fullerton Language Test for Adolescents, Second Edition

Full Scale Score Total (FSST)

Functional Ambulation Categories

Functional Assessment Inventory

Functional Communication Profile (FCP)

Functional Fitness Assessment for Adults over 60 Years

Functional Life Scale (FLS)

Functional Limitation Profile

Functional Linguistic Communication Inventory

Functional Needs Assessment (FNA)

Functional Performance Record (FPR)

Functional Status Index (FSI)

Functional Status Questionnaire (FSQ)

Functional Systems Scale (FSS)

Functional Time Estimation Questionnaire (FTEQ)

Fundamental Achievement Series

Fundamental Interpersonal Relations Orientation-Behavior (FIRO-B)

Fundamental Interpersonal Relations Orientation-Feelings (FIRO-F)

Funkenstein test

Galveston Orientation and Awareness Test (GOAT)

Gamblers Anonymous 20 Questions

Gambling Symptom Assessment Scale (G-SAS)

GAP Reading Comprehension Test, Third Edition

Gardner Analysis of Personality Survey (GAP)
GARF scale
Gastrointestinal Symptom Rating Scale
Gates-MacGinitie Reading Tests
Gates-MacGinitie Reading Tests, Third Edition
Gates-McKillop-Horowitz Reading Diagnostic Test
Gates-McKillop-Horowitz Reading Diagnostic Test, Second Edition
General Ability Measure for Adults
General Aptitude Test Battery (GATB)
General Aptitude Test Battery, Canadian Edition
General Clerical Test (GCT)
General Cognitive Index (GCI)
General Health Questionnaire (GHQ)
General High Altitude Questionnaire (GHAQ)
General Processing Inventory
General Well-Being Index
Generalized Contentment Scale (GCS)
George Washington University Series
Geriatric Depression Scale
Gerontological Apperception Test (GAT)
Gesell Child Development Age Scale (GCDAS)
Gesell Developmental Schedule
Gesell Infant Scale
Gesell Preschool Test
Gesell School Readiness Test
G-F-W Battery
Gibson Spiral Maze, Second Edition
Gifted and Talented Scale
Gifted and Talented Screening Form
Gifted Evaluation Scale (GES)
Gifted Evaluation Scale, Second Edition
Gifted Program Evaluation Survey
Gilliam Autism Rating Scale
Glasgow Assessment Schedule
Glasgow Coma Scale (GCS)

Global Assessment of Functioning Scale (GAF)
Global Assessment of Relational Functioning Scale (GARF)
Global Assessment Scale (GAS)
Global Clinical Judgments Scale
Global Deterioration Scale
Global Obsessive Compulsive Scale
Global Severity Index (GSI)
Global Sexual Satisfaction Index (GSSI)
Global Tic Rating Score
Global Ward Behavior Scale (GWBS)
Goal Attainment Scale (GAS)
GOALS: A Performance-Based Measure of Achievement
Goldberg Index
Goldman-Fristoe Test of Articulation (G-FTA)
Goldman-Fristoe-Woodcock Auditory Skills Test Battery
Goldman-Fristoe-Woodcock Test
Goldscheider test
Goldstein-Scheerer Cube Test (The)
Goldstein-Scheerer Tests of Abstract and Concrete Thinking
Golombok Rust Inventory of Sexual Satisfaction
Golombok-Rust Inventory of Marital State (GRIMS)
Good and evil test
Goodenough Animal Test
Goodenough Draw-A-Man Test
Goodenough Draw-A-Person Test
Goodenough-Harris Drawing Test
Goodenough Intelligence Test
Goodman Lock Box
Gordon Diagnostic System Test
Gordon Occupational Checklist-II (GOCL-II)
Gordon Personal Inventory (GPI)
Gordon Personal Profile Inventory (GPPI)
Gottfries-Brane-Steen Rating Scale for Dementia

Gottschalk-Gelser Content Analysis Scales

Graded Naming Test

Graded Word Spelling Test

Graduate and Managerial Assessment

Graduate Record Examination (GRE)

Graduate Record Examination Aptitude Test (GREAT)

Grammar Language Quotient

Grandparent Strengths and Needs Inventory

Grassi Basic Cognitive Evaluation (GBCE)

Grassi Block Substitution Test

Gray Oral Reading Test (GORT)

Gray Oral Reading Test, Third Edition (GORT-3)

Gray Oral Reading Tests, Diagnostic

Gregorc Style Delineator

G Response including entire inkblot

Grid Test of Schizophrenic Thought Disorder (GTSTD)

Grief Experience Inventory (GEI)

Grief Measurement Scale

Grooved Pegboard Test

Group Achievement Identification Measure

Group Diagnostic Reading Aptitude and Achievement Tests, Intermediate Form

Group Embedded Figures Test (GEFT)

Group Encounter Scale (GES)

Group Encounter Survey

Group Environment Scale (GES)

Group Environment Scale, Second Edition

Group Inventory for Finding Creative Talent

Group Literacy Assessment

Group Mathematics Test, Second Edition

Group Reading Test (GRT)

Group Reading Test, Fourth Edition

Group Styles Inventory (GSI)

Group Tests of Musical Ability

Guidance Centre Classroom Achievement Tests

Guide to the Assessment of Test Session Behavior for the WISC-III and the WIAT

Guidelines for Adolescent Preventive Services (GAPS)

Guilford-Zimmerman Aptitude Survey (GZAS)

Guilford-Zimmerman Interest Inventory (GZII)

Guilford-Zimmerman Personality Test (GZPT)

Guilford-Zimmerman Temperament Survey (GZTS)

Hachinski Ischemia Scale

Hahnemann Elementary School Behavior Rating Scale

Hahnemann High School Behavior Rating Scale

Hall Occupational Orientation Inventory (HOOI)

Hall-Tonna Inventory of Values

Halstead and Reitan Batteries

Halstead Aphasia Test (HAT)

Halstead Category Test

Halstead Impairment Index

Halstead Modified Technique

Halstead-Russell Neuropsychological Evaluation System (HRNES)

Halstead-Reitan Battery (HRB)

Halstead-Reitan category subtest

Halstead-Reitan Neurological Battery and Allied Procedures

Halstead-Reitan Neuropsychological Test Battery (HRNTB)

Halstead-Wepman Aphasia Screening Test

Hamburg Obsession-Compulsion Inventory

Hamburg Obsessional-Compulsion Inventory-Short Form

Hamburg-Wechsler Intelligence Test for Children (HAWIC)

Hamilton Anxiety Rating Scale (HARS)

Hamilton Depression Inventory

Hamilton Depression Rating Scale (HDRS)

Hamilton Depression Scale (HAM-D)

Hamilton Depression Score

Hamilton Rating Scale for Anxiety (HAM-A)

Hammill Multiability Achievement Test

Hammill Multiability Intelligence Test (HAMIT)

Hand Test, Revised

Hand Test, Revised 1983

Handedness Questionnaire

Hanfmann-Kasanin Concept Formation Test

Haptic Intelligence Scale (HIS)

Harding Stress-Fair Compatibility Test

Hare Psychopathy Checklist, Revised

Hare Psychopathy Checklist: Screening Version

Harrington-O'Shea Career Decision-Making System, Revised

Harris Tests of Lateral Dominance

Harris-Lingoes Subscales—MMPI

Harrison Antinarcotic Act

Harter Self-Perception Profile for Children

Harvard Group Scale of Hypnotic Susceptibility (HGSHS)

Hassles and Uplifts Scales, Research Edition

Hausa Speaking Test

Hawaii Early Learning Profile Checklist

Haws Screening Test for Functional Articulation Disorders

Hay Aptitude Test Battery

Hay Aptitude Test Battery, Revised

Hazelden Family Guide

Health and Daily Living

Health Assessment Questionnaire (HAQ)

Health Attribution Test

Health Behavior Scale (HBS)

Health Care Questionnaire

Health Problems Checklist

Health Systems Agency (under A-Z)

Healy Pictorial Completion Test

Hearing Measurement Scale

Hebrew Speaking Test

Hebrew University Depression Database Questionnaire (HUDD-Q)

HELP Checklist

Henderson-Moriarty ESL/Literacy Placement Test

Henmon-Nelson Ability Test, Canadian Edition

Henmon-Nelson Tests of Mental Ability (The)

Hereford Parental Attitude Survey (HPA)

Herrmann Brain Dominance Instrument

Herrmann Brain Dominance Instrument, Revised

Hess School Readiness Scale (HSRS)

Heston Personality Index (HPI)

Heterosexual Attitudes Toward Homosexuality (HATH)

High School Career-Course Planner (HSCCP)

High School Personality Questionnaire (HSPQ)

High School Subject Test

High/Scope Child Observation Record for Ages 2½-6

Hill Interaction Matrix (HIM)

Hill Performance Test of Selected Positional Concepts

Hillside Akathisia Scale

Hilson Adolescent Profile

Hilson Personnel Profile/Success Quotient (HPP/SQ)

Hiskey-Nebraska Test of Learning Aptitude (HNTLA)
HIV Risk Assessment Battery
Hodder Group Reading Tests
Hodkinson Mental Test (HMT)
Hogan Development Survey
Hogan Personality Inventory
Hogan Personality Inventory, Revised
Hogan Personnel Selection Series
Hoge 10-Item Intrinsic Religiosity Scale
Holden Psychological Screening Inventory
Hollingshead-Redlich scale
Holmes-Rahe questionnaire
Holtzman Inkblot Technique (HIT)
Home Environment Questionnaire
Home Observation for Measurement of the Environment
Home School Situations Questionnaire-Revised
Home Screening Questionnaire
Hooper Visual Organization Test
Hopelessness Scale
Hopkins Symptom Checklist (HSCL)
Hopkins Symptom Checklist-90 (HSCL-90)
Hopkins Verbal Learning Test (HVLT)
Horn Art Aptitude Inventory
Horn-Hellersberg Drawing Completion Test
Hospital Anxiety and Depression Scale (HADS)
Hostility and Direction of Hostility Questionnaire (HDHQ)
House-Tree-Person and Draw-A-Person as Measures of Abuse in Children: A Quantitative Scoring System
House-Tree-Person Technique
House-Tree-Person Test
House-Tree Test (HT)
Houston Test for Language Development

Houston Test for Language Development, Revised
How a Child Learns
How Supervise?
Howell Prekindergarten Screening Test
How-I-See-Myself Scale (HISMS)
Human Figure Drawing (HFD)
Human Information Processing Survey
Hundred Pictures Naming Test (HPNT)
Hunt-Minnesota Test for Organic Brain Damage
Hutchins Behavior Inventory (HBI)
Hymovich Chronicity Impact and Coping Instrument (CICI)
Hypnotic Induction Profile (HIP)
I.P.I Aptitude-Intelligence Test Series
IDEA Oral Language Proficiency Test II
I-E Scale of Rotter
Illinois Children's Language Assessment Test
Illinois Test of Psycholinguistic Ability (ITPA)
Illness and Symptom History Schedule
Illness Behavior Checklist (IBC)
Illness Behavior Questionnaire (IBQ)
Imagined Process Inventory (IPI)
Impact Message Inventory (IMI)
Impact of Events Scale (IES)
Impairment Rating Score
Improving Writing, Thinking and Reading Skills test
Impulsive Nonconformity Scale
Inattention/Overactivity With Aggression Conners scale
incomplete pictures test
incomplete sentence blank test
Incomplete Sentences Survey
Incomplete Sentences Task
Independent Living Behavior Checklist
Index of Adjustment and Values
Index of Potential Suicide
Index of Primitive Thought

Index of Spouse Abuse
Index of Well-Being (IWB)
Index of Work Satisfaction (IWS)
indirect survey
Individual Career Exploration (ICE)
Individual Learning Disabilities
    Classroom Screening Instrument
    (ILDCSI)
Individualized Criterion Reference
    Testing Mathematics (ICRTM)
Individualized Criterion Reference
    Testing Reading (ICRTR)
Individualized Criterion Referenced
    Testing (ICRT)
Infant Behavior Questionnaire
Infant Reading Test
Infant/Toddler Environment Rating
    Scale (ITERS)
Informal Reading Comprehension
    Placement Test
Injury Severity Score (ISS)
inkblot test (IBT)
Inpatient Multidimensional Psychiatric
    Scale (IMPS)
Insight and Treatment Attitudes
    Questionnaire (ITAQ)
Insight to Treatment Questionnaire
Institute for Behavioral Genetics
Institute for Behavioral Healthcare
Institute of Educational Research Test
Institute of Personality and Ability
    Testing (IPAT)
Institutional Functioning Inventory
    (IFI)
Institutional Goals Inventory (IGI)
Instructional Leadership Evaluation and
    Development Program (ILEAD)
Instructional Leadership Inventory
Instrument Timbre Preference Test
Integrated Assessment System (IAS)
Integrated Child Development scheme
    (ICDS)
Integration Test

intelligence quotient (IQ)
intelligence test
interest checklist
Interest Determination, Exploration and
    Assessment System, Enhanced
    Version
interest survey
Intermediate Booklet Category Test
Intermediate Personality Questionnaire
    (IPQ)
Internal State Scale (ISS)
International Personality Disorder
    Examination (IPDE)
International Pilot Study of
    Schizophrenia (IPSS)
International Primary Factors (IPF)
International Primary Factors Test
    Battery
International Test for Aphasia
International Version of the Mental
    Status Questionnaire
Interpersonal Behavior Survey (IBS)
Interpersonal Communication Inventory
    (ICI)
Interpersonal Language Skills and
    Assessment (ILSA)
Interpersonal Perception Scale (IPS)
Interpersonal Reaction Test (IPRT)
Interpersonal Style Inventory
Inter-Person Perception Test (IPPT)
interviewer-administered self-report
    questionnaire
Intimacy Potential Quotient (IPQ)
Intra- and Interpersonal Relations Scale
intracorporeal pharmacological testing
Intrex Questionnaire
Inventory for Counseling and
    Development (ICD)
Inventory of Anger Communication
    (IAC)
Inventory of Complicated Grief
Inventory of Individually Perceived
    Group Cohesiveness

Inventory of Peer Influence on Eating Concern

Inventory of Perceptual Skills (IPS)

Inventory of Psychosocial Development (IPD)

Inventory of Suicidal Orientation-30 (ISO-30)

Inventory to Diagnose Depression

Inwald Personality Inventory (IPI)

Iowa Algebra Aptitude Test (IAAT)

Iowa Conners Rating Scale

Iowa Pressure Articulation Test (IPAT)

Iowa Structured Psychiatric Interview (IPSI)

Iowa Stuttering Scale

Iowa Tests of Basic Skills

Iowa Tests of Educational Development, Forms X-8 and Y-8

IPAT Anxiety Scale

IPAT Depression Scale

IPF Test Battery

Irish Study of High-Density Schizophrenia Families

Irresistible Impulse Test

Irritability/Depression and Anxiety Scale

It Scale for Children (ITSC)

Item Counseling Evaluation Test

48-Item Counseling Evaluation Test (ICET)

15-Item Memorization Test

Jackson Evaluation System

Jackson Personality Inventory (JPI)

Jackson Vocational Interest Survey

Jail Suicide Assessment Tool (JSAT)

James Language Dominance Test

Jansky Screening Index (JSI)

Jarman Underprivileged Area

Jenkins Activity Survey (JAS)

Jenkins Non-Verbal Test

Jesness Behavior Checklist (JBC)

Jesness Inventory (JI)

Jette Functional Status Index

Jevs Work Sample Battery

Job Attitude Scale (JAS)

Job Description Index (JDI)

Job Seeking Skills Assessment

Johns Hopkins Functioning Inventory

Johnson-Kenney Screening Test (JKST)

Johnston Informal Reading Inventory (JIRI)

Joint Commission on Mental Health of Children (JCMHC)

Joint Commission on Mental Illness and Mental Health

Jordan Left-Right Reversal Test (JLRRT)

Joseph Pre-School and Primary Self-Concept Screening Test

Jourad Self-Disclosure Questionnaire (JSDQ)

Judgment of Occupational Behavior-Orientation

Jung association test

Junior Eysenck Personality Inventory (JEPI)

Kahn Intelligence Test (KIT)

Kahn Test of Symbol Arrangement (The) (KTSA)

Kaiser-Meyer-Olkin Measure

Karolinska Scales of Personality

Kasanin-Hanfmann Concept Formation Test

Katz Adjustment Scale (KAS)

Katz ADL Index

Kaufman Adolescent and Adult Intelligence Test (KAIT)

Kaufman Assessment Battery for Children (K-ABC)

Kaufman Brief Intelligence Test (K-BIT)

Kaufman Development Scale

Kaufman Infant and Preschool Scale

Kaufman Survey of Early Academic and Language Skills (K-SEALS)

Kaufman Test of Educational Achievement

K-corrected raw score
Keirsey Temperament sorter
Kendrick Cognitive Tests for the
  Elderly
Kenny Self-Care Evaluation
Kent E-G-Y Test
Kent Infant Development Scale
Kent-Rosanoff Test
Kent Series of Emergency Skills
KeyMath Revised: A Diagnostic
  Inventory of Essential Mathematics
Khatena-Torrance Creative Perception
  Inventory
Kindergarten Auditory Screening Test
  (KAST)
Kindergarten Language Screening Test
  (KLST)
Kindergarten Readiness Test (KRT)
Kinetic Family Drawing (KFD)
Knowledge of Occupations Test (KOT)
Knox Cube Test
Kohnstamm Test
Kohs Block Design Test
Kolbe Conative Index (KCI)
Koppitz Scoring System for Organicity
Kuder General Interest Survey, Form E
Kuder Occupational Interest Survey
Kuder Preference Record
Kuder Preference Record-Vocational
  (KPR-V)
Kuhlman-Anderson Intelligence Tests
Lambeth Disability Screening
  Questionnaire
Language Modalities Test for Aphasia
  (LMTA)
Language Processing Test
Language Sampling, Analysis and
  Training
Language Screening Test
Language-Structured Auditory
  Retention Span (LARS)
Laterality Preference Schedule
Leader Behavior Analysis II (LBAII)

Leader Behavior Description
  Questionnaire (LBDQ)
Leadership Ability Evaluation
Leadership Evaluation and Department
  Scale
Leadership Evaluation and
  Development Scale (LEADS)
Leadership Opinion Questionnaire
  (LOQ)
Leadership Practices Inventory (LPI)
Leadership Skills Inventory
Learning Accomplishment Profile
Learning and Study Strategies
  Inventory (LASSI)
Learning Disability Evaluation Scale
  (LDES)
Learning Disability Rating Procedure
Learning Efficiency Test-II (LET-II)
Learning Inventory of Kindergarten
  Experiences (LIKE)
Learning Style Profile (LSP)
Learning Styles Inventory
Least Preferred Coworker Score
Leatherman Leadership Questionnaire
  (LLQ)
Leeds Anxiety Scale
Leeds Scales for the Self-Assessment of
  Anxiety and Depression
Lehman Quality of Life Interview
Leisure Activities Blank (LAB)
Leisure Diagnostic Battery
Leisure Interest Inventory (LII)
Leiter Adult Intelligence Scale (LAIS)
Leiter International Performance Scale-
  Revised (LIPS-R)
Leiter Recidivism Scale
"Let's Talk" Inventory for Adolescents
Level of Functioning Scale
Levine-Pilowsky Depression
  Questionnaire
Levy Draw-and-Tell-a-Story Technique
Leyton Obsessive Inventory (LOI)
Liebowitz Social Anxiety Scale (LSAS)

Life Change Rating Scale
Life Event Scale Adolescents
Life Event Scale Children
Life Experiences Checklist (LEC)
Life Experience Survey (LES)
Life History of Aggression
    Assessment
Life Interpersonal History Enquiry
    (LIPHE)
Life Satisfaction Index (LSI)
Life Skills, Forms 1 & 2
Life Skills Program
Life Skills Profile
Life Skills Profile Index
Life Span Study
Life Study Sample (LSS)
Likert scale
Limon Self-Image Assessment
Lincoln-Oseretsky Motor Performance
    Test (LOMPT)
Lindamood Auditory Conceptualization
    Test (LACT)
Linguistic Analysis and Remediation
    Procedure
Linguistic Analysis of Speech Samples
    (LASS)
Listening Comprehension Test (LCT)
Lock Wallace Short Marital Adjustment
    Scale
Locus of Control of Behavior Scale
Loevinger's Washington University
    Sentence Completion Test
Lollipop Test: A Diagnostic Screening
    Test of School Readiness
Lombard voice-reflex test
London Psychogeriatric Scale (LPS)
Longitudinal Interval Follow-up
    Evaluation
Lorge-Thorndike Cognitive Abilities
    Test
Lorge-Thorndike Intelligence Test
Lorr Scale
LOTE Reading and Listening Test

Louisville Behavior Checklist
Luborsky Health-Sickness Rating
    Scale
Luria test
Luria-Nebraska Neuropsychological
    Battery (LNNB)
Luria's Neuropsychological
    Investigation
Maastricht History and Advice
    Checklist-Revised (MAAS-R)
Maastricht Interview for Vital
    Exhaustion
MacAndrew Addiction Scale (MAS)
MacArthur
MacArthur Competence Assessment
    Tool (Mac-CAT)
MacArthur Competence Assessment
    Tool-Proxy (Mac-CAT-P)
MacArthur Perceived Coercion Scale
Mach Scale
Machover Draw-A-Person Test
    (MDAP)
Macmillan Graded Word Reading Test
MacQuarrie Test for Mechanical
    Ability
Major Role Adjustment Scale II
Major Symptoms of Schizophrenia
    Scale
Make-a-Picture Story
Management Appraisal Survey (MAS)
Management Development Profile
Management Inventory on Leadership,
    Motivation and Decision-Making
    (MILMD)
Management Philosophies Scale
Management Philosophies Scale (I-V)
    (MPS)
Management Position Analysis Test
Management Readiness Profile
Management Styles Inventory
Management Transactions Audit
    (MTA)
Manager Profile Record

Managerial Style Questionnaire (MSQ)

Mandel Social Adjustment Scale (MSAS)

Mandsley Personality Inventory (MPI)

Mania "9" Scale

Mania Rating Scale (MRS)

Manic-State Rating Scale

Manifest Anxiety Scale (MAS)

Manipulative Aptitude Test (MAT)

Mann-Whitney U Test

Mantel-Haenszel Test for Linear Trend

Marital Attitudes Evaluation (MATE)

Marital Communication Scale

Marital Satisfaction Inventory

Marital Satisfaction Scale (MSS)

Marks-Sheehan Phobia Scale

Marlowe-Crowne Scale (MCS)

Marlowe-Crowne Scale of Social Desirability

Marriage Adjustment Inventory (MAI)

Marriage and Family Attitude Survey

Marriage Skills Analysis (MSA)

Martin Suicide-Depression Inventory (MSDI)

Martinez Assessment of the Basic Skills

Maryland Parent Attitude Survey

Maslach Burnout Inventory (MBI)

Massachusetts Gambling Screen (MAGS)

Matching Familiar Figures Test (MFFT)

Maternal Attitude Scale (MAS)

Maternal Trait Anxiety Score (MTAS)

Mathematics Anxiety Rating Scale (MARS)

Mathematics Anxiety Rating Scale-Adolescents (MARS-A)

Matrix Analogies Test

Mattis Dementia Rating Scale

Mattis Organic Mental Status Syndrome Examination (MOMSSE)

Mattis-Kovner Scale

Maudsley Obsessional Compulsive Inventory (MOCI)

Maudsley Personality Inventory (MPI)

Maxfield-Buchholz Social Maturity Scale for Blind Preschool Children

McAndrew Addiction Scale

McAndrew Alcoholism Scale (MAC)

McAndrew Alcoholism Scale, Revised

McCarthy Scales of Children's Ability (MCSA)

McCarthy Screening Test

McGill Pain Assessment Questionnaire (MPAQ)

McGill Pain Questionnaire

McMaster Family Assessment Device

McMaster Health Index Questionnaire

McMaster Structured Interview of Family Functioning

Measurement of Language Development

Measures of Musical Ability

Measure of Parental Style

Measures of Psychosocial Development (MPD)

Medical Investigation of Neurodevelopmental Disorders (MIND)

Medical Outcomes Study Short Form-36

Medical Outcomes Study Short-Form General Health Survey Physical Functioning Scale

Meeting Street School Screening Test (MSSST)

Meffill-Palmer Scale

Meier Art Judgment Test (The)

Memorial Symptom Assessment Scale

Memory Assessment Scales (MAS)

Memory-for-Designs Test

Menstrual Distress Questionnaire (MDQ)

Mental Alteration Test (MAT)

Mental Deterioration Battery (MDB)

Mental Illness Needs Index (MINI)

Mental Measurements Yearbook (MMY)

Mental Status Questionnaire (MSQ)

Merrill-Palmer Scale

Merrill-Palmer Scale of Mental Tests (MPSMT)

Mertens Visual Perception Test (MVPT)

Methamphetamine Experience Questionnaire

Methodology for Epidemiology in Children and Adolescents (MECA)

Metropolitan Achievement Test (MAT)

Metropolitan Achievement Test, Seventh Edition (MAT7)

Metropolitan Language Instructional Test

Metropolitan Readiness Tests (MRT)

Meyer-Kendall Assessment Survey (MKAS)

Michigan Alcoholism Screening Test (MAST)

Michigan Alcoholism Screening Instrument-Geriatric Version (MASI-GV)

Michigan English Language Assessment Battery

Michigan Picture Inventory

Michigan Picture Stories

Michigan Picture Test (MPT)

Michigan Picture Test-Revised (MPT-R)

Michigan Screening Profile of Parenting

Michigan Vocabulary Profile Test

Military Environment Inventory

Mill Hill Vocabulary Scale

Miller Analogies Test (MAT)

Miller Assessment for Preschoolers

Miller-Yoder Language Comprehension Test

Millon Adolescent Clinical Inventory (MACI)

Millon Adolescent Personality Inventory (MAPI)

Millon Behavioral Health Inventory (MBHI)

Millon Clinical Multiaxial Inventory (MCMI)

Millon Clinical Multiaxial Inventory II (MCMI-II)

Milwaukee Academic Interest Inventory (MAII)

Mini International Neuropsychiatric Interview

Mini Inventory of Right Brain Injury (MIRBI)

Mini-Mental State Examination (MMSE)

Minimum Essentials Test (MET)

Minnesota Child Development Inventory (MCDI)

Minnesota Clerical Aptitude Test

Minnesota Clerical Assessment Battery (MCAB)

Minnesota Clerical Test (MCT)

Minnesota Cocaine Craving Scale (MCCS)

Minnesota Differential Diagnosis of Aphasia (MDDA)

Minnesota Engineering Analogies Test (MEAT)

Minnesota Importance Questionnaire (MIQ)

Minnesota Impulsive Disorder Interview Model for Compulsive Buying

Minnesota Impulsive Disorders Interview

Minnesota Infant Development Inventory

Minnesota Job Description Questionnaire (MJDQ)

Minnesota Mechanical Assembly Test (MMAT)

Minnesota Multiphasic Personality Inventory (MMPI)

Minnesota Multiphasic Personality Inventory, Adolescent (MMPI-A)

Minnesota Multiphasic Personality Inventory, Second Edition (MMPI-2)

Minnesota Occupational Classification System (MOCS-III)

Minnesota Paper Form Board Test (MPFBT)

Minnesota Percepto-Diagnostic Test (MPDT)

Minnesota Preschool Scale

Minnesota Rate of Manipulation Test

Minnesota Satisfaction Questionnaire (MSQ)

Minnesota Satisfaction Scale (MSS)

Minnesota Scholastic Aptitude Test (MSAT)

Minnesota Spatial Relations Test (MSRT)

Minnesota Speed of Reading Test for College Students

Minnesota Teacher Attitude Inventory (MTAI)

Minnesota Test for the Differential Diagnosis of Aphasia (MTDDA)

Minnesota Twin Family Study

Minnesota Vocational Interest Inventory (MVII)

Minnesota-Hartford Personality Assay (MHPA)

Miskimins Self-Goal-Other Discrepancy Scale

Mississippi Scale for Combat-Related Posttraumatic Stress Disorder

Missouri Auditory Learning Test

Missouri Children's Picture Series (MCPS)

Missouri Kindergarten Inventory of Developmental Skills

Modern Language Aptitude Test

Missouri Occupational Card Sort

Modern Occupational Skills Test (MOST)

Modified Autonomic Perception Questionnaire

Modified Health Assessment Questionnaire (MHAQ)

Modified Simpson-Angus Rating Scale

Modified Simpson Dyskinesia Scale

Modified Vigotsky Concept Formation Test

Modified Word Learning Test (MWLT)

Monitoring Basic Skills Progress (MBSP)

Monotic Word Memory Test (MWMT)

Montgomery-Asberg Depression Rating Scale (MADRS)

Mood and Physical Symptoms Scale (MPSS)

Mood Disorder Questionnaire

Mooney Faces Closure Test

Mooney Problem Checklist (MPCL)

Mooney Test

Moos Family Environment Scale

Moos Menstrual Distress Questionnaire (MMDQ)

Morbid Anxiety Inventory (MAI)

Morgan-Russell scale

Mosaic Test

Mother-Child Relationship Evaluation (MCRE)

Mother/Infant Communication Screening (MICS)

Mother's Assessment of the Behavior of Her Infant (MABI)

Motivation Analysis Test (MAT)

Motivational Patterns Inventory

Motor Impersistence Test (MIT)

Motor Steadiness Battery

Motor-Free Visual Perception Test (MVPT)

Movement Disorder Questionnaire

Movement Scale

Mullen Scales of Early Learning (MSEL)

Multiaxial Evaluation Report Form

Multidimensional Aptitude Battery

Multidimensional Assessment of Gains in School (MAGS)

Multidimensional Assessment of Philosophy of Education (MAPE)

Multidimensional Pain Inventory (MPI)
Multidimensional Perfectionism Scale
Multidimensional Scale for Rating
  Psychiatric Patients (MSRPP)
Multidimensional Self Concept Scale
  (MSCS)
Multifactor Leadership Questionnaire
  (MLQ)
Multilevel Informal Language Inventory
Multilingual Aphasia Examination
  (MAE)
Multiphasic Environmental Assessment
  Procedure (MEAP)
Multiphasic Personality Inventory (MPI)
Multiple Affect Adjective Checklist
  (MAACL)
Multiple Aptitude Test
Multiple Sleep Latency Test (MSLT)
Multiscore Depression Inventory (MDI)
Multivariate Personality Inventory (MPI)
Murphy-Meisgeier Type Indicator for
  Children (MMTIC)
Music Achievement Test (1–4) (MAT)
Musical Aptitude Profile (MAP)
Myers-Briggs Type Indicator (MBTI)
Myokinetic Psychodiagnosis Test
Names Learning Test (NLT)
Narcotic Addict Treatment Act
National Adult Reading Test (NART)
National Alliance for Research on
  Schizophrenia and Depression
  (NARSAD)
National Alliance for the Mentally Ill
  (NAMI)
National Association for Children of
  Alcoholics
National Association of Alcoholism and
  Drug Abuse Counselors
National Association of Children of
  Alcoholics
National Association of State Mental
  Health Program Directors (NASMHPD)

National Association of State Mental
  Health Program Directors Research
  Institute
National Attention Test (NAT)
National Educational Development Test
National Institute of Mental Health
  Diagnostic—Interval Schedule
National Institute of Mental Health
  Work Group on Culture, Diagnosis,
  and Care
National Institute of Mental Health-
  Global Obsessive Compulsive Scale
  (NIMH-OC)
National Occupation Competency
  Testing (NOCT)
National Police Officer Selection Test
  (POST)
Natural Process Analysis
Naylor-Harwood Adult Intelligence
  Scale (NHAIS)
Naylor-Harwood Intelligence Scale
  (NHIS)
need-a-sentence test
Need for Cognition Scale
needs-assessment survey
NEO (neuroticism, extroversion,
  openness to experience) Personality
  Inventory-Revised (NEO PI-R)
NEO Five-Factor Inventory
Neonatal Behavioral Assessment Scale
  (NBAS)
Neonatal Behavioral Assessment Scale
  with Kansas Supplements (NBAS-K)
NEO Personality Inventory–Revised
NEO personality questionnaire
Neurobehavioral Cognitive Status
  Examination
Neurological Dysfunctions of Children
Neuropsychiatric Inventory (NPI)
Neuropsychiatric Inventory/nursing
  home version (NPI/NH)
Neuropsychiatric Rating Schedule

Neuropsychological Screening
Examination
Neuropsychological Status Examination
Neurotic Personality Factor Test (NPFT)
Neuroticism Scale Questionnaire (NSQ)
Neuroticism-Extroversion-Openness to
Experience Personality Questionnaire
Neuroticism-Extroversion-Openness
Personality Inventory
New Haven Schizophrenia Index
New Jersey Test of Reasoning Skills
New Mexico Attitude Toward Work
Test (NMATWT)
New Mexico Career Planning Test
(NMCPT)
New Mexico Job Application
Procedures Test (NMJAPT)
New Mexico Knowledge of
Occupations Test (NMKOT)
New Sucher-Allred Reading Placement
Inventory
New York University Parkinson
Disease Scale
NIH Stroke Scale
NIMH Global Obsessive-Compulsive
Scale
Non-Language Learning Test
Non-Language Multi-Mental Test
Non-Reading Aptitude Test Battery
(NATB)
Non-Reading Intelligence Test, Levels
1–3 (NRIT)
Nonverbal Ability Test (NAT)
Normative Adaptive Behavior Checklist
Norris Educational Achievement Test
(NEAT)
North American Adult Reading Test
(NAART)
North American Association for the Study
of Obesity (NAASO) (under A-Z)
North American Depression Inventories
for Children and Adults

Northwestern Syntax Screening Test
(NSST)
Northwestern University Children's
Perception of Speech Test
Northwick Park Index of Independence
in ADL
Nottingham Extended ADL Index
Nottingham Health Profile
Nottingham Ten-Point ADL Scale
Numeracy Progress Tests
Numerical Ability
Numerical Attention Test (NAT)
Nurses Global Impressions Scale
Nurses Observations Scale for Inpatient
Evaluation (NOSIE)
NYLS Adult Temperament
Questionnaire
OARS Multidimensional Functional
Assessment Questionnaire (OMFAQ)
Object Classification Test (OCT)
Object Relations Technique
Object Sorting Scale (OSS)
Object Sorting Test (OST)
Objective Analytic Battery
Objective Opiate Withdrawal Scale
object test (OT)
objective test (OT)
O'Brien Vocabulary Placement Test
Obsessive-Compulsive Drinking Scale
(OCDS)
Obsessive-Compulsive Drinking Scale-
Modified for Pathological Gambling
(OCDS-PG)
Obsessive-Compulsive Personality
Disorder Subscale from Millon
Clinical Multiaxial
Obsessive-Compulsive Subscale of the
Comprehensive Psychopathological
Rating Scale
Occupational Check List
Occupational Environment Scales,
Form E-2

Occupational Interests Explorer (OIE)
Occupational Interests Surveyor (OIS)
Occupational Roles Questionnaire (ORQ)
Occupational Stress Indicator (OSI)
Occupational Test Series-Basic Skills Test
O'Connor Wiggly Block Test
Offer Parent-Adolescent Questionnaire
Offer Self-Image Questionnaire (OSIQ)
Offer Self-Image Questionnaire for Adolescents
Ohio Vocational Interest Survey (OVIS)
Ohio Work Values Inventory (OWVI)
OISE Picture Reasoning Test (PRT)
Oliphant Auditory Discrimination Memory Test (OADMT)
Oliphant Auditory Synthesizing Test (OAST)
Omnibus Personality Inventory (OPI)
One Word Receptive Picture Vocabulary Test
Oral and Written Language Scale (OWLS)
Oral Language Sentence Imitation Diagnostic Inventory (OLSIDI)
Oral Language Sentence Imitation Screening Test (OLSIST)
Oral Verbal Intelligence Test (OVIT)
Oral-Motor/Feeding Rating Scale
Ordinal Scales of Psychological Development
Organic Integrity Test (OIT)
Organizational Climate Index
Organizational Culture Inventory (OCI)
Organizational Value Dimensions Questionnaire (OVDQ)
Organization Health Survey
Orleans-Hanna Algebra Prognosis Test
O'Rourke Mechanical Aptitude Test
Otis Group Intelligence Scale
Otis Quick Scoring Mental Abilities Test

Otis Self-Administered Tests of Mental Ability
Otis-Lennon Mental Ability Test (OLMAT)
Otis-Lennon School Ability Test
Ottawa School Behavior Checklist (OSBCL)
Overcontrolled Hostility Scale (OHS)
Overt Aggression Scale
Oxford STA scale
Paced Auditory Serial Addition Test (PASAT)
PACG Inventory
Pachon test
Pain Apperception Test (PAT)
Pain Perception Profile (PPP)
Pair Attraction Inventory (PAI)
Panic Control Treatment-Adolescents (PCT-A)
Panic Disorder Severity Scale
Panic-Agoraphobic Spectrum Questionnaire
Pantomime Recognition Test (PRT)
Paranoia "6" Scale
Paranoid Sensitivity Profile
Parent as a Teacher Inventory (PAAT)
Parent Attachment Structured Interview
Parent Attitude Scale (PAS)
Parent Awareness Skills Survey (PASS)
Parent Bonding Instrument (PBI)
Parent Daily Report
Parent Interview for Child Syndrome (PICS)
Parent Opinion Inventory
Parent Perception of Child Profile (PPCP)
Parent Rating of Student Behavior
Parent-Adolescent Communication Scale
Parental Acceptance-Rejection Questionnaire
Parental Bonding Instrument

Parental Stressor Scale
Parental Stressor Scale: Neonatal Intensive Care Unit (PSS:NICU)
Parenting Stress Index
Parent-Teacher Questionnaire (PTQ)
Partner Relationship Inventory (PRI)
Past History Schedule
PA subtest
Pathologic Laughing and Crying Scale (PLACS)
Pathological Gambling Signs Index
Patient Rated Anxiety Scale (PRAS)
Patient Rated Disability Scale
Patient Rated Impairment Scale
Patient Rated Overall Life Impairment
Patient Satisfaction Questionnaire-III
Patrick test
Pattern Misfit Scale
Patterns of Individual Change Scale (PICS)
Paykel Life Events Scale
PDI Employment Inventory
Peabody Developmental Motor Scales and Activity Cards
Peabody Individual Achievement Test (PIAT)
Peabody Mathematics Readiness Test
Peabody Picture Vocabulary Test (PPVT)
Peabody Picture Vocabulary Test–Revised
Peabody Vocabulary Test (PVT)
Pediatric Behavior Scale (PBS)
Pediatric Early Elementary Examination
Pediatric Examination of Educational Readiness at Middle Childhood
Pediatric Extended Examination at Three (PEET)
Pediatric Speech Intelligibility Test
Peer Nomination Inventory of Depression
Peer Profile
Penn State Worry Questionnaire

Perceived Social Support Scale (PSS)
Perception of Ability Scale for Students (PASS)
Perception of Illness Scale
Perception-of-Relationships-Test (PORT)
Perceptual Maze Test
Perceptual Organization Deviation Quotient (PODQ)
Performance Assessment of Syntax Elicited and Spontaneous (PASES)
Performance Efficiency Test
Performance Intelligence Quotient
Performance IQ Score
Performance Levels of a School Program Survey
Performance Scale Scores
Periodic Evaluation Record (PER)
Peritraumatic Dissociation Index
Perkins-Binet Test of Intelligence for the Blind
Perley-Guze Hysteria Checklist
Personal Adjustment and Role Skills (PARS)
Personal and Role Skills (PARS)
Personal Assessment for Continuing Education (PACE)
Personal Assessment of Intimacy in Relationships (PAIR)
Personal Attributes Questionnaire (PAQ)
Personal Experience and Attitude Questionnaire (PEAQ)
Personal Experience Screening Questionnaire (PESQ)
Personal Inventory
Personal Inventory of Needs
Personal Orientation Inventory (POI)
Personal Preference Scale (PPS)
Personal Problems Checklist (PPC)
Personal Problems Checklist for Adolescents (PPC)
Personal Relationship Inventory (PRI)

Personal Resource Questionnaire (PRQ)
Personal Strain Questionnaire (PSQ)
Personal Style Inventory (PSI)
Personal Values Abstract (PVA)
Personal Values Inventory (PVI)
Personality Adjective Check List
    (PACL)
Personality Assessment Inventory (PAI)
Personality Diagnostic Questionnaire
    (PDQ)
Personality Diagnostic Questionnaire-
    Revised (PDQ-R)
Personality Disorder Examination
    (PDE)
Personality Factor Questionnaire (PFQ)
16 Personality Factor Questionnaire (16
    PF)
Personality Index (PI)
Personality Inventory (PI)
Personality Inventory for Children (PIC)
Personality Rating Scale (PRS)
Personality Research Form (PRF)
Personnel Reaction Blank
Personnel Security Preview (PSP)
Personnel Selection Inventory
Personnel Tests for Industry (PTI)
Phelps Kindergarten Readiness Scale
    (PKRS)
Philadelphia Head Injury Questionnaire
    (PHIQ)
Philadelphia Multilevel Assessment
    Instrument
Phillips Scale
Phobic Attitude Evaluation
Photoarticulation Test (PAT)
Physical and Architectural Features
    Checklist
Physical Self-Maintenance Scale
Physical Tolerance Profile (PTP)
Physician's Questionnaire
Physiognomic Cue Test (PCT)
Picha-Seron Career Analysis
Pickford Projective Picture (PPP)

Pictorial Test of Intelligence (PTI)
Picture Anomalies Test
Picture Articulation and Language
    Screening Test (PALST)
Picture Identification for
    Children–Standardized Index
Picture Identification Test (PIT)
Picture Interest Exploration Survey
    (PIES)
Picture Interpretation Test
Picture Reasoning Test (PRE)
Picture Story Language Test (PSLT)
Picture World Test
Piers-Harris Children's Self-Concept
    Scale
Pimsleur Language Aptitude Battery
Pinter-Paterson Performance Test
Pitowsky Illness Behavior
    Questionnaire
Pittsburgh Sleep Quality Index
Planning Career Goals (PCG)
Pleasant Events Schedule (PES)
Policy and Program Information Form
Politte Sentence Completion Test
Polyfactorial Study of Personality
Porch Index of Communicative Ability
    (PICA)
Porch Index of Communicative Ability
    in Children (PICAC)
Porteus Maze Test (PMT)
Position Analysis Questionnaire (PAQ)
Positive and Negative Stroke Scale
    (PANSS)
Positive and Negative Symptom Scale
Positive and Negative Symptoms of
    Schizophrenia Scale
Positive and Negative Syndrome Scale
    (PANSS)
Positive and Negative Syndrome Scale
    Excited Component
Positive Attention Behavior
Positive Humanitarian Subscale
Positive Military Subscale

Posttraumatic Stress Disorder Symptom Scale
Potential for Addiction Index
Practical Math Assessment
Pragmatics Profile of Early Communication Skills
Pragmatics Screening Test
Predictive Ability Test (PAT)
Predictive Screening Test of Articulation
Preliminary Diagnostic Questionnaire
Premarital Communication Inventory (PCI)
Premenstrual Assessment Form (PAF)
Premorbid Social Adjustment Scale
Pre-Professional Skills Test
Pre-Reading Expectancy Screening Scale (PRESS)
Preschool and Kindergarten Interest Descriptor
Preschool Behavior Questionnaire (PBQ)
Preschool Development Inventory
Preschool Language Scale (PLS)
Preschool Language Screening Test
Preschool Screening Test
Preschool Speech and Language Screening Test
Prescriptive Reading Inventory (PRI)
Present State Examination (PSE)
Prevocational Assessment and Curriculum Guide (PACG)
Prevocational Assessment Screen (PAS)
Primary Mental Abilities Test (PMAT)
Primary Self-Concept Inventory (PSCI)
Primary Test of Cognitive Skills (PTCS)
Primary Visual Motor Test (PVMT)
Printing Performance School Readiness Test (PPRST)
Priority Counseling Survey (PCS)
Problem Experiences Checklist
Problem-Oriented Screening Instrument for Teenagers (POSIT)

Problem Solving Inventory
Process Diagnostic (PD)
Process for the Assessment of Effective Student Functioning
Process Skills Rating Scale (PSRS)
Professional and Administrative Career Evaluation/Examination
Professional Employment Test (PET)
Professional Sexual Role Inventory (PSRI)
Proficiency Assessment Report (PAR)
Profile of Adaptation to Life (PAL)
Profile of Mood States (POMS)
Profile of Mood States, Vigor
Profile of Nonverbal Sensitivity (PONS)
Profile of Out-of-Body Experiences (POBE)
Prognostic Scale
Program for Assessing Youth Employment Skills
Progress Assessment Chart of Social and Personal Development (PAC)
Progressive Achievement Tests of Listening Comprehension (PATLC)
Progressive Achievement Tests of Reading
Progressive Deterioration Scale (PDS)
Projective Assessment of Aging Method
Projective Human Figure Drawing Test
proverb interpretation test
proverbs test
PSI Basic Skills Test for Business, Industry and Government
Psychasthenia "7" Scale
Psychiatric Diagnostic Interview
Psychiatric Diagnostic Screening Questionnaire (PDSQ)
Psychiatric Epidemiology Research I Interview-Demoralization Scale (PERI-D)
Psychiatric Epidemiology Research Interview (PERI)
Psychiatric Evaluation Form (PEF)

Psychiatric Evaluation Profile (PEP)
Psychiatric Knowledge and Skills Self-Assessment Program (PKSAP)
Psychiatric Status Rating Scale
Psychiatric Status Schedule (PSS)
psychoacoustic test (PAT)
Psycho-Educational Evaluation
Psychoeducational Profile (PEP)
Psycho-Epistemological Profile (PEP)
Psychogeriatric Dependency Rating Scale
Psycholinguistic Rating Scale
Psychological Distress Inventory
Psychological Screening Inventory (PSI)
Psychopathic Deviance "4" Scale
Psychopathological Rating Scale
Psychopathy Checklist-Revised
Psychosis Screening Questionnaire
Psychosocial Adjustment to Illness Scale (PAIS)
Psychosocial Assessment of Childhood Experiences (PACE)
Psychosocial History Screening Questionnaire (PHSQ)
Psychosocial History Screening Test (PHST)
Psychotherapy Competence Assessment Schedule (PCAS)
Psychotherapy Supervisory Inventory
Psychotic Inpatient Profile (PIP)
Psychotic Reaction Profile (PRP)
PTSD Symptom Scale
Pupil Rating Scale (PRS)
Pupil Rating Scale: Screening for Learning Disabilities
Pupil Record of Education Behavior (PREB)
Purdue Industrial Mathematics Test
Purdue Pegboard Dexterity Test
Purdue Perceptual-Motor Survey (PPMS)
Purdue Student-Teacher Opinionnare (PSTO)

Purdue Teacher Opinionnaire (PTO)
Purdue Teacher Questionnaire (PTQ)
Purpose in Life Test
Q sort
Quality of Crisis Support scale
Quality of Life Enjoyment and Satisfaction Questionnaire
Quality of Life Interview (QOLI)
Quality of Life Inventory (QOLI)
Quality of Life Questionnaire (QLQ)
Quality of Life Scale
Quality of Well-Being Scale
Queckenstedt-Stookey test
Questionnaire of Basic Personality Support
Questionnaire on Resources and Stress for Families with Chronically Ill or Handicapped
Quick Picture Vocabulary Test (QPVT)
Quick Screening of Mental Development
Quick Word Test
Quick-Score Achievement Test
Racial Perceptions Inventory (RPI)
Rand Functional Limitations Battery
Rand Patient Satisfaction Questionnaire
Rand Physical Capacities Battery
Rand Social Health Battery
Random Letter Test
Random Letter Test Raskin Severity of Depression Scale
Rape Aftermath Symptom Test
Raskin Severity of Depression Scale
Rated Anxiety Scale
Rated Overall Life Impairment
Rathus Assertiveness Test
Rating Inventory for Screening Kindergartners
Rating Scale of Communication in Cognitive Decline (RSCCD)
Raven Colored Progressive Matrices Test (RCPMT)
Raven Progressive Matrices

Raven Standard Progressive Matrices (RSPM)
Raven Test
raw Q score
RBH Test of Learning Ability
Reaction to Loss Inventory
Readiness Scale—Self Rating and Manager Rating Forms
Reading Achievement
Reading Comprehension Battery for Aphasia
Reading Comprehension Inventory
Reading-Free Vocational Interest Inventory (RFVII)
Reading Grade Equivalent
Reading Grade Rating
Reading Miscue Inventory (RMI)
Reading Sight Vocabulary Standard Score
Reality Check Survey (RCS)
Reasons for Living Inventory (RLI)
Receptive One-Word Picture Vocabulary Test (ROWPVT)
Receptive-Expressive Emergent Language scale (REEL)
Receptive-Expressive Observation Scale
Recognition Memory Test
Reductions in Eating Attitudes Test
REEL scale
Rehabilitation Client Rating Scale (RCRS)
Rehabilitation Indicator (RIs)
Reid Report
Reitan Evaluation of Hemispheric Abilities and Brain Improvement Training
Reitan-Indiana Aphasia Screening Test (RIAST)
Reitan-Indiana Neuropsychological Test Battery for Adults
Reitan-Indiana Neuropsychological Test Battery for Children
Reitan-Klove Lateral Dominance Examination

Reitan-Klove Sensory Perceptual Evaluation
Reitan-Klove Sensory Perceptual Examination
Reitan-Klove Tactile Form Recognition Test
Relative Aspects of Potential (RAP)
Relative Value Scale
Remote Associates Test (RAT)
Repeated Test of Sustained Wakefulness (RTSW)
Repertory Grip Technique
Repertory Test
Research Diagnostic Criteria (RDC)
Resident and Staff Information Form
Resource-Based Relative Value Scale (RBRVS)
Responsibility and Independence Scale for Adolescents (RISA)
Retirement Descriptive Index (RDI)
Revised Behavior Problem Checklist
Revised Childhood Experiences Questionnaire (CEQ-R)
Revised Children's Depression Scale (RCDS)
Revised Children's Manifest Anxiety Scale
Revised Denver Prescreening Development Questionnaire (R-PDQ)
Revised Diagnostic Interview for Borderlines
Revised Edinburgh Functional Communication Profile
Revised Evaluating Acquired Skills in Communication
Revised NEO Personality Inventory
Revised Ontario Child Health Study Scale
Revised Physical Anhedonia Scale (PAS)
Revised Token Test
Revised Ways of Coping Checklist
Rey and Taylor Complex Figure Test
Rey Auditory Verbal Learning Test (RAVLT)

Rey Complex Figure Test

Reynell Developmental Language Scales

Reynell-Zinkin Scales: Developmental Scales for Young Handicapped Children

Reynolds Adolescent Depression Scale (RADS)

Reynolds Adolescent Scale

Reynolds Child Depression Scale (RCDS)

Rey-Osterreith Complex Figure Test

Rey-Osterrieth Complex Figure Copy and Delayed Recall Test

Rey-Osterrieth Complex Figure Design

Rhode Island Pupil Identification Scale (PIPIS)

Right-Left Orientation Test (RLO)

Right-Wing Authoritarianism Scale

Riley Articulation and Language Test (RALT)

Riley Inventory of Basic Learning Skills (RIBLS)

Riley Motor Problems Inventory

Riley Preschool Developmental Screening Inventory (RPDSI)

Ring and Peg Tests of Behavior Development

Risk Assessment Battery

Risk Behavior Index

Risk of AIDS Behavior Scale

Risk-Taking, Attitude, Values Inventory (RTAVI)

Ritvo-Freeman Real Life Rating Scale for Autism

Rivermead ADL Test

Rivermead Behavioral Memory Test (RBMT)

Rivermead Mobility Index (RMI)

Rivermead Motor Assessment

Rivermead Perceptual Assessment Battery

Robert Apperception Test for Children (RATC)

Roeder Manipulative Aptitude Test

Rogers Criminal Responsibility Scale

Rokeach Value Survey (RVS)

Role Construct Repertory Test

Rorschach Content Test (RCT)

Rorschach Index of Primitive Thought

Rorschach Inkblot Test

Rorschach test

Rosen Drawing Test

Rosenberg Draw-a-Person Technique/Test

Rosenberg Draw-a-Person Test

Rosenberg Self-Esteem Scale (RSES)

Rosenzweig Picture-Frustration Study

Ross Information Processing Assessment

Ross Test of Higher Cognitive Processes

Rothwell-Miller Interest Blank

Rotter Incomplete Sentences Blank (RISB)

Rotter Sentence Completion Test (RSCT)

Rucker-Gable Educational Programming Scale (RGEPS)

Rule Eleven Psych Evaluation

Russell Version Wechsler Memory Scale

Rust Inventory of Schizotypal Cognitions

Rutler-Graham Psychiatric Interview

Rutter Child Behaviour Questionnaire

Rutter-B Questionnaire

Safran Student's Interest Inventory (SSII)

Salamon-Conte Life Satisfaction in the Elderly Scale (LSES)

Sales Attitude Check List (SACL)

Sales Personality Questionnaire (SPQ)

Salience Inventory (SI)

Sarason General Anxiety and Test Anxiety Scale

SCAL scale

Scale for Assessment of Thought, Language, and Communication

Scale for Emotional Blunting (SEB)

Scale for the Assessment of Negative Symptoms (SANS)

Scale for the Assessment of Positive Symptoms (SAPS)
Scale for the Assessment of Unawareness of Mental Disorder (SUMD)
Scale of Independent Behavior
Scale of Social Development
Scale to Assess Unawareness of Mental Disorder (SUMD)
Scaled Curriculum Achievement Levels Test (SCALE)
Scales of Creativity and Learning Environment (SCALE)
SCAN survey
SCAN-TRON Reading Test
Schaie-Thurstone Adult Mental Abilities Test
Schedule for Affective Disorders and Schizophrenia (SADS)
Schedule for Affective Disorders and Schizophrenia-Change (SADS-C)
Schedule for Affective Disorders and Schizophrenia for School-Age Children (KIDDIE-SADS)
Schedule for Affective Disorders and Schizophrenia for School-Age Children-Epidemiologic Version (K-SADS-E)
Schedule for Affective Disorders and Schizophrenia for School-Age Children-Present Episode (K-SADS-P)
Schedule for Affective Disorders and Schizophrenia Lifetime Version
Schedule for Affective Disorders and Schizophrenia-Lifetime (SADS-L)
Schedule for Assessment of Insight (SAI)
Schedule for Attitudes Toward Hastened Death
Schedule for the Assessment of Negative Symptoms
Schedule of Affective Disorders
Schedule of Growing Skills
Schedule of Recent Experience (SRE)

Schedules for Clinical Assessment in Neuropsychiatry (SCAN)
Schizophrenia "8" Scale
Schizophrenia-Mania Rating Scale
Scholastic Abilities Test for Adults (SATA)
Scholastic Aptitude Test (SAT)
School Ability Test (SAT)
School Administrator Assessment Survey
School and College Ability Tests (SCAT)
School and College Ability Tests (SCAT) and Sequential Tests of Educational Progress (STEP)
School and College Ability Tests (SCAT) and Sequential Tests of Educational Progress (STEP) (Form 1c)
School Apperception Method
School Assessment Survey (SAS)
School Atmosphere Questionnaire (SAQ)
School Attitude Survey (SAS)
School Attitude Test (SAT)
School Climate Inventory
School Environment Preference Survey
School Handicap Condition Scale (SEH)
School Interest Inventory
School Library/Media Skills Test
School Motivation Analysis Test (SMAT)
School Problem Screening Inventory (SPSI)
School Readiness Screening Test
School Readiness Survey
School Situation Survey
School Social Skills Rating Scale
Schubert General Ability Battery
Schwab and England Activities of Daily Living Scale
Schwaback Test
SCID Interview
Science Research Associates Mechanical Aptitude
Scott Mental Alertness Test
Screen for Child Anxiety-Related Emotional Disorders

Screening Assessment for Gifted Elementary Students, Primary (SAGES-P)

Screening Children for Related Early Educational Needs

Screening for Learning Disabilities

Screening for Learning Disabilities, Pupil Rating Scale

Screening Instrument for Targeting Educational Risk (SIFTER)

Screening Inventory

Screening Kit of Language Development (SKOLD)

Screening Questionnaire

Screening Test for Auditory Comprehension of Language (STACL)

Screening Test for Educational Prerequisite Skills (STEPS)

Screening Test for the Assignment of Remedial Treatment (STaRT)

Screening Test of Academic Readiness

Screening Test of Adolescent Language

Screening Tests for Young Children and Retardates (STYCAR)

S-D Proneness Checklist

SDI-Learning Abilities Test: Screening Form for Gifted

SEARCH: A Scanning Instrument for the Identification of Potential Learning Disability

Seashore Rhythm Test (SRT)

Seasonal Pattern Assessment Questionnaire (SPAQ)

Seattle Longitudinal Study

SEC scale

Seeking of Noetic Goals Test

Selective Reminding Test

self-administered alcohol screening test (SAAST)

Self-Administered Dependency Questionnaire (SADQ)

Self-Assessment Depression (SAD)

Self-Assessment Depression Scale

Self-Assessment in Writing Skills

Self-Concept and Motivation Inventory (SCAMI)

Self-Concept as a Learner (SCAL)

Self-Concept as a Learner scale

Self-Concept Scale

Self-Consciousness Scale

Self-Control Inventory

Self-Control Scale (SCS)

Self-Description Inventory

Self-Description Questionnaire II (SDQII)

Self-Esteem Index (SEI)

Self-Esteem Inventory (SEI)

Self-Esteem Questionnaire

Self-Perception Inventory (SPI)

Self-Perception Profile for Children

Self-Rating Anxiety Scale (SAS)

Self-Rating Depression Scale (SDS)

Semi-Structured Assessment for the Genetics of Alcoholism

Senior Apperception Technique (SAT)

Senior Apperception Test (SAT)

Senoussi Multiphasic Marital Inventory (SMMI)

Sensation-Seeking Scale (SSS)

Sense of Coherence Questionnaire

Sensory Integration and Praxis Tests (SIPT)

Sentence Closure Test

Sentence Completion Test (SCT)

Separation Anxiety Symptom Inventory (SASI)

Sequenced Inventory of Communication Development (SICD)

Sequenced Inventory of Language Development (SILD)

Sequential Assessment of Mathematics Inventories: Standardized Inventory

Sequential Tests of Educational Progress, Series III (STEP-III)

Sequential Tests of Educational Study (STEP)

Series of Emergency Scales

Severity of Psychiatric Illness Scale
Severity of Psychosocial Stressors Scale
Sex Knowledge and Attitude Test (SKAT)
Sexual Abuse Interview
Sexual and Physical Abuse
  Questionnaire
Sexual Compatibility Test (SCT)
Sexual Experiences Questionnaire
Sexual Functioning Index (SFI)
Sexual Risk Index
Sexuality Preference Profile (SPP)
Shapes Analysis Test (SAT)
Shedler-Western Assessment
  Procedure-200 (SWAP-200)
Sheehan Disability Scale
Sheltered Care Environment Scale
Shipley Abstraction Test
Shipley Institute of Living Scale (SILS)
Shipley Institute of Living Scale for
  Measuring Intellectual Impairment
Shipley Personal Inventory (SPI)
Shipley-Hartford Scale
Shipman Anxiety Depression Scale
  (SADS)
Short Category Test
Short Employment Tests
Short Form-36 General Health Survey
  (SF-36)
Short Form Test of Academic Aptitude
  (SFTAA)
Short Imaginal Processes Inventory
  (SIPI)
Short Increment Sensitivity Index (SISI)
Short Michigan Alcoholism Screen Test
  (SMAST)
Short Michigan Alcoholism Screening
  Test (SMAST)
Short Portable Mental Status
  Questionnaire (SPMSQ)
Short Term Auditory Retrieval and
  Storage (STARS)
Short Test for Use with Cerebral Palsy
  Children

Shortened Edinburgh Reading Tests
Sickness Impact Profile (SIP)
Similarities Test of Verbal Abstract
  Reasoning
Simpson Scale
Simpson-Angus Rating Scale
Singer-Loomis Inventory of Personality
  (SLIP)
Single and Double Simultaneous
  Stimulation Test
Situational Attitude Scale (SAS)
Six-Hour Retarded Child
Sixteen Personality Factor Questionnaire
Skill Scan for Management
  Development
Slavson Activity Interview Therapy
Sleep and Breathing Problems Scale
Sleep Screening Questionnaire for
  Parents
Sleepiness Scale
Slingerland Screening Tests (SST)
Slosson Children's Version Family
  Environment Scale
Slosson Drawing Coordination Test
Slosson Intelligence Test-Primary
  (SIT-P)
Slosson Intelligence Test-Revised (SIT-R)
Slosson Test of Reading Readiness
  (STRR)
Smith-Johnson Nonverbal Performance
  Scale
Smoking Behavior Questionnaire (SBQ)
Snaith-Hamilton Pleasure Scale
Social Adaptation Status (SAS)
Social Adequacy Index (SAI)
Social Adjustment Scale
Social Adjustment Scale II
Social Adjustment Self-Report
  Questionnaire
Social Adjustment Self-Report Scale
  (SASRS)
Social and Occupational Functioning
  Assessment Scale (SOFAS)

Social and Prevocational Information Battery (SPIB)

Social Avoidance and Distress Scale

Social Behavior Assessment Inventory (SBAI)

Social Behavior Assessment Schedule

Social Climate Scale (SCS)

Social Constraints Scale (SCS)

Social Disability Scale

Social Function Index (SFI)

Social Intelligence Test

Social Interaction Scale

Social Maladjustment Schedule

Social Phobia Inventory

Social Problem-Solving Inventory-Revised, Short Form

Social Readjustment Rating Scale (SRRS)

Social Reintegration Scale

Social Relations Test (SRT)

Social Reticence Scale

Social Security Disability

Social Skills Rating System (SSRS)

Social Support Questionnaire

Social Support Scale

Social Thoughts and Beliefs Scale (STABS)

Social-Emotional Dimension Scale

SOI-Learning Abilities Test: Screening Form for Gifted

Somatic "3" Scale

Somatic Inkblot Series

Sorting of Figures Test (SOFT)

South Oaks Gambling Screen (SOGS)

South Oaks Gambling Screen-Revised (SOGS-R)

South Oaks Gambling Screen-Revised for Adolescents (SOGS-RA)

Southern California Postrotary Nystagmus Test

Southern California Sensory Integration Tests

Space Relations

Spadafore Diagnostic Reading Test

SPAR Spelling and Reading Test

Spatial Orientation Memory Test (SOMT)

Special Aptitude Test Battery (SATB)

Specific Aptitude Test Battery

SPECTRUM-I: A Test of Adult Work Motivation

Speech and Language Screening Questionnaire (SLSQ)

Speech Questionnaire

Speech with Alternating Masking Index (SWAMI)

Speech-Language Pathology Evaluation Assessment

Speech-Sounds Perception Test

spell-a-word-backwards test

Spelling Grade Equivalent

Spelling Grade Rating

Spelling Scale

spider's web test

Spielberger Anxiety Inventory

Spielberger State-Trait Anger Expression Inventory

Spielberger State-Trait Anxiety Inventory

Spiritual Well-Being Scale (SWBS)

Spondee Picture Test (SPT)

S-R Inventory of Anxiousness

SRA Arithmetic Test

SRA Pictorial Reasoning Test

SRA Reading Test

SRA Verbal

St. George Anxiety Questionnaire

St. Paul-Ramsey Scale

Staff Burnout Scale for Health Professionals

Standard Progressive Matrices

Standardized Assessment of Depressive Disorders (SADD)

Standardized Test of Computer Literacy (STCL)

Stanford Achievement Test (SAT)

Stanford Acute Stress Reaction Questionnaire
Stanford-Binet Intelligence Scale (SBIS)
Stanford-Binet Profile
Stanford-Binet Scale
Stanford-Binet Scale-Revised
Stanford-Binet test
Stanford-Binet, Fourth Edition (SB-IV)
Stanford Diagnostic Arithmetic Test
Stanford Diagnostic Reading Test (SDRT)
Stanford Early School Achievement Test
Stanford Hypnotic Clinical Scale and Children
Stanford Hypnotic Susceptibility Scale (SHSS)
Stanford Sleepiness Scale
Stanton Survey
State-Trait Anger Expression Inventory (STAXI)
State-Trait Anger Scale (STAS)
State-Trait Anxiety Index
State-Trait Anxiety Inventory (STAI)
State-Trait Anxiety Inventory for Children (STAIC)
State-Trait Anxiety Inventory for Stein Sentence Completion test
State-Trait Personality Inventory (STPI)
Stein Sentence Completion (SSC)
Stenger Test
Stephens Oral Language Screening Test (SOLST)
Steps Up Developmental Screening Program
Stimulus Recognition Test
Stoelting Brief Intelligence Test (S-BIT)
Stone and Neale Daily Coping Assessment
Strauss-Carpenter scale
Street Survival Skills Questionnaire
Strength of Grip Test
Stress Evaluation Inventory
Stress Impact Scale (SIS)
Stress Response Scale

Strong-Campbell Interest Inventory (SCII)
Strong Vocational Interest Blank
Stroop Color-Word Test
Stroop Color Interference Test
Stroop Color-Word Interference Test
Structure of Intellect Learning Abilities Test, From P
Structured and Scaled Interview to Assess Maladjustment (SSIAM)
Structured Clinical Interview for DSM-III-R (SCID)
Structured Clinical Interview for DSM-III-R Dissociative Disorders (SCID-D)
Structured Clinical Interview for DSM-III-R Non-Patient Edition (SCID-NP)
Structured Clinical Interview for DSM-III-R Personality Disorders (SCID-II)
Structured Clinical Interview for DSM-III-R Psychotic Disorders (SCID-PD)
Structured Clinical Interview for DSM-III-R-Patient Version (SCID-P)
Structured Clinical Interview for DSM-IV (SCID)
Structured Clinical Interview for DSM-IV Axis I Disorders: Clinician Version (SCID-CV)
Structured Clinical Interview for DSM-IV Axis II Personality Disorders (SCID-II)
Structured Clinical Interview for DSM-IV Dissociative Disorders (SCID-D)
Structured Clinical Interview for DSM-IV Patient Edition
Structured Clinical Interview for the Panic-Agoraphobic Spectrum
Structured Composite International Diagnostic Interview for Psychological Disorders
Structured Interview of Reported Symptoms (SIRS)
Structured Photographic Expressive Language Test-II (SPELT-P)

Structured Trauma Interview
Student Adaptation to College
  Questionnaire (SACQ)
Student Adjustment Inventory (SAI)
Student Disability Survey
Student Orientation Survey
Student Opinion Inventory (SOI)
Student Reactions to College (SRC)
Student Talent and Risk Profile
Students Against Drunk Driving (SADD)
Study Attitudes and Methods Survey
  (SAMS)
STYCAR Hearing Test (SHT)
STYCAR Language Test (SLT)
STYCAR Vision Test (SVT)
Style of Leadership Survey
Style of Management Inventory
Style of Mind Inventory (SMI)
Subject Treatment Emergent Symptom
  Scale
Subjective High Assessment Scale
Subjective Opiate Withdrawal Scale
Subjective Response Questionnaire
Subjective Symptoms Scale
Subjective Treatment Emergent Side
  Effects Scale
Subjective Units of Distress Scale (SUDS)
Substance Abuse and Mental Health
  Administration (SAMHA)
Substance Abuse Problem Checklist
Substance Abuse Questionnaire (SAQ)
Substance Abuse Subtle Screening
  Inventory (SASSI)
Suicide Intent Scale
Suicide Intervention Response
  Inventory
Suicide Opinion Questionnaire (SOQ)
Suicide Probability Scale
Suicide-Depression Proneness Checklist
  (SDPC)
Suinn Test Anxiety Behavior Scale
  (STABS)
Supervisory Practices Inventory

Supervisory Practices Test (SPT)
Supervisory Profile Record
Supplemental Security Income (SSI)
Suprathreshold Adaptation Test (STAT)
Survey of Employee Access (SEA)
Survey of Interpersonal Values
Survey of Personal Values
Survey of School Attitudes
Survey of Study Habits and Attitudes
  (SSHA)
Survey of Work Values, Revised, Form U
Surveys of Achievement
suspected child abuse/neglect survey
Swanson, Nolan, and Pelham Rating
  Scale
Swinging Story Test
Symbol Digit Modalities Test (SDMT)
Symbolic Play Test (SPT)
Symptom Checklist 90-Revised Global
  Severity Index
Symptom Checklist-90 (SCL)
Symptom Checklist-90-Revised
  (SCL-90-R)
Symptom Rating Scale (SRS)
Synthetic Sentence Identification Test
System for Interaction Guidance
  Information (SIGI)
System for Testing and Evaluation of
  Potential
System of Multicultural Pluralistic
  Assessment (SOMPA)
Systematic Assessment for Treatment
  of Emergent Events (SAFTEE)
Systematic Treatment Enhancement
  Program for Bipolar Disorder
  (STEP-BD)
Szondi Test
Tactile Finger Recognition Test (TFRT)
Tactile Form Recognition Test (TFRT)
Tactile Perception Test
Tactile Performance Test (TPT)
Talbieh Brief Distress Inventory (TBDI)
Tanner sexual maturity rating

Tanner stage
TARC Assessment System
Task Assessment Scale
Task Force on Nicotine Dependence
Taylor Manifest Anxiety Scale (TMAS)
Taylor-Johnson Temperament Analysis
Teacher and Parent Separation Anxiety
  Rating Scales for Preschool Children
Teacher Assessment of Social Behavior
  (TASB)
Teacher Evaluation Scale (TES)
Teacher Feedback Questionnaire
Teacher Opinion Inventory
Teacher School Readiness Inventory
  (TSRI)
Teacher's Reading Global Improvement
  (TRGI)
Teacher Stress Inventory
Teaching Style Inventory
Team Effectiveness Survey (TES)
Teen Addiction Severity Index (T-ASI)
Tell-Me-A-Story (TEMAS)
Temperament and Character Inventory
  (TCI)
Temperament and Values Inventory
Temperament Assessment Battery for
  Children
temperament survey
Tennessee Self-Concept Scale (TSCS)
Test Anxiety Profile
Test Anxiety Scale
Test for Auditory Comprehension of
  Language (TACL)
Test for Examining Expressive
  Morphology (TEEM)
Test of Adolescent Language (TOAL)
Test of Adolescent/Adult Word Finding
  (TAWF)
Test of Articulation Performance—
  Diagnostic (TAP-D)
Test of Articulation Performance,
  Screen (TAP-S)
Test of Attentional Style

Test of Attitude Toward School (TAS)
Test of Auditory Discrimination (TAD)
Test of Cognitive Style in Mathematics
  (TCSM)
Test of Concept Utilization (TCU)
Test of Creative Potential
Test of Early Language Development
  (TELD)
Test of Early Language Development,
  Second Edition (TELD-2)
Test of Early Mathematics Ability,
  Second Edition (TEMA-2)
Test of Early Reading Ability, Second
  Edition (TERA-2)
Test of Early Written Language, Second
  Edition (TEWL-2)
Test of Economic Literacy (TEL)
Test of Functional Health Literacy in
  Adults (TOFHLA)
Test of Kindergarten/First Grade
  Readiness Skills (TKFGRS)
Test of Language Competence (TLC)
Test of Language Competence for
  Children (TLC-C)
Test of Language Development-
  Intermediate, Second Edition
  (TOLD-I:2)
Test of Language Development-
  Primary, Second Edition (TOLD-P:2)
Test of Language Development
  (TOLD)
Test of Listening Accuracy in Children
  (TLAC)
Test of Memory and Learning
  (TOMAL)
Test of Nonverbal Auditory
  Discrimination (TENVAD)
Test of Nonverbal Intelligence (TONI)
Test of Nonverbal Intelligence-3
  (TONI-3)
Test of Pragmatic Language (TOPL)
Test of Problem Solving
Test of Social Inferences (TSI)

Test of Variables of Attention
Test of Visual Motor Integration
Test of Visual Perception
Test of Word Finding (TWF)
Test of Word Finding in Discourse
  (TWFD)
Test of Work Competency and Stability
  (TWCS)
Test of Written Language (TOWL)
Test of Written Language-3 (TOWL-3)
Test of Written Spelling
Testing-Teaching Module of Auditory
  Discrimination (TTMAD)
Tests for Auditory Comprehension of
  Language-Revised (TACL-R)
Tests of Basic Experience (TOBE)
Tests of Fundamental Abilities in
  Visual Art
Tests of Mechanical Comprehension
Tests of Perception of Scientists and
  Self (TOPOSS)
Texas Revised Inventory of Grief
Thackray Reading Readiness Profile
  (TRRP)
The Goldstein-Scheerer Cube Test
The Henmon-Nelson Tests of Mental
  Ability
The Instructional Environment Scale
  (TIES)
The Kahn Test of Symbol Arrangement
The Mega Test
The Meier Art Judgment Test
The Primary Language Screen (TPLS)
The Wide Range Achievement Test
The Wiggley Block
Thematic Apperception Test (TAT)
Thematic Aptitude Test (TAT)
Thematic Content Modification
  Program (TCMP)
Thinking Creatively in Action and
  Motion
Thinking Creatively with Sounds and
  Words

Thinking Good Profile
This I Believe (TIB)
Thorndike Handwriting Scale
Thought Disorder Index
Three-Minute Reasoning Test
Three-Dimensional Block Construction
  Test
Three-Factor Eating Questionnaire
Three-Item Delirium Scale
Three-Stage Command Test
Thurstone scale
Thurstone Attitude Scale
Thurstone Interest Schedule
Thurstone Temperament Schedule
Time Perception Inventory
Time Problems Inventory
Time Sense Test
Time Use Analyzer
Timed Stereotypes Rating Scale
Tinker Toy Test
TLC-Learning Preference Inventory
TOEFL Test of Written English
Token Test for Aphasia
Token Test for Children
Token Test for Receptive Disturbances
  in Aphasia
Tomkins-Horn Picture Arrangement
  Test
Toronto Alexithymia Scale (TAS)
Toronto Functional Capacity
  Questionnaire (TFCQ)
Torrance Tests of Creative Thinking
  (TTCT)
Tourette Syndrome Global Scale
Tourette Syndrome Questionnaire
Tourette Syndrome Severity Scale
Tourette Syndrome Symptom List
Trail Making Test
Trail of Nonpharmacologic
  Interventions in the Elderly Study
Trainer's Assessment of Proficiency
  (TAP)
Trait Evaluation Index

Transactional Analysis Life Position Survey (TALPS)
Transition Behavior Scale (TBS)
Transitional Object Questionnaire
Trauma Symptom Checklist for Children Ages 8–15
Traumatic Antecedents Questionnaire
Treatment Alternatives to Street Crime (TASC)
Tridimensional Personality Questionnaire
Trites Neuropsychological Test Battery
Twenty Statements Test (TST)
Unified Psychogeriatric Biopsychosocial Evaluation and Treatment (UPBEAT)
Uniform Determination of Death Act
University Residence Environment Scale (URES)
Unpleasant Events Schedule (UES)
Utah Test of Language Development (UTLD)
Uzgiris-Hunt Scale
Valpar Work Sample Battery
Values Inventory for Children (VIC)
Vane Evaluation of Language Scale (VELS)
Verbal and Oral Language Ability
Verbal Comprehension Deviation Quotient (VCDQ)
Verbal Fluency Test
Verbal Intelligence Quotient (VIQ)
Verbal IQ Score
Verbal Language Development Scale
Verbal Meaning Test
Verbal Scale Scores
Verbal-Auditory Screen for Children (VASC)
Verbalizer-Visualization Questionnaire (VVQ)
Verdun Depression Rating Scale (VDRS)
Verdun Target Symptom Rating Scale (VTSRS)

Vigotsky Concept Formation Test, Modified
Vigotsky Test
Vineland Adaptive Behavior Scale
Vineland Social Maturity Scale (VSMS)
Visual Form Discrimination Test (VFDT)
Visual Memory Score (VMS)
Visual Motor Test
Visual Neglect Test
Visual Pattern Completion test
Visual Perception Test
Visual Retention Test
Visual Search and Attention Test (VSAT)
Visual-Auditory Screen for Children (VASC)
Visual-Motor Gestalt Test (VMGT)
Visual-Motor Integration Test (VMIT)
Visual-Motor Sequencing Test (VMST)
Visual-Tactile System of Phonetic Symbolization
Vocabulary Comprehension Scale
Vocational Apperception Test (VAT)
Vocational Evaluation and Work Adjustment (VEWA)
Vocational Interest and Sophistication Assessment (VISA)
Vocational Interest Blank (VIB)
Vocational Interest Inventory
Vocational Interest Inventory and Exploration Survey
Vocational Interest, Experience, and Skill Assessment (VIESA)
Vocational Interest Questionnaire (VIQ)
Vocational Interest Survey
Vocational Learning Styles (LSV2)
Vocational Opinion Index (VOI)
Vocational Planning Inventory (VPI)
Vocational Preference Inventory (VPI)
Voc-Tech Quick Screener (VTQS)
Vulpe Assessment
Wachs Analysis of Cognitive Structures

Wada test
Wahler Physical Symptoms Inventory
Wahler Self-Description Inventory (WSDI)
WAIS-R Block Design Test
Wakefield Self-Assessment Depression Inventory
Waldrop Scale
Walker-McConnell Scale of Social Competence and School Adjustment
War Zone Exposure Subscale
Ward Atmosphere Scale (WAS)
Ward Behavior Rating Scale (WBRS)
Waring Intimacy Questionnaire (WIQ)
Washington Speech Sound Discrimination Test (WSSDT)
Washington University Sentence Completion Test (WUSCT)
Watson-Glaser Critical Thinking Appraisal (WGCTA)
Ways of Coping Scale
Weak Opiate Withdrawal Scale (WOWS)
Weber Advanced Spatial Perception (WASP)
Weber test
Wechsler Adult Intelligence Scale (WAIS)
Wechsler Adult Intelligence Scale-Revised
Wechsler Individual Achievement Test (WIAT)
Wechsler Individual Achievement Test-second edition (WIAT-II)
Wechsler Intelligence Scale
Wechsler Intelligence Scale for Children (WISC)
Wechsler Intelligence Scale for Children–Revised (WISC-R)
Wechsler Intelligence Scale for Children, Revised Version and Version III
Wechsler IQ Scale
Wechsler Memory Scale (WMS)

Wechsler Memory Scale, Russell Version
Wechsler Memory Scale, Standard and Russell versions
Wechsler Memory Scale/Memory Quotient (WMS-MQ)
Wechsler Preschool Primary Scale of Intelligence (WPPSI)
Wechsler-Bellevue Scale (WBS)
Weiss Comprehensive Articulation Test
Weiss Intelligibility Test
Weller-Strawser Scales of Adaptive Behavior for the Learning Disabled
Welsh Figure Preference Test
Wender Utah Rating Scale
Wepman Auditory Discrimination Test
Wesman Personnel Classification Test
Western Aphasia Battery (WAB)
Western Personality Inventory
What I Like to Do: An Inventory of Students' Interest (WILD)
Whitaker Index of Schizophrenic Thinking (WIST)
Who Are You? Technique
Who Are You? Test
WHO Handicap Scale
Wide Range Achievement Test (WRAT)
Wide Range Achievement Test-Revised (WRAT-R)
Wide Range Achievement Test, Third Edition (WRAT-3)
Wide Range Assessment of Memory and Learning (WRAML)
Wide Range Employment Sample Test (WREST)
Wide Range Intelligence and Personality Test (WRIPT)
Wide Range Interest-Opinion Test (WRIOT)
Wide Range Vocabulary Test
Wiggins Content Scale (WCS)
Wiggly Block Test

Wilson-Patterson Attitude Inventory (WPAI)

Wing Negative Symptom Scale

WISC-III Companion

WISC-III Compilation: What to Do Now That You Know the Score

WISC-III Compilation: What to Do Now that You Know the Score (Computer)

Wisconsin Card-Sorting Test (WCST)

Wisconsin Psychosocial Pain Inventory

Wisconsin Scoring Test

Within Session Rating Scale for Cocaine

Wittenborn Psychiatric Rating Scale (WITT)

Wittenborn Psychiatric Rating Scale Test

Wood Assessment Scale

Woodcock Language Proficiency Battery

Woodcock Reading Mastery Test

Woodcock-Johnson Achievement Test (WJAT)

Woodcock-Johnson Psycho-Educational Test Battery, Revised (WJPB-R)

Word Association Test

Word Finding Test

Word Fluency Test

Word Intelligibility by Picture Identification (WIPI)

Word Processing Test

Word Processor Assessment Battery

Word Recognition Test

Word-in-Context Test

Work and Social Adjustment Scale

Work Attitudes Questionnaire (WAQ)

Work Environment Preference Schedule (WEPS)

Work Environment Scale (WES)

Work Information Inventory (WII)

Work Interest Index

Work Motivation Inventory (WMI)

Work Sample Battery

Work Skills Series Production (WSS)

Work Values Inventory (WVI)

World of Work Inventory (WWI)

Worry Scale for Children

Worse Premorbid Adjustment Scale

Wortman Social Support Scale

Writing Skills Test

Written Language Assessment

Yale-Brown Obsessive Compulsive Scale (Y-BOCS)

Yale-Brown Obsessive Compulsive Scale, Modified for Pathological Gambling (PG-YBOCS)

Yale Global Tic Severity Scale

Yale Revised Developmental Schedule

Yale Schedule for Tourette Syndrome and Other Behavioral Disorders

Yale Schedule for Tourette Syndrome and Other Behavioral Disorders, Hebrew Version

Yale Tic Severity Scale

Yale-Brown Obsessive Compulsive Scale (YBOCS)

Yerkes-Bridges Test (YBT)

Young Adult Behavior Checklist

Young Mania Rating Scale (YMRS)

Ziegler Mania Rating Scale

Zimmerman Personality Test

Zulliger Test

Zung Anxiety Scale

Zung Depression Scale (ZDS)

Zung Self-Rating Anxiety Scale

Zung Self-Rating Depression Scale

Drugs by Indication

ACETAMINOPHEN POISONING
Mucolytic Agent
  acetylcysteine
  Acys-5®
  Mucomyst®
  Parvolex® (Can)

ALCOHOLISM
Aldehyde Dehydrogenase Inhibitor
  Agent
  Antabuse®
  disulfiram
Phenothiazine Derivative
  mesoridazine
  Serentil®

ALCOHOL WITHDRAWAL
Alpha-Adrenergic Agonist
  Apo®-Clonidine (Can)
  Catapres® Oral
  Catapres-TTS® Transdermal
  clonidine
  Dixarit® (Can)
  Duraclon™ Injection
  Novo-Clonidine (Can)
  Nu-Clonidine (Can)
Antihistamine
  Apo®-Hydroxyzine (Can)
  Atarax®
  hydroxyzine
  Hyzine® Injection
  Novo-Hydroxyzin (Can)
  PMS-Hydroxyzine (Can)
  Restall® Injection
  Vistacot® Injection
  Vistaril®
Benzodiazepine
  alprazolam
  Alti-Alprazolam (Can)

Apo®-Alpraz (Can)
Apo®-Chlordiazepoxide (Can)
Apo®-Clorazepate (Can)
Apo®-Diazepam (Can)
Apo®-Oxazepam (Can)
chlordiazepoxide
clorazepate
Diastat® Rectal Delivery System
Diazemuls® Injection
diazepam
Diazepam Intensol®
Dizac® Injectable Emulsion
Gen-Alprazolam (Can)
Gen-XENE®
Librium®
Novo-Alprazol (Can)
Novo-Clopate (Can)
Novo-Poxide (Can)
Nu-Alpraz (Can)
oxazepam
Serax®
Tranxene®
Valium® Injection
Valium® Oral
Vivol® (Can)
Xanax®
Beta-Adrenergic Blocker
  Apo®-Atenol (Can)
  Apo®-Propranolol (Can)
  atenolol
  Gen-Atenolol (Can)
  Inderal®
  Inderal® LA
  Nu-Atenol (Can)
  Nu-Propranolol (Can)
  propranolol
  Taro-Atenol® (Can)
  Tenolin (Can)
  Tenormin®
Phenothiazine Derivative

Apo®-Thioridazine (Can)
Mellaril®
thioridazine

ALZHEIMER DISEASE
Acetylcholinesterase Inhibitor
Aricept®
Cognex®
donepezil
Exelon®
rivastigmine
tacrine
Acetylcholinesterase Inhibitor (Central)
galantamine
Reminyl®
Cholinergic Agent
Exelon®
rivastigmine
Ergot Alkaloid and Derivative
ergoloid mesylates
Germinal®
Hydergine®
Hydergine® LC

AMMONIA INTOXICATION
Ammonium Detoxicant
Acilac (Can)
Cephulac®
Cholac®
Chronulac®
Constilac®
Constulose®
Duphalac®
Enulose®
Evalose®
Heptalac®
Kristalose™
lactulose
Lactulose PSE®
Laxilose (Can)
PMS-Lactulose (Can)

ANTIFREEZE POISONING
Antidote

Antizol®
fomepizole

ANXIETY
Antianxiety Agent
BuSpar®
buspirone
Antianxiety Agent, Miscellaneous
Apo®-Meprobamate (Can)
Equanil®
meprobamate
Miltown®
Antidepressant/Phenothiazine
amitriptyline and perphenazine
Etrafon®
Triavil®
Antidepressant, Tetracyclic
Ludiomil®
maprotiline
Novo-Maprotiline (Can)
Antidepressant, Tricyclic (Secondary Amine)
amoxapine
Asendin® (Can)
Antidepressant, Tricyclic (Tertiary Amine)
Alti-Doxepin (Can)
amitriptyline and chlordiazepoxide
Apo®-Doxepin (Can)
doxepin
Limbitrol® DS 10–25
Novo-Doxepin (Can)
Sinequan® Oral
Zonalon® Topical Cream
Antihistamine
Allerdryl® (Can)
AllerMax® Oral [OTC]
Allernix® (Can)
Apo®-Hydroxyzine (Can)
Atarax®
Banophen® Oral [OTC]
Belix® Oral [OTC]
Benadryl® Injection

Benadryl® Oral [OTC]
Benadryl® Topical
Ben-Allergin-50® Injection
Benylin® Cough Syrup [OTC]
Bydramine® Cough Syrup [OTC]
Compoz® Gel Caps [OTC]
Compoz® Nighttime Sleep Aid [OTC]
Dihyrex® Injection
Diphenacen-50® Injection [OTC]
Diphen® Cough [OTC]
Diphenhist [OTC]
diphenhydramine
Dormarex® 2 Oral [OTC]
Dormin® Oral [OTC]
Genahist® Oral
Hydramyn® Syrup [OTC]
hydroxyzine
Hyrexin-50® Injection
Hyzine® Injection
Maximum Strength Nytol® [OTC]
Miles Nervine® Caplets [OTC]
Nordryl® Injection
Nordryl® Oral
Novo-Hydroxyzin (Can)
Nytol® Oral [OTC]
Phendry® Oral [OTC]
PMS-Diphenhydramine (Can)
PMS-Hydroxyzine (Can)
Restall® Injection
Siladryl® Oral [OTC]
Silphen® Cough [OTC]
Sleep-eze 3® Oral [OTC]
Sleepinal® [OTC]
Sleepwell 2-nite® [OTC]
Sominex® Oral [OTC]
Tusstat® Syrup
Twilite® Oral [OTC]
Uni-Bent® Cough Syrup
Vistacot® Injection
Vistaril®
Winks® [OTC]
Barbiturate
  butabarbital sodium

Butalan®
butalbital compound and codeine
Buticaps®
Butisol Sodium®
Fiorinal®-C (Can)
Fiorinal® With Codeine
Tecnal C (Can)
Benzodiazepine
alprazolam
Alti-Alprazolam (Can)
Alti-Bromazepam (Can)
Apo®-Alpraz (Can)
Apo®-Bromazepam (Can)
Apo®-Chlordiazepoxide (Can)
Apo®-Clorazepate (Can)
Apo®-Diazepam (Can)
Apo®-Lorazepam (Can)
Apo®-Oxazepam (Can)
Apo®-Temazepam (Can)
Ativan®
bromazepam (Canada only)
chlordiazepoxide
clorazepate
Diastat® Rectal Delivery System
Diazemuls® Injection
diazepam
Diazepam Intensol®
Dizac® Injectable Emulsion
Gen-Alprazolam (Can)
Gen-Bromazepam (Can)
Gen-Temazepam (Can)
Gen-XENE®
halazepam
Lectopam® (Can)
Librium®
lorazepam
Novo-Alprazol (Can)
Novo-Bromazepam (Can)
Novo-Clopate (Can)
Novo-Lorazem (Can)
Novo-Lorazepam (Can)
Novo-Poxide (Can)
Novo-Temazepam (Can)

Nu-Alpraz (Can)
Nu-Bromazepam (Can)
Nu-Loraz (Can)
Nu-Temazepam (Can)
oxazepam
Paxipam®
PMS-Temazepam (Can)
Restoril®
Riva-Lorazepam (Can)
Serax®
temazepam
Tranxene®
Valium® Injection
Valium® Oral
Vivol® (Can)
Xanax®
General Anesthetic
Actiq® Oral Transmucosal
Duragesic® Transdermal
fentanyl
Fentanyl Oralet®
Sublimaze® Injection
Neuroleptic Agent
Apo®-Methoprazine (Can)
methotrimeprazine (Canada only)
Novo-Meprazine (Can)
Nozinan® (Can)
Phenothiazine Derivative
Apo®-Trifluoperazine (Can)
Stelazine®
trifluoperazine
Sedative
Alti-Bromazepam (Can)
Apo®-Bromazepam (Can)
bromazepam (Canada only)
Gen-Bromazepam (Can)
Lectopam® (Can)
Novo-Bromazepam (Can)
Nu-Bromazepam (Can)

ARSENIC POISONING
Chelating Agent
BAL in Oil®

dimercaprol

ATTENTION-DEFICIT/HYPERACTIVITY DISORDER (ADHD)
Amphetamine
Desoxyn®
Dexedrine® Spansule®
Dexedrine® Tablet
dextroamphetamine
Dextrostat®
methamphetamine
Central Nervous System Stimulant,
Nonamphetamine
Concerta™
Cylert®
Metadate® CD
Metadate™ ER
Methylin™
Methylin™ ER
methylphenidate
PemADD®
PemADD CT®
pemoline
PMS-Methylphenidate (Can)
Riphenidate® (Can)
Ritalin®
Ritalin-SR®

AUTISM
Antipsychotic Agent, Butyrophenone
Apo®-Haloperidol (Can)
Haldol®
Haldol® Decanoate
haloperidol
Novo-Peridol (Can)
Peridol (Can)
PMS-Haloperidol LA (Can)

BARBITURATE POISONING
Antidote
Actidose-Aqua® [OTC]
Actidose® With Sorbitol [OTC]
CharcoAid® [OTC]

charcoal
Charcocaps® [OTC]
Charcodote Aqueous (Can)
Liqui-Char® [OTC]

BENZODIAZEPINE OVERDOSE
Antidote
  Anexate® (Can)
  flumazenil
  Romazicon®

BIPOLAR DEPRESSION DISORDER
Anticonvulsant
  Alti-Valproic (Can)
  Apo®-Divalproex (Can)
  Apo®-Valproic (Can)
  Depacon™
  Depakene®
  Depakote® Delayed Release
  Depakote® ER
  Deproic® (Can)
  Epival® (Can)
  Gen-Valproic (Can)
  Novo-Divalproex® (Can)
  Nu-Divalproex® (Can)
  Nu-Valproic (Can)
  PMS-Valproic Acid (Can)
  Rhoxal-valproic (Can)
  valproic acid and derivatives
Antimanic Agent
  Carbolith™ (Can)
  Duralith® (Can)
  Eskalith®
  Eskalith CR®
  lithium
  Lithobid®
  PMS-Lithium Carbonate (Can)
  PMS-Lithium Citrate (Can)
Antipsychotic Agent
  Clopixol-Acuphase® (Can)
  Clopixol® (Can)

Clopixol® Depot (Can)
zuclopenthixol (Canada only)

BROMIDE INTOXICATION
Diuretic, Loop
  Edecrin®
  ethacrynic acid

CACHEXIA
Antihistamine
  cyproheptadine
  Periactin®
Progestin
  Apo®-Megestrol (Can)
  Lin-Megestrol (Can)
  Megace®
  megestrol acetate
  Nu-Megestrol (Can)

CURARE POISONING
Cholinergic Agent
  edrophonium
  Enlon®
  Reversol®
  Tensilon®

CYANIDE POISONING
Antidote
  cyanide antidote kit
  methylene blue
  sodium thiosulfate
  Urolene Blue®
Vasodilator
  amyl nitrite

DEMENTIA (ALSO SEE ALZHEIMER DISEASE)
Acetylcholinesterase Inhibitor
  Aricept®
  donepezil
Antidepressant, Tricyclic (Tertiary Amine)
  Alti-Doxepin (Can)
  Apo®-Doxepin (Can)
  doxepin

Novo-Doxepin (Can)
Sinequan® Oral
Benzodiazepine
diazepam
Valium® Injection
Valium® Oral
Vivol® (Can)
Ergot Alkaloid and Derivative
ergoloid mesylates
Germinal®
Hydergine®
Hydergine® LC
Phenothiazine Derivative
Apo®-Thioridazine (Can)
Mellaril®
thioridazine

DEPRESSION

Antidepressant
Celexa™
citalopram
Antidepressant, Alpha-2 Antagonist
mirtazapine
Remeron®
Remeron® SolTab™
Antidepressant, Aminoketone
bupropion
Wellbutrin®
Wellbutrin® SR
Zyban™
Antidepressant, Miscellaneous
nefazodone
Serzone®
Antidepressant, Monoamine Oxidase
Inhibitor
Alti-Moclobemide (Can)
Apo®-Moclobemide (Can)
isocarboxazid
Manerix® (Can)
Marplan®
moclobemide (Canada only)
Nardil®
Novo-Moclobemide (Can)

Nu-Moclobemide (Can)
Parnate®
phenelzine
tranylcypromine
Antidepressant, Phenethylamine
Effexor®
Effexor-XR®
venlafaxine
Antidepressant/Phenothiazine
amitriptyline and perphenazine
Etrafon®
Triavil®
Antidepressant, Selective Serotonin
Reuptake Inhibitor
Alti-Fluoxetine (Can)
Alti-Fluvoxamine (Can)
Apo®-Fluoxetine (Can)
Apo®-Fluvoxamine (Can)
Apo®-Sertraline (Can)
fluoxetine
fluvoxamine
Gen-Fluoxetine (Can)
Luvox®
Novo-Fluoxetine (Can)
Novo-Fluvoxamine (Can)
Novo-Sertraline (Can)
Nu-Fluoxetine (Can)
Nu-Fluvoxamine (Can)
paroxetine
Paxil™
PMS-Fluoxetine (Can)
PMS-Fluvoxamine (Can)
Prozac®
Prozac® Weekly™
Sarafem™
sertraline
Zoloft®
Antidepressant, Tetracyclic
Ludiomil®
maprotiline
Novo-Maprotiline (Can)
Antidepressant, Triazolopyridine
Alti-Trazodone (Can)

Apo®-Trazodone (Can)
Desyrel®
Gen-Trazodone (Can)
Novo-Trazodone (Can)
Nu-Trazodone (Can)
PMS-Trazodone (Can)
trazodone
Trazorel (Can)
Antidepressant, Tricyclic (Secondary Amine)
Alti-Desipramine (Can)
amoxapine
Apo®-Desipramine (Can)
Apo®-Nortriptyline (Can)
Asendin® (Can)
Aventyl® Hydrochloride
desipramine
Norpramin®
nortriptyline
Novo-Desipramine (Can)
Nu-Desipramine (Can)
Pamelor®
PMS-Desipramine (Can)
protriptyline
Triptil® (Can)
Vivactil®
Antidepressant, Tricyclic (Tertiary Amine)
Alti-Doxepin (Can)
amitriptyline
amitriptyline and chlordiazepoxide
Apo®-Amitriptyline (Can)
Apo®-Doxepin (Can)
Apo®-Imipramine (Can)
Apo®-Trimip (Can)
doxepin
Elavil®
imipramine
Limbitrol® DS 10–25
Novo-Doxepin (Can)
Novo-Tripramine (Can)
Nu-Trimipramine (Can)
Rhotrimine® (Can)

Sinequan® Oral
Surmontil®
Tofranil®
Tofranil-PM®
trimipramine
Vanatrip®
Benzodiazepine
alprazolam
Alti-Alprazolam (Can)
Apo®-Alpraz (Can)
Gen-Alprazolam (Can)
Novo-Alprazol (Can)
Nu-Alpraz (Can)
Xanax®

DRUG DEPENDENCE (OPIOID)

Analgesic, Narcotic
Dolophine®
levomethadyl acetate hydrochloride
Metadol™ (Can)
methadone
Methadose® (Can)
ORLAAM®

INSOMNIA

Antihistamine
Allerdryl® (Can)
AllerMax® Oral [OTC]
Allernix® (Can)
Apo®-Hydroxyzine (Can)
Atarax®
Banophen® Oral [OTC]
Belix® Oral [OTC]
Benadryl® Injection
Benadryl® Oral [OTC]
Benadryl® Topical
Ben-Allergin-50® Injection
Benylin® Cough Syrup [OTC]
Bydramine® Cough Syrup [OTC]
Compoz® Gel Caps [OTC]
Compoz® Nighttime Sleep Aid [OTC]
Dihyrex® Injection

Diphenacen-50® Injection [OTC]
Diphen® Cough [OTC]
Diphenhist [OTC]
diphenhydramine
Dormarex® 2 Oral [OTC]
Dormin® Oral [OTC]
Genahist® Oral
Hydramyn® Syrup [OTC]
hydroxyzine
Hyrexin-50® Injection
Hyzine® Injection
Maximum Strength Nytol® [OTC]
Miles Nervine® Caplets [OTC]
Nordryl® Injection
Nordryl® Oral
Novo-Hydroxyzin (Can)
Nytol® Oral [OTC]
Phendry® Oral [OTC]
PMS-Diphenhydramine (Can)
PMS-Hydroxyzine (Can)
Restall® Injection
Siladryl® Oral [OTC]
Silphen® Cough [OTC]
Sleep-eze 3® Oral [OTC]
Sleepinal® [OTC]
Sleepwell 2-nite® [OTC]
Sominex® Oral [OTC]
Tusstat® Syrup
Twilite® Oral [OTC]
Uni-Bent® Cough Syrup
Vistacot® Injection
Vistaril®
Winks® [OTC]
Barbiturate
  amobarbital
  amobarbital and secobarbital
  Amytal®
  butabarbital sodium
  Butalan®
  Buticaps®
  Butisol Sodium®
  Luminal®
  Nembutal®

pentobarbital
phenobarbital
secobarbital
Seconal™
Tuinal®
Benzodiazepine
  Apo®-Diazepam (Can)
  Apo®-Flurazepam (Can)
  Apo®-Lorazepam (Can)
  Apo®-Temazepam (Can)
  Apo®-Triazo (Can)
  Ativan®
  Dalmane®
  Diastat® Rectal Delivery System
  Diazemuls® Injection
  diazepam
  Diazepam Intensol®
  Dizac® Injectable Emulsion
  Doral®
  estazolam
  flurazepam
  Gen-Temazepam (Can)
  Gen-Triazolam (Can)
  Halcion®
  lorazepam
  Novo-Lorazem (Can)
  Novo-Lorazepam (Can)
  Novo-Temazepam (Can)
  Nu-Loraz (Can)
  Nu-Temazepam (Can)
  PMS-Temazepam (Can)
  ProSom™
  quazepam
  Restoril®
  Riva-Lorazepam (Can)
  Somnol® (Can)
  temazepam
  triazolam
  Valium® Injection
  Valium® Oral
  Vivol® (Can)
Hypnotic
  Apo®-Zopiclone (Can)

Gen-Zopiclone (Can)
Imovane® (Can)
Nu-Zopiclone (Can)
Rhovane® (Can)
zopiclone (Canada only)
Hypnotic, Nonbarbiturate
  Ambien™
  Aquachloral® Supprettes®
  chloral hydrate
  ethchlorvynol
  Placidyl®
  PMS-Chloral Hydrate (Can)
  zolpidem
Hypnotic, Nonbenzodiazepine
  (Pyrazolopyrimidine)
  Sonata®
  Starnoc® (Can)
  zaleplon

IRON POISONING
Antidote
  deferoxamine
  Desferal® Mesylate

MANIA
Anticonvulsant
  Alti-Valproic (Can)
  Apo®-Divalproex (Can)
  Apo®-Valproic (Can)
  Depacon™
  Depakene®
  Depakote® Delayed Release
  Depakote® ER
  Deproic® (Can)
  Epival® (Can)
  Gen-Valproic (Can)
  Novo-Divalproex® (Can)
  Nu-Divalproex® (Can)
  Nu-Valproic (Can)
  PMS-Valproic Acid (Can)
  Rhoxal-valproic (Can)
  valproic acid and derivatives

Antimanic Agent
  Carbolith™ (Can)
  Duralith® (Can)
  Eskalith®
  Eskalith CR®
  lithium
  Lithobid®
  PMS-Lithium Carbonate (Can)
  PMS-Lithium Citrate (Can)
Phenothiazine Derivative
  Chlorpromanyl (Can)
  chlorpromazine
  Largactil® (Can)
  Thorazine®

METHANOL POISONING
Pharmaceutical Aid
  alcohol (ethyl)
  Lavacol® [OTC]

METHOTREXATE POISONING
Folic Acid Derivative
  leucovorin
  Wellcovorin®

MUSCARINE POISONING
Anticholinergic Agent
  Atropair®
  atropine
  Atropine-Care®
  Atropisol®
  Isopto® Atropine
  I-Tropine®
  Sal-Tropine™ Oral

NARCOTIC DETOXIFICATION
Analgesic, Narcotic
  Dolophine®
  Metadol™ (Can)
  methadone
  Methadose® (Can)

OBSESSIVE-COMPULSIVE DISORDER (OCD)

Antidepressant, Selective Serotonin
  Reuptake Inhibitor
  Alti-Fluoxetine (Can)
  Alti-Fluvoxamine (Can)
  Apo®-Fluoxetine (Can)
  Apo®-Fluvoxamine (Can)
  Apo®-Sertraline (Can)
  fluoxetine
  fluvoxamine
  Gen-Fluoxetine (Can)
  Luvox®
  Novo-Fluoxetine (Can)
  Novo-Fluvoxamine (Can)
  Novo-Sertraline (Can)
  Nu-Fluoxetine (Can)
  Nu-Fluvoxamine (Can)
  paroxetine
  Paxil™
  PMS-Fluoxetine (Can)
  PMS-Fluvoxamine (Can)
  Prozac®
  Prozac® Weekly™
  Sarafem™
  sertraline
  Zoloft®
Antidepressant, Tricyclic (Tertiary
  Amine)
  Anafranil®
  Apo®-Clomipramine (Can)
  clomipramine
  Gen-Clomipramine (Can)
  Novo-Clopamine (Can)

OPIOID POISONING

Antidote
  Depade®
  nalmefene
  naloxone
  naltrexone
  Narcan®
  Revex®
  ReVia®

PANIC ATTACKS [ALSO SEE PANIC DISORDER (PD)]

Benzodiazepine
  alprazolam
  Alti-Alprazolam (Can)
  Apo®-Alpraz (Can)
  Apo®-Temazepam (Can)
  Gen-Alprazolam (Can)
  Gen-Temazepam (Can)
  Novo-Alprazol (Can)
  Novo-Temazepam (Can)
  Nu-Alpraz (Can)
  Nu-Temazepam (Can)
  PMS-Temazepam (Can)
  Restoril®
  temazepam
  Xanax®

PANIC DISORDER (PD)

Antidepressant, Selective Serotonin
  Reuptake Inhibitor
  paroxetine
  Paxil™

PREMENSTRUAL DYSPHORIC DISORDER (PMDD)

Antidepressant, Selective Serotonin
  Reuptake Inhibitor
  Alti-Fluoxetine (Can)
  Apo®-Fluoxetine (Can)
  fluoxetine
  Gen-Fluoxetine (Can)
  Novo-Fluoxetine (Can)
  Nu-Fluoxetine (Can)
  PMS-Fluoxetine (Can)
  Prozac®
  Prozac® Weekly™
  Sarafem™

PSYCHOSES

Antipsychotic Agent
  Clopixol-Acuphase® (Can)
  Clopixol® (Can)
  Clopixol® Depot (Can)
  olanzapine
  quetiapine
  Seroquel®
  zuclopenthixol (Canada only)
  Zyprexa®
  Zyprexa® Zydis®
Antipsychotic Agent, Benzisoxazole
  Risperdal®
  risperidone
Antipsychotic Agent, Butyrophenone
  Apo®-Haloperidol (Can)
  droperidol
  Haldol®
  Haldol® Decanoate
  haloperidol
  Inapsine®
  Novo-Peridol (Can)
  Peridol (Can)
  PMS-Haloperidol LA (Can)
Antipsychotic Agent, Dibenzoxazepine
  Apo®-Loxapine (Can)
  Loxapac® (Can)
  loxapine
  Loxitane®
  Nu-Loxapine (Can)
  PMS-Loxapine (Can)
Antipsychotic Agent, Dihydroindoline
  Moban®
  molindone
Phenothiazine Derivative
  Apo®-Perphenazine (Can)
  Apo®-Thioridazine (Can)
  Apo®-Trifluoperazine (Can)
  Chlorpromanyl (Can)
  chlorpromazine
  Compazine®
  fluphenazine
  Largactil® (Can)

Mellaril®
mesoridazine
Modecate® (Can)
Neuleptil® (Can)
Nu-Prochlor (Can)
pericyazine (Canada only)
Permitil® Oral
perphenazine
PMS-Fluphenazine Decanoate (Can)
prochlorperazine
Prolixin Decanoate® Injection
Prolixin Enanthate® Injection
Prolixin® Injection
Prolixin® Oral
promazine
Serentil®
Stelazine®
Stemetil® (Can)
thioridazine
Thorazine®
trifluoperazine
triflupromazine
Trilafon®
Vesprin®
Thioxanthene Derivative
  Navane® Capsule
  thiothixene

PYRIMETHAMINE POISONING

Folic Acid Derivative
  leucovorin
  Wellcovorin®

SCHIZOPHRENIA

Antipsychotic Agent
  Clopixol-Acuphase® (Can)
  Clopixol® (Can)
  Clopixol® Depot (Can)
  Fluanxol® Depot (Can)
  Fluanxol® Tablet (Can)
  flupenthixol (Canada only)
  olanzapine

quetiapine
Seroquel®
zuclopenthixol (Canada only)
Zyprexa®
Zyprexa® Zydis®
Antipsychotic Agent, Benzisoxazole
Risperdal®
risperidone
Antipsychotic Agent, Dibenzodiazepine
clozapine
Clozaril®
Neuroleptic Agent
Apo®-Methoprazine (Can)
Majeptil® (Can)
methotrimeprazine (Canada only)
Novo-Meprazine (Can)
Nozinan® (Can)
thioproperazine (Canada only)
Thioxanthene Derivative
Fluanxol® Depot (Can)
Fluanxol® Tablet (Can)
flupenthixol (Canada only)

SMOKING CESSATION
Antidepressant, Monoamine Oxidase
Inhibitor
Alti-Moclobemide (Can)
Apo®-Moclobemide (Can)
Manerix® (Can)
moclobemide (Canada only)
Novo-Moclobemide (Can)
Nu-Moclobemide (Can)
Smoking Deterrent
Habitrol™ Patch
NicoDerm® Patch
Nicorette® DS Gum
Nicorette® Gum
Nicorette® Plus (Can)
nicotine
Nicotrol® Inhaler
Nicotrol® NS Nasal Spray
Nicotrol® Patch [OTC]
ProStep® Patch

TOXICITY (NONSPECIFIC) [TREATMENT]
Antacid
magnesium hydroxide
magnesium oxide
Mag-Ox® 400 [OTC]
Maox® [OTC]
Phillips'® Milk of Magnesia [OTC]
Uro-Mag® [OTC]
Antidote
Actidose-Aqua® [OTC]
Actidose® With Sorbitol [OTC]
CharcoAid® [OTC]
charcoal
Charcocaps® [OTC]
Charcodote Aqueous (Can)
ipecac syrup
Liqui-Char® [OTC]
Diuretic, Osmotic
mannitol
Osmitrol® Injection
Resectisol® Irrigation Solution
Electrolyte Supplement, Oral
Fleet® Enema [OTC]
Fleet® Phospho®-Soda [OTC]
sodium phosphates
Laxative
Citro-Mag (Can)
magnesium citrate

VALPROIC ACID POISONING
Dietary Supplement
Carnitor® Injection
Carnitor® Oral
levocarnitine
VitaCarn® Oral

Phobias Listed by Clinical Name

Fear is a feeling that is experienced by all humans at one time or another. Phobias take fear a step further than the normal feeling of anxiety one gets when faced with a new adventure, or when one comes face-to-face with something unpleasant. The definition of specific phobia summarizes phobias in general.

"specific phobia: (1) a persistent pattern of significant fear of a social or performance situation, manifesting in anxiety or panic on exposure to the situation or in anticipation of it, which the person realizes is unreasonable or excessive and which interferes with the person's functioning; (2) a DSM diagnosis that is established when the specific criteria are met." (Source: *Stedman's Medical Dictionary,* 27th Edition)

There is a clinical name for almost every fear. The following pages list phobias in alphabetical order by clinical name and by the fear itself.

CLINICAL NAMES	ABNORMAL FEAR OF
acarophobia	mites or ticks on the skin
acerophobia	sourness
achluophobia	darkness
acousticophobia	sounds
acrophobia	heights
aeroacrophobia	high open places
aerodromophobia	airports
aerophobia	air
agoraphobia	being in open spaces; leaving one's home
agyiophobia	streets
aichmophobia	knives; points
ailurophobia, aelurophobia	cats
albuminurophobia	albumin in urine as sign of kidney disease
alcoholophobia	alcoholism
alektorophobia	chickens
algophobia	pain
amathophobia	dust
amaxophobia	riding in vehicles
amychophobia	being scratched; scratches
androphobia	men; dislike of males
anemophobia	wind; drafts
anginophobia	sore throat; choking
anglophobia	England or dislike of anything English
anthophobia	flowers

anthropophobia	people
antlophobia	floods
anuptophobia	remaining single
apeirophobia	infinity
aphephobia	being touched
apiphobia	bees
aquaphobia	bathing; swimming in a body of water
arachibutyrophobia	peanut butter on roof of mouth
arachnephobia	spiders
asthenophobia	weakness
astraphobia, astrapophobia	lightning
astrophobia	the stars
ataxophobia, ataxiophobia	disorder
atelophobia	imperfection
atephobia	ruin
aulophobia	flutes or similar wind instruments
aurophobia	gold
auroraphobia	northern lights
autodysosmophobia	offensive personal body odor
automysophobia	being dirty
autophobia	self; aloneness; solitude
aviophobia	flying
bacillophobia	bacilli
ballistophobia	missiles
barophobia	gravity
basiphobia, basophobia; basistasiphobia, basistasophobia	walking
bathophobia	depths
batophobia	high objects
batrachophobia	reptiles; frogs
belonephobia	needles; sharp objects
bibliophobia	books
blennophobia	slime; mucus
bogyphobia	demons and goblins
botanophobia	plants and flowers
bromidrosiphobia	having an unpleasant personal body odor
brontophobia	thunder; thunderstorms
cainophobia, kainophobia	novelty
cancerophobia, carcinophobia	cancer; malignancy
cardiophobia	heart disease
carnophobia	meat
catagelophobia, katagelophobia	ridicule; being made fun of
cathisophobia, kathisophobia	sitting down

catoptrophobia	mirrors
celtophobia	Celts or dislike of anything Celtic
cenotophobia	anything new
chaetophobia	hair
cheimaphobia	cold
cherophobia	gaiety
chionophobia	snow
cholerophobia	cholera
chrematophobia	money; wealth
chromatophobia, chromophobia	colors
chronophobia	time
cibophobia	food
claustrophobia	confinement; closed spaces
climacophobia	stairs; climbing
clinophobia	going to bed
clithrophobia	being locked in
cnidophobia	stings
coitophobia	sexual intercourse
cometophobia	comet
coprophobia	excrement
counterphobia	seeking out that which is feared
cremnophobia	precipices; cliffs
cryophobia	ice
crystallophobia	glass
cymophobia	sea swells
cynophobia	dogs; rabies
cypridophobia, cypriphobia	venereal disease; sexual intercourse
decidophobia	making decisions
defecalgesiophobia	defecating due to pain
deipnophobia	dining; dinner conversation
demonophobia, daemonophobia	demons; the devil
demophobia	crowds
dendrophobia	trees
dermatophobia, dermatopathophobia, dermatosiophobia	skin disease
dextrophobia	objects to the right
diabetophobia	diabetes
didaskaleinophobia	school
dikephobia	justice
dinophobia	whirlpools
diplopiaphobia	double vision
dipsophobia	drinking

domatophobia	houses
doraphobia	fur; skin of animals
dromophobia	crossing streets
dysmorphophobia	deformity
ecclesiophobia, ecclesiaphobia	churches
ecophobia	home environment
eisoptrophobia	termites
electrophobia	electricity
eleutherophobia	freedom
emetophobia	vomiting
enosiophobia	committing the unpardonable sin
entomophobia	insects
eosophobia	dawn
equinophobia	horses
eremiophobia, eremophobia	stillness; being alone
ergasiophobia	work
ergophobia	hatred of work
eroticophobia	erotica
erotophobia	sexual love or physical expression
erythrophobia, ereuthophobia	blushing; red
eurotophobia	female genitals
febriphobia	fever
felinophobia	cats
francophobia	France or dislike of anything French
galeophobia	sharks
gallophobia	France of dislike of anything French
gamophobia	marriage
gatophobia	cats
geniophobia	chins
genophobia	sex
gephyrophobia	crossing bridges
gerascophobia	growing old
germanophobia	Germany or dislike of anything German
gerontophobia	old age
geumaphobia	tastes
glossophobia	speaking in public
graphophobia	writing
gringophobia	white strangers in Latin countries
gymnophobia	nakedness
gynephobia, gynophobia	women
hadephobia	hell
hagiophobia	saints; holy people
hamartophobia	sin; error

hamaxophobia	vehicles
haptephobia, haphephobia	being touched
harpaxophobia	robbers
hedonophobia	pleasure
heliophobia	sunlight
hellenologophobia	cumbersome pseudoscientific words
hellenophobia	Greece or dislike of anything Greek
helminthophobia	worm infestation
hemophobia, hematophobia	blood
herpetophobia	reptiles; amphibians
hierophobia	sacred things
hippophobia	horses
hodophobia	travel
homichlophobia	fog
homilophobia	sermons
homophobia	homosexuals
hormephobia	shock
hyalophobia, hyelophobia	glass
hydrophobia	water
hydrophobophobia	hydrophobia; rabies or water
hygrophobia	dampness; moisture; liquids
hylophobia, hylephobia, hylophobia	forests; wood
hypengyophobia	responsibility
hypnophobia	sleep
hypsiphobia, hypsophobia	high places
iatrophobia	doctors
ichthyophobia	fish
iconophobia	worship
ideophobia	ideas
iophobia	poisons
isolophobia	being alone
isopterophobia	termites
japanophobia	Japan or dislike of anything Japanese
judeophobia	Jews or dislike of anything Jewish
kainotophobia, kainophobia, cainotophobia, cainophobia	anything new; change; novelty
kakorrhaphiophobia	failure; defeat
katagelophobia	ridicule
kenophobia, cenophobia	barren space; emptiness
keraunophobia, ceraunophobia	thunder and lightning
kilobytophobia	computers
kinesophobia	motion

kleptophobia; cleptophobia	stealing; thieves
koniophobia	dust
kopophobia	having a physical or mental exam
lalophobia, laliophobia	speaking; stuttering
leprophobia; lepraphobia	leprosy
levophobia	objects to the left
limnophobia	lakes
linonophobia	strings
logophobia	words
lyssophobia	insanity
maieusiophobia	pregnancy; childbirth
maniaphobia	insanity
mastigophobia	flogging; being beaten
mechanophobia	machinery
megalophobia	large objects
melissophobia	bees
meningitophobia	meningitis; brain disease
merinthophobia	being bound
metallophobia	metals
meteorophobia	meteors
microbiophobia	microorganisms; germs
microphobia	small or minute objects
molysmophobia; molysomophobia	contamination; infection
monopathophobia	definite disease
monophobia	aloneness; being alone
motorphobia	motor vehicles
musicophobia	music
misophobia, mysophobia	contamination; filth
musophobia	mice
mythophobia	myths; stories
myxophobia	slime; mucus
nebulaphobia	clouds
necrophobia	corpses; death
neophobia	anything new; change; novelty
nephophobia	clouds
noctiphobia	night
nomatophobia	names
nosemaphobia	illness
nosophobia	disease
nostophobia	returning home
nucleomitaphobia	death from nuclear war
nudophobia, nudiphobia	nudity
nyctophobia	darkness; night

ochlophobia	crowds
ochophobia	vehicles
odontophobia	teeth; dental surgery
odynophobia; odynephobia	pain
oecophobia, oikophobia	home environment
oenophobia	wine (or dislike for)
oikophobia, oikiophobia, oechophobia	home or home surroundings
olfactophobia	odors
ombrophobia	rain
ommatophobia	eyes
oneirophobia	dreams
onomatophobia	hearing certain words or names
ophidiophobia	snakes
optophobia	opening one's eyes
ornithophobia	birds
osmophobia	odors
osphresiophobia	odors
ouranophobia	heaven
pagophobia	eating
panphobia, panophobia, pantophobia	everything
papaphobia	the Pope
paralipophobia	neglect; omission of duty
paraphobia	sexual perversion
parasitophobia	parasites
parthenophobia	girls
parturiphobia	getting pregnant
pathophobia	disease
patriophobia	heredity; hereditary disease
peccatiphobia, peccatophobia	sinning
pediculophobia	lice
pediophobia, pedophobia, paedophobia	dolls; children
pellagraphobia	pellagra
peniaphobia	poverty
phagophobia	eating
phallophobia	the penis
pharmacophobia	medicine
phasmophobia	ghosts
phengophobia	daylight
philosophobia	philosophy; philosophers
phobophobia	fearing; phobias
phonophobia	sounds; voices
photangiophobia	eye pain caused by light

photaugiophobia	bright light
photophobia	light (increased sensitivity to light)
phronemophobia	thinking
phthiriophobia	lice
phthisiophobia	tuberculosis
placophobia	tombstones
pneumatophobia	air
pnigerophobia	smothering
pnigophobia	choking; sore throats
pogonophobia	beards
poinephobia	punishment
politicophobia	politicians
polyphobia	many things
ponophobia	work; fatigue
porphyrophobia	the color purple
potamophobia	rivers
potophobia	drinking
proctophobia	the rectum; rectal disease
proteinphobia	protein foods (or extreme dislike of)
pseudohydrophobia	dogs; rabies
psychophobia	the mind
psychrophobia	cold climates or temperatures
pteronophobia	feathers
pyrexiophobia	fever
pyrophobia	fire
radiophobia	radiation; x-rays
rectophobia	the rectum; rectal disease
rhabdophobia	being beaten; flogging
rhypophobia, rypophobia, rupophobia	filth
russophobia	Russia or dislike of anything Russian
satanophobia	the devil; Satan
scabiophobia	scabies
scatophobia	excrement; obscene language
scelerophobia	bad men; burglars; thieves; robbers
scholionophobia	school
sciophobia, sciaphobia	shadows
scoleciphobia	worms
scopophobia, scoptophobia	being stared at
scotophobia	darkness
selaphobia	flash
selenophobia	the moon
siderodromophobia	railroad; train travel
siderophobia	stars

sinophobia	China or dislike of anything Chinese
sitophobia, sitiophobia	food
spectrophobia	phantoms
spermatophobia, spermophobia	semen (or loss of)
spheksophobia	wasps
stasibasiphobia	standing up and walking
stasiphobia	standing up
stenophobia	narrow spaces
stygiophobia	hell
symbolophobia	symbolism
syphilophobia, syphiliphobia	syphilis
tabophobia	wasting sickness
taeniophobia	tapeworms
taphephobia, taphophobia	being buried alive
tapinophobia	small things
taurophobia	bull
technophobia	technology
telephonophobia	telephones
telophobia	teleology
teratophobia	bearing a deformed child; monsters
testophobia	taking a test
teutophobia, teutonophobia	Germany or dislike of anything German
thaasophobia	sitting
thalassophobia	the sea; ocean
thanatophobia	death
theatrophobia	theaters
theophobia	God
thermophobia	heat
tocophobia	childbirth
tomophobia	surgical operations
tonitrophobia; tonitruphobia	thunder; thunderstorms
topophobia	certain places; performing
toxiphobia, toxicophobia, toxophobia	poison
traumatophobia	physical injury; war
tremophobia	trembling
trichinophobia	trichinosis
trichopathophobia, trichophobia	hair
tridecaphobia; triskaidekaphobia	the number 13
tropophobia	moving; making change
trypanophobia	inoculation
tuberculophobia	tuberculosis
tyrannophobia	tyrants
uranophobia	heaven

urophobia	passing urine
vaccinophobia	vaccination
venereophobia	venereal disease
vermiphobia	worm infestation
xenophobia	strangers; foreigners
xerophobia	arid climates, deserts; dryness
zelophobia	jealousy
zoophobia	animals

Phobias Listed by Abnormal Fear

ABNORMAL FEAR OF	CLINICAL NAMES
air	aerophobia; pneumatophobia
airports	aerodromophobia
albumin in urine as sign of kidney disease	albuminurophobia
alcoholism	alcoholophobia
aloneness	monophobia
amphibians	herpetophobia
animals	zoophobia
anything new	cenotophobia
anything new; change; novelty	kainotophobia, kainophobia, cainotophobia, cainophobia; neophobia
arid climates, deserts; dryness	xerophobia
bacilli	bacillophobia
bad men	scelerophobia
barren space; emptiness	kenophobia, cenophobia
bathing; swimming in a body of water	aquaphobia
beards	pogonophobia
bearing a deformed child	teratophobia
bees	apiphobia, melissophobia
being alone	isolophobia; eremiophobia; autophobia; eremophobia; monophobia
being beaten	rhabdophobia; mastigophobia
being bound	merinthophobia
being buried alive	taphephobia, taphophobia
being dirty	automysophobia
being in open spaces; leaving one's home	agoraphobia
being locked in	clithrophobia
being made fun of	katagelophobia; catagelophobia
being scratched	amychophobia
being stared at	scopophobia, scoptophobia
being touched	aphephobia; haptephobia, haphephobia
birds	ornithophobia
blood	hemophobia, hematophobia
blushing; red	erythrophobia, ereuthophobia
books	bibliophobia
brain disease	meningitophobia
bright light	photaugiophobia

bulls	taurophobia
burglars	scelerophobia
cancer	cancerophobia, carcinophobia
cat	ailurophobia, aelurophobia; felinophobia, gatophobia
Celts, or dislike of anything Celtic	celtophobia
certain places; performing	topophobia
chickens	alektorophobia
childbirth	tocophobia
China, or dislike of anything Chinese	sinophobia
chins	geniophobia
choking	anginophobia; pnigophobia
cholera	cholerophobia
churches	ecclesiophobia, ecclesiaphobia
clouds	nebulaphobia; nephophobia
cold	cheimaphobia
cold climates or temperatures	psychrophobia
color purple	porphyrophobia
colors	chromatophobia, chromophobia
comets	cometophobia
committing the unpardonable sin	enosiophobia
computers	kilobytophobia
confinement; closed spaces	claustrophobia
contamination; filth	misophobia, musophobia, mysophobia
contamination; infection	molysmophobia, molysomophobia
corpses; death	necrophobia
crossing bridges	gephyrophobia
crossing streets	dromophobia
crowds	ochlophobia; demophobia
cumbersome pseudoscientific words	hellenologophobia
dampness; moisture; liquid	hygrophobia
darkness	achluophobia; scotophobia
darkness; night	nyctophobia
dawn	eosophobia
daylight	phengophobia
death	thanatophobia
death from nuclear war	nucleomitaphobia
defecating due to pain	defecalgesiophobia
definite disease	monopathophobia
demons and goblins	bogyphobia
demons; the devil	demonophobia, daemonophobia
dental surgery	odontophobia

depths	bathophobia
devil; Satan	satanophobia
diabetes	diabetophobia
dining; dinner conversation	deipnophobia
disease	nosophobia; pathophobia
dislike of gold	aurophobia
disorder	ataxophobia, ataxiophobia
doctors	iatrophobia
dogs; rabies	pseudohydrophobia; cynophobia
dolls; children	pediophobia, pedophobia, paedophobia
double vision	diplopiaphobia
dreams	oneirophobia
drinking	potophobia; dipsophobia
dust	amathophobia; koniophobia
eating	pagophobia, phagophobia
electricity	electrophobia
England, or dislike of anything English	anglophobia
endlessness	apeirophobia
erotica	eroticophobia
error	hamartophobia
everything	panphobia, panophobia, pantophobia
excrement	coprophobia
excrement; obscene language	scatophobia
eye pain caused by light	photangiophobia
eyes	ommatophobia
failure; defeat	kakorrhaphiophobia
fatigue	kopophobia
fearing; phobias	phobophobia
feathers	pteronophobia
female genitalia	eurotophobia
fever	febriphobia; pyrexiophobia
filth	rhypophobia, rypophobia, rupophobia
fire	pyrophobia
fish	ichthyophobia
flash	selaphobia
flogging	mastigophobia; rhabdophobia
floods	antlophobia
flowers	anthophobia
flutes, or similar wind instruments	aulophobia
flying	aviophobia

fog	homichlophobia
food	sitophobia, sitiophobia; cibophobia
foods high in protein	proteinphobia
forests; wood	hylophobia, hylephobia
France, or dislike of anything French	francophobia; gallophobia
freedom	eleutherophobia
frogs	batrachophobia
functioning	ergasiophobia
fur; skin of animals	doraphobia
gaiety	cherophobia
Germany, or dislike of anything German	teutophobia, teutonophobia; germanophobia
getting pregnant	parturiphobia
ghosts	phasmophobia
girls	parthenophobia
glare	photaugiaphobia
glass	hyalophobia, hyelophobia; crystallophobia
God	theophobia
going to bed	clinophobia
gravity	barophobia
Greece, or dislike of anything Greek	hellenophobia
growing old	gerascophobia
hair	chaetophobia, trichopathophobia, trichophobia
hatred of work	ergophobia
having a physical or mental exam	kopophobia
hearing certain words or names	onomatophobia
heart disease	cardiophobia
heat	thermophobia
heaven	ouranophobia
heaven	uranophobia
heights	acrophobia
hell	hadephobia; stygiophobia
heredity; hereditary disease	patriophobia
high objects	batophobia
high open spaces	aeroacrophobia
high places	hypsiphobia, hypsophobia
home environment	oecophobia, oikophobia, oechophobia; ecophobia
homosexuals	homophobia
horses	equinophobia, hippophobia
houses	domatophobia

human companionship	anthropophobia; phobanthropy
humankind	anthropophobia
humiliation	katagelophobia, catagelophobia
ice	cryophobia
ideas	ideophobia
illness	nosemaphobia
imaginary body deformity	dysmorphophobia
imperfection	atelophobia
infinity	apeirophobia
inherited illness or disease	patroiophobia, patriophobia
inoculation	trypanophobia
insanity	lyssophobia, maniaphobia
insects	entomophobia
Japan, or dislike of anything Japanese	japanophobia
jealousy	zelophobia
Jews, or dislike of anything Jewish	judeophobia
justice	dikephobia
knives; sharp points	aichmophobia
lakes	limnophobia
large objects	megalophobia
leprosy	leprophobia, lepraphobia
lice	pediculophobia; phthiriophobia
light	photophobia
lightning	astraphobia, astrapophobia
machinery	mechanophobia
making decisions	decidophobia
malignancy	cancerophobia; carcinophobia
many things	polyphobia
marriage	gamophobia
meat	carnophobia
medicine	pharmacophobia
men; dislike of males	androphobia
meningitis	meningitophobia
metals	metallophobia
meteors	meteorophobia
mice	musophobia
microorganisms; germs	microbiophobia
mind	psychophobia
mirrors	catoptrophobia
missiles	ballistophobia
mites or ticks on the skin	acarophobia
money; wealth	chrematophobia
monsters	teratophobia

moon	selenophobia
motion	kinesophobia
motor vehicles	motorphobia
movement	kinesophobia
moving; making change	tropophobia
music	musicophobia
myths; stories	mythophobia
nakedness	gymnophobia; nudophobia
names	nomatophobia
narrow spaces	stenophobia
needles; sharp objects	belonephobia
neglect; omission of duty	paralipophobia
new things	neophobia; kainophobia,
	cainophobia; kainophobia
nudity	nudophobia, nudiphobia
number 13	tridecaphobia; triskaidekaphobia
objects to the left	levophobia
objects to the right	dextrophobia
odors	olfactophobia; osmophobia,
	osphresiophobia
offensive personal body odor	autodysosmophobia;
	bromidrosiphobia
old age	gerontophobia
opening one's eyes	optophobia
pain	algophobia; odynophobia,
odynephobia	
parasites	parasitophobia
passing urine	urophobia
peanut butter on the roof of the mouth	arachibutyrophobia
pellagra	pellagraphobia
penis	phallophobia
people	anthropophobia
phantoms	spectrophobia
philosophy; philosophers	philosophobia
physical injury; war	traumatophobia
pins	belonephobia
plants and flowers	botanophobia
pleasure	hedonophobia
points; pointed objects	aichmophobia
poison	toxiphobia, toxicophobia; iophobia
politicians	politicophobia
the Pope	papaphobia
poverty	peniaphobia

precipices; cliffs	cremnophobia
pregnancy; childbirth	maieusiophobia
punishment	poinephobia
rabies; water	hydrophobophobia
radiation	radiophobia
railroads; train travel	siderodromophobia
rain; rainstorms	ombrophobia
rectum; rectal disease	proctophobia; rectophobia
remaining single	anuptophobia
reptiles	herpetophobia; batrachophobia
responsibility	hypengyophobia
returning home	nostophobia
ridicule	katagelophobia, catagelophobia
riding in vehicles	amaxophobia
rivers	potamophobia
robbers	scelerophobia
ruin	atephobia
Russia, or dislike of anything Russian	russophobia
sacred things	hierophobia
saints; holy people	hagiophobia
scabies	scabiophobia
school	scholionophobia; didaskaleinophobia
scratches	amychophobia
sea or ocean	thalassophobia; nautophobia
sea swells	cymophobia
seeking out that which is feared	counterphobia
self; aloneness; solitude	autophobia
semen, or the loss of it	spermatophobia, spermophobia
sermons	homilophobia
sex	genophobia
sexual intercourse	coitophobia
sexual love; physical expression	erotophobia
sexual perversion	paraphobia
shadows	sciophobia, sciaphobia
sharks	galeophobia
shock	hormephobia
sin; error	hamartophobia
sinning	peccatiphobia, peccatophobia
sitting	thaasophobia
sitting down	cathisophobia, kathisophobia
skin disease	dermatophobia, dermatosiophobia, dermatopathophobia

sleep	hypnophobia
slime; mucus	myxophobia; blennophobia
small or minute objects	microphobia
small things	tapinophobia
smothering	pnigerophobia
snakes	ophidiophobia
snow	chionophobia
sore throats	anginophobia; pnigophobia
sounds; voices	acousticophobia; phonophobia
sourness	acerophobia
speaking in public	glossophobia
speaking; stuttering	lalophobia, laliophobia
spiders	arachnephobia
stairs; climbing	climacophobia
standing up	stasiphobia
standing up and walking	stasibasiphobia
stars	astrophobia; siderophobia
stealing; thieves	kleptophobia, cleptophobia
stillness; being alone	eremiophobia, eremophobia; isolophobia; autophobia; monophobia
stings	cnidophobia
strangers; foreigners	xenophobia
streets	agyiophobia
strings	linonophobia
sunlight	heliophobia
surgical operations	tomophobia
symbolism	symbolophobia
syphilis	syphilophobia, syphiliphobia
taking a test	testophobia
tapeworms	taeniophobia
tastes; flavors	geumaphobia
technology	technophobia
teeth	odontophobia
teleology	telophobia
telephones	telephonophobia
termites	isopterophobia; eisoptrophobia
theaters	theatrophobia
thieves	harpaxophobia; scelerophobia
thinking	phronemophobia
thunder	brontophobia
thunder and lightning	keraunophobia, ceraunophobia
thunder; thunderstorms	tonitrophobia, tonitruphobia

time	chronophobia
tombstones	placophobia
travel	hodophobia
trees	dendrophobia
trembling	tremophobia
trichinosis	trichinophobia
tuberculosis	phthisiophobia; tuberculophobia
tyrants	tyrannophobia
vaccinations	vaccinophobia
vehicles	amaxophobia
venereal disease	venereophobia
venereal disease; sexual intercourse	cypridophobia, cypriphobia
vomiting	emetophobia
walking	basiphobia, basophobia, basistasiphobia, basistasophobia
wasps	spheksophobia
wasting sickness	tabophobia
water	hydrophobia
weakness	asthenophobia
whirlpools	dinophobia
white strangers in Latin countries	gringophobia
wind; drafts	anemophobia
wine	oenophobia
women	gynephobia, gynophobia
words	logophobia
work	ergasiophobia
work; fatigue	ponophobia
worm infestation	helminthophobia; vermiphobia
worms	scoleciphobia
worship	iconophobia
writing	graphophobia
x-rays	radiophobia